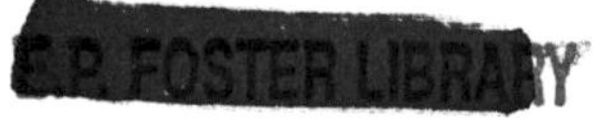

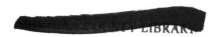

MEN LIKE US

MEN LIKE US

The GMHC Complete Guide to Gay Men's Sexual, Physical, and Emotional Well-being

Daniel Wolfe

BALLANTINE BOOKS • NEW YORK

A Ballantine Book
The Ballantine Publishing Group

www.randomhouse.com/BB/

Photo and illustration credits can be found on page 613.

LIBRARY OF CONGRESS CATALOGING-IN-PUBLICATION DATA
Wolfe, Daniel.
Men Like Us : The GMHC complete guide to gay men's sexual, physical, and emotional well-being / Daniel Wolfe. — 1st ed.
p. cm.
ISBN 0-345-41496-9 (alk. paper)
Gay men—Health and hygiene. 2. Gay men—Sexual behavior.
Safe sex in AIDS prevention. 4. Gay men—Mental health. I. Gay Men's Health Crisis, Inc. II. Title.
RA777.8.W65 2000
613'.086'642—dc21 99-28583

Trade Paperback ISBN 0-345-41495-0

Art direction by Amy Steiner
Illustrations by Ellen Forney
Text design by H Roberts Design
Cover photos front cover (top to bottom): Alexis Rodriguez-Duarte, Peter Lien/LNP, Lisa Ross, Laurence Monneret/Tony Stone Images, Linda Palotta/Impact Visuals
Cover photos back cover (top to bottom): Kate Rudin, Chantal Regnault, Anja Hinrichsen, Tom McKitterick/Impact Visuals

Manufactured in the United States of America

First Edition: April 2000

10 9 8 7 6 5 4 3 2 1

To Richard, whose life remains

the deepest and best source I've found on gay health,

love, and possibility.

Contents

Writers

This book would not have been possible without the contributions of a number of talented writers. Their contributions, made for free or close, brought focus, clarity, and humor to subjects too often rendered as lifeless and somber. Among the contributors:

David Barr	Chapter 9
Michael Bettinger, MSW	Chapter 11
Marc Boisclair	Chapters 6, 10, sidebars
Susan Carleton	Chapters 7, 10
David France	Chapter 6
Wayne Hoffman	Sidebars
Tim Horn	Chapters 9, 10
Patrick Letellier	Chapter 12
Ed Mickens	Chapter 8
Tim Murphy	Chapters 3, 5, 8
Eva Pendleton	Chapters 1, 3, 4, sidebars
Tamar Schreibman	Chapter 10, sidebars
Michael Shernoff, MSW	Chapter 12
Don Shewey	Chapter 13
Cherry Smyth	Sidebars
Karen Timour	Chapter 7
Robert Vickerman	Chapter 10, sidebars
David Wetter	Chapter 5
Ron Winchel, MD	Chapter 11

Acknowledgments

Books of this scope owe much to many. Billy Goldstein and literary agent Barbara Lowenstein helped bring the project to life, and to GMHC. Benjamin Dreyer helped make the proposal concrete. GMHC Executive Directors Mark Robinson and Ana Oliveira, Board President David Hollander, and the many members of the GMHC review committee put the power of years of experience behind it. Our editorial team at Ballantine—Peter Borland and Emily Grayson—kept the book on track with unfailing astuteness and unflagging humor. Amy Steiner spent long hours finding pictures worth the many words, Greg Lugliani and David Nimmons read the book particularly closely and critically, and Michael Lipson—a brilliant writing coach—helped me picture it from start to finish.

But perhaps the largest debt is owed the skeleton staff who shepherded this project from babble to book, particularly Eva Pendleton and Robert Vickerman. Both performed huge amounts of research, revisions, interviewing, writing, and proofreading, and joined forces with interns and volunteers offering virtually unlimited support. John Wang and Regina McNamara stand out among this group, but thanks are also due to volunteers David Hopson and David Woolwine, Erich(a) DeWald and Ann Waters, Glenn Miller and Bryan Crystal. Derry Duncan in GMHC's volunteer department worked both to recruit help for the project and help herself, and was a support throughout. Others of the many GMHC staff to whom special thanks are due include Larry Abrams, Bob Bergeron, Daniel Castellanos, Frank Cevasco, Susan Dooha, Lorne Feldman, Marla Hassner, James E. Miles Jr., and Robert Bank. Part-timers who helped make the project work included Chan Casey, Chris Cochrane, Jen Higgins, David Levine, Paul Mueller, Alison Redick, and Anthony Viti.

Many people outside of and within GMHC also worked to enhance the text and ensure its accuracy. Any errors that remain are not theirs. Many of the insights are. Among those kind enough to review part or all of the manuscript:

Larry Abrams
Joe Amico, M.Div.
Daniel Bao
Bob Bergeron
Karl Beutner, MD
Gregg Bordowitz
George Carter
Daniel Castellanos
Douglas Crimp, Ph.D.
Gary Dowsett
Richard Elovich
Jeffrey Escoffier
Cade Fields-Gardner, MS, RD
David France
Beth Gery, MD
Stephen Goldstone, MD
Lester Gottesman, MD
Howard Grossman, MD
Christine Hannema, MS, RD
Peter Hawley, MD

David Hollander
Damien Jack
Michael Lipson, Ph.D.
Mark Litwin, MD
Franklin Lowe, MD
Greg Lugliani
Ken Mayer, MD
Loring McAlpin
Scott McCallister, MD
Stephen McFadden, CSW
Thomas Morgan, III
Jack Morin, Ph.D.
David Nimmons
Jeff Nunokawa, Ph.D.
Charles Rosenberg, MS, CN
Jeffrey Roth, MD
John Sealy, MD
Charles Silverstein, Ph.D.
Fred Tripp, MS, RD, CDN
Val Ulstad, MD
Bill Vayo
John Weis
Deborah Wexler, MD
Michael Warner, Ph.D.
Dan William, MD
Todd Yancey, MD

Many not quoted in these pages, and some who are, helped with referrals, suggestions, and observations drawn from their own experiences. Among those to whom we owe special thanks:

Steve Ball, CSW
Jay Best
Steve Boswell, MD
Bert DaFonte
Robert Dostis, MS, RD
David Fleischer
Peter Goldblum, Ph.D.
Doug Goldschmidt, MSW
Tim Hammond
Jill Harris
Robert Hawkins, Ph.D.
Robert Kertzner, MD
Julie Macredy
Rob McHugh
James E. Miles Jr.
Laura Pinsky, MSW
Gabriel Ramirez, MD
Justin Richardson, MD
Sue Rochman
Michael Scarce
Pepper Schwartz, Ph.D.
Philip Spivey, Ph.D.
Rena Steinhauer
Patti Sullivan
Kathy Tennert
Barbara Warren, Psy.D.
Renee Westmoreland

Finally, this book owes an enormous debt to gay men all over the country. Hundreds provided their assistance, offering their insights in one-on-one interviews, via mailed questionnaires, through a yearlong Internet survey, in workshops, and over dinner tables. Their contributions have given structure and direction to every chapter. Many of these men are quoted, often with their names changed by request, throughout. The variety of their stories captures the full and complicated lives we lead better than any one can. For that, and for the tremendous support gay men have provided over the nearly twenty years of our history, Gay Men's Health Crisis (GMHC) is tremendously grateful.

The information in this book is not intended to substitute in any way for health care advice from a trained professional. All health matters, including highly personal ones such as sexual practices and recreational drug use, require medical supervision. This book is a supplement to, but not a replacement for, medical advice on any and all health concerns.

The authors, medical advisers, and publisher urge you to seek that advice from a physician or other trained health professional, and disclaim any liability arising directly or indirectly from the use of this book.

Models appearing on these pages may have been paid. Inclusion of their image, likeness, or photograph is not meant to imply anything about their sexual orientation or about the status of their health.

Gay Men's Health Crisis (GMHC), is the nation's oldest and largest AIDS service organization. Founded by six gay men in 1981, the agency has helped thousands of gay men infected and affected by HIV since the start of the epidemic. Our AIDS hotline and Buddy program were the world's first. Today, GMHC serves thousands of men, women, and children with HIV, educates the public about HIV prevention and treatment, and advocates for hundreds of thousands nationwide.

For information, or to help support the work of GMHC, please contact the GMHC AIDS Hotline at 800/AIDS-NYC (TDD: 212/645-7470 for the hearing impaired) or see the GMHC Web site: www.gmhc.org.

Introduction

In the early 1970s, shortly after Stonewall put them squarely in the public eye, gay men gathered again: not for protest, this time, but for exploration. From Manhattan to Montana, Berkeley to Boston, gay doctors, nurses, and men on the street took a page from the feminist health movement and started talking about how we could know our bodies better. Sexually transmitted diseases and how to avoid them were the start of the discussions, which ranged in some cities to peer counseling, encounter groups, love-ins, martial arts trainings, whole foods preparation, sharing of coming out stories, and other unfamiliar pleasures. "There was a national excitement about working on issues that health care professionals had never dared discuss with each other," says Mark Behar, a physician's assistant who—along with a flight instructor, a Certified Public Accountant, and several nurses—was among the founders of the Gay People's Union VD clinic in Milwaukee, Wisconsin. "Particularly since, in those days, going into a regular doctor's office and saying you were gay was in itself likely to be a serious risk to your health."

Then came AIDS. In the face of the ravages of HIV, other sexually transmitted diseases seemed like minor details. Staples of consciousness raising—talk of coming out, growing older, or good lovemaking techniques—were suddenly beside the point. Who could discuss aging when so many obviously wouldn't survive the decade? Why talk of living well when so many of us wouldn't be living at all? While some of the early gay health efforts refocused to cope with AIDS, many disappeared in the wake of a new generation of programs dedicated specifically to fighting the new "gay plague."

The first of the new organizations—Gay Men's Health Crisis—was formed in 1981, back when AIDS was still called "Gay Related Immune Deficiency." GMHC's tools—a reliance on volunteers, fierce gay pride, and a commitment to combining medical expertise with wisdom gained from first-hand experience—were similar to those of earlier gay health efforts. The organization's growth and intensity—like that of the epidemic it was fighting—was unprecedented. Volunteers stepped forward to staff hot lines, run buddy programs, and lead workshops on safer sex. As the full scope of the epidemic became known, GMHC—with "gay" still in its name and mission—expanded to serve men, women, and children with HIV and those who cared for them. A decade after GMHC's founding, more than a million Americans—and thousands upon thousands of gay men—had come for services, joined a GMHC workshop or advocacy effort, or helped raise money for the fight.

Even as the epidemic magnified the strength of our community, it underscored the weakness of simple notions of who "we" were. The spread of HIV gave us a way to mark what was true before AIDS and will likely be true after it is over: that for men who have sex with other men, there is no single "gay identity." A teacher in Chelsea might feel like a full-fledged, full time member of the gay community; for a teacher in a Minneapolis suburb or another New York neighborhood, that feeling might be more of an in-the-bar-on-the-weekends-with-friends-and-then-only-sometimes sort of thing. Black and Latino and Asian men who have sex with men, even those who are out and proud, talk often of feeling torn between communities, and resting securely in none. Young gay men—some of whom may have never known a person with HIV or a time when there were no gay magazines or celebrities—talk of the differences between their world and those of older men who lost half of their youth to the closet and half their friends to AIDS. In fact, for most of us, talk of "men like us" raises the question "who is us?" and the suspicion that whoever it is, we are probably not included. "Sure, there are bars and magazines everywhere, but for most of the big challenges of my life, I feel like I'm on my own," said one of the hundreds of men interviewed for this book, summing up a feeling expressed by many others.

This book is an effort to close that gap, to have that gay part of you, however you define it, speak to the gay part of someone else. Like gay men themselves, the subjects covered in these pages vary widely, from scabies to spirituality, disclosing your HIV status to disposing of love handles. The basics of HIV are covered here, but so are many issues that have been overshadowed by AIDS: heart disease, cholesterol, prostate cancer, testicular cancer, and other health problems particular to men. Insights from and experiences with women, too, are included—gay porn notwithstanding, few of us live lives that are all-male, all the time. Even if you do, women have much to teach gay men about self-knowledge, mutual support, and community health.

Why would GMHC—an AIDS organization—write a book as broad as this one? Because nearly two decades of experience with gay men have shown that issues raised by HIV are much bigger than condoms to stop the virus or pills to treat it. For gay men, effective HIV prevention and treatment has meant grappling with the full scope of issues raised by how we live and love: how we think about ourselves and others, sexual communication, relationships, spirituality, and aging. These pages try to communicate some of that wisdom, and recognize how important it is to build on it as the lives of gay men with HIV—and the lives of gay men who don't have the virus—stretch into the new millennium.

Almost twenty years after AIDS, this book is a bridge between the spirit of the earlier, broad gay health movement and the hard-won lessons of the epidemic. Like the AIDS movement, this book recognizes that health—involving mind, body, and spirit—is not always the same as being illness-free. These pages include advice on how to cope with insurance, Medicaid, hospitals, and serious illness, drawing often on the legacy of many who—even as it undermined their bodies—refused to let AIDS take away their personhood.

Like the gay health movement, this book recognizes the power of the personal, the importance of drawing on our collective experience as well as on the expertise of trained professionals. Issues of gay pleasure and well-being, unfortunately, are not yet required reading in most medical schools or therapy textbooks. Men interviewed for this project talked—in the twenty-first century—of doctors telling them not to put things "up there" if they wanted to stay healthy, or therapists who told them nonmonogamy was sick. It's tempting, even in our own communities, to label sex that involves no risk of HIV or social criticism as "good" and other sex as "bad," making health a kind of Trojan Horse concealing easy moral judgements.

This book includes the wisdom of doctors, lawyers, and therapists, many of them gay themselves. It also relies—heavily—on the lived experiences of "ordinary" men across the country. The voices included don't always agree: premature ejaculation depends on your definition, and one man's graceful aging is another's descent into the underworld of the lonely old queen. Safer sex depends on your idea of pleasure and risk. Spirituality has at least as many forms as Jesus had disciples, or Krishna had incarnations.

Those looking for the single answer—is anal sex good?—may be disappointed. This book sometimes tells you more about what you *could* do than about what you should do. Most people recognize that spirituality, for example, or aging, do not come with a single prescription. Neither does treatment of HIV, or depression. Sex—as reassuring as it is to have rules to live by—changes with time and circumstance. What worked for you in the first year of your relationship may not be as compelling three years later. What you're willing to do may depend on how you feel about the person with whom you're doing it.

As wide-ranging as it is, this book will leave some men wanting more. Those just finding themselves as gay men and talking about that may want additional advice: while other books cover the process of coming out in greater detail, this one assumes that step is largely behind you. Those not wishing to be confined as "gay"—particularly bisexuals—may wish that the section on sex with women were longer, or may feel excluded by references to "men like us." And those whose lives do not fit neatly into the category "men"—especially transgendered women, men, or those choosing to live somewhere in between—will have some unanswered questions. Though the resources here offer a start, a whole book on transgender health concerns—from hormone use to genital reassignment surgery to how to discuss transitions with lovers, friends, and family—is badly needed.

But if gay man describes you well enough—whether you are single in Savannah or coupled in Boca Raton, twenty-eight or eighty-two, wearing wedding rings or nipple rings (or both), this book should have something for you. It is meant for all of us who are used to reading between the lines to find the homosexuality, or who have spent too long searching other health guides and encyclopedias for definitions and descriptions of our lives. As the disclaimer in the front points out, it's no substitute for medical advice from a trained professional. Think of it as more *Our Bodies, Ourselves* than *Merck Manual,* a homosexual counterpart to the endless books, television shows, magazine articles, and advice columns that help heterosexual America learn to hook up, get off, and live to tell about it.

There are many different stories here—of friends and boyfriends, major health struggles and minor bouts of embarrassment, old patterns and news ways of looking at them. The variety is testament to what the mainstream media and medical professionals often forget: that there are many men like us, with many different approaches to well-being. I hope these pages—even as they return us to some questions long displaced by AIDS—open a window onto what has always been at the heart of gay pride in the era of the epidemic: the incredible ways that gay men—in all our diversity—care for ourselves and each other.

Daniel Wolfe

PART 1

SEX BASICS

CHAPTER 1

The Anatomy of Pleasure

Nipples • Penis • Foreskin • Penis Size • Erection and Penile Pleasure • Balls and Beyond • Anal Pleasure • Anal Health • Prostate Health • Kegels • What's Up Down There? A Troubleshooting Guide

You may be working out in a gym in West Hollywood, or working a beer-bellied-bear look in rural Vermont. Perhaps you're feeling super hot and ready for sex, or too burned by past experiences to try to have it at all. You might see yourself as a craggy, cigar-smoking daddy, a svelte sophisticate, a B-boy built for nonstop lovemaking, or a man unsuited for such crude categorizations. Gay men have all kinds of bodies and all kinds of ways of thinking about them.

And yet when we do get unsuited, unshirted, and unshorted—for all our celebration of physical variety—it's common to have questions about basics. Even the buffest, most gym-friendly among us has been known to contemplate his naked body in the mirror and wonder if there's something lacking. You've paged through porn magazines or stared deeply and comparatively at the asses or crotches around you in the locker room. For one thing, seeing the hidden revealed is endlessly fascinating. Perhaps nowhere is our bodily interest—and that nagging suspicion of insufficiency—more pronounced than when it comes to the parts of the body we use for sex.

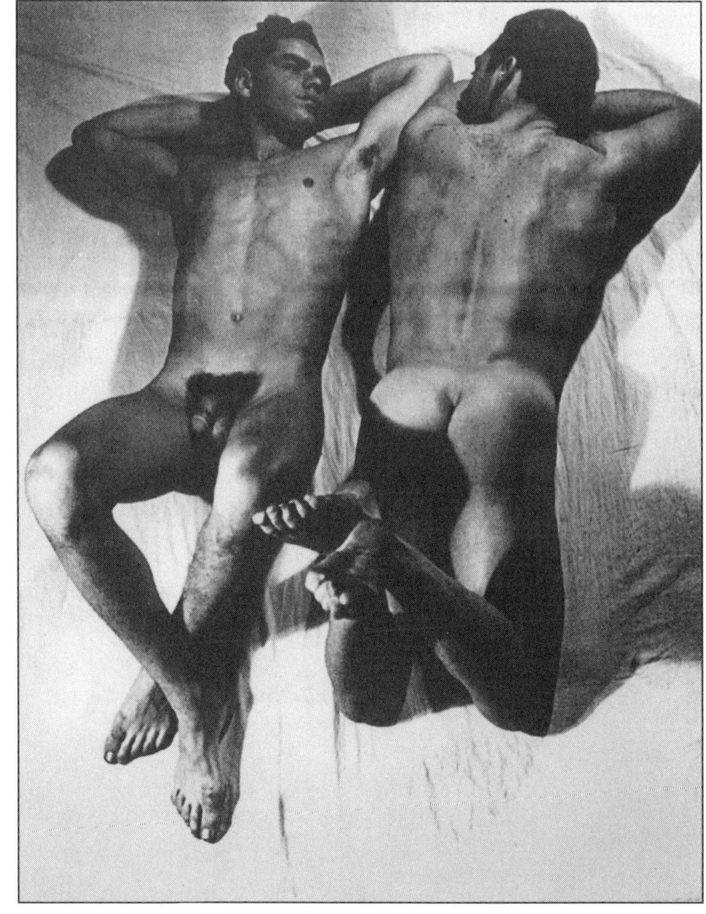

Some people say that problems start right there, with a focus on body parts instead of the whole person. That could be. There's no question that gay men are more than the sum of our private parts, and that the mythic eight-inch penis (and six-pack abs, and chiseled chest) are standards that can only leave most of us feeling short of the mark. There's no question that focusing on your genitals without considering your mind is reductive, and that looking good and feeling good are not synonymous, no matter what the adult-moviemakers, cigarette companies, or fashion advertisers try to sell or tell you.

And there's also no question that in today's

movie-minded, media-mad, ad-filled society, it's human to feel the pull of glossy pictures and the inner conflict they produce. If you're like most men, gay or straight, you at some point have put dick to ruler to see how you measure up. You've looked at a smooth bubble butt in a magazine and lamented your own soft and hairy one, or pondered Marky Mark's chest on a billboard and wished yours stopped traffic that effectively.

The truth? While you can't escape the hype, you don't have to live by it. Satisfaction and health both begin with knowing your own body: its appearance, how it feels on different days, how it changes, how to make it feel good, or how to help it if it hurts. Whether you're thin or heavy, hairy or smooth, not getting any from your boyfriend or happily contending for slut-of-the-month club, your body's built for pleasure. Another truth? Most of us could use a little help to find it.

Every gay man's pleasure points are different. This first chapter offers a top-to-bottom review of the anatomy of a few of the most prominent—nipples, penis, balls, anus, and prostate. The next chapters look at what we do with them: the complicated interplay of bodies and minds better known as sex.

Nipples

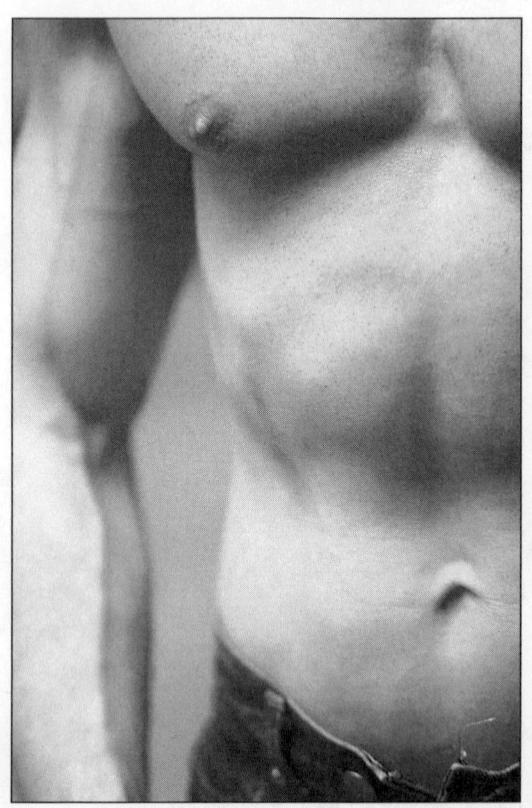

I hadn't really paid any attention to my nipples since summer camp, when "titty twisters" were something boys did to punish each other. But I found a boyfriend, when I was nineteen, who was also a nipple freak. At first I was like, "What's he doing?" Then a few minutes later, oh, God! It totally turned my world upside down.

Why do men have nipples? Some years ago, renowned scientist Stephen Jay Gould reported that this question was the one most often asked by readers of his column in the magazine *Natural History*. A number of recent male health books—and dozens of postings to Internet discussion groups—show the question to be very much alive today. Apparently scientific minds are used to thinking of bodies in terms of what they do to help a species feed and multiply. Since men don't nurse, what is the purpose of the two little bumps on our chests? "It is probably easier for the body to produce nipples in men than to eliminate them," suggests a not-so-helpful posting from a company that helps train science teachers in elementary schools. "All embryos develop as female until the male genes kick into action," explains another, this one from the library of the National Museum of Science and Industry in London. "Hence a rudimentary and vestigial nipple remains on the male, a useless reminder of our feminine past."

Nipples? Useless? Feminine past? It's a straight thing. We might not understand.

Gay men have had our own answer to the nipple question for years. Sex researchers Masters and Johnson, who made 1960s history by inviting heterosexual and homosexual couples into their research rooms and watching them have sex, were struck by how nipple play marked the difference between homo and hetero sex. Nearly 75 percent of the gay couples Masters and Johnson observed began their lovemaking by nipple stimulation, with frequent penile erections resulting. Heterosexual women, by contrast, rarely stimulated their partner's nipples at all; when they did, they met with few hard-ons in response. Have things changed since the sixties? Probably for increasing numbers of straight folks, who have found out what they're missing.

Nipples come in all sizes. Whether big as quarters or smaller than dimes, with tiny points or flesh plugs that measure nearly an inch in length, the sensitive, soft flesh is shot through with nerve endings. For many of us, confronted with mental or physical stimulation, the nipples swell to erection like the much more talked-about penis. Unlike the penis, which we can place strategically to give pleasure even as we get it, our nipples keep us on the receiving end. It is this that makes nipples a delight or, for those who'd rather stay firmly in the driver's seat of sexual pleasure, a threat. To hear men tell it, it is not a question of masculine or feminine, active or passive; even big ol' self-described "tops" may buck and beg when you play with their chests.

Many describe being taught about their nipples by another, though you can also teach yourself. Take it slow until you figure out what level of stimulation suits you best. For some, a simple grazing with moistened fingertips is enough; others crave harder pulling of the nipples, or tugging on the chest hair that sometimes surrounds them. Sadly, there's no real way to suck on your own nipples. Since this chapter is about examination of one's own body, we'll leave oral pleasures for the next.

Many have found that the more they play with their nipples, the more there is to play with. Piercing, for example (see page 7), increases sensitivity. Consistent pulling, or the use of weights and clamps, can give nipples an enlarged, worked look and enhance stimulation. The tiny-titted among us, and those who play with them, have found that the smallest suction cup from snakebite kits (see "Toys and Tools," in Chapter 2) can pull the nipple out temporarily and enhance sensitivity. Applying a lubricant can also help bring a resistant nipple to erection; if, later, the lube keeps seeking fingers from finding their target, try grasping with a tissue or, for a rough thrill, a paper towel. Find the right way to do it and nipple pleasure for some men can be enough to cause orgasm all by itself.

Care of the nipple and breast is relatively simple. The appearance of any unusual lump in the breast should be checked out by a doctor, though cancerous growths are rare. Only 1,600 cases of breast cancer are reported annually among American men. Nipple soreness, or even bleeding, is much more common, the result of the chafing that can occur from an evening of stimulation, the rubbing of a mustache or goatee, or the friction of a starched shirt or sweaty tee against a bare chest. A daily application of baby oil, and taking a break for a week or so, can soothe; if your exercise routine is the cause, try putting a little baby oil or Vaseline, or a strategically applied Band-Aid, on each nipple before starting your workout. Intense nipple play, particularly with toys, can cause bruising (which fades on its own), fluid-filled blisters that can break open, and bleeding. For broken skin, an antibacterial ointment such as Neosporin usually does the trick. As with all open cuts, keep these from contact with another's bodily fluids to protect yourself from HIV or other kinds of infection, and see a doctor if it doesn't seem to be healing.

Somewhere around a third of us will experience breast growth in our lifetimes, and not

WRITTEN ON THE BODY

It's a way to claim ownership of your body, mark an important moment, heighten sexual sensitivity, and express your individuality. It's also a great excuse to accessorize. Whatever the motivation, piercing and tattooing are extremely popular among gay men, be they leathermen or skate punks, drag queens, circuit queens, or all the rest of us.

As with anything involving needles, body fluids, or sexual activity, piercing and tattooing carry health considerations ranging from minor infections to HIV. Make sure your tattooer or piercer is vigilant about safety, and that he or she uses disposable needles, an autoclave to sterilize other equipment, and surgical steel or other sterile rings and rods for piercing. Once it's done, be equally vigilant about keeping your new addition clean: Salt water and witch hazel are the best cleaners, and antibacterial creams should be used sparingly. Avoid hydrogen peroxide, which burns sensitive tissue. And remember that tattoos and piercings both are open cuts until they heal, so keep other people's body fluids away. That includes saliva, which won't give you HIV but may transmit hepatitis or other infections. If you already have a weak immune system, healing may take longer.

Finally, there's the most important consideration of all: what to decorate. Many places won't tattoo above the neck or below the wrists or ankles, but just about any body part can be pierced. Logger, a piercing legend in the gay community of Washington, DC, says, "You pick it, I'll poke it." Below, find only a few of the more popular and erotic piercing options.

EAR

Piercing for beginners, it's the least shocking, fastest healing, and least painful option.

VARIETY Traditional (low on the lobe) or more daring (farther up the ear). Or both. Conventional wisdom holds that pierced right ears are for gay boys. In reality, it's not which ear is pierced, it's how fabulous your earrings are.

SAFETY Don't use a piercing gun at a cheap mall shop; the guns are difficult to sterilize, and you don't want hepatitis. Healing takes a few weeks. And watch out when you put on a sweater.

NOSE

Popular with trendy alternateens and hardened sadomasochists alike.

VARIETY Glam (through a nostril, à la Joan Osborne) or butch (through the septum: either a cavemanesque bone straight across, or a bull-ring so other guys can lead you around).

SAFETY Takes a couple of months to heal. Blow your nose gently and clean the hole with a Q-Tip.

TONGUE/LIPS

You might have to adjust the way you eat, talk, and do other things with your mouth. Then again, you survived braces just fine. Some people report chipped teeth.

VARIETY Barbells through the tongue, the kind you can't stop playing with. A librette goes through the lower lip.

SAFETY Not as painful as it sounds, and quicker to heal than some other piercings—a month or two. During the healing process, you must be fastidious with oral hygiene, rinsing with germ-killing mouthwash constantly (the American Dental Association opposes the whole idea, warning of infection or possible nerve damage). While the piercing is fresh, you should avoid heavy kissing and oral sex, since they're risky for hepatitis and HIV transmission. Can you really last a month?

NAVEL

This'll draw attention to your abs, so you'd better be proud of them.

VARIETY Typically a vertical ring through the top of the navel. Doesn't work if you're an outie.

SAFETY Healing can take several months, and this piercing is the one most commonly infected. Seek expert advice before removing jewelry; doing so often makes infection worse. Try salt water and antibiotic ointment.

NIPPLE

Once kinky, now it's so mainstream that straight guys are doing it.

VARIETY Barbells or rings, in varying gauges. Nipple piercings also echo the hanky code: left for tops, right for bottoms—but this distinction is getting blurred.

SAFETY Healing can take months, so be careful with heavy tit play for a while. Expect an initial period of soreness; avoid wearing scratchy shirts (unless you're into that). Most guys report increased sensitivity, but a few notice a decrease. If the pierced area oozes or weeps, it could mean they struck a gland, so have it checked out by a doctor ASAP.

SCROTUM

Heightened sensitivity could make you the belle of the balls.

VARIETY Either through the scrotum itself, or a guiche, just behind the scrotum through the perineum.

SAFETY While these can be extremely stimulating—especially a guiche, with a bit of weight added—they also take several months to heal and are easily irritated, causing rejection or migration from their original placement. Perspiration, friction from clothing, and inadequate ventilation are the main culprits, so wear cotton underwear and loose pants, and soak the piercings in salt water to help the healing.

PENIS

No, they usually won't set off airport metal detectors, provoking embarrassing yet strangely erotic scenes with security guards.

VARIETY Plenty. The famous Prince Albert, or PA, is a ring that goes in the urethra and out through a piercing in the frenulum. An *ampalling* is a rod through the head side to side, while an *apadravya* runs through the head back to front. Uncut guys can pierce their foreskins. There are also simple frenulum piercings—rings through the underside of the shaft.

SAFETY These can bleed heavily for several days after piercing, and most take several weeks to heal. Avoid getting sucked while the hole is fresh—it could be risky for both of you in terms of hepatitis and perhaps HIV. Some guys worry that their PA will tear condoms, but this is rare. Ampallings and apadravyas are the hardest on condoms, and they also take much longer—up to a year—to heal completely. Don't worry about your own urine infecting the piercing; urine is nearly sterile and actually may help keep the holes clean.

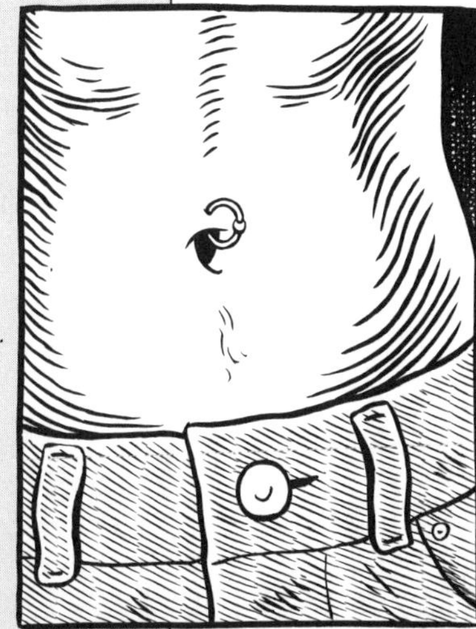

Navel pierce

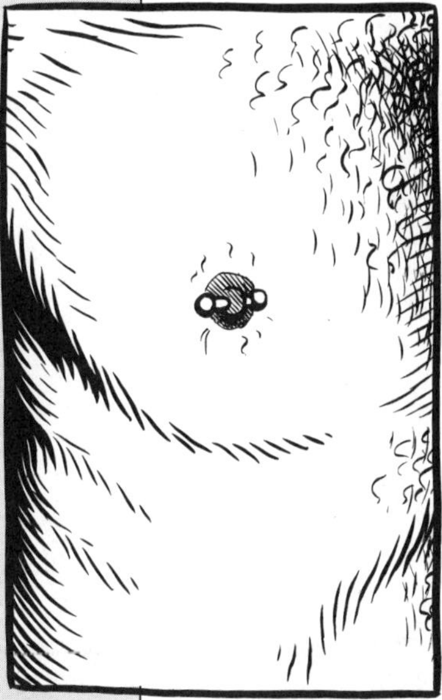

Nipple pierce

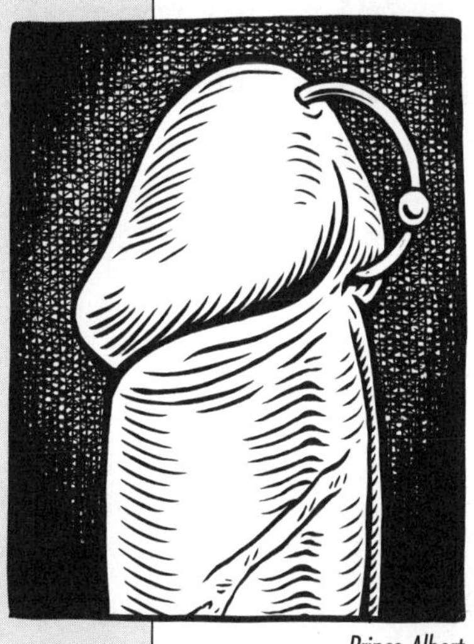

Prince Albert

the kind that comes from bench presses. Men over fifty are especially prone to the condition. Liver problems, heavy drinking, or prostate-shrinking drugs that increase the amount of the hormone estrogen in your body are among the causes, though in overweight men simple weight gain can produce a similar symptom. There is rarely any serious health risk associated with the condition, but the medical name—*gynecomastia,* Latin for "woman's breast"—speaks to some of men's anxieties about the unmanliness of it all. Whether big breasts have less sexual potential than huge hard pecs will be for you, and fashion, to decide. In the meantime, a change of medication or, if it really bothers you, plastic surgery may reverse the enlargement.

PENIS

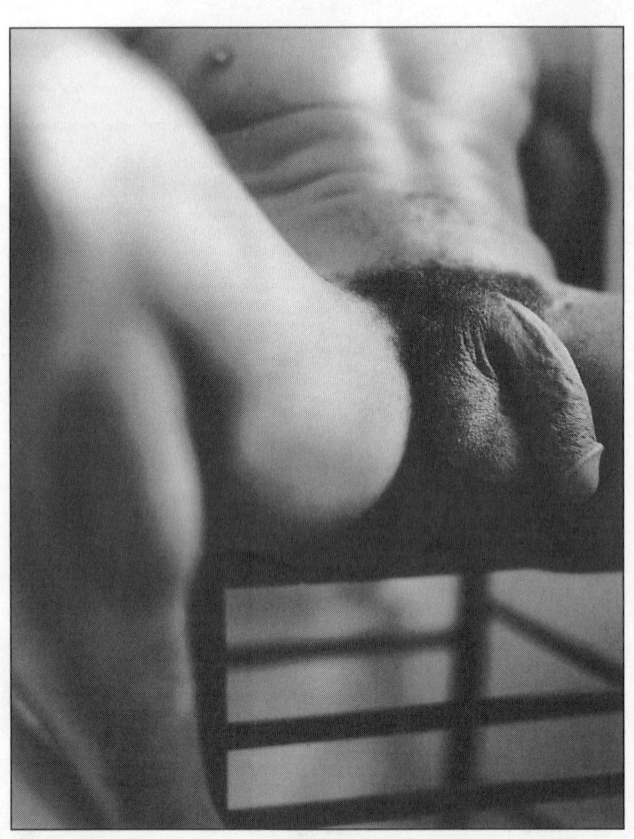

Gay men talk and think a lot about penises. In that regard, we share plenty with men in general. Men throughout history have been obsessed with the subject, giving their own penises special names or making up more general ones to describe the category: the seeker (Arabic), the arrow of love (Tantric), the monster (dreamers from all countries). Men boast about our dicks, compare them to others', and worry about length, width, angle, and bent. We carefully guide them down one pant leg or another (if we wear pants), pierce them or douse them in cologne, shield them from view or parade them around the gym shower. We buy pictures of penises in porn magazines and videos, write of them endlessly in novels and magazines, and advertise their dimensions in personal ads and on computer bulletin boards and phone sex lines. More than a few of us can reel off the particulars—"eight inches, cut, big head, pretty fat"—as if giving directions to an often-traveled destination.

But for all that, what don't we say? For one thing, that penises come in a wide variety, and that not all of them are fat, hard, and eight or more inches long. Some men have hair on their penises, while others don't; some penises are wrinkly, others smooth; some are the same color as the rest of the body, and some are lighter or darker. Some penises have heads partially covered by foreskin; others may have an inch of overhang. For those who are circumcised, the scar and amount of loose skin on the shaft may vary from very visible to not at all noticeable.

Why do we focus so on our penises? Political thinker Herbert Marcuse saw it as a capitalist ploy: by isolating the genitals as sites of pleasure, the rest of our bodies can be put to work in the service of industry. Feminist men and women both have argued that it has to do with a reductive masculinity, a constant need to affirm male power at women's expense. Some gay men speak of penile preoccupation as a natural law, attributing to their penises an almost numbing power. "For years my life has been shaped by a my-penis-made-me-do-it attitude," says a New York office manager whose name, appropriately enough, is Peter.

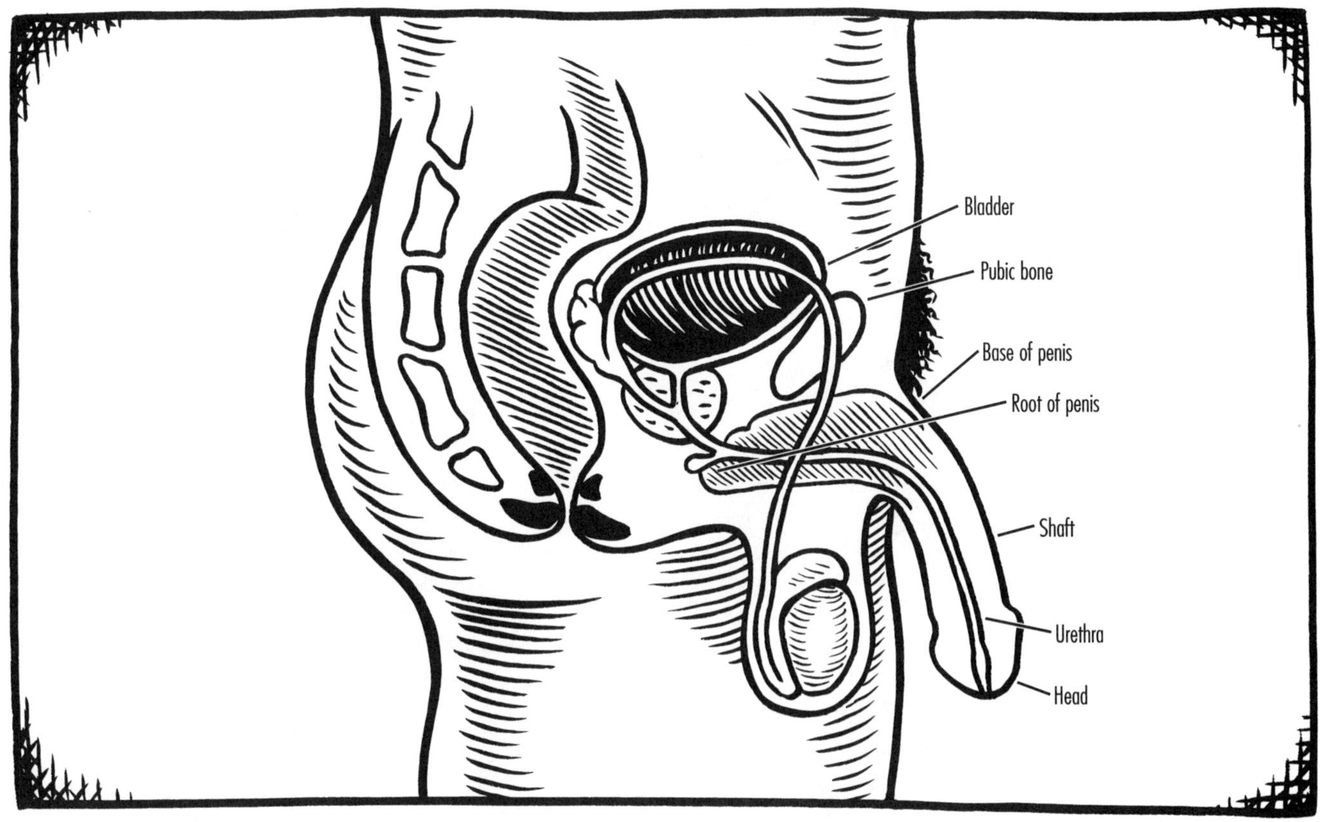

Penis

Reactions to the penis, of course, exist in context. Those of us in countries where men pee standing up touch our dicks daily, mostly without the stimulation of the sexual. Stand next to someone at a men's room urinal, however, and you may feel a tension or a charge. Rush to get dressed for work and the penis is ignorable. Undress for a first session of lovemaking, and you may find yourself conscious of each curve or emerging wrinkle.

It's a good idea to take your penis in hand every once in a while, not just for sex but to feel how things are going. Considering how much pulling and prodding we put it through, the penis is a pretty resilient body part: Serious penile problems, such as cancer, are relatively rare. Many of us have a number of tiny, pearly bumps on the skin of our penises. Known as "pearly penile papules," these are harmless. Also relatively common are minor cases of itching, irritation from a fungus, or sores or warts caused by a sexually transmitted disease (see Chapter 4).

More delicate is the urethra, the tube that carries urine and semen through the penis and out of the body. The mucous membranes that line the urethra are sensitive, so the introduction of anything foreign—any kind of object, shampoo, soap, whatever—is quick to cause stinging, burning, or worse. "There have always been idiots who will shove anything up their dicks that will fit—pencils, wires, ballpoint pens, glass tubes, you name it!" writes Larry Townsend in *The Leatherman's Handbook II* (Masquerade Books, 1997) in a bit of S/M observation echoed by urologists. Danger of infection and tearing makes it important not to put anything inside your penis without strict and careful precautions. Burning in the urethra, discharge, or blood in the urine can be signs that something is amiss with the urethra, kidneys, prostate, or other internal organs.

If you do find a physical problem with your penis—bumps, burning upon urination, discharge, or pain—see the chart on page 42. Since self-treatment is a tricky business, you should also see a medical professional.

HINTS FROM THE HOMO SUTRA: *PENILE HOT SPOTS*

You know them already, but do you know what to call them? Whether you are attempting to gain an erection, stimulate the one you have, or just find your way around, certain pleasure points on the penis should not be missed. Happily, these are quickly grasped—many of them at the same time—by your hand or someone else's.

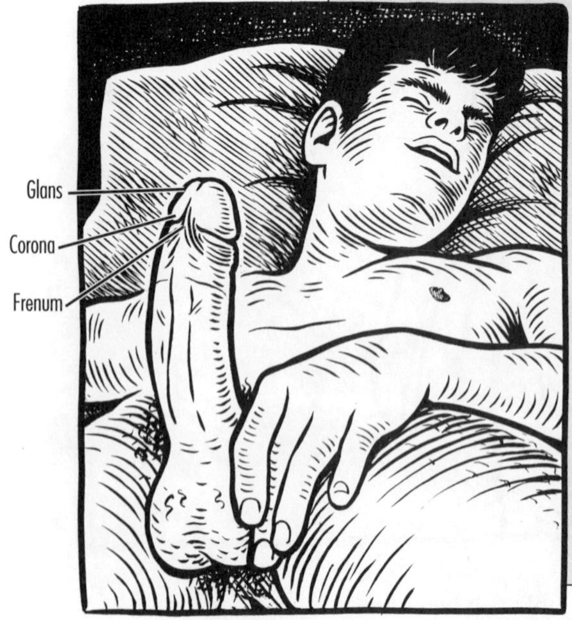

• *Gratify the glans,* which means "acorn" in Latin. In English it refers to the head of the penis, one of its most sensitive parts. The whole glans fills with blood during erection, making it primed for touch.

• *Caress the corona,* the fancy name for the edge of the head, and another of the penis's hot spots. In uncircumcised men, the corona may not be completely visible until or even during erection, but it's still highly sensitive to the way the foreskin slides over it. It often deepens in color as men become highly aroused, leading an astute observer to be able to predict oncoming orgasm.

• *Finger the frenulum.* Trace a finger around the corona until you reach the underside. That's the frenulum (also known as the frenum), the little Y-shaped membrane on the "throat" of the penis just under the head. On uncircumcised men, it's what attaches the foreskin to the shaft. On circumcised men, it's smaller or gone entirely, replaced by a highly sensitive ridge of skin or scar tissue. Many are able to ejaculate just by continued stimulation of this small spot with hand or tongue.

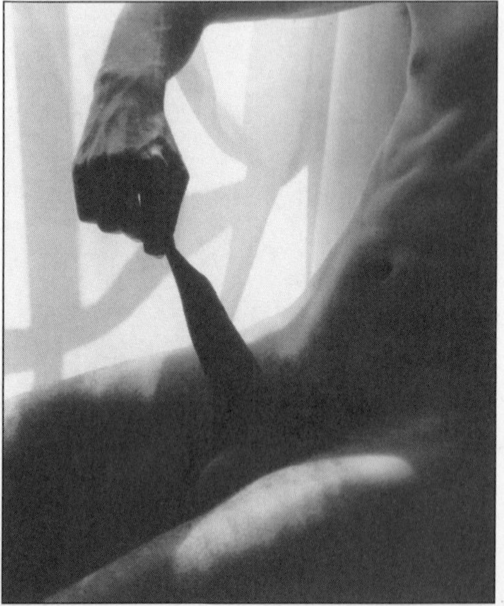

FORESKIN

Erotics and Realities

You can touch it with the skin up or the skin down. You can nibble and bite it. With apologies to my cut brothers, I have to say that all that extra skin means extra fun.

It stretches enough for me to pull it over the head of somebody else's dick and masturbate us both into the hottest orgasm ever.

My foreskin is a part of me, like my hairy legs, the way I smell, the curve of my chest.

Before I take off my clothes, I always skin it back so no one sees it. I don't have any overhang, so, if I do it quickly, no one can even tell.

I had a boyfriend who was really into it, but a lot of guys look at me like, "Is that thing clean?"

Circumcision—removal of the prepuce, or foreskin, that covers the head of the penis—is a hotly debated issue among urologists, pediatricians, and parents in America, and a different kind of hot topic for adult gay men. Many of us find circumcised penises a turn-on because of the familiar nature of their beauty (an estimated two-thirds of men in America are circumcised) or because of cultural associations: Jews and Muslims are traditionally circumcised. Others see those same kinds of erotic resonances in a Latino or Italian uncut penis, or swear the smell and silky feel of a foreskin promises pleasures unobtainable from a cut cock. Medical "experts" have recognized the mysterious allure of the foreskin since the late 1800s, arguing for circumcision as a cure for "masturbatory insanity," transmission of syphilis, and even homosexuality. By the 1940s, in a tradition carried forward until today, those arguments were replaced by more clinical appeals to cleanliness and the avoidance of cancer, sexually transmitted diseases, or a tightness of foreskin that might necessitate circumcision later in life.

Nonsense, respond the proud owners and admirers of intact penises, the most fervent of whom liken the head of a circumcised penis to the callused foot of someone who has gone without shoes for years. While penile cancer is virtually unknown among circumcised men, it's among the rarest of any cancers among any men at all, afflicting one in a hundred thousand Americans. Recent studies have refuted the old claim that uncircumcised men are more likely to contract STDs, and most gay men don't need to worry about reports that women whose partners are uncircumcised experience higher rates of cervical cancer. All in all, say some skin-folk, the increased sensitivity of life with foreskin is more than worth the simple daily maintenance—retracting the hood of skin and washing underneath—that prevents most infections.

Some uncircumcised men report discomfort with even their healthy foreskins, though, and surveys show that uncut men are less likely to feel comfortable masturbating or receiving oral sex. Whether that has to do with embarrassment or other cultural or economic factors is none too clear. Other men revel in what they describe with phrases such as the "crowning experience of total sexual stimulation," the way in which their foreskin, acting as a self-lubricating, moveable sheath, gives an added caress to the glans with every thrust of the penis. Some even welcome the accumulation in themselves or their sexual partners of a little bit of smegma, a creamy or cheesy substance under the foreskin of an unwashed penis. The delights of "cheesehounds" aside, that accumulation can be the cause of health problems. To fully enjoy the foreskin—and the extra nerve endings that come along with it—it makes sense to put in the extra time to keep the head of the penis clean.

Somewhat alarming, though also not fully explored, are a number of studies that found that sexually active uncircumcised gay men faced as much as twice the risk of HIV infection, even after adjusting for factors such as race, history of injection drug use, or sexually transmitted diseases. One theory is that the motion of the foreskin may create tiny cuts or abrasions that facilitate the transfer of HIV. Still, condoms go on penises with foreskins and without. If you wish to be circumcised, it need not be a safer-sex decision.

Tips for Uncut Tips

My mother took me to be circumcised at age twelve because I couldn't skin my foreskin back. Later I found out that it can take that long for the foreskin to naturally separate from the head. The operation went fine, but I still wonder if it was necessary or just an expression of her discomfort with my growing awareness of my sexuality.

• *Use a mild soap, or none at all.* The damper, moister head of the uncircumcised penis is exquisitely sensitive and does not do well with parching, irritating soaps. A foreskin also has a smell, which Jim Bigelow, Ph.D., foreskin expert and author of *The Joy of Uncircumcising!,* says is one of the main reasons people insist that it should be scrubbed. "In America, people think the body should smell like perfume or nothing at all," says Bigelow. "In fact, the foreskin is an internal organ, and washing it with harsh soap is no more advisable than washing out your mouth with soap and water." Ironically, scrubbing your foreskin in the name of health may in fact cause more sensitivity and inflammation. A hypoallergenic soap, or just warm water, can often do the trick.

Balanitis is an inflammation of the head of the penis and foreskin most commonly caused by a yeast infection, contact with rough fabric, sensitivity to detergent, or an allergic reaction to latex or other irritants. Washing with clear water and careful drying—perhaps using a hair dryer set on "warm"—should relieve the problem. In the event that it persists, says Mark Litwin, MD, assistant professor of urology at the University of California, Los Angeles, topical treatment—an antifungal cream for a yeast infection or cortisone cream for more generalized skin irritation—should clear it quickly. To get the right cream for the job, see a doctor.

• *Stretch yourself.* If you are experiencing phimosis, the tightness of the foreskin that prevents easy retraction over the head of the penis, try stretching your boundaries. One process involves sparing use of nonsteroidal or steroid creams applied to the head of the penis, says George C. Denniston, MD, president of Doctors Opposing Circumcision (D.O.C.) and an assistant professor in the University of Washington's Family Medicine Department. A more organic approach, to be done in consultation with a doctor but achieved at home, is a do-it-yourself stretching program. Soak your penis in warm water, grease the head with a mild, non-irritating lubricant, and apply gentle pressure with your index fingers to dilate the foreskin. This is a gradual process, writes *Men's Private Parts* author James Gilbaugh, MD, and should be discontinued if there is any pain or hint of tearing. Men who can't even get their fingers in to start the process report that small plastic speculums, like the kind used to look into a baby's nose, can be inserted to dilate the skin. While you're at the medical supply store that sells such items, you might also want to pick up a small plastic bulb and syringe used for a baby's nostrils. These can be filled with mild saline solution and used to clean the glans and under the foreskin until it is more stretchable.

How stretched a foreskin is desirable depends on who's doing the desiring, with some men dilating theirs to be big enough to encompass the head of somebody else's penis. Other men are happy with a foreskin that retracts enough to clean the glans when they're soft, but stays halfway over the head when they're hard.

If you are stretching at home, don't pull your foreskin all the way back over the head until it seems wide enough to slide back in the other direction. In the event that your foreskin does get stuck behind your glans, a condition called paraphimosis, don't just leave it there, and don't panic. Dr. Denniston suggests lubricating your glans and foreskin, then squeezing the blood out of the head of the penis by pressing it firmly between your thumb and first two fingers. In many cases the skin will slide back. If it doesn't, seek immediate medical attention, says Dr. Denniston, since you can cause yourself serious damage, or even gangrene, within hours of cutting off circulation.

FORESKIN RESTORATION

I always used to push the head of my penis back toward my body in the bathtub at age six. One day I looked in the dictionary and saw an illustration with a dotted line pointing to the foreskin. I still remember looking at my own penis and seeing that I didn't have one.

It was actually Jewish athletes in 330 B.C. who started the tradition. In those days, though athletes competed naked, revealing the head of the penis was considered improper by the Greeks. More than a few Jewish contenders in the Greco-Roman games figured out ways to stretch the skin on their penis forward until it could cover the head. Two thousand years later, in the 1970s, gay porn star Al Parker again raised the profile of the issue, and a few eyebrows, by undergoing surgical re-creation of the foreskin on his rather public penis. Today, thousands of men who feel circumcision left them missing something important are using a variety of methods, most of them nonsurgical, to urge the loose skin of their penis over their glans. "I grew up as a boy believing that I was the only one in the world pushing my glans back toward my body or wishing I hadn't been circumcised," says Jim Bigelow, Ph.D., the California-based psychotherapist who restored his own foreskin in the mid-eighties. His *Joy of Uncircumcising!* (Hourglass, 1995), which includes resource lists, bibliographies, extensive medical analysis, and personal testimonies, has become a kind of bible for the restoration movement. Written with the zeal of the converted—Bigelow is a former evangelical minister—and blurbed by doctors around the world, the book has also established itself as a handbook for care of the uncircumcised man.

The restoration process, done in consultation with a doctor but performed at home, involves a gradual stretching, using first-aid tape to hold the skin in place and straps or small weights to create the necessary amount of tension. The resulting foreskin often passes for original. Judging by the many letters published by Bigelow, and the dozens of Internet and in-person support groups around the world, the restoration, which can take up to two years, is an emotional process as well as a physical one.

One Internet site, Paul's Foreskin Restoration Diary (http://net.indra.com/~shredder/restore/diary.html) offers a bird's-eye view, chronicling one man's restoration experience in intimate detail, including photos of the process and diary entries at various stages. NORM, the National Organization of Restoring Men (www.norm.org), has information and referrals.

A few men, even after stretching, find it difficult to retract the foreskin over the head and want to change that. A few others may feel a tightness at the frenulum, at the underside of the head where the foreskin attaches, or experience tearing or bleeding there during vigorous sex. In both cases, circumcision is a surgical option, though not usually the only option. Some phimosis can often be relieved by making a small incision in the foreskin, known as a z-plasty, and then resewing in a way that relieves the pressure.

If you and your doctor decide circumcision is necessary, it is a straightforward surgery. It does involve cutting and sewing, though, and it should not be attempted by anyone except a trained professional. Sure, you've heard stories about do-it-yourself success stories or hot S/M scenes. But you don't want to live with a ragged edge or the complications of infection or massive bleeding. In a doctor's office, says UCLA's Mark Litwin, MD, circumcision is an outpatient procedure, in most cases remarkably painless and requiring about three weeks to heal. "When I do it, it's a three-visit scenario," says Litwin, "one visit to talk about the procedure, another to perform it, and a third to make sure it has healed properly."

If possible, find a doctor who has some experience with uncircumcised penises before you seek treatment for any of these complaints. Circumcision is so accepted as the default mode of medical intervention in most medical schools and literature that many doctors may get unnecessarily snippy. NORM, the National Organization of Restoring Men (www.norm.org), maintains a list of foreskin-friendly doctors.

As for those gay Americans, circumcised or not, who are into boys with a hood, the West is the best: According to government estimates, national averages in that part of the country (we're talking Pacific Standard Time here) are reversed, with more than two-thirds of males born there leaving the hospital intact.

Penis Size

Big Talk

If I sleep with White boys, I can't get over the sense that they're going to be disappointed—that somehow, no matter what they say, they're still expecting me to have a big Black sausage between my legs.

I try to "fluff" before I go to shower. Lots of guys at the gym do it. You want to be hard enough to look big, but not so hard you look sleazy.

Bob, my first boyfriend, was totally relaxed. "I'm not badly endowed," he said, "and I get a kick of looking around at other guys." Actually, I always thought his penis looked quite small, but he was so relaxed it made him great in bed.

I, for one, love being pounded by a tiny tool, or being with someone whose penis I can easily get in my mouth.

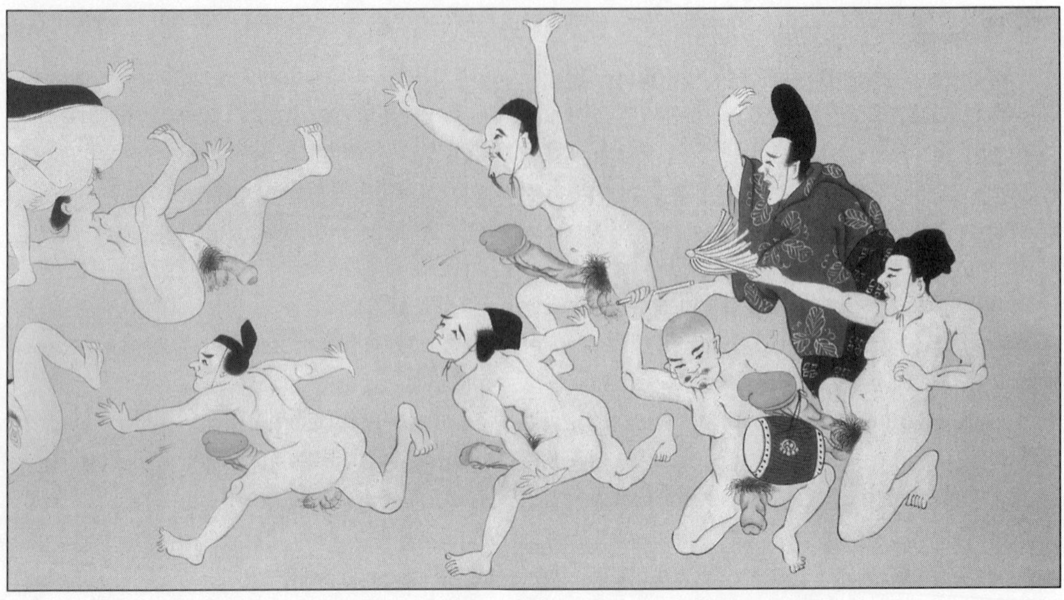

Sometimes, looking at your penis, it's easy to forget that it's connected to your head, and to a whole system of thought that in various ways equates penises and power. That equation isn't simple for any man, but for those seen as outside the majority—gay men, Black men, Latino men, or those of us who belong to more than one of those categories—it gets especially complicated. If many of us feel contradictory things about our penises and what we do with them, the contradictions don't all come from within. On one hand, critics accuse gay men of being dick-crazy, pointing to our penises and our failure to control them as a source of AIDS and powerlessness. On the other hand, there's the school locker room scenario, where gay men are made fun of as unmanly, sissies, pussies. Growing up in America, a stream of nearly constant jokes and locker room banter reinforces the idea that the bigger the penis, the bigger the man. Look at the euphemisms for the penis in gothic romances or those great gay pulp novels of the 1970s, where someone is at long last allowed the pleasure of touching the hero's "sex," his "manhood," or his "member," and you get the idea about how your penis is supposed to stand in for all kinds of issues relating to masculinity, power, and belonging.

And then, of course, we're gay, which means we may think even more than other men about how others' penises look, and whether ours looks good, too. Some of us think about it a lot, or admit to a special fascination with the big ones. The perfect-sized penis, though, resides primarily in the imagination. The reality, as any honest observer of his own penis knows, is that size varies: not only from person to person, but from hour to hour. Your penis shrinks and expands according to the temperature, what you're wearing, or how you're feeling.

For centuries researchers have delighted in asking subjects to shuck their pants and put their penises on the line. French colonial doctor Jacobus Sutor marched through Africa and the Middle East, measuring men in every village he passed through. Pioneering entomologist-turned-sexologist Alfred E. Kinsey got 3,500 men to mark a postcard with their dick length and return it by mail. California urologist Jack McAninch, MD, injected an erection inducer into his willing subjects and then measured for himself. In the process, studies have debunked most of the penis mythologies, finding no strong correlation between foot size and penis size, nose size and penis size, or African descent and penis size. Nonetheless, the myths persist. People delight in fantasizing about what lies behind the clothing. Lots of us even delight in imagining the research done to figure penis size out.

"What a tiresome obsession it's become!" writes Charles Silverstein, Ph.D., author of *The New Joy of Gay Sex* (HarperCollins, 1993), on the question of penis size. "The man with the big cock feels he's valued by his appendage alone. The man with a small cock is embarrassed by it and feels that he's spurned because of it." Dr. Silverstein's impatience comes from decades of work as a psychotherapist with gay men. "Often," says Silverstein, "cock size becomes a cover for other insecurities."

Happily, not everyone worries. Two-thirds of the ten thousand gay men surveyed by *The Advocate* in 1995 said they would like a "bigger penis." That doesn't say much; the question, a little like "Would you like to be richer?" is easy to answer in the affirmative. Project Sigma, a groundbreaking research project working with gay men in England, found that two-thirds of those they asked worried rarely or not at all about their penis size, though they did find the topic of great interest. Ever resourceful in recognizing the something-for-everyone nature of the sexual marketplace, some gay men have joined together in informal clubs and associations with other men of similar endowment. J. Meisler, director of Small Etc., New York's association for gay men short in stature or penile length (and the men who love them), says that hundreds of men from around the country pay a $20 membership fee not just to list their personal ads, but for camaraderie and advice. Among Small Etc.'s offerings: formfitting condoms made especially for the smaller-endowed man (Bikini Fit, $7 a dozen), videos, and porn stories that feature men with small penises in "a positive light, as proof that small is beautiful." "Letters pour in from men looking for partners with small dicks," says Meisler. "They say Michelangelo's David is their ideal, and since David had a small penis, that's what they're looking for in their partners."

Pump It Up!, on the other hand, a quarterly publication full of personals, fiction, and ads for various sex toys and equipment, bills itself as "a publication for men into size." If a magazine for men who like 'em big seems like an unnecessary attempt to make a "special interest" out of the majority, consider that this is a particular kind of size, brought about by the use of vacuum pumps or other procedures on penis, testicles, and nipples. Numerous doctors, while prescribing vacuum pumps to treat erection problems, have judged claims of penis enlargement to be false, and many of the companies in *Pump It Up!* sell their products with the dubious but obviously self-protective tag lines "Sold as a novelty only" or "Not intended for use." Numerous pictures attest, however, to the fact that men do use vacuum mechanisms to draw fluid into the penis or nipples, sometimes for hours at a time, and that their genitals are definitely enlarged. The confusion about whether enlargement is possible may be due to the limitations of language, since the spongy, fluid-filled, but fattened penis of the hard-core pumper looks no more like a regular penis than Arnold Schwarzenegger's pecs look like a regular chest. The language of desire from *Pump It Up!* personals—including words like *bloated, grotesque,* and *monster*—captures some of the particular appeal. Some men even use a saline drip to infuse their scrotums with up to a quart or more of solution, making their balls look like water balloons until the fluid seeps out and is reabsorbed by the body. "Gotta be crazy," warns E. Douglas Whitehead, MD, assistant professor of urology at Albert Einstein College of Medicine and director of New York City's Association for Male Sexual Dysfunction. "Anytime you inject something into the scrotum you risk infection, and we could be talking about one rip-roaring infection." UCLA's Dr. Mark Litwin raises concerns about cellular damage from prolonged pumping, as well as the danger of infection from scrotal infusion.

Big Truths

It's a cliché, but it's the biggest of big truths: It's not the meat, it's the motion. From the perspective of the sexual partner, penis size doesn't seem to have much to do with satisfaction: Masters and Johnson's interviews found that men with erections of two inches were still able to satisfy their partners, and they didn't even talk to people who especially loved being pounded by petite penises. Or, as the authors of the straight but savvy *Sex: A Man's Guide* (Rodale Press, 1997) put it: If you want to measure something, measure the pleasure.

If you feel like all that's a line you can't buy, then consider a few other big truths.

1. Don't Believe Everything You Hear

Men are notoriously bad at evaluating their own or others' penises. According to a 1989 study by researchers at the Kinsey Institute, 30 percent of American men had the wrong idea about how long the average penis is, with the vast majority of those believing it to be eight to twelve inches long. Since gay men see more erections than the average straight man, you'd think we'd be better at gauging. Not necessarily so, say researchers in the know, at least not when we're making big claims for ourselves. "All of the subjects who initially claimed an erect cock length of ten inches or more turned out on re-estimation to have a considerably smaller cock length," noted Project Sigma's study. One self-proclaimed eleven-incher, for example, actually measured six and a half.

2. A Soft Penis Is Not Indicative of How It Will Look at Full Mast
Careful investigation has found that guys with relatively short limp penises gain much more in erection—almost twice as much, proportionately—than their longer counterparts.

3. It's the Variations That Are Small
There are a very few men who have a condition called micropenis and an erect length of less than two inches, and a very few men who have penises that top the eight-inch mark. Around 85 percent of guys measure within only a few inches of each other when they get hard. That magic average, confirmed by study after study? Five to seven inches long when erect, measuring along the top (from tip of penis to where a ruler pushes into the abdomen). Average circumference is 4.9 inches around.

Hard Sell? Penile Enlargement Surgery

For as long as man has wanted a bigger, harder penis, there have been people offering inches for money. The latest entry in that arena is penile enlargement surgery, whose ads now jockey for space with those for vacuum pumps and baldness remedies in the magazines for men between twenty and fifty who are the procedure's largest consumers. Common enlargement efforts involve one of several different surgical procedures. The first involves snipping the ligament that anchors the penis to the pubic bone, freeing the several inches of the organ that ordinarily remain hidden inside the body. The second involves the grafting or injection of fat—liposuctioned from belly or thighs, for those who want to take care of two issues at once—onto the shaft of the penis to make it wider.

At as much as $6,000 a clip (or is that "a shot"?) for the combination, the procedures are neither cheap nor without detractors. "None of the men I've seen who've wanted it have had anything less than normal penis size," says Jack W. McAninch, MD, professor of urology at the University of California, San Francisco, and past president of the American Urological Association. "But surgeons wanting to make money are quick to take advantage of a moment of emotional weakness." Gary Alter, MD, an assistant clinical professor of plastic surgery at the University of California, Los Angeles, performs the surgery and has made headlines fixing up botched jobs. Still, he cautions that men who believe ligament surgery means they can just cut and run should think about the extensive follow-up and commitment. "Most length is gained after the operation, with the patient consistently wearing weights to stretch the penis," says Dr. Alter. "You have to wear heavy weights, eight, ten, twelve pounds, twice a day for ten minutes a day, for months."

Those willing to go to those elaborate lengths can expect to gain a little of their own—somewhere between one and two inches when soft. To the surprise of some men who have had the surgery but no adequate explanation beforehand, their *erect* penises gain much less, perhaps as little as three-tenths of an inch. Nor do their "new" erections get as high, since the penis's support system has been severed.

Fat injections, while less involved than ligament surgery, get even worse reviews from doctors and recipients alike. Many men report gradual and uneven reabsorption of the fat, which leaves a dick noticeably lumpy without follow-up injections as often as every six months. "I think that practitioners who do it should be shot," says New York City urologist Franklin C. Lowe, MD, after seeing a number of the lumpy, bumpy results. Newer technology involves grafting strips of fat and skin taken from the buttock or groin, increasing penile width by as much as a third and diminishing the chance of reabsorption. This is more extensive surgery, says New York's Dr. E. Douglas Whitehead, lasting up to several hours and requiring surgical dressings for three weeks and no penetrative sex for six. For uncircumcised men, agreeing to the graft also means agreeing to circumcision, since swelling under the foreskin can take months to subside. Nonetheless, says Dr. Whitehead, the operation leaves only "moderate to minimal scarring" and yields "a very nice result."

Practitioners of these surgeries, and those suspicious of them, agree on one point: They will do nothing to enhance your sexual skills. "It's a psychological thing, but it won't do anything to make you a better lover," says Dr. Whitehead. Dr. McAninch, in San Francisco, asserts that "these operations have a lot more to do with what's between your ears than what's between your legs," and says patients are often better served by a doctor willing to explain the unproven nature of the surgery and the range of normal penis size.

If you are considering penile enlargement, make sure you choose your surgeon carefully, asking to talk to patients and look at pictures. "This is a new field, and numbers are less important than skill," says Alter. "Just because the doctor says he's done a whole lot of penile enlargements doesn't mean he's been doing them well." McAninch urges men to get a second opinion rather than rushing for a resolution that will leave them unsatisfied.

As for the men themselves? Hard to know, since many don't want to advertise their new enhancements. San Francisco–based therapist Randy Klein, Ph.D., surveyed fifty-eight men, 20 percent of whom were gay or bisexual, about their experiences after surgery. All of them had soft penises over 2.6 inches in length before they started, and most cited a better self-image as their motivation. Apparently that wasn't so easy to find. Less than half were happy with the width of their "improved" penises, more than two-thirds were disappointed with the length, and a whopping 80 percent were dissatisfied with the aesthetics of their penis due to scarring, curvature, or lumpiness. Sexual satisfaction among the men dropped significantly after the operations, as did masturbation. Not exactly what the doctor ordered.

Erection and Penile Pleasure

First of all, contrary to popular belief, erection and penile pleasure are not one and the same. While plenty of men feel self-conscious about their soft penises, not enough of us take the time to enjoy them. The loose skin of a penis, rolled gently between your own fingers, is a special pleasure. There are as many nerve endings capable of transmitting impulses to the brain in a soft penis as in a hard one. And though the billion-dollar impotence industry is unlikely to let you know, orgasm and ejaculation are both possible without becoming totally hard.

Men's experience of penile pleasure can be as varied as the shapes of their dicks: staying strong, solid, and without much distinction between beginning and end; tapering off; or swelling to a head. It's common in the course of ongoing stimulation for penises to rise and fall, even if you're still turned on. Stimulation can also mean different things to different people. Dick and ball torture, for example, can send shudders of discomfort and revulsion down the spines of some; for others, those are shivers of delight.

Be that as it may, there's no question about it: An erection is something to enjoy. "A hard-on isn't everything," says Joseph, forty-four, from Atlanta, "but it's sure not nothing, either."

Forty years later, I still remember Mark B.'s cock from gym class. I thought about that boy's dick nightly. As for my own, it would start to stiffen each time I had to change in the locker room. I used to hide it with my hands and look away, as if by not paying any attention to it I could conceal my secret.

For gay men who grew up concealing their sexual desire, the hard-on is a moment of self-revelation tinged with delight and danger. Many of us remember the combination of intense desire and intense fear experienced in high-school locker rooms, men's rooms, or other places where men open their pants together. The idea that your hard-on says things you don't dare to remains for some of us a lifelong pleasure. In certain kinds of sex—the public, silent kind—a hard-on's worth a thousand words, revealing without revealing too much that you're aroused and ready for further stimulation. In a bedroom, certain kinds of dirty talk—urging your partner to "suck that dick," or asking if he likes "that cock"—offer a different appeal, separating penis from person in a way that lets us get hot without being too bothered about the fact that it's we who are asking for the pleasure.

In other contexts, though, showing our hard penis is something we do only when revealing our softest, most private parts: thoughts we've never told anyone, deeply intimate feelings about ourselves, whom we love, and what makes up our fantasies. When things are good, hard-ons and those feelings combine into explosive, ecstatic sex and orgasm. Other times, the penis wilts even as we come together with someone we are very conscious of wanting.

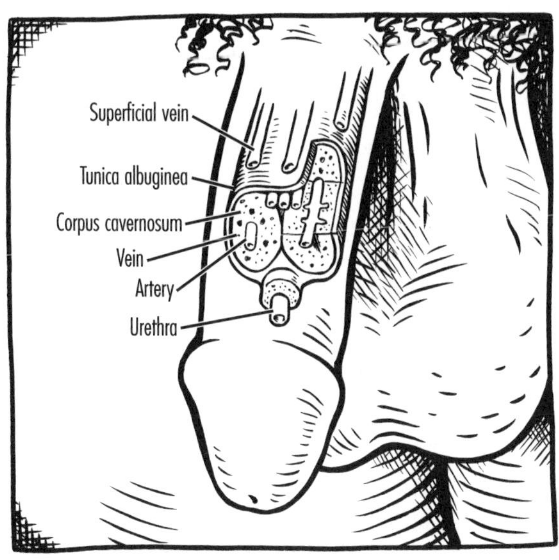

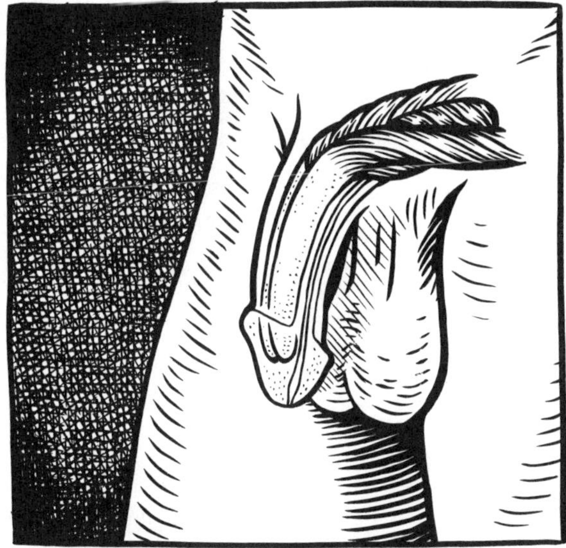

Penis: Two internal views

BAD BREAKS . . . Rough riders beware. Though an erection is built to withstand quite a bit of pressure, it can break. More precisely, you can rupture the tunica albuginea, the sheath that gives shape and rigidity to an erection, or the ligament that runs from the penis back to the pubic bone. "Forcing your way into a nondilated, nonlubricated anus can be a cause," says New York City urologist Franklin C. Lowe, MD, though what the medical professionals call *coitus inversus*—intercourse with the receptive partner on top—is the more common cause. The ordinarily gentle position goes awry if the person astride falls backward, or pulls up and off and then comes down wrong. You'll know by the loud popping sound, sudden loss of your erection, swelling, and pain. Should you be unlucky enough to experience this, proceed to an emergency room immediately, says Dr. Lowe. Medical attention is needed to restore and retain proper functioning.

Physically, blood flow is the key to what makes a hard-on hard. The veins that often snake down the middle of the penis, while beautiful to behold, are only one part of the secret. Equally crucial is a complicated network of smaller blood vessels and reservoirs, invisible to the eye, that are flooded with blood when stimulated by the brain's response to a sexy thought, image, or the right kind of touch. Central to the penis and the process are the corpus cavernosa, two columns of spongy material that run from just under the glans all the way down the shaft. At the appropriate signal, these columns are flooded with blood, their sponge-like cells swelling up and pressing against a rigid sheath, the tunica albuginea, that gives your erection shape and form. That pressure, in turn, presses closed the veins that carry blood away from the penis. The effect, when working properly, is like filling a balloon: With the blood trapped inside, the penis rises up hot, full, and ready for action. The erection remains firm until the brain sends a signal to slow down blood flow and release the pressure, which usually happens after ejaculation, or after the stimulus is removed.

If yours bends downward or lists a little to one side as it fills, fear not: Erections curve often, veering leftward about five times as often as they turn to the right. They also vary widely in their angle, jutting straight out, pointing down, or arching up toward the belly. According to Kinsey, whose famous sexuality surveys included extensive documentation of states of arousal and orgasm, the average angle of dangle is somewhere between 5 and 30 degrees above horizontal. That lift decreases as we age, and changes with the size of your penis. The bigger the "burden," the slighter the rise.

Erection Enhancement

For centuries, the specter of the soft penis has moved men to, well, extraordinary lengths. Bear paw, rhino horn, tiger penis, and the beetle known as Spanish fly are only a few of the remedies tried by men throughout history anxious to get and stay hard. Today, men are more likely to turn to the technological than to the animal, using Viagra, vacuum pumps, cock rings, or creams and potions. Drugstores and tobacconists sell a host of over-the-counter preparations whose benefits—despite names such as Linger Longer, Sta-Hard, and Stud 100—are primarily the power of suggestion, as well as a little local desensitization (to prevent early ejaculation).

Every inch as important, unless a physical problem is causing your erectile dysfunction, is the power of the mind. Experience a failure to get an erection, and you can generalize it into an

. . . AND BENDS

Some men, particularly men between the ages of forty and sixty, may experience a severe and painful bending of the erection, or wake up one morning to find their hard-ons of extremely irregular hardness. This condition, called Peyronie's disease, may transform an ordinarily upstanding erection into an hourglass shape that looks like it has an invisible belt around the middle, for example, or something that is hard at the bottom and floppy on top. In some cases the penis actually bends up to 90 degrees, causing sharp pain or making intercourse impossible. The cause of Peyronie's disease is not definitively known, though many suspect it to be the result of a tiny tear in the tunica albuginea (see "Bad Breaks . . . "). The tear itself is not the problem; some men are not even aware that they have experienced such a rupture. When the tear heals, though, the scar tissue, or plaque, that forms there is too rigid to bend, causing one side of the penis to buckle around the immovable spot when you get an erection.

Among the best treatments for Peyronie's is a year's worth of patience, says Mark Litwin, MD, assistant professor of urology at the University of California, Los Angeles. The body often clears the condition itself, and in any case you want to make sure it has developed fully before attempting surgical correction. During the waiting period, many patients are understandably anxious to try other treatments, and many doctors are more than willing to deliver them: topical applications of vitamins E, A, or B, and injections of everything from steroids to gout medication to calcium channel blockers to an enzyme called collagenase. None of these treatments has won approval by the FDA or the confidence of many doctors, leaving the National Institutes of Health to deem surgery "the best option."

anxiety for the next time, and the time after that. Give men a sugar pill—a placebo—and tell them it will help, and we experience as much as a 30 percent improvement in hardness.

None of which is to say that if you are having hard-on problems, your mind is the matter. In fact, about 80 percent of the inability to gain or keep an erection is now thought to have at least some physical component, often relating to our decreasing blood flow as we age. If you're among the one in three men over forty who have hard-on problems, self-help may not be enough. A discussion of the range of medical and physical hard-on helpers can be found in Chapter 4 (see page 169).

For the rest, with good luck and a few of the steps below, you can expect to have erections well into your nineties.

Erection Enhancement Basics

• *Stop smoking.* According to the Centers for Disease Control in Atlanta, men who smoke are nearly twice as likely as nonsmokers to develop erectile difficulties. Not only does nicotine mess with your nervous system, but it also clogs the blood vessels you need to fill to get hard.

• *Eat low-fat.* Fatty foods clog arteries, including those in your penis. The more clogged they are, the less oxygen-rich blood gets through them, and the softer you remain.

• *Exercise aerobically.* What's good for your heart is good for your part.

Balls and Beyond

The testicles—the firm, egg-shaped masses of tubes that hang below the penis and are better known as balls—are the site of production for the male hormone testosterone and for sperm. They are also supersensitive sexual barometers, filling with blood and growing in size when we

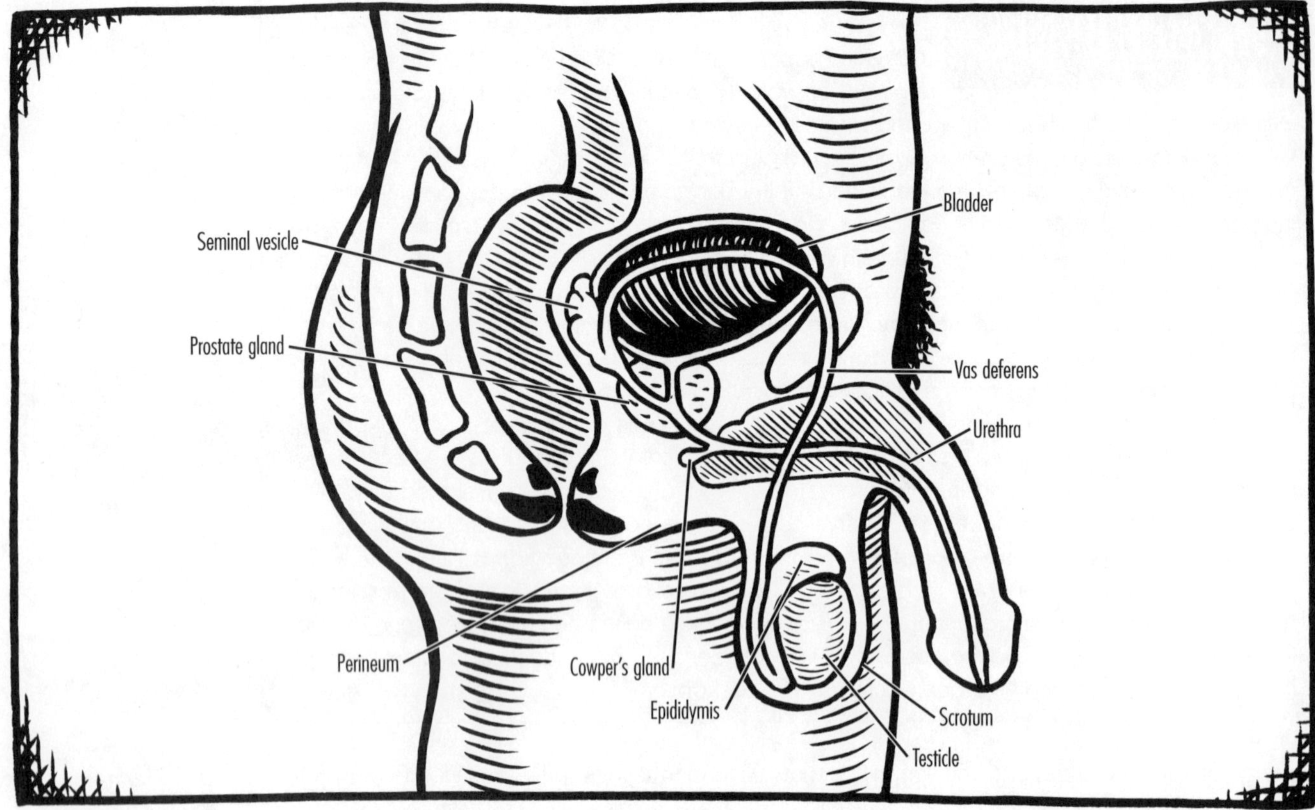

Balls and beyond

are aroused, and rising up toward or even into our body as orgasm approaches. The scrotal sac, the wrinkled pouch of skin in which the testicles hang, is pure skin, nerves, muscle, and blood vessels. No other part of the body except the eyelid has so little fat, leaving the scrotum highly sensitive to touch. Small wonder that Romans and other men of yore used to put their hands between each other's thighs when one was "testifying" to a particularly important point.

Today's men are also keen on putting their hands on their balls, but more for sexual stimulus. Some men find that shaving their ball sac makes it so sensitive that "balljacking"—slow manipulation of the balls and scrotum, ignoring the penis—can bring them to orgasm. Still others like their balls to be pulled or tugged lightly during lovemaking, or find that balls stretched away from their body, using ball spreaders, can both enhance sensitivity and delay ejaculation.

Less entertaining, but even more important, is doing a testicular self-examination once a month to monitor for growths that might be cancerous. Those few minutes can make a major difference in the course of your health and your life. If you're not familiar with the testicular exam, particularly if you're under forty, turn immediately to page 300 in the "Five Tests and Vaccines No Gay Man Should Go Without," section of Chapter 7.

Pain in the testicles, at times for no apparent reason, is common. Being the production site for sperm, the testicles are connected to a network of sensitive internal vessels and organs that work to produce and eject the fluid that shoots out of the penis during ejaculation. While testicular pain that lasts for only a minute or two is neither uncommon nor cause for alarm, more persistent aches or pains may be the result of inflammation or infection and are cause for a visit to the doctor. Most aren't serious. Following is a list of those that are seen frequently.

TIPS FROM THE HOMO SUTRA: *PRIVILEGE THE PERINEUM*

"Highway to heaven" is what some call that strip between scrotum and anus, full of supersensitive nerve endings. Press a finger into the soft area and note that your erection jumps slightly, moved by the sheet of muscle that connects tail and pubic bones. Stroke the perineum and feel the exquisite impulses that run to the brain. Why "highway to heaven"? Inch your finger up (and read the "Seven Solo Steps toward Anal Awareness" section on page 25 before you answer.

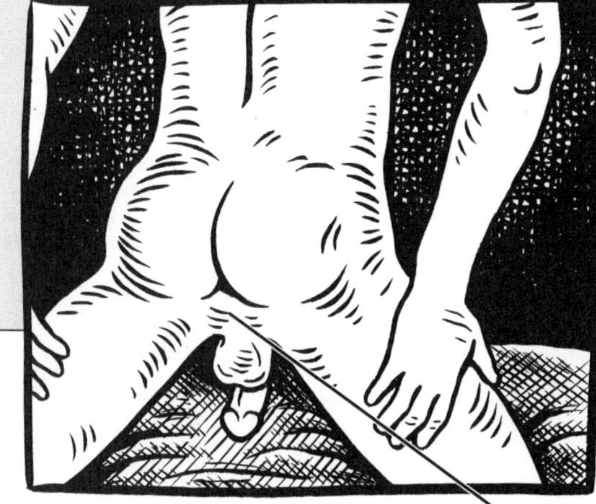

Epididymitis

Epididymitis is an inflammation of the epididymis, the bumpy, soft tube on the back of your testicle that stores sperm. Your epididymis feels like a squiggly tube when you slide your testicle around in your hand, but an inflamed one will feel swollen and painful. Caused by sexually transmitted infections, epididymitis, and the fever and swelling that sometimes accompany it, are treatable by oral antibiotics if attended to early, but may require IV antibiotics in advanced cases. Untreated, epididymitis can cause sterility.

Hernia (Inguinal)

It's what the doctor was looking for when he held your balls and told you to cough when you were growing up. The word *hernia* literally means "rip" or "break"—in this case, in the thin layer of abdominal tissue above the groin area—though with men at thirty times greater risk for the condition (and in a nod to our feminist sisters), *hisnia* might be a better name for the condition. Tears in the muscle sheet can be caused by anything from heavy lifting to a genetic predisposition to the natural weakening of the muscle due to age.

The most common form of hernia is when the intestine pushes through the tear in the abdomen into the inguinal canal, the passageway around your spermatic cord. This shows itself outside as a bulge or lump in the groin or scrotum when you strain or cough, or a swelling that decreases or disappears when you lie down. If the blood supply to the protruding bit of intestine is cut off (strangulated), this can be both painful and dangerous; other times, you may be able to gently guide the tissue back where it came from without pain. In most cases, surgery is recommended, the most common involving a simple stitching of the tear. While an expert surgeon can do this with little risk of recurrence—the Shouldice Clinic in Toronto, reputed to be the world's best, reports less than a 1 percent failure rate—less skilled surgeons report that as many as 10 to 15 percent open up again. More consistent results often come from patching the hole with a kind of surgical mesh that reinforces surrounding tissue and prevents recurrences. In both cases, you can expect to be out of the hospital the same day and home from work for at least a couple more, though it'll hurt when you laugh for weeks to come.

Hydrocele

The scrotum contains a slight amount of fluid that bathes each testicle, cushioning it. A hydrocele, or "bag of water," forms when too much fluid is produced, causing liquid to accumulate in a sac within your sac. This condition is usually harmless and painless. If you want to remove it, says Litwin, there are two options: drawing the fluid out, in which case "it will definitely return," or surgery to remove the pouch itself. It's an outpatient procedure.

Spermatocele

An enlargement of the spermatic tubes in the epididymis, this sometimes feels like a grape under the skin. If it's not painful, no treatment is usually required, though removal of the sac can be aesthetically pleasing.

Varicocele

It's pronounced "va-ri-koh-ceel," like varicose vein, which is in essence what it is—enlarged veins of the scrotum. A varicocele feels and looks like a bunch of tangled-up veins, usually massed above the left testicle, and is most common in tall men. The condition usually requires no treatment unless it's painful or suspected in infertility, which it can cause by throwing off the temperature in the testicle. A heavy feeling in your ball is often the most noticeable effect. If surgery is required or desired, it's an outpatient procedure that can be done in an afternoon, including prep time.

Other Conditions

Other pains in the testicles come from outside. Kicks in the balls, or other blows or collisions there, cause swelling, bruising, and pain that can last for a day or longer, as well as an accumulation of blood. Torsion—twisting of the spermatic cord, which provides blood to the testicles—can be the result of way too vigorous ball play during sex, or a genetic predisposition (some men's testicles are looser in the scrotum than others). Mild torsion, where the cord twists and untwists, causes pain that can last only a few minutes. If the cord remains twisted, you know it: pain, nausea, and vomiting are among the results. Cock rings that are too tight can also produce this result. "Torsion is one of the genuine urological emergencies," says Dr. Litwin, "and if not immediately corrected can lead to removal of the testicle." If you're experiencing that kind of intense pain, get to a doctor, who can untwist you, and in some cases place a simple stitch to prevent the event from recurring.

Finally, there is the famous "blue balls"—the dull ache that comes from long periods of sexual stimulation without ejaculation. The cure is simple, and has long been used to treat problems ranging from boredom to tension to insomnia: Take things in hand, and make yourself come.

Anal Pleasure

You recline that magnificent pair of buttocks
Against the wall . . . why tempt the stone, which is incapable?
—*Strato, translated by Teddy Hogge*

Male lust for the ass—or more precisely, someone else's ass—is a classic. And never mind those stereotypes: Between 25 and 40 percent of married heterosexual couples, according to the Kinsey Institute, have experimented with anal intercourse. Define the term more broadly, as we should—including fingers, say, and tongues—and the percentage of people who have received anal pleasure shoots skyward, rising as fast as the penises of the many men who, though they don't talk about it, have found a definite erotic boost from a deftly placed digit or a little lapping at their hole.

Why, then, do so few speak up? Instead of praises for the anus and all its rich nerve endings, we grow up with schoolyard insults: "asshole," "ass-wipe," "ass-lick," "anal retentive," and the like. To give someone the finger is to disrespect them. Freudians reduce the pleasures of the anus to the level of the "immature"; religious leaders and lawmakers declare them unnatural and illegal. Sex therapists tend to know less about these pleasures, too, accepting unexamined claims from straight MDs that anal sex is hazardous by definition. The fact that AIDS is passed primarily by anal intercourse among gay men has reinforced that sense of danger, though it did not cause it. The sphincter, after all—the muscle that controls the anal opening—takes its name from the same root as the Sphinx, the silent, mysterious force in Greek mythology that asked a riddle and then crushed to death all those who could not answer it.

The anal pleasure riddle, though, is solvable if you are interested. "Everyone has the potential to have the anus be the source of the most exquisite experience you can imagine," says Collin Brown, director of the Body Electric School in Oakland, California. "Unfortunately, a lot of us got turned off by an early experience, or were never told that we had another sexual organ besides our penis." Body Electric's workshops—including their weeklong exploration of the land down under, affectionately known as "butt camp"—have drawn more than ten thousand gay men interested in moving beyond bodily taboos to explore erotic energy, massage, and spirituality.

Some might argue that the taboo is the thrill—the thing that makes anal sex dirty in the best of senses. Other men will tell you that they don't need to think about their ass, since no one's putting anything up there while they have anything to say about it. Neither naughty lovers nor the anally averse need worry. Looking more closely at your anus will neither erase the thrill of practices society thinks of as forbidden nor require you to enjoy them. Self-examinations can, however, help you learn more about anal health and pleasure. What sensations can you get from touching outside? Inside? How deep feels best?

Ready, A.I.M., F.I.R.E.! Seven Solo Steps Toward Anal Awareness

I'd been operating under the premise that, physically, I can't do this. So when I went for a physical, I asked the doctor, can you please look to see if there's anything wrong? When he said I was fine, I realized that anal sex probably had to do with trust, and that maybe I didn't even trust myself. I went to the Pleasure Chest, walked in, and announced to the salesman that I wanted a dildo because I was going to teach myself to get fucked. He was extremely helpful, though of course I insisted on one that turned out to be way too large and had to go back later and get another one. I practiced, thinking that if I'm able to do this with myself, I'll be

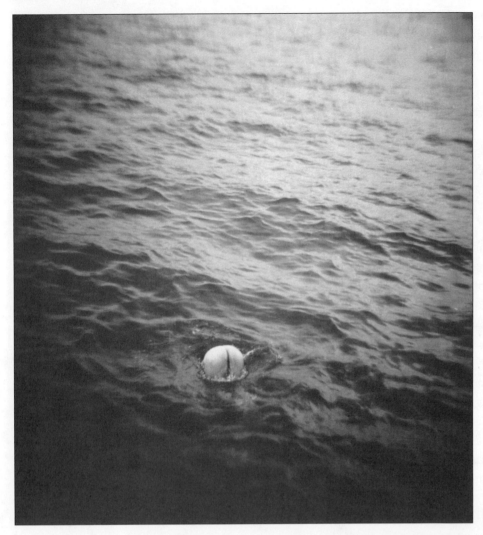

able to do this with someone else. It's not like I would get out the dildo and just cram it up me. I would set aside the time, and make myself comfortable, and play nice music, light candles, and experiment. Later, I must say, it panned out, because I was able to work up to the larger dildo and then be fucked very easily and very fulfillingly.

Fingers, yes, absolutely. Dildo? Penis? Not a chance.

I remember when I was twelve I found this stone in the field near my house, and it was kind of in the shape of a penis, and I used it as a dildo and had this fantasy that it had fallen from an ancient, powerful statue of God.

Anal awareness always happens overnight in storybooks (porn magazines are a kind of storybook, aren't they?). You know: "I told him I couldn't take it, but he pressed on, and with one push he was in, pain turned into pleasure, and I felt myself thrusting back on his full ten inches." In real life, anal pleasure is often an acquired taste, something that you build to over time. Following are some steps to help you get there that you can do alone, culled from sex experts, doctors, and laymen who have done a lot of laying and playing with their anuses. You may go only for step one, or decide that you're beyond the entire introductory program.

If you're just starting, don't be one of those who skips right to the dildo so that they can feel as though they know "how to take it" with somebody else. Tips on anal sex with another person are in the next chapter. And as powerful as it can be to be "overwhelmed" or taken over during anal intercourse, knowing your limits and comforts can make the difference: between safer sex and a risky encounter, between anxiety and awesome anal awareness, and between feeling oh-so-saddle-sore or simply opened up like a flower. Some rosebuds have been closed for years. Let them blossom slowly.

Phase I: A-I-M: Acquaint Yourself, Insert a Finger; Masturbate with Anal Involvement

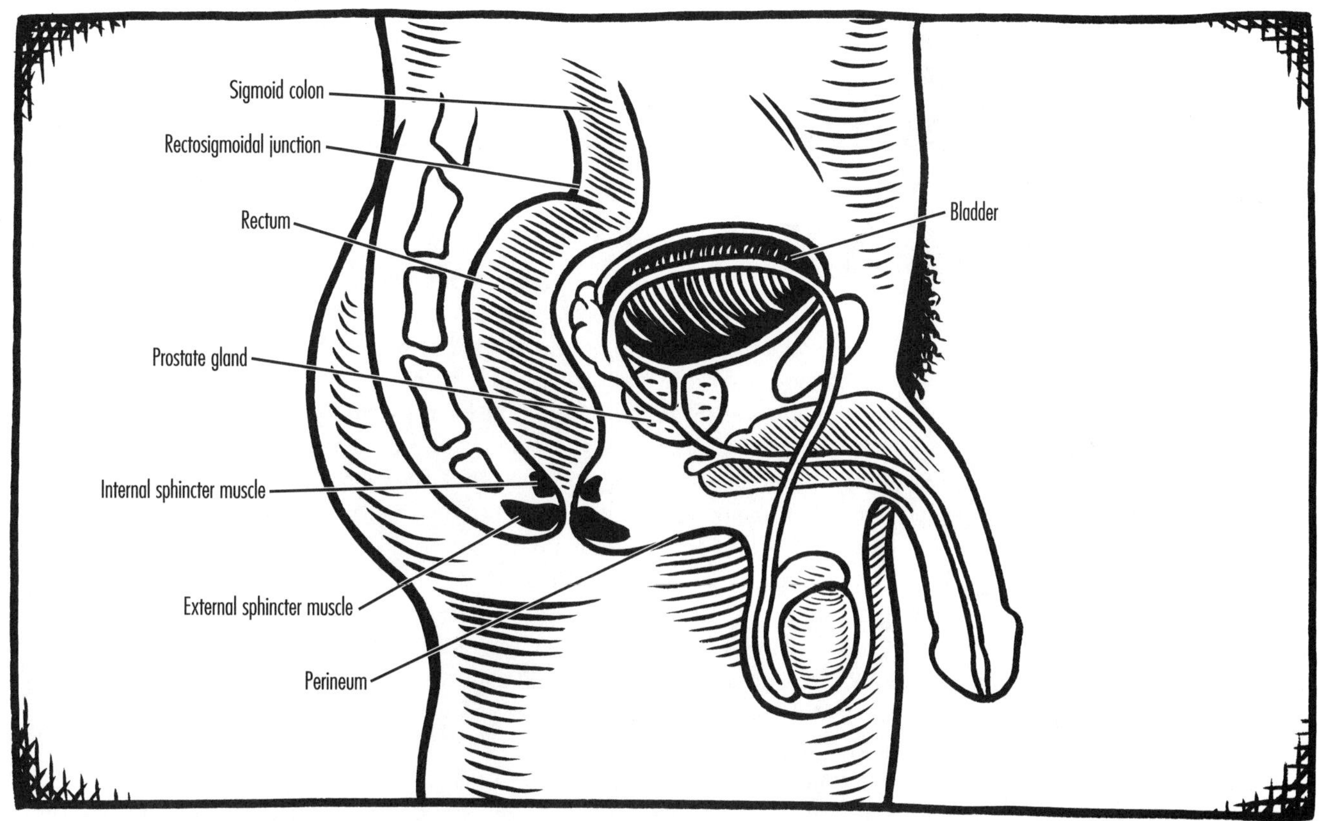

Anus, rectum, and surroundings

STEP 1: ACQUAINT YOURSELF

Making your anus's acquaintance means sensing how it changes with your mood or situation. Jack Morin, Ph.D., therapist, author, and researcher on anal pleasure (see sidebar on page 28), suggests taking a few moments at various points during the day to close your eyes, breathe deeply, and feel your anus. Does it feel tense? Relaxed? Contract and release it.

As part of the acquaintance process, pay attention to your bowel movements. Do you need to strain and push, or does the process seem to happen naturally? Ordinarily, bowel movements are achieved through rhythmic waves of muscle movement known as peristalsis, without straining. If you can, try to follow your body's natural urges, going to the toilet as soon as you feel a readiness, and allowing the process to take place without pushing or hurry. If the urge passes and you have not moved your bowels, return to your normal activities and wait for it to come again.

Finally, take a look at yourself. The women's health movement recognized the value of self-examination years ago: Having spent so much time in the dark with people trying to stick things inside them, women found there to be something freeing about seeing for themselves. The same proves true for gay men, says Chris Bartlett, coordinator at the AIDS Information Network in Philadelphia and facilitator of a workshop entitled "Anything Butt." "Virtually none of the men in our groups had ever looked at themselves in the mirror," he says, "but guys who did that for 'homework' came in talking about how it got them in touch with all kinds of feelings," not to mention a new understanding of what their butthole looked like on a good (or bad) day.

After a bath or shower is often a good time to examine yourself. Since bending over and sticking your head between your legs isn't so comfortable, some men find it useful to squat over a hand mirror, using a flashlight to illuminate if necessary. Note the shape of your anus,

ANAL PLEASURE PRINCIPLES

San Francisco–based psychotherapist Dr. Jack Morin has worked with men and women for years to find ways to enhance their erotic lives. His book *Anal Pleasure and Health* (Down There Press, 1998), as timeless as the *Joy of Cooking*, presents a complete and nuanced program of anal awareness for men and women. Here he offers some of the major pleasure principles.

• ***Anal sex is much more than intercourse.*** "This is a big problem in a culture that's really intercourse-oriented," says Morin. "There's a wide range of anal sex, of which intercourse is probably the least practiced of all. A lot of people get turned off to the whole idea because they don't feel comfortable being penetrated by a penis."

• ***Anal penetration doesn't have to hurt.*** "There's a misconception that you've got to endure the pain to get to the pleasure," says Morin. "If you want to put some effort into having more enjoyable anal experiences, make an agreement with yourself never to go ahead when it hurts. Even if you're into being dominated as part of anal sex, you can find ways to make sure that you have comfort and safety. Then you can let go and be ravished."

• ***Don't deny the power of the anal taboo.*** Most people will encounter strong feelings of shame or taboo during anal exploration. "We're taught: Don't be conscious there, don't look there, don't put your fingers there, don't put your attention there," says Morin. "The result is that too many of us end up groping in the dark, pretending we know exactly what we're doing and ignoring strong feelings of discomfort." Deny these feelings and you'll make yourself more tense.

• ***Know the landscape.*** There are two anal sphincters—an internal one and an external one—that hold your anus closed. The outside muscle you control; the inside one, only a quarter of an inch away, is autonomous, meaning it—like your heart or your breathing—operates independently. The internal sphincter tightens as it senses gas or fecal matter coming down from above or a penis or finger coming up from below. While practice can make autonomous responses amenable to suggestion—yogis can slow their heartbeats or direct blood to certain parts of the body—patience is the key for those of us who are less disciplined. The inner sphincter, like any muscle, remains tensed for only so long before it relaxes. If you have a problem getting past, wait thirty seconds or so. Remember also that the rectum is not a straight tube: it takes a slight curve toward your navel and another toward your back. "It's easy to get in a couple of inches or so, and then some people just start ramming," says Morin. Round those curves gently, and see the illustration on page 33.

• ***Explore.*** "One of the best favors you can do for yourself is put your finger in your butt every day," says Morin. "Not just for sex, but for health. Many people start this process because they had a bad case of hemorrhoids. Self-exploration and relaxation not only can help with these problems, but can help prevent them."

the delicate tissues that surround the opening. Still watching, touch the sensitive tissue. Don't put your finger inside, even if you've done that, or more, before. Stroke your anus. Do you note pain? Pleasure? Tension, much of which we store in the anus, is also common. Don't try to get rid of it; just try to keep your focus.

This stage may last a few weeks, or a lifetime. Even when you have a partner explore your ass, it is not necessary for him to go inside. Chris Bartlett names a number of methods that win praise from men in his groups: massage, spanking, light whipping, teasing with the fingertips. "It's easy to fall into the trap of believing that the only good cock is a hard cock and the only good butt-play is penetration," says Body Electric director Collin Brown. "There are incredible sensations to be had just by working with the outside of the anus."

Step 2: Insert Your Finger

After getting acquainted, invite yourself in. Lubricant will definitely make this easier—since you're doing this yourself, and no condoms are involved, either water-, oil-, or silicone-based is fine. In general, for anal play, avoid lotions (they are absorbed too quickly and often contain irritating scents) as well as gloppy oil-based lubes like Vaseline (they cover up pores in your rectum, get stuck in hair, and so on). Water-based lubes wash up more quickly, and silicone-based lubricants stay wet longer. Take a look to make sure your fingernail is smoothly trimmed, so as not to snag any of the sensitive tissue inside.

Start slowly, repeating the touching exercise above. Then lubricate your finger and your anal opening, breathe deeply, and insert the tip of your finger into your anus as you exhale. Even a quarter inch at first may be fine. Patience is critical—trying to force things will make you tense, as will sudden withdrawal. Stay with it. Try massaging around the opening with your other fingers to relax and open the anus. If the sensation hurts, then you're going too fast; as you breathe and relax, you should feel yourself opening more. "A hungry butthole is a happy butthole when it comes to penetration," says Collin Brown.

If you can, move your finger around gently in a circle. Press up or down you will feel the walls of the anal canal—a small tube about an inch in length. You may also feel, about a quarter of an inch apart from each other, the two sphincter muscles: the outer sphincter you use to keep your ass closed, as well as the inner sphincter muscle, which operates more independently to close the entrance to the rectum.

As you relax, you will be able to put two fingers in, or even three, and move them deeper. When extraordinarily relaxed—as happens in surgical procedures, or with those few people who have practiced fisting—the canal and inner sphincter can open wide enough to accommodate an arm. Much more common, though, is for even a finger to encounter resistance, or a feeling of trying to expel the object, at the inner sphincter. Try to stay curious rather than deciding right away how it feels, advises Morin. "Imagine that you're going back to being a twelve-year-old kid who's just exploring," agrees Brown. "Give yourself that innocence."

Step 3: Masturbate with Anal Involvement

Since how we relate to anal penetration is so much about control—control of your bowels, control of your embarrassment, control of your masculine position in the world—self-love is especially appropriate for the new anal explorer. Choose a place and position that allows you to be relaxed: on your back with your legs spread, or with your knees raised to your side. If music or a porn video helps set the mood, then feel free to use them. Don't feel as though you have to go right for your target—run your hands over your whole body instead. Make sure to play with your perineum, the space between your ass and balls, and tease your penis. When the moment is right, breathe deeply, then slip a greased finger of one hand inside yourself and continue to play with your penis with the other.

Don't get too worried about orgasm or hard-on; it's quite common with anal penetration for your erection to fall as a finger or a penis moves inside you. Forget about how much you're supposed to be able to feel, or what you imagine you "should" be doing. If you have fantasies, go with them; if not, go with the sensation. Your goal for the moment is just to get used to the pairing of anal attention and penile stimulation.

If you do build toward erection and orgasm, see if you note any changes in anal tension as you do so. The same increased blood flow that is causing your penis to respond to arousal

COMING CLEAN: *The Dirt on Anal Douching and the Shit Taboo*

I remember the first time someone stuck his finger up my ass. I didn't feel anything except, "Oh, my God, what if he pulls it out and there is some turd stuck to it?" It still makes me nervous.

For me, it became a part of the Saturday-night routine: shower, douche, do my hair, and shave. Not that I always ended up finding someone to go home with, but I felt prepared.

From toilet training on, we've learned that even our own shit is dirty, that we should go into a room with a locked door to deal with it, that we should wipe it away and wash our hands as soon as possible. It's common, especially at first, to find the whole idea of exploring our own or someone else's anus tinged with that fear of dirtiness. There are real health risks from someone else's shit—hepatitis and parasites are among the illnesses transmitted by fecal matter—but the intensity of our reaction even to self-exploration says more about our mind-set than our bodily functions. With the exception of just before bowel movements, and you know when those are, little fecal matter is usually stored in what doctors evocatively call "the vault," the anal canal and that part of the lower rectum within reach of a finger. When stools are healthy and well-formed, they tend to pass with little trace. And even if there is a trace, it's probably worth it to think through the repulsion to a more rational response. "Relatively few people are ever going to like fecal matter—a few people love it—but it is realistic for most of us to be able to let go of that intense revulsion reaction," says Dr. Morin. "Yes, there are dead and live bacteria in shit, and it has a smell. But it's part of the digestive process, not poison."

Still, a little washing up (emphasis on up) can make you feel a lot more comfortable during any kind of anal play. Douching—the washing out of the rectum and/or lower colon, also referred to as an enema—can remove anxiety, as well as the small amount of shit that may irritate your tissues as something longer than a finger moves in and out of your ass. It may also unfortunately remove the protective oils produced by your anal glands and cause some irritation of its own. If you do douche, you don't need to go for a whole hot-water-bottleful, though for some those belly-swelling enemas can be highly erotic. Also, avoid commercially available vaginal douches, whose

is filling up the tissues in your anus, making it more sensitive and receptive Some people find it useful to wait until they are sexually excited before approaching their anus at all. Again, don't force anything. If you ejaculate while your finger is inside you, feel the contractions that accompany the pulsing of the penis. Be conscious, also, that after orgasm the anus tightens up—when you pull out, do it slowly.

Phase II: F-I-R-E: Find Your Prostate, Insert a Vibrator or Butt Plug, Relax, Enjoy

For some men, external stimulation of the anus is enough. Some find a finger pleasurable but decline to receive bigger guests. For many of us, the pleasure of penetration is heightened by an added treat: massage of the prostate gland, which, pressed right, makes our penises leak and our bodies groan with pleasure. It's a male thing (women don't have a prostate). It's a good thing. And for some of us, it's a key to anal ecstasy.

Step 4: Find Your Prostate

The prostate, the little doughnut-shaped gland that surrounds the urethra, produces the majority of the liquid that makes up your ejaculate. Many men never even know they have a prostate until, later in life, a doctor tells them it's enlarged, inflamed, or in need of removal.

scented liquid may be especially irritating, going instead for a modest Fleet enema from your local pharmacy. Tap water also works just fine, though if your T-cell count is less than 200, either boil it first (and let it cool) or use distilled water to keep yourself safer from microorganisms. Whatever you use, make sure you allow enough time to drain yourself completely: It's common, especially for men on the go, for there to be some seepage later. If you're looking for a means of cleaning, there are a number of inexpensive devices to get the liquid where it needs to go:

- *Turkey baster.* Pharmacies call it a bulb and syringe because it sounds more clinical. In any event, this is a $1.29 item at any grocery store, and holds enough water to clean you out just fine. Take a nail file to the seam down the middle and lube well to avoid scratchiness, and do your roommates a favor and don't put it back in the drawer with the wooden spoons.
- *Shower tube.* Large pharmacies often stock this item, a small metal cylinder with holes in it, attached to a flexible steel tube. The tube screws right into your bathtub faucet, which means you need no extra gadgets to wash out. Use very low water pressure (a little goes a long way) and check the temperature before you start—hot in this context can be seriously painful.
- *Douche bag.* This is the red rubber staple of the seventies gay bathroom, now less visible but still available at any pharmacy. Essentially, it's a hot-water bottle with a long tube and tapered plastic nozzle. Fill it with water, hang it from the shower knob or shower curtain rod, stick in the lubed nozzle, and let it flow.
- *Ear syringe.* The choice for the man on the run, this small bulb is really designed for cleaning a different erotic orifice. Still, it fits nicely in your backpack, can be filled more or less discreetly in the sink of a public bathroom, and provides enough water for a quick refresher. Get the kind with the tapered end.

If you're douching in preparation for being fucked, and don't want to risk getting HIV inside you, you've got to make sure he uses a condom. Placing a nozzle up your butt may cause small cuts or abrasions; as noted above, douching and scrubbing can also irritate the mucous membranes that line the rectum. All of this may increase your risk of HIV. For the same reasons, douching in the event of condom breakage—a home remedy tried by some gay men—is not a good idea, and is actually likely to place you at greater risk of infection.

Some people, understandably, confuse it with *prostrate,* which means lying facedown (or ass up). But those who know how to find (and spell) their prostate are certain of one thing: That first *p* is for *pleasure* (see box on page 32).

Step 5: Introduce a Dildo, Vibrator, or Other Stimulus

Penis-shaped vibrators are often hard. Softer, more forgiving latex dildos, or the even more flexible and more expensive silicone models, are more comfortable for many. A small vibrator, a butt plug, a dildo, or anal beads (see "Toys and Tools," page 75) all work well for anal exploration, as does a good old carrot provided it's washed. Skip the candles—they're overly brittle—and save the big fat cucumbers for advanced sessions. If you're new to it, slow and slimmer wins the race.

Crucial to good vibrator use—and good anal intercourse—is understanding the curves and byways of the rectum. It makes intuitive sense to most of us that the lower part of the rectum runs toward the belly button. Less appreciated is the fact that, about three inches in, it takes a curve in the opposite direction, toward your back. If you're in the right position and relaxed, the curve straightens out somewhat to allow free passage. Ignore it, or have someone ignore it for you, and whatever you are trying to put up yourself runs smack into the wall.

MAKING FRIENDS WITH YOUR PROSTATE

1. ***Get in touch.*** When you have an erection, slide your finger inside your anus about two inches, then head up toward the navel. The prostate's between your finger and your belly button, and is normally about the size of a walnut. When you're aroused, it (like many other good body parts) increases in size, swelling to almost the size of a golf ball, which is why it's easier to find when things are hot. The gland, when you find it, feels a little like the edge of a plum. Press gently, and you may feel a fullness, a pressure, and a sensation that seems to be pressing something out your penis. Actually, since your prostate secretes much of the fluid you ejaculate, that's exactly what's happening. If you are prone to pre-cum, this move may urge a little more out of you. Some men find that prostate massage gives them an immediate urge to pee.

2. ***Don't poke, stroke.*** The prostate is actually two different lobes, wrapped up in a thin layer of tissue. Some men claim a special sensitivity to the seam running down the middle, stimulatable by moving your finger up and down that tiny ridge. "If I find it, it's like pressing the button on the Bikini Atoll," crows Howard, thirty-seven, from Michigan. "Blastoff!" Insistent jabbing, on the other hand, can range from irritating to excruciating. Approach tenderly.

3. ***Kegel it.*** The exercises allow you to squeeze the muscles that surround the prostate, giving it a little mini-massage, and are described at the end of this chapter.

4. ***Share with others.*** The truth is, unless you're very flexible, it's much easier for someone else's hand to find your prostate than it is for your own. Let them try it. You may like it.

5. ***Come along.*** Stimulate the prostate enough, and it often induces a particular kind of orgasm. "Deep," "physical," and "delightfully unavoidable" are a few of the words men use. "It's like I don't have to do anything, it just happens to me," enthuses David, a thirty-eight-year-old waiter. "Mechanical," "soulless," and "like pressing toothpaste out of a tube," offer opponents. Some men can't tolerate prostate stimulation at all. There's no one road to pleasure.

6. ***If it hurts, don't ignore it.*** As with the anus, prostate pain should not be part of the package during sex. More than the anus, the prostate is prone to different kinds of ailments, some serious. If you are experiencing lower abdominal pain, or frequent trouble urinating, see a doctor, and the prostate health section on page 39.

Much of the pain associated with bad experiences of anal intercourse comes from trying to force your way by this wall, rather than readjusting to get in more easily. With enough pushing, you or he can probably force your way by. You can also get a tear, better known as a fissure, or a deeply unpleasant pain. Much better to figure out how to line things up so they can move in more smoothly.

Some like to learn with objects that have flared bases, like butt plugs or dildos with balls at the base, to make sure that the sex toy won't slip inside. Tales of the hungry anus grabbing things out of your hands are mostly tantalizing fiction; much more common is the feeling that your muscles are going to push the dildo out as it rounds that first curve in the rectum. Still, don't push a straight object inside you up to the very end.

If a dildo or other sex toy does go up inside you beyond reach, squat and bear down slightly: the object will probably come down on its own. If it doesn't appear within an hour, says Provincetown surgeon Lenny Alberts, MD, seek medical attention from an emergency room. Take a friend; even though the ER has seen it all before, there's something to having a little support in the face of the inevitable snickering nurse.

The great thing about solo sex-toy use is that you control the pace. Go as slowly as you need to, try to breathe deeply and easily, and dispense with the idea that you have to get it

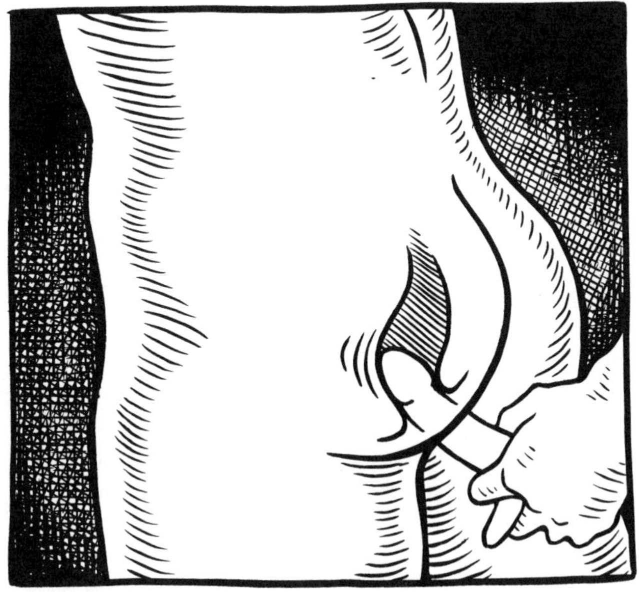
Dildo inserted incorrectly

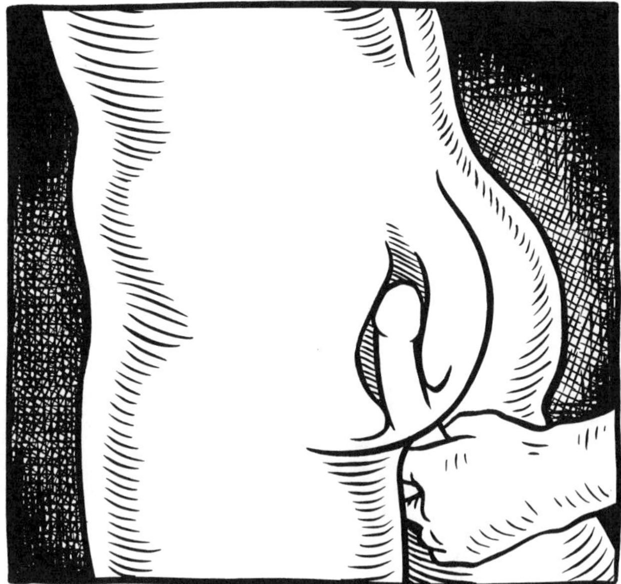
Dildo inserted correctly

"all the way in." If you encounter resistance at the first curve, try pulling out a little, adjusting the angle, and moving in again. When you find an angle that works, make a mental note of it for future use. Some men use dildos with suction cup bases that stick to the wall, finding it hotter and easier to move their bodies into the dildo than the other way around, and liking to leave their hands free for better masturbation.

You are likely, say the experts, to experience new sensations once an object is inside your rectum. "I've seen crying, rage, disbelief at how good it can feel, and people having memories of someone trying to rape or force them to have sex," says Body Electric director Collin Brown. "Anything Butt" facilitator Chris Bartlett says that men in his workshops are able to recall, with great clarity, early toilet training experiences, being shamed about shit, or a gentle and experienced lover who was their first teacher.

Though there's no need to dash to the sink, make sure to wash your dildo or vibrator clean when you're done. If you haven't douched and are using something six inches long or more, be warned that some fecal matter may be in evidence, though nothing a baby wipe—or soap and water—can't easily handle. If you find yourself sharing a sex toy with another person, either put a fresh condom on before each entry or wash with hot water and soap, wipe down with a disinfectant like Betadine, and dry thoroughly between uses.

The general advice about anal play is particularly pertinent here: As you experience a new sensation, try to figure out if it is uncomfortable or simply unfamiliar. If you are unable to get in at all, find it too painful, or feel worried that you are going to inadvertently move your bowels, try the step below. Whether moving in or moving out, move slowly.

Step 6: Relax (and Relocate if You Need To)

Often, as you insert something longer than a finger into your ass, your internal sphincter tightens just as it would if some fecal matter or gas were tickling it from above. The result is the familiar though not necessarily welcome (at that moment) feeling of having to move your bowels. Feelings, as the old self-help saying goes, are not facts. Breathing through the muscle's reflexive tightening can help loosen it, as can the realization, usually born of experience, that you are not really about to move your bowels and so don't need to be as tense. Some people find it useful to introduce themselves to deeper anal exploration in the bathtub, or on a sheet, where the idea of "an accident" seems less scary.

STEP 7: ENJOY

From light stroking of the external anal area to impaling yourself on a life-size replica of a porn man's monster (Jeff Stryker, John Holmes, Kris Lord, and four or five others have been cast in plastic), there's pleasure there somewhere. Take the time. Half the nerve endings in your pelvic region deserve more than a glancing swipe of toilet paper.

ANAL HEALTH

If you find a bit of bright red on your toilet paper that looks suspiciously like blood, feel pain during a bowel movement, or find yourself squatting over a mirror and contemplating a piece of puffy or painful tissue, you may have one of a number of common anal ailments. The medical establishment has come up with a nifty acronym—BAD, or benign anorectal disorders—to describe these, which range from the easily treated hemorrhoid to the less talked-about fissure, abscess, and fistula. Some go away quickly, almost on their own; others can require surgical intervention. Even though all these disorders are labeled "benign," you should never leave them unaddressed. A few simple measures can go a long way toward relieving the discomfort caused by most of these and facilitate the healing process. But because BADs share some of the symptoms of colorectal cancer, which is anything but benign, you should consult your doctor if symptoms persist for more than a few days.

BAD, of course, is also how some of us feel about having a doctor look inside our asses, especially if we think we brought the problem on ourselves. "The biggest message I want to send when I see gay men for a hemorrhoid or fissure is: Anal sex didn't do this to you," says New York City's Stephen Goldstone, MD, a gay surgeon specializing in rectal disorders. "The vast majority of problems of this kind are related to bowel movements—straining, constipation, tearing—not to what someone did with his boyfriend a week ago." Provincetown surgeon Lenny Alberts, MD, while acknowledging that anal sex without enough lube can lead to tears or fissures, adds that gay men who are comfortably anal receptive are actually *less* likely to develop these problems. "Learn how to control your sphincter," he says, "and you don't tend to have the kinds of tension and spasms that can lead to trouble." As for those of us who fear that a trip to the doctor's office will reveal the Bottom within, rest easy. "Generally speaking, unless someone's into fisting, a clinical exam won't tell you whether someone's had anal sex," says Dr. Goldstone. "And straight men also get warts, hemorrhoids, and all the rest."

Warts are sexually transmitted (see Chapter 4), but hemorrhoids, fissures, and the like have less to do with what you put in your ass than with what's coming out. The quality of your stool and the frequency of your bowel movements can tell you a lot about a rectal problem or the likelihood that you'll develop one. In this context, there is such a thing as too hard. Bowel movements may not happen every day—anywhere from twice a day to three times a week may be normal—but they should be regular, firm, and pass easily. Spending lots of time on the toilet straining to push boulders through your butt may give you more time to

THE FIBER FACTOR

"An apple a day keeps the doctor away," wherever that came from, may have really been a fiber reminder. When it comes to health of the colon and rectum, fiber—of which apples are one excellent source—is a key to intestinal and anal health. According to the National Cancer Institute, your colon should get between 20 and 30 grams of fiber per day in order to keep things moving along smoothly. Unfortunately, most of us in the United States eat only about half that amount.

All fiber comes from plants, but it's not all the same. Optimally, says New York City nutritionist Maria Baldo, MS, RD, your body needs a balance of two kinds of fiber: soluble and insoluble. The difference relates to the fiber's ability to absorb water. "Soluble fiber—whose sources include oatmeal, cooked barley, and bananas, among others—helps absorb water in the digestive process, reducing diarrhea," says Baldo. "Insoluble fiber—including raw fruits and vegetables, bran, and whole grains—provides firmness, improving transit time and reducing constipation." Fiber also aids in cholesterol reduction, offers a protective effect against certain kinds of diabetes, heart disease, and high blood pressure, and may help prevent colon cancer.

Twenty to thirty grams of fiber daily might take a whole new way of being, but you can get most of the way there with a little effort. Order whole-wheat instead of Wonder bread, go for fresh fruits instead of juice, and pour yourself a big bowl of whole-grain cereal in the morning. Have some rice and beans for lunch, leave the skins on your potatoes, and hit the salad bar instead of the egg salad for lunch.

If your eating habits are just too hard to break or remake, you can always supplement your diet with psyllium (a soluble fiber, aka Metamucil), oat bran capsules (insoluble fiber), or other supplements available in drug, health food, and grocery stores. Supplements, though, will make you gassy or constipated if you don't drink enough water. Take them with meals if at all, and gradually increase the dosage over a couple of weeks until you reach your target. As with vitamins, it's best to get your fiber directly from food sources. If the fiber is still in the food, so are many nutrients. And the more fiber you eat, the less room you'll have for all those fatty, high-cholesterol snacks.

read *Entertainment Weekly,* but beware the consequences: You may wind up with a BAD-ass problem. Constant diarrhea, too, can lead to a BAD end. So if you think the solution to constipation is to dose yourself with laxatives, or if you were just planning on riding out weeks of the runs, consider dietary changes instead (see box above, and Chapter 6).

Hemorrhoids

It's as if the Preparation H commercials so many of us grew up with have become a stand-in for the hemorrhoid itself, widely experienced but little discussed. The Mayo Clinic in Minnesota estimates that 75 percent of Americans will have hemorrhoidal symptoms at least once in their lifetime. The vast majority of those suffer in shame and silence, embarrassed by the idea that our asses could spontaneously produce anything but the bowel movements we supposedly learned to deal with in childhood.

Ironically, toilet training—or, more precisely, the rush to get it all out that the training sometimes inspired—is one of the biggest causes of anal problems. "Technically speaking, everyone has hemorrhoids, which is just a word for the blood vessels lining the anus and rectum," says Lester Gottesman, MD, a colon and rectal surgeon at St. Luke's–Roosevelt Hospital in New York City. If you push and strain, though, pumping blood into those vessels, they cause problems by filling with small blood clots or becoming permanently swollen. In simplest terms, hemorrhoids are probably best described as varicose veins of the anus.

Veins on the outside, at the entrance to the anus, sometimes get a small clot inside: these are known as external hemorrhoids, and look like small purple balloons that feel mildly to seriously painful. Other hemorrhoids are internal, in the anus and lower rectum: unless internal hemorrhoids are prolapsed (falling out of the opening of the anus), you don't usually see them. They may, however, be the source of blood on your toilet paper or in your toilet bowl, and, if prolapsed, can soil your underwear or get irritated and painful.

Sadly, the old girls' tale—that a good screw can fix an internal hemorrhoid—is fiction. Some internal hemorrhoids come out during a bowel movement and can be pushed in with either finger or penis, but that does not make them go away. Practice in anal relaxation, which may or not be achieved through receptive anal sex, can help with prevention of BADs in general, and may also have some mild effect on healing.

Self-Help for Hemorrhoids

Follow these, and many external hemorrhoids just go away. The first four are also a hemorrhoid-prevention plan.

1. *Diet.* Make sure you're getting your fiber, and avoid spicy or acidic foods (including wine), and caffeine.

2. *Soak.* Warm baths, regular or just bun-deep, ease discomfort and get the blood flowing. Skip the scented bath oils, which may further irritate your troubled tush.

3. *Hydrate.* Drink lots and lots of water (at least eight large glasses per day) to help things pass easily. Doing so will also give your complexion that dewy, youthful glow.

4. *Mild exercise, yes. Heavy lifting, no.* Weight lifting, jogging, aerobics, or other activities where you are bearing down are all likely to increase blood flow, pressure, and swelling. Moderate exercise (such as walking), on the other hand, is good, aiding blood flow and decreasing constipation. At the very least, try not to sit for hours at a time; that weight on your rear is pressing your hemorrhoid, giving it little chance to disappear.

5. *Try a stool softener.* These—ranging from docusate sodium gel-caps (brand name Colace) to mineral oil—make your stool slip out more easily. Unlike stimulant laxatives such as Ex-Lax, they won't cause dependence or damage to intestinal nerves.

6. *Pamper yourself—but not with baby wipes.* These overclean, drying out and irritating the anal area. Scented toilet papers, bubble baths, and harsh soaps all increase irritation, as can rasping and grasping with regular toilet paper. Try medicated pads such as Tucks, or the cheaper folk favorite—witch hazel on a cotton ball. As for Preparation H, Dr. Gottesman dismisses it as good for some relief of itching, but little else. He recommends a mineral oil mixture sold under the name of Balneol, which he dubs "the Clinique of asshole creams."

Medical Help

So there I am, butt in the air, when this nurse with a voice like a three-pack-a-day smoker leans over me. "Don't worry, honey," she croaks. "When this is over, you'll be just like a virgin again."

External hemorrhoid problems usually go away after a couple of days and a little TLC (see "Self-Help for Hemorrhoids," above), which is why people mistake the minor relief provided by over-the-counter hemorrhoid creams for a genuine cure. If your hemorrhoid is a keeper, though, or you don't have patience for the pain, removing an external hemorrhoid takes a matter of minutes. Some doctors apply a local anesthetic, make a small cut in the swollen vessel, and break up the blood clot that is at the center of the little balloon. Better still, says New York City's Dr. Stephen Goldstone, is removal of the hemorrhoid altogether, to prevent the little skin tag left over after the clot is extracted from swelling up again later. You may get sent home with a maxipad between your cheeks to protect your underwear, and the warning that bowel movements will hurt for a few days. Buy a stool softener on your way home—because of temporary tightness, pain, and straining during bowel movements, an estimated 10 percent of patients get fissures (see below).

Medical intervention for internal hemorrhoids depends on the severity of the hemorrhoid. Unless it's falling out of you and causing great pain, best is rubber-band ligation, where the doctor wraps a rubber band tightly around the hemorrhoid to cut off the blood flow, and then leaves it to wither away. A few days off work are definitely in order here, though a week and a minimal amount of pain later, you should be hemorrhoid-free. Other surgical techniques include sclerotherapy, where a chemical solution is injected around the blood vessel to shrink the hemorrhoid, and laser or infrared surgery, which burns the hemorrhoid away.

For seriously prolapsed or painful internal hemorrhoids, you may need a hemorrhoidectomy: complete surgical removal of the hemorrhoid. While the surgery usually solves the problem, an unskilled surgeon will leave you with a narrower, tighter anal canal. This sounds a lot hotter than it is; make sure you choose a surgeon who has lots of experience, and who's able to discuss (if you are) the idea that your anal canal is something you want to leave open for future pleasure. If you can talk to a few of his or her patients, ideally gay patients, so much the better. Even with a good doctor, it will be at least three to four weeks after surgery before you can experience anal penetration or a bowel movement without serious pain.

Anal Fissures

Anal fissures are less common than hemorrhoids, though symptoms are often the same: blood covering the stool, on toilet paper, or in the toilet. Like hemorrhoids, fissures—small tears in the anal canal, which sometimes look like a tiny cut at the opening or just inside—are usually caused by constipation or straining. Once the skin is torn, any subsequent hard edge, including the edge of a bowel movement coming out or a penis or finger coming in, can worsen the tear and the pain. It's a vicious circle: the pain and irritation of the tear cause protective tightening of the internal sphincter, and the tightening of the internal sphincter makes passage of anything solid in either direction more disruptive and damaging. Treatment of a fissure, in fact, revolves around various ways of relaxing the internal muscle, usually by cutting it or dilating it under anesthesia.

The exact cause of anal fissures is not known, although anecdotal evidence from doctors and patients suggests that stress causes the sphincter to tighten, increasing pressure, and eventually, creating a tear. "The expression 'tight ass' doesn't come from nowhere," says Stephen Gorfine, MD, a New York City colon and rectal specialist. Many fissure patients are type A, highly stressed personalities, or those whose stress is peaking at various times. "The accountant gets his fissure in April, the student around exam time," says Dr. Gorfine. "Someone else might get a fissure if their boyfriend or mother is in the hospital."

The first line of treatment for fissures are the same home remedies as for hemorrhoids: warm baths, dietary changes, moderate exercise, and patience (see "Self-Help for Hemorrhoids," page 36). Don't use stool softeners or suppositories, advises Dr. Gottesman—the first can make fissures worse, and suppositories are usually pushed past the fissure and the point where they can do any good. Follow the other self-help tips, and some 50 to 75 percent of fissures will heal on their own, though the process can take anywhere from several weeks to several months. A great resource and reality check is the Anal Fissure Self-Help Page (www.boardsailor.com/jack/af), full of links to medical articles and personal accounts of treatment successes and failures. The accounts of anal problems tend toward the hetero ("nothing more soothing than a wife that you love and that loves you") and are full of the completely interesting and unsubstantiated claims that accompany most individually maintained Internet health sites. Still, the people posting there are courageous enough to share all they have learned since their butts started acting up.

One extremely promising, nonsurgical fissure treatment discussed on the site, and increasingly in medical journals, is topical nitroglycerin therapy. Nitroglycerin (aka NTG) acts to relax the internal anal sphincter, allowing the fissure to heal. One study of thirty-eight patients published in *The Lancet* found that NTG healed nearly seven of ten patients of their fissures in eight weeks. A major side effect was headaches. A major benefit was nearly immediate pain relief.

Dr. Gorfine, who has researched and published on NTG treatment, says doctors unfamiliar with it can make headaches worse by prescribing it in the 2 percent concentration generally used for cardiac patients. The optimal dosage is still being worked out, but appears to be closer to 0.2 percent, a tenth of the cardiac dose. It has to be mixed specially for you at the pharmacy, but the headache at the drugstore will spare you the many more intense ones that are a side effect of putting the 2 percent cream into your anal canal. Use the ointment sparingly after each bowel movement, and two or three other times a day, and wipe off any excess. The longer you've had a fissure, the longer it takes to heal. Some will take up to twelve months. **If you're using Viagra, the erection-enhancing pill (see page 170), do not use NTG at the same time. You could risk a fatal drop in blood pressure.**

Another nonsurgical treatment for fissures is botulinum toxin, injected into the sphincter. Like nitroglycerin, the botulinum toxin heals the fissure by relaxing the clenched muscle. It's the same treatment plastic surgeons use to smooth the wrinkle between your eyebrows, conjuring up all kinds of high-school humor about people who have their heads up their asses and the like. More seriously, it doesn't provide the pain relief that nitroglycerin does, and may relax the muscle so completely that you have a few months of incontinence: You go to pass gas and let go of liquid instead.

Incontinence is also the major risk of surgery for fissures. If you do decide on surgery, the state-of-the-art treatment is lateral sphincterotomy, an incision made in the sphincter to relieve pressure and allow the fissure to heal. "The cure rate for this surgery is between 95 percent and 98 percent, and with a deft surgeon, incontinence rates should run less than 1 percent," says Dr. Gottesman. Trouble telling when you're going to fart is common right after surgery, but that, like gas, passes quickly. Ask the doctor about his experience, and make sure you are not entrusting your delicate anal canal to an inexperienced hand. Even with a good surgeon, expect to spend as much as a week or two recovering quietly at home. "My doctor told me I'd be back at work in two days," says Neville, thirty-four, from Atlanta. "Two weeks later, I was still hobbling around, wincing and farting every time I coughed. You don't realize how often you use your sphincter muscle until it's been snipped." Pain relievers can help, but may also throw you into yet another vicious circle of the sphincter: They make you constipated, and straining causes you more pain. Fiber is your friend.

Abscesses and Fistulas

The glands just inside your anal opening secrete a little bit of oil to keep things moist and flexible. If bacteria or foreign matter get inside them and cause infection, though, they swell with pus, causing an anal abscess. Symptoms of abscesses include throbbing pain that increases gradually over several days, fever, and occasionally a white discharge.

As an abscess drains, about half the time it creates a second unpleasant phase, known as a fistula. The fluid from the abscess burrows its way out of the anal canal through the flesh, causing inflammation and a tiny tunnel joining two ordinarily unconnected areas, such as your anal canal and the skin of your buttocks. It may take weeks, months, or even years to know if you have a fistula, since they can develop long after the abscess appears to have drained.

Abscesses can sometimes be drained in a doctor's office, though deep ones may require general anesthesia and hospitalization. Fistulas usually need a surgical solution, though be careful about having the two operations simultaneously: Since fistulas take a while to appear, you may be wasting your time. Again, drinking lots of water, eating lots of fiber, taking warm baths, and having a doctor who's experienced can help you recover more quickly, and stay open to future anal pleasures.

Prostate Health

Sitting just below the bladder as it does, producing fluid that is part of semen, with direct access to the urethra and right near the sheet of muscle that stretches almost from penis to anus, the prostate is at the center of the action of the urogenital system. Many gay men have found the pleasure potential of that central location (see "Seven Solo Steps Toward Anal Awareness," page 25). When the prostate hurts or swells because of infection, age, or something more serious, it makes itself felt in different ways: pain in the lower back or abdomen, trouble with urination, erection or anal sex, discharge from the penis, and chills and fever, to name only a few. For young men, most prostate problems are infections, caused by anything from a sexually transmitted disease to too much abstinence. Near forty, though, the gland begins to grow, with complications—including benign tumors, infections, or cancer—not infrequently following behind. Chapter 8, "Coming of Age," describes these problems, and their diagnosis, in greater detail.

Prostatitis is the general name given to conditions that can occur at any age, and range from acute bacterial infection that lands you in the hospital to milder, chronic inflammations without a clearly identifiable source. Only about 10 percent of prostatitis cases come from bacterial causes, while closer to 90 percent of the cases fall into the more nebulous and hard-to-treat nonbacterial variety. "People think of prostatitis as an infection, but in these cases it's more like arthritis or bursitis—a chronic inflammation," says UCLA's Dr. Mark Litwin. If you have prostatitis, or its even-harder-to-diagnose, more chronic cousin prostatodynia, a prostate exam is in order. The process, where a doctor slides a greased, gloved finger up your ass, doesn't last long, shouldn't hurt much if at all, and is described and illustrated in Chapter 8. If you want to help your healing, or prevent prostatitis in the first place, try the self-help steps on the next page.

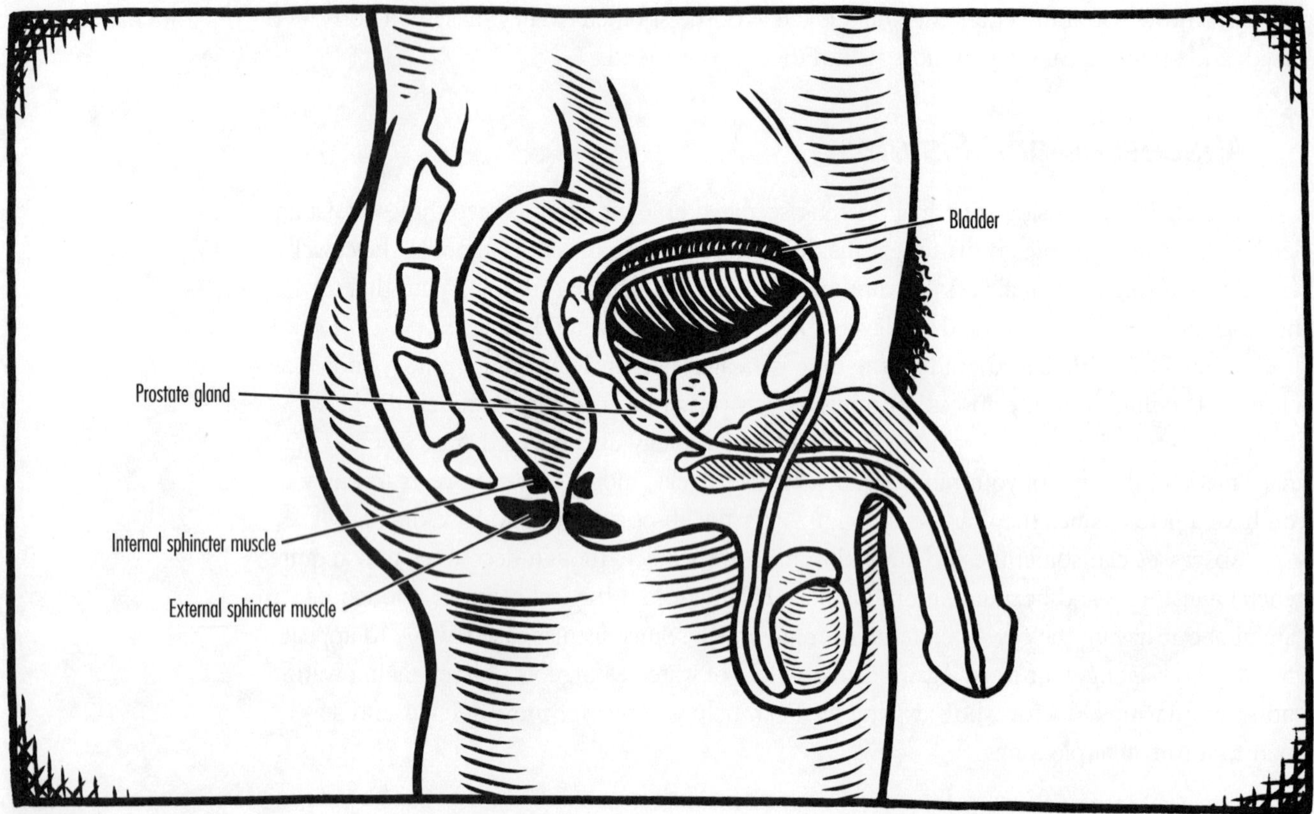

Prostate

PROSTATE SELF-HELP

• *Come again* . . . Go too long without ejaculation and you risk congestion and pain of the prostate. "Priest's disease" and "sailor's disease" are two names for this kind of prostatitis, so called because of those fellows' tendency to build up a backlog. Truck drivers, motorcycle cops, and others who get a lot of genital vibrations without the same amount of release also suffer congestion. Sounds like an ailment some of us would be happy to help cure.

• . . . *but not too often.* Overstress the prostate, which produces most of your ejaculate, and it may get cranky. Age can sometimes be a factor here, since the refractory period, the time you need to rest between orgasms, increases as you get older. If you need to, give it a rest.

• *Water it down.* Once again, drinking water helps your health. In this case it dilutes concentrated urine, which can irritate the prostate. Green tea, too, is a prostate helper, though its benefits have been studied more in connection with prostate cancer (see Chapter 8).

• *Keep it mild.* Avoidance of the same foods that irritate your intestinal tract, such as caffeine, spicy foods, and alcohol, will help. So will avoiding stress, or finding ways to relieve it (see Chapter 11).

• *Work globally.* Once again, the systemic approach helps. Those who get regular aerobic exercise and eat less fat have fewer prostate problems.

• *Act locally.* It's Kegel time (see next section). Actually, most doctors say these are better for recovery from prostate surgery than for preventive health, but they definitely won't hurt. Read on.

KEGELS

Anal awareness. Multiorgasmic potential. Stronger erections. Faster recovery from prostate surgery. Better bladder control. It can all be yours after you start paying attention to what sex therapists and obstetricians have long known as the Kegel exercise. An obstetrician who worked with women to help them improve bladder control after giving birth, Kegel discovered that those who did the exercise not only had less leakage, but increased sexual sensation and vaginal control. Other doctors, coming after, found that Kegels increased men's ability to experience their anuses, and enhanced their own and others' pleasure during anal lovemaking. Modern Taoists, Tantrists, and a host of other students of spirituality and sex say the Kegel is a key to stronger orgasmic control and, in some cases, to the multiple male orgasm (see page 112). Whew! Why don't they teach this exercise at the gym?

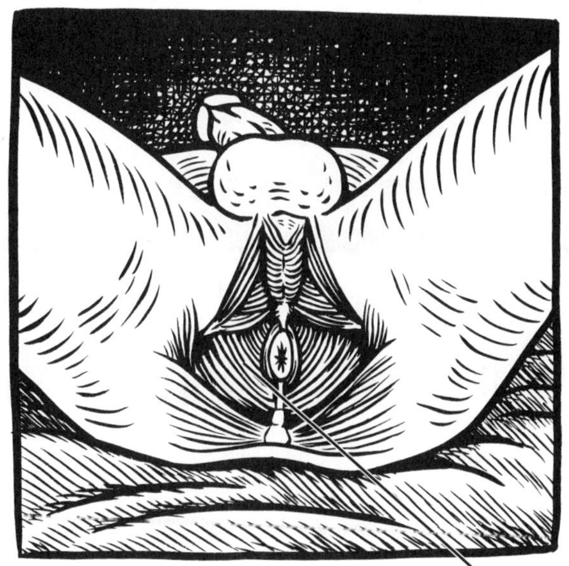

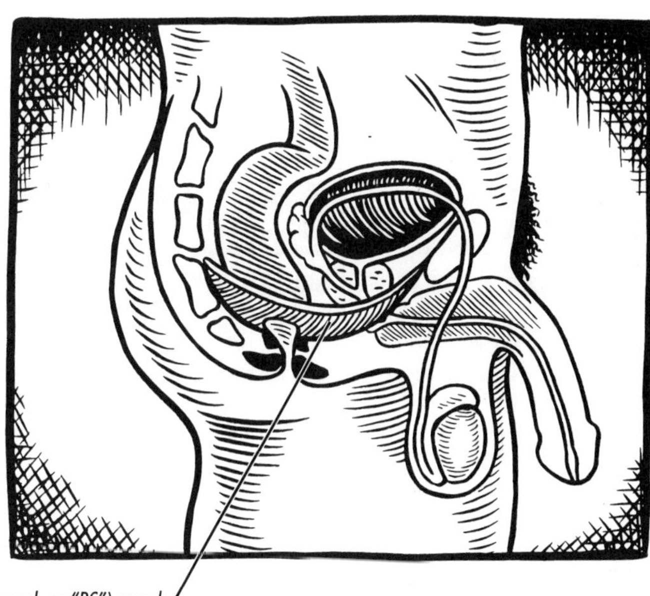

"Kegel (pubococcygeal, or "PC") muscle

Actually, though they do make a Kegelciser, or "vaginal barbell," for women, you need no equipment (except your own). At the heart of the Kegel is your PC, which stands, refreshingly, neither for personal computer nor political correctness, but rather for the pubococcygeal muscle. As you can guess from its name, the PC muscle extends from the pubic bone in the front of your body to the coccyx, or tailbone, in the back. It's a thin sheet of muscle, almost like a hammock, through which the prostate and the urethra pass, and which adjoins a number of smaller muscles at the entrance to your anus. The points at which your penis attaches to your pubic bone, too, adjoin the PC muscle. Work the muscle, in other words, and you touch a whole bunch of points in the pleasure system.

Doing your first Kegel is simple. Simply imagine yourself peeing, and squeeze your urethra shut as if blocking an imaginary flow of urine. That contraction is the basic PC exercise. If you can't find the muscle that way, start while actually peeing (if it stings at first, that's normal, and should go away quickly). Some men start and stop their urine flow as many as five or ten times during a pee just to practice.

One of the beauties of Kegels is that once you've got the hang of it, you can practice anywhere: waiting for the subway, sending a fax, sitting in traffic or in a boring meeting. Afraid people will be able to tell? Ask your friends to look into your eyes and see if they can tell whether or not you're Kegeling. It's also a guaranteed conversation starter at a local bar, if you're daring. People's natural PC strength varies, though most men seem to be able to hold for about ten seconds when first beginning. Practice makes the muscle, and too much practice makes you sore. Sex therapists recommend two kinds of exercises. The first involves inhaling deeply and clenching the Kegel muscle, then relaxing as you exhale. The second involves doing a series of shorter, faster contractions in sets of five or so. Many recommend about ninety long contractions daily, and anywhere between twenty and fifty of the shorter kind.

As for its effect on sex, try it and see. Many men find their erections jump up and get a little firmer when they squeeze their PC muscles as they are penetrating someone's mouth or ass. Those being anally penetrated can use the contraction to grasp or massage whatever's inside them. And whether with someone else or alone, squeezing the PC muscle can prolong pleasure and intensify orgasm, holding the contractions that are the beginning of ejaculation at bay until you build up to a tremendous release.

WHAT'S UP DOWN THERE? A TROUBLESHOOTING GUIDE

SYMPTOM	AMONG THE POSSIBLE CAUSES	SELF-HELP? [As an addition to, not a substitute for, consultation with a doctor]	MEDICAL TREATMENT
PENIS: INTERNAL			
Persistent burning when you pee	Bladder infection	Cranberry juice, extra fluids to flush out system	Antibiotics
	Gonorrhea or nongonococcal urethritis (NGU)		Antibiotics (see pages 161–162)
Frequent urge to urinate, dribbling, weak stream	Bladder infection Gonorrhea NGU	Cranberry juice, extra fluids	Antibiotics
	Prostatitis (inflammation of the prostate)	Avoid caffeine, alcohol, spicy foods, stress; zinc supplements and lots of fluids may help	Antibiotics helpful in some cases (see page 39)
	Prostate enlargement (BPH) if you're over 40	Saw palmetto, African plum, beta sitosterol, green tea (see Chap. 8)	Medication and/or surgical treatment
Dark urine	Liver problems (hepatitis)	Avoid alcohol, drugs (prescription or non-); consider dandelion root, milk thistle, schizandra, and alphalipoic acid	Doctor's visit for diagnosis and treatment (see pages 154–159)
Blood in urine	Bladder infection Cancer of urinary tract Kidney problems	Cranberry juice, extra fluids	Doctor's visit for diagnosis and treatment
	Prostatitis	Zinc and lots of fluids. Avoid caffeine, alcohol, spicy or fatty foods, stress	
Milky or creamy or other discharge (not semen)	Prostatitis	See entry above	See above (see page 39)
	Gonorrhea, NGU		Antibiotics

WHAT'S UP DOWN THERE? A TROUBLESHOOTING GUIDE

SYMPTOM	AMONG THE POSSIBLE CAUSES	SELF-HELP? [As an addition to, not a substitute for, consultation with a doctor]	MEDICAL TREATMENT
PENIS: EXTERNAL			
Tiny white bumps	Pearly penile papules	None needed	None needed
Tiny white or pink bumps, dented center	Molluscum	Vitamin E applications	Scraping, chemical removal, freezing (see page 149)
Inflamed or irritated center vein	Blood clot, often from rough oral sex	Warm packs, penile rest	Doctor's visit if it persists
Itching on shaft or at base, with white, gray, and/or dark red specks visible	Crabs (pubic lice)	Removal of eggs and critters with fine comb or fingernails (get a friend to help)	Over-the-counter anti-pubic-lice shampoo, prescription medication (see page 150)
Itching on shaft or at base, with rash and/or wavy lines on skin	Scabies (mites)		Prescription lotion (see page 151)
Itching or inflammation on head or foreskin, sometimes with chapping or pus	Balanitis or postbalanitis (yeast infection, or irritation from soap or clothes)	Change soap or detergent brands, wear loose-fitting underwear, eat live-culture yogurt	Antifungal or cortisone cream (see page 12)
	Gonorrhea		Antibiotics
Bump under the skin, appearing and disappearing	Broken blood vessel or swollen lymph node	Penile rest	Usually none needed; if painful, doctor's visit
Itching or tingling sensation, followed by eruption of sores	Herpes	Try aloe vera compresses, cornstarch on sores, or oral lysine or licorice root; avoid stress, sun, cold, and foods containing arginine (see page 145)	Antiviral drugs can reduce pain, itching, and frequency of outbreaks (see page 143)
Sores with swelling of genital region or groin	LGV (lymphogranuloma venereum), GI (granuloma inguinale)		Antibiotics
One red or open sore, hard surface; may be painless or weep clear liquid	Syphilis		Antibiotics (see page 159)
One or more painful, red, or open sores, soft surface	Chancroid		Antibiotics
Bumpy, painless growths on shaft or head	Genital warts (HPV)	Vitamin E application	Removal with chemicals, freezing, or topical solution (see page 145)
Bite with broken skin	Fellatio		Antibiotics
Caught in zipper	Not wearing underwear when you're in a hurry	Oil to loosen skin; snipping of bar at bottom of zipper that holds two sides together	Immediate medical visit if self-help measures fail
Foreskin can't come back off head or is too painful to retract	Phimosis	Cleansing with saline solution, gentle stretching after consultation with doctor	Doctor's visit, topical steroid cream, maybe circumcision (see page 12)
Foreskin stuck behind head	Paraphimosis	Lubricate head, squeeze blood out, and slide skin back	Immediate medical attention if self-help measures fail (see page 12)
ERECTIONS			
Bend, no pain	Natural	None needed	None needed
Sharp bend, pain	Peyronie's disease	Wait for natural resolution in consultation with doctor	Corrective surgery (see page 21)

WHAT'S UP DOWN THERE? A TROUBLESHOOTING GUIDE

SYMPTOM	AMONG THE POSSIBLE CAUSES	SELF-HELP? [As an addition to, not a substitute for, consultation with a doctor]	MEDICAL TREATMENT
ERECTIONS (cont'd)			
Cracking sound, pain, swelling	Tear in the penile sheath (tunica albuginea)		Immediate emergency room visit (see page 20)
No erection at all, once in a while	Natural	Relax and move on	None needed
No erection or soft erection, consistently	Physical causes: medications, high cholesterol, diabetes, low testosterone, neurological problems, medications Psychological causes: anxiety, depression, stress	Yohimbine (prescription in some states), gingko biloba, arginine, vacuum pump	Doctor's visit to determine cause and explore treatment options (see page 162)
Erection that won't subside (priapism)	Impotence medications, certain antidepressants	Cold packs on inner thighs	If more than four hours, go to emergency room (see box on page 172)
BALLS (TESTICLES AND SCROTUM)			
Short, sharp pain after twisting or tugging	Normal	None needed	None needed
Persistent pain after twisting or use of a cock ring	Twisting of the spermatic cord or blocking of artery (torsion)		Immediate emergency room visit
One testicle, usually left one, hanging lower	Normal	None needed	None needed
Redness, pain, possible fever	Epididymitis (inflammation of tube at back of testicle)		Antibiotics
Accumulation of fluid (flashlight shines through)	Hydrocele (accumulation of fluid around testicle), spermatocele (cyst of the epididymis)		None needed, or if painful, surgery
Small, squiggly, tubular mass at back of each testicle	Normal: it's the epididymis	None needed	None needed
Larger, squiggly mass enlarging scrotum	Varicocele (varicose vein in scrotum)		If painful, surgery, though none needed
Solid mass, pea-sized or larger (no light shines through)	Testicular cancer, benign growth		Doctor's visit for diagnosis and treatment
EJACULATION			
No sperm comes out	Retrograde ejaculation (into the bladder)		Usually none needed
Blood in semen	Strain from exercise, broken blood vessel in urethra, prostatitis, kidney problems, non-specific	None needed for exercise strain or broken blood vessel; for others, need to determine cause	None needed for exercise strain, broken blood vessel, or non-specific; for others, doctor's visit necessary
Pain on ejaculation	Prostatitis	Zinc, plenty of liquids; avoid caffeine, spicy foods, stress	Antibiotics may help
Take a very long time to, or can't, ejaculate	Psychological, antidepressant side effect	Gingko biloba, arginine, exercises with partner	Change or addition of medication if on antidepressants
Take a very short time to ejaculate	Usually psychological, though "short" is a relative term.	Kegel exercises, work with partner	Sex therapy, medication

WHAT'S UP DOWN THERE? A TROUBLESHOOTING GUIDE

SYMPTOM	AMONG THE POSSIBLE CAUSES	SELF-HELP? [As an addition to, not a substitute for, consultation with a doctor]	MEDICAL TREATMENT
ANUS AND RECTUM: INTERNAL			
Blood from anus or on stool (bright red)	Hemorrhoid, warts, postsex soreness, anal cancer	Baths, stool softener, high-fiber diet	Doctor's visit if it persists after a few days (see page 34)
Bright blood on stool with intense pain on bowel movements	Fissure	Baths, high-fiber diet	Doctor's visit if it persists after a few days (see page 37)
Blood in stool (dark or brown)	Colitis, polyps, colon cancer		Doctor's visit to determine cause
Mucus discharge from anus or on stool	Postsex soreness, gonorrhea, colitis, abscess, fistula, syphilis	Baths, stool softeners for abscess and fistula, dietary changes for colitis	Doctor's visit if no relief after a few days
Throbbing pain, made worse with bowel movements	Abscess, fissure	Baths, high-fiber diet	Doctor's visit
Diarrhea, bloating, cramping, gas	Parasites, flu, postsex soreness, numerous gastrointestinal ailments, reaction to medication, food bacteria	Short-term, try the BRATT diet (bananas, rice, applesauce, weak tea, toast); avoid spicy foods, caffeine; drink lots of water to rehydrate	If symptoms persist more than three days, see doctor
Sharp stabbing pain, vomiting, fever, and shivers	Internal injury, gastrointestinal disturbance		Immediate medical attention
ANUS AND RECTUM: EXTERNAL			
Small flap of skin outside of hole	Skin tag, maybe caused by scratching or former hemorrhoid		None needed unless really unsightly
Bumpy, painless growths outside of hole	Genital warts		Removal with outpatient surgery
Open sore	Chancroid, syphilis, fistula, herpes		Antibiotics, and for fistula, surgery
Itching around anus	Pruritus	Change detergents, soaps, and/or diet (cut spicy and acidic foods and juices, alcohol and excess fluids) Keep yourself dry, trade in toilet paper for Tucks and Balneol, and don't scrub	Doctor's visit if it persists
	Impending herpes outbreak		
	Gonorrhea		
	Hemorrhoid	Baths, stool softener, high-fiber diet	
Hard lump, or painless protruding tissue that can be pushed in	Hemorrhoid	See entry above	Surgical procedure if self-help fails

FURTHER READING

Bechtel, Stefan, et al. (1997) *Sex: A Man's Guide*. Emmaus, PA: Rodale Books. Straight, but savvy.

Bigelow, Jim. (1995) *The Joy of Uncircumcising!* Aptos, CA: Hourglass Book Publishing. Everything you always wanted to know and then some.

Coxon, Anthony P. M. (1996) *Between the Sheets: Sexual Desire and Gay Men's Sex in the Era of AIDS*. London and New York: Cassell. Sex, sexual organs, and how gay men feel about them in AIDS-era England.

Goldstone, Stephen, MD. (1999) *The Ins and Outs of Gay Sex.* New York: Dell. A gay surgeon's expert advice on anal health, STDs, and more.

Morin, Jack. (1998) *Anal Pleasure & Health: A Guide for Men and Women*. San Francisco, CA: Down There Press. As classic, and as necessary to your bookshelf, as the *Joy of Cooking*.

Reinisch, June M., with Ruth Beasley. (1992) *Kinsey Institute New Report on Sex*. New York: HarperPerennial. Questions, answers, and insight from the institute that made sex research famous in America.

CHAPTER 2

Sex Acts and Facts

Notes on Normal • Sex Acts and Facts • Flying Solo: Masturbation • Fantasy • Touching • Mutual Masturbation • Oral Sex • Anal Sex • Sex with Women • Water Sports • Scat • S/M • HIV Risk in the New Millennium • Toys and Tools • Beyond Condoms • Free at Last?

My boyfriend and I had just been out drinking and were engaged in a passionate, though drunk, act of lovemaking. It was a little awkward, on the floor, and I couldn't seem to keep up with him. When he flipped me over onto my stomach, I wasn't expecting it, and the delicious Mexican food I had just had for dinner came back for a visit, this time in a less solid, gas form. In his face. And what a man I have—he just kept going. (I could have died.)

I was in this club and this very hot guy with no shirt on was standing across from me. Our eyes locked and I went over to him, kind of tentative, and started running my hands very lightly across his chest. "What's the matter," he says, "don't you have a mouth?" So I immediately started kissing his chest, lapping at his nipple with my tongue. He pushed me away. "No," he said, "I mean, what's your name?"

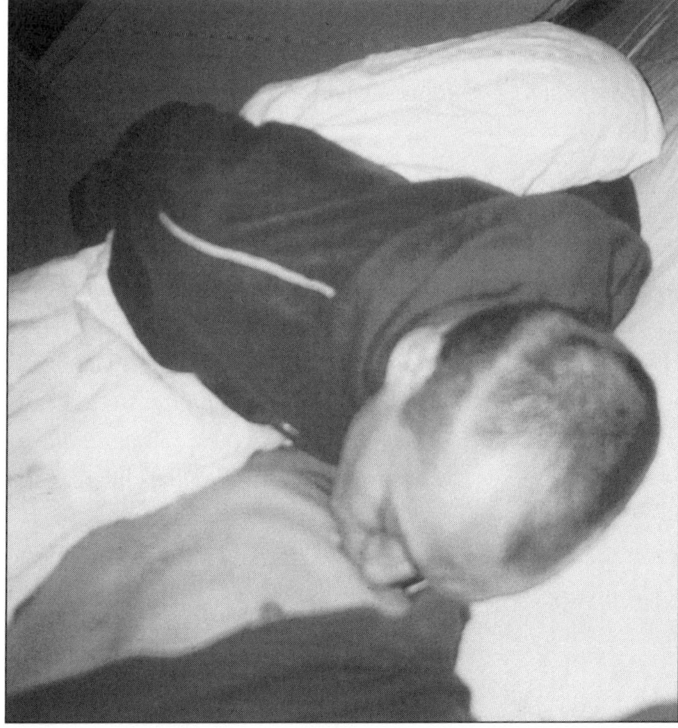

Never lose your sense of humor. Sex is more comic—and complicated—than most of us like to admit, though it's often worth it. While many gay men protest rightly that our lives are more than just our sex lives, few can dispute the transformative, affirming potential of sexuality. Think of the earth-stopping power of your last great orgasm, or the soul-melting memory of your first romantic kiss. In the face of a society that would squelch lust, love, or even affection between men, gay sex can be an affirmation of courage and creativity, a means of escape and communion uniting Republicans and Democrats, Black men and White, older gentlemen and younger leathermen, and all the rest of us. At least when it's good.

What's good sex? It's as varied as gay men ourselves. Some of us love feet, or ass play, or taking charge of a handsome man we've never spoken to and working his penis with hand or mouth. Still others thrill to serial seduction, quick runs to the bathhouse with our lovers, romantic courtship, or saving our bodies for the one to whom we've given our hearts.

Notes on Normal

I haven't let anyone inside me in years—except in my fantasy life, where I'm completely submissive and serving.

It's like that T-shirt says: Monosexuality bores me. I'm only with one person at a time, but I've never felt comfortable having to choose whether it's going to be a man or a woman.

For almost two years I've been celibate—consciously gay, and consciously focusing on other things beside my sexual drive.

I consider myself a dominant bottom. My ex is an exclusive top who liked to get his ass eaten. For me, I guess top and bottom have less to do with butt sex and more to do with who gets serviced and who services. Even then, it doesn't quite work. A friend said to me, "Oh, John, you know you're a big bottom," and I just felt uncomfortable, like that didn't capture it.

As a woman, I was interested in women and would never have looked twice at a man. Transitioning from female to male, I find my gaze lingering on anything that moves. I think it's hormonal. Since taking the testosterone I'm a teenage boy. At least I feel like one.

All of us—young and old, sick and well, disabled or not, coupled or single—feel the power of sexuality. How we express it—and the complicated ways that change in response to circumstances within and without—make it nearly impossible to simply categorize and describe. Even the language of sex reflects the limits. The scientific terms, such as *receptive oral intercourse* (sucking) and *aniobrachic intercourse* (fisting), range from the awkward to the absurd. *Penis, anus,* and *semen* sound stilted; *dick, ass,* and *cum* seem embarrassing or crude. The categories of our own creation—*top* and *bottom, fuck buddy, daddy, boy,* or *lover*—are more descriptive of desire but do not quite get at the way our roles or feelings change over a lifetime or even a single night. When one man rims another, who's the top? Is your sexuality different in your twenties, when guys assume your slender butt is ripe for plucking, than when you're forty-something, hairy, heavy, and look the daddy part? What word describes the end of the relationship between you and a man you've seen only for sex for the last year? How about that college crush you once had awkward sex with years ago, and who is now a close and treasured friend?

This book uses a mixture of language, both crude and clinical. Expressing your own gay sexuality, though, means a certain amount of creativity and self-invention. Anyone who's been through teenage taunting, parental disapproval, or any of the other various forms of homosexual hassle—meaning any man who grew up gay in America—knows that men who want sex with men get a double dose of the country's already negative feelings about sex. While TV shows, pop songs, movies, and high-school health classes offer heterosexuals dozens of different scripts, however limited, on how to combine sex and social life, men who want sex with other men learn early to "take it outside," going away from friends and family for action or advice. At the same time, searching out territory that is more gay-friendly often means entering a world where gay meeting places and cruising spaces can seem synonymous, where competition can overwhelm cooperation, where gay and proud looks suspiciously like young, fit, and White, and where comfort with sexual freedom is assumed much faster than it is achieved. Figuring out how to fit into the world of gay sex, or whether you want to, is a struggle that continues long after men hit the dating and mating trail.

The biggest obstacle to sexual well-being may be the nagging idea of the normal, the faint but persistent hope that by seeing how we stack up against others we can figure out if we're "doing it right." Yet classification and quantification, no matter how precise, aren't really up to the task of capturing the complications of gay lives. Are we all talking about the same thing when we say "gay"? Lots of men who have sex with men, or want to, may call themselves bisexual, or prefer to use no term at all. What word describes gay men who prefer sex with men who aren't gay? For that matter, what do you mean by men? Increasing numbers of people are messing with the monolith of masculinity, coming out—regardless of their genitalia—as transgendered people "transitioning" from man to woman, or woman to man.

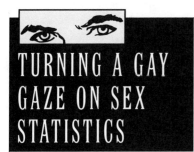

KNOW-IT-ALLS DON'T

Surveys of gay sex, like surveys of gay men in general, should be taken with a healthy dose of skepticism. Sex surveys face the obvious obstacle of getting gay men to talk honestly to strangers, or even finding a sample random and wide enough to represent the spectrum of our relationships and desires. Not that the rest of America really wants to know. The biggest and best sexuality survey in recent years, published under the title *Sex in America* (Warner Books, 1994), had its federal funding blocked for years by lawmakers afraid of what asking such questions might reveal. When the researchers finally got private money, it wasn't enough to give them strong data about how many partners gay men had or how we met each other, or even a realistic assessment of our "sexual preferences and practices." That's a lot of question marks.

CONSIDER THE SOURCE

Smaller or less random studies—and there have been many—tend to suffer from the problem that what you find depends on where you look. Poll in bars and you find that gay men drink a lot before they have sex. Recruit in therapists' offices and you conclude we need a lot of therapy. Get us from mail order companies and gay magazine subscription rolls and you find that few of us are homeless and that we have money to spend on things such as fashion, aerobics classes, and magazines. Study after study—from Kinsey in 1948 to *The Advocate* in 1995—has largely undercounted Black, Asian, and Hispanic men and then been quoted to speak for gay men as a whole.

NOTES ON NORMAL: THE SOCIAL

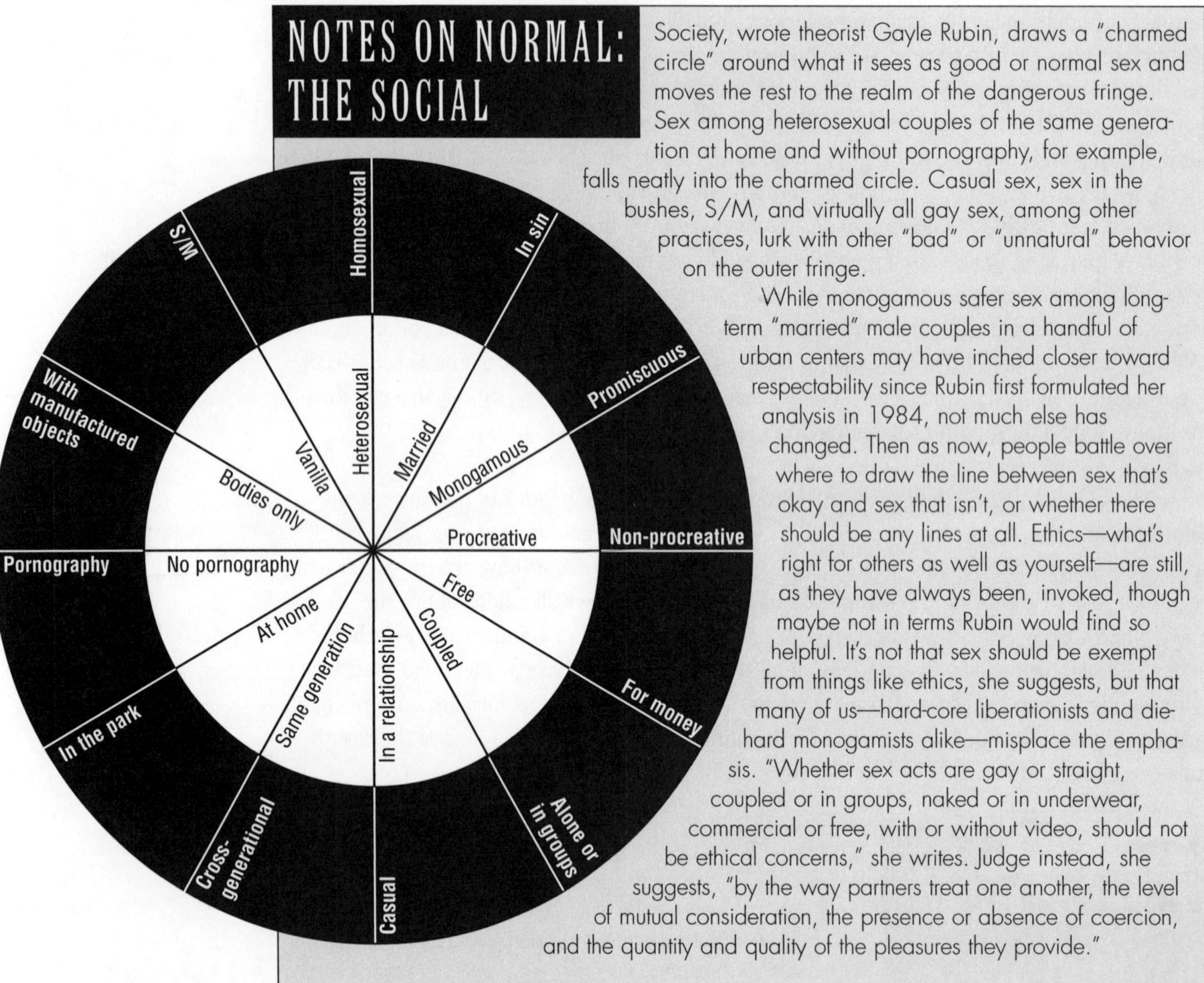

Society, wrote theorist Gayle Rubin, draws a "charmed circle" around what it sees as good or normal sex and moves the rest to the realm of the dangerous fringe. Sex among heterosexual couples of the same generation at home and without pornography, for example, falls neatly into the charmed circle. Casual sex, sex in the bushes, S/M, and virtually all gay sex, among other practices, lurk with other "bad" or "unnatural" behavior on the outer fringe.

While monogamous safer sex among long-term "married" male couples in a handful of urban centers may have inched closer toward respectability since Rubin first formulated her analysis in 1984, not much else has changed. Then as now, people battle over where to draw the line between sex that's okay and sex that isn't, or whether there should be any lines at all. Ethics—what's right for others as well as yourself—are still, as they have always been, invoked, though maybe not in terms Rubin would find so helpful. It's not that sex should be exempt from things like ethics, she suggests, but that many of us—hard-core liberationists and die-hard monogamists alike—misplace the emphasis. "Whether sex acts are gay or straight, coupled or in groups, naked or in underwear, commercial or free, with or without video, should not be ethical concerns," she writes. Judge instead, she suggests, "by the way partners treat one another, the level of mutual consideration, the presence or absence of coercion, and the quantity and quality of the pleasures they provide."

Forget all that, you say, and focus on the millions of us genetic men who love and sleep with other men and say we're gay. That works to an extent; studies will tell you, for example, that somewhere between 60 and 90 percent of us have tried anal intercourse in our lives, and that about two-thirds of those have tried it in the past year. What numbers won't tell is what the experience felt like, what actually happened, and with whom. Numbers won't tell you about what you'll do to have sex with someone who looks like the fantasy man you always thought was inaccessible, or how that may feel different from the sex you have with your partner of twenty years. Numbers don't say much about how we decided which man was worth what risk or how much we worried about it afterward, or what you were thinking as you pulled down your pants or pulled out a condom.

Given all the options, what "should" you be doing? It's a question you'd think would make gay men, long used to being told that no gay sex is natural, suspicious. "Traditional thinking makes all kinds of assumptions about the meaning of sex: that nature gives it meaning, biology gives it meaning, that there's such a thing as normal sex," says John Gagnon, Ph.D., a sociologist and one of the authors of *Sex in America*. "The question is, normal where, when, and to whom?" Variety in the garden of desire is vast, and beauty is in the eye of the beholder. "Flowers," says Dr. Gagnon, "are just weeds you like."

Different kinds of sex, though, have different consequences. Figuring out what makes you blossom in bed (or wherever else)—and how to stay healthy and well while doing it—is never simple. Though we often talk about our individual favorite modes and methods, most sex is relational, changing in response to feedback from the men we're with (whether we're with them for an hour, a month, or a lifetime). Though we often claim it to be private, sex is social, shaped by whether we're having it while looking over our shoulder for a police officer, a group of men who might bash us, or the approval of a family who thinks all of us is wonderful except for the part that sleeps with other men.

And then there's AIDS. Gay men have changed the course of public health history, working and organizing and fighting on every level to beat back AIDS. But no matter how fast we have pushed for treatment advances, no matter how much we have done to care for the sick and support the well, no matter how successful we have been at creating and continuing the safer-sex practices that have kept us alive, HIV continues to deform gay men's sexual landscapes. It is natural after almost twenty years and some good treatment news to want to believe that AIDS is over. But in some age or social groups, as many as a third of us may be infected with HIV. Even those of us who have no direct experience of AIDS illness and death, or who have managed to push it to a tiny corner of our consciousness, still feel the epidemic's anxious legacy, the stigma and silences that keep us wondering if gay sex and sickness are somehow the same. Our challenge is to rework that tired old equation, protecting mind and body as we find something more expansive and exuberant.

Sex Acts and Facts

Listen closely and the phrase "sex acts" rings wrong. An act sounds simple, clear, and bounded—Act I, curtain down. Sex, though, has as much to do with what's going on *behind* the curtain, the meanings in our minds, as with our bodies. We may talk about it as though it's as simple as going to the movies or buying clothes, but sex says much more to us about who we are or want to be. As for sex facts, there's really only one: The things you find sexiest are completely uninteresting to someone else, and someone else's fantasy may not appeal to you at all. It's nice to think there is a recipe—and this chapter has more than a few how-to tips you may find useful—but the fact is that your mind is always cooking, consciously and unconsciously taking ingredients from the people around you and stewing up your own special tastes for sexual pleasure.

Flying Solo: Masturbation

I lie naked in a dark room, no covers, hands at my side. Then I begin to create every detail of whom I want touching my body. If I really concentrate, I can bring myself off without touching myself.

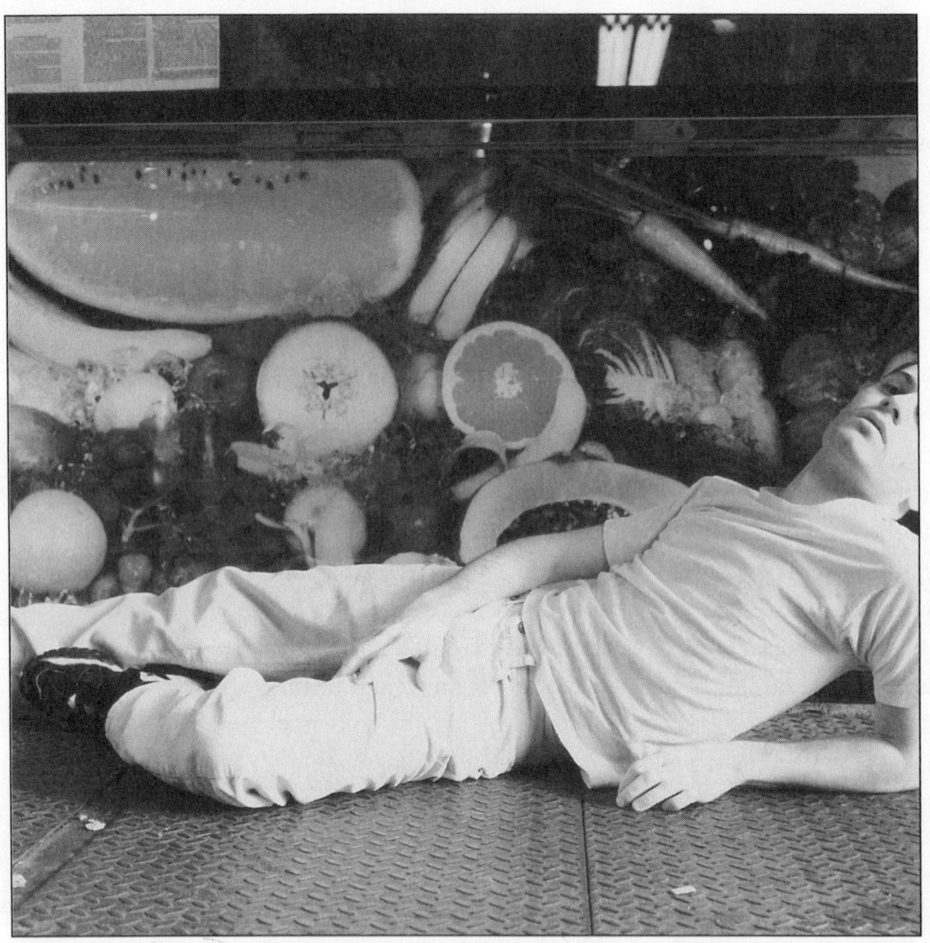

The Pleasures

Doctors will tell you what a body part does, not how it feels. Religion may set out rules for use. Biological texts inform us how organs function "in nature," which when it comes to sexual organs usually translates to what they do for reproduction. But when it comes to which touch or tingle gets your heart racing and blood flowing and cheeks flushing, clarity begins at home.

The higher your education level, say researchers, the more you're likely to masturbate, but advanced pleasure doesn't require an advanced degree. Many of us have a favorite method: dry or wet, rubbing a single spot below the head of the penis or all along the shaft, fondling our balls with one hand or humping the pillow with no hands at all. For many, the way we have an orgasm in masturbation—the different strokes and strengths, the buildup and release of pressure—becomes a blueprint for how we come during sex with others. Masturbation's a work in progress: If old patterns seem confining, or just boring, try opening yourself up to new possibilities. And though we think of it as solo sex, in masturbation you're rarely alone. Just look at your fantasies, the men you spend time with in your mind.

The Risks

Masturbation won't expose you to HIV or any other diseases, but it does come with serious risks: Do it wholeheartedly enough and it can open up mind and body, revealing new pleasures and a dangerous sense of independence. No wonder U.S. Surgeon General Joycelyn Elders was fired for talking up the subject in public.

Some men, or our partners, feel worried that masturbation means taking something away from their sexual partners. That's true only when it's true. Masturbation is easier than sex with someone else, but plenty of people manage to do both happily. If you feel as though masturbation alone is detracting from your sex life with your partner, then see about stopping for a while, or including him in the action. If you can't or don't want to do that, the issue is probably a deeper one (see "Relight My Fire," page 130).

HINTS FROM THE HOMO SUTRA: *SELF-CULTIVATION*

"I have nothing against quickies, but if that's all you do, you're ignoring a great part of your sexuality," says Betty Dodson, Ph.D., author of *Sex for One* (Crown, 1997), and veteran leader of masturbation workshops for men and women. Try, at least once, to spend a whole hour on what masturbation mavens sometimes call "self-cultivation." Lose your roommate. Tell your partner you'll make it up to him later. Choose a time and place where you won't be interrupted: a bedroom or bathroom, someplace warm and soft enough to linger. If you have a full-length mirror there, so much the better. Make the mood romantic—light a candle, burn some incense, put on whatever music gets you going, have lubricant at hand. "You're getting ready to receive the man of your dreams," suggests Dr. Dodson, "and for this moment, that man is you."

And then just look at yourself. Resist the impulse to get lost in worrying about where there's too much this or not enough that, focusing instead on what parts of your body you feel good about. Spread your cheeks. Lift your arms. Let your hands and gaze linger on your pleasure points, the spots that get you going. All of them—perhaps the inside of your ear, the tender flesh between your toes, or your buttocks—may not be visible. Think about them anyway. Sense them. Most men find our eyes and hands lingering on the fine instruments of indulgence between our legs. Look and do touch, but avoid using the same old strokes you always do. If a certain piece of porn gets you going, by all means use it, but again, allow your focus to move to new sensations.

Breathe deeply; it opens your mind and body. Lubricant can be a great sensation stimulator. So can a finger or dildo, especially if you've practiced Chapter 1's anal pleasure hints. Let the session last a full hour at least, as long as you might spend with a wonderful lover. Create a dialogue, with your hands and mind offering something and your body responding. Orgasm need not be your goal, but if it is, savor its approach. Note the buildup of tension in your thighs, legs, and feet, and experiment with consciously relaxing them to make yourself last longer. Your balls have to rise up toward your body before you come, and some men intentionally interrupt the process by pulling them down toward their feet, or use a Kegel exercise (see page 41) to cause a tantalizing delay. If you decide to cum, relish the sensation and its aftermath for a few moments before rushing to clean up. Just as with any lover, time after orgasm can be precious, full of openness and relaxation.

FANTASY

The Pleasures

I imagine myself at the mercy of a group of organized, masculine men: high-school athletes, firemen, army buddies. I am being disciplined—forced to service them—though my erection shows them I really love it. As I attend to them, they attend—roughly, almost without noticing—to me, caressing my penis and nipples until I explode in an orgasm over the hand of one of them. He makes me lick it off. I love these fantasies because in them I don't have any choice or indecision or ambivalence. My body is speaking for me.

After fifteen years with my lover, I think of him sometimes as someone else when we're in bed. You know, your mind drifts and it's Keanu Reeves who's with you. Not all the time; just for a flash.

For me, it's more images than stories: very young men with useless soft dicks who give me their asses.

I imagine myself as a Black woman with a handsome Black man as a lover who licks and caresses my body until I am washed away in a wave of pleasure.

Most of us had fantasies about sex with other men before we had the opportunity to enjoy it physically. Long after we have become sexually active, and no matter how active we are, our sexual fantasies speak to us in a language outside of language, offering images and feelings as powerful and hard to spell out as dreams. Fantasies can be stories or pictures, fleeting images or fully fleshed-out narratives, based on an old lover, a porn story, or someone we saw riding the bus to work.

My life partner, whom I love, is a hairy, manly man with a slight potbelly. My fantasy is of younger, feminine men who look like women.

My fantasies usually involve forbidden things, specifically straight men and unprotected sex. I fantasize about being the host of a gang bang for about ten straight men. I find a woman for them, and watch them strip off their clothes and get hard. I've never had sex with a woman, so for me, straight sex is "kinky." I love the idea of straight men being naked around each other, with hard-ons. I watch them take turns getting blow jobs and fucking the woman. My only request is that they pull out and dump the loads in my mouth. I swallow each of them.

Getting comfortable with our fantasies means giving up on the idea that they need to reflect something particular about reality. The gap between the fantastic and the real is what makes fantasies fantastic. Use them as secret erotic fuel, drawn upon quietly to warm things up, or share them with a friend to tap into good role playing. Choose your confidants wisely: Like dreams, fantasies are deeply personal, and easily disrupted by a negative response.

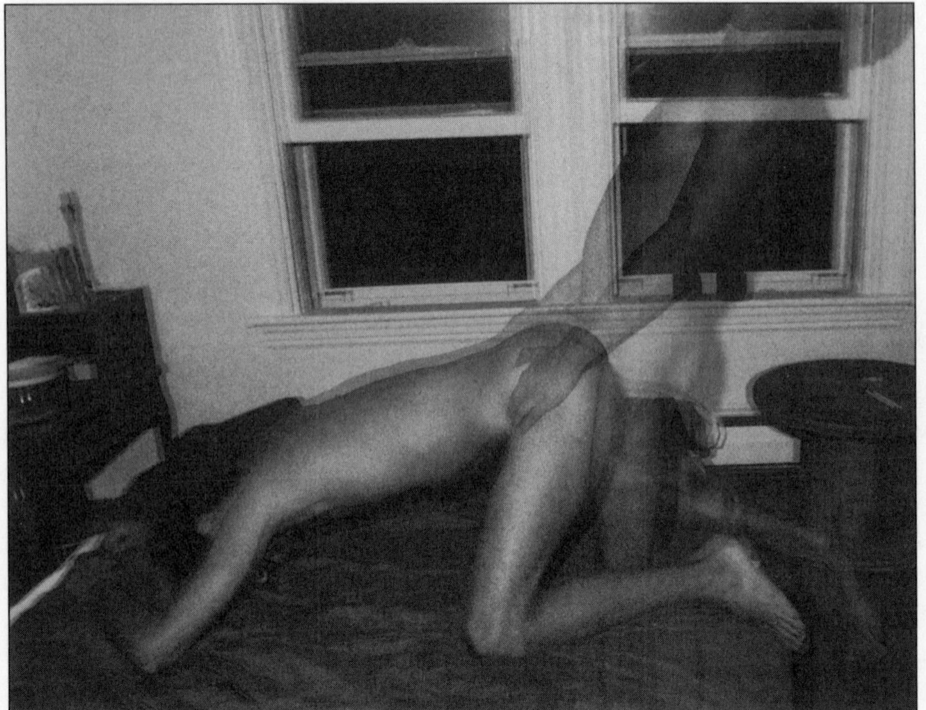

The Risks

Acting out your fantasies—just as with all sex—comes with all the complications of the real world. There are definitely things to consider before letting four policemen tie you up, and having sex with your boyfriend's brother will almost certainly not end up pretty. Imaginary unsafe sex is much different from sex that leaves you with HIV in your body. For some of us, pursuit of a certain fantasy can also have a blinding intensity that leaves us feeling bored or blocked by other sexual situations. If that's the case and it's making you unhappy, it's wise to find some safe place to talk about it (see "Dr. Love: Finding a Sex Therapist," in Chapter 4).

In the realm of the imagination, though, there's no such thing as a thought crime. Cherish your fantasies. Spend some time with them. Look at their themes and common threads, the messages they whisper about your deep erotic longings.

Touching

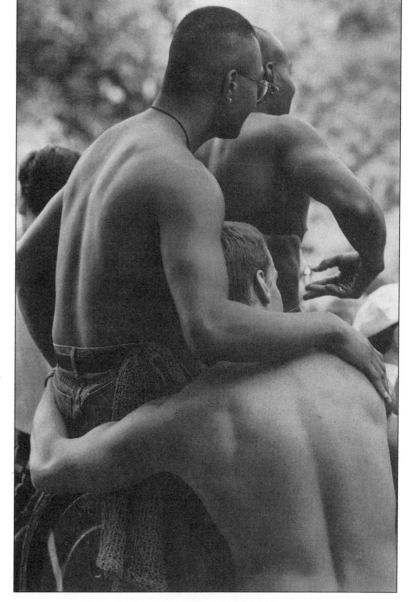

Some of the best parts of making love for me are just holding my partner, being held, feeling his back and shoulders tense as he nears orgasm and then feeling him relax. More than cumming, sometimes I just like the physical contact, the way only a man can hold me.

This guy's body was incredible, but it was his hands—his incredibly sensitive, responsive hands—that made the night for me. We spent the whole night tracing each other's arms and shuddering at the sensations.

The Pleasures

Touch—a slow, deep massage, the heat of thigh against thigh, the feel of a forearm on your chest—is among the most basic and important of animal pleasures. Babies who aren't touched wither away and get sick; sick people who aren't touched often heal less quickly; healthy men who aren't touched have been known to act like babies, or pretend to be sick, in search of manual ministrations. Touch doesn't have to be genital to be sexy: In *The Advocate*'s survey of gay men, 85 percent rated hugging, caressing, and snuggling as the "sex acts they loved most." Touch doesn't have to be sexy to be lovely: Look at how good it feels to get a warm, deep hug from a friend. Touch needn't be divided into sexy or not: Think of all those bare-chested boys swaying with their arms around each other's shoulders at every Pride event, or the brush of your thigh against the stranger's in that busy subway car.

The Risks

Aside from a few sexually transmitted diseases whose seriousness is somewhere on the order of the common cold (see Chapter 4), nongenital touching has only the risk of bringing you closer. For touch involving genitals, or mouths and genitals, read on.

Mutual Masturbation

The Pleasures

We sit with legs around each other's waists, facing each other, naked and well-lubed, hands in each other's laps. We try breathing in sync, even putting our mouths over one another's and trading breaths for a while. Usually we stare into each other's eyes, though one of us will throw his head back when it gets to be too much. I don't even have to look down to know when he's going to come.

A complete stranger sat next to me in a movie theater (and not a porno one—we're talking Cineplex Odeon). He took a chance and started nudging my knee with his, and we ended up jerking each other off before the movie was a third over! Very unexpected and very hot.

I love to watch, from across the shower stall at the gym, and see who has a chubby. I know the tricks: touch your own to get things going, look often but not too intently. Nothing else has to happen, but I go away charged.

Playing with each other's penises is among the most adored and adaptable of gay sexual acts. Equally achievable in bedrooms and steam rooms, standing up in an airplane bathroom or

DIFFERENT STROKES—TWO MASTURBATION RESOURCES

"Get it up, get it off, and go to sleep tends to be the mode we learn early," says Collin Brown, of the Body Electric School in Oakland, California. Body Electric—with workshops, videos, and an array of massage strokes with names like Twist and Shout (pull the skin tight on the lower third of a well-lubricated penis with one hand and slide the other hand like a corkscrew up the shaft and around the head)—seeks to use erotic massage with a partner (and usually without ejaculation) as a way of waking body and spirit. Breathing together, slow stimulation, and atunement to the erotic delight of masturbatory male brotherhood (or recently, in women's workshops, female sisterhood) are among the school's basic building blocks, which they extend to include other sexual acts as well. Body Electric is at 6527 Telegraph Avenue, Oakland, CA 94609, tel. (510) 653-4991; www.bodyelectric.org.

Celebrate the Self, like Body Electric, takes its name from that icon of brotherly love, the poet Walt Whitman. This phrase is the title of a black-and-white bimonthly journal for men—gay, straight, transgender, you name it—highlighting the many pleasures of masturbation alone and with a friend. *CTS* includes book reviews, poems, essays on the body and spirit, and testimony from readers all over the country and spectrum of sexual tastes. *Celebrate the Self*, Factor Press, Box 8888, Mobile, AL 36689.

lying down in a field of flowers, this can be an arousing appetizer or a main course. If you are uncircumcised and have a loose enough foreskin, pulling your skin over the top of his penis (it's called "docking") can be a special pleasure.

A long, slow masturbation of someone else can tease him to a state of distraction or satisfaction. Joint jerk-offs are also great for achieving one of the greatest erotic treats, the simultaneous orgasm. Try kissing as you fondle each other, twining tongues and pleasures until you both burst. Or masturbate him as a teaser, tracing his penis through his underpants or slipping a hand inside as you undress him. Pre-cum may appear at the tip of the penis as he grows harder—it's a natural lubricant and will enhance sensation if you smear it around. Heft his balls in your hand, rolling them gently (or roughly, if he likes it). Jerking off leaves you freer than most sex acts to look at each other, to see how his chest heaves or legs tighten, or to appreciate how your own body shudders and stiffens. With practice, or close observation, you may feel you see his inner state as well, knowing just when you have him on the edge, or how to push him over.

Looking can make jerking off together something you do without touching at all, from across a gym shower or in adjoining booths at the adult bookstore, next to your partner in bed or with twenty partners at a JO party. Masturbating yourself in front of someone can also be a way to release your sexual tension when he's tired, already done, or not in the mood. Even when together, many men feel more comfortable finishing themselves off with their own hand. Watch while they do it, to see what you can learn for the future.

Rubbing bodies against each other—also called frottage, the Princeton rub, and belly fucking—can be combined with hand play or be its own art form. The Greeks—famous for fucking—actually used a modified version of frottage, a man slipping his penis between the smooth, hairless thighs of his boy beloved. Or try cupping his oiled penis and yours together with your hand as you both lie, belly to belly, and thrust toward blastoff.

The Risks

There is virtually no risk of getting or giving HIV from mutual masturbation or rubbing bodies. Anxieties about getting his cum in your paper cut, or about the occasional shot in the eye, are common. Getting HIV that way is definitely not. It is possible, though rare, to get a sexually transmitted infection in your eye or your penis, usually from rubbing them after you've touched your or someone else's open sore. And before you wank every old skank, remember that you can get warts, herpes, or a minor but unwelcome case of crabs through mutual masturbation or bodily contact.

ORAL SEX

The Pleasures

When it comes to sexual centers of the body, the mouth stands out. It gives and receives, forming the words that let someone know what you want or need, the gasps and breaths that tell of orgasm approaching or a caress gone wrong. The warm, wet caresses of tongue to tongue or mouth to penis aren't bad, either. Small wonder that surveys of gay men's sex, however imperfect, consistently find oral pleasures at the top of the list.

HINTS FROM THE HOMO SUTRA: *This Is No Gag*

Long before "don't ask, don't tell," notes author Robert Gluck, the U.S. armed services experimented with a different gauge of homosexuality: a tongue depressor. New recruits in the 1940s had their tonsils touched; those who gagged, the army decided, weren't gay. While science has moved swiftly on, our worries haven't always done the same. Many are the men who feel guilty, or less than gay, for gagging.

First, a silver lining. You may not like it, but he might. While throwing up on your partner (it's happened) is a definite no-no, a little retch may make him feel big and powerful. But if you want to avoid gagging and give a blow job that'll blow his mind, here are some suggestions drawn from Internet postings and interviews from men who claim they know.

1. ***Look before you lick.*** "I hold his penis in my hand and look at it," advises one devotee of the art. "Carefully, like I'm preparing to worship. What parts look tastiest? How does it curve or bend? Does it look like I can fit it all in my throat, or will I need to use my hand as well? The attention alone is likely to get him hard and ready."

2. ***Keep breathing.*** "I wish someone had told me this years ago," says Mike, a New York City therapist. "Breathing is the single most crucial thing if you don't want to gag. It's like swimming—get your air on the upstroke. I try to blow my nose first, since things can get a little runny. Also, practice in the morning, when your gag reflex is at its weakest."

3. ***Use your hands and tongue.*** "If he's too big for comfort, I curl my hand around the bottom third of his dick and move it up and down in time with my mouth," advises Perry, a waiter in Tucson, Arizona. "It keeps him from getting too deep as he thrusts, but so long as I've slicked him down good beforehand, it feels like an extension of my wet, warm mouth." David, a planner in Washington, DC, offers an addendum: "Tapping your tongue at that little spot on the underside, right where the head meets the shaft, drives him wild."

4. ***Vary your rhythm.*** "Keep varying your strokes—shallow and deep, slow and speedy, with your hands stroking his thighs or balls," offers Bill, an architect. "When I make him moan, I make a note of it for later and keep experimenting. Also, make sure to pace yourself: Once you've started with the super friction, licking and nibbling won't feel like much. When I want to draw things to a close, I gently slide a lubed finger up his ass. Nine times out of ten, he'll blow."

5. ***Wet, yes. Rough, no.*** "I get as much spit going as I can," says Sam, a Democratic campaign organizer. "I think it probably keeps me safer [though saliva does inhibit HIV activity, there's little scientific support for this idea] and it definitely makes him hotter. I suck and slobber over his balls, too. And I never use my teeth or my beard unless asked. They both hurt."

6. ***Try different positions.*** "The length from mouth to throat is four or five inches, and the length of his dick is likely to be longer," says one would-be sex advisor on the Internet. "Which means you need to find a way to open your throat for easy access. I like hanging my head over the side of a couch or bed, so that my throat is more open, and get him to thrust. Otherwise, I skip the deep throating—you don't need it—and use other techniques." Among the oft-mentioned favorites is kneeling in front of him as he sits in a chair, letting his balls rest on your tongue, and giving him long, slow, and repeated licks up the balls, up the underside of the shaft, and up over the head.

7. ***Brush up?*** "My gag reflex used to be out of control, and I trained myself to control it with my toothbrush," says Mike. "I'd just brush a little closer to the back of my throat every day. It worked, I swear. Okay, I admit it, I also practiced a little on bananas."

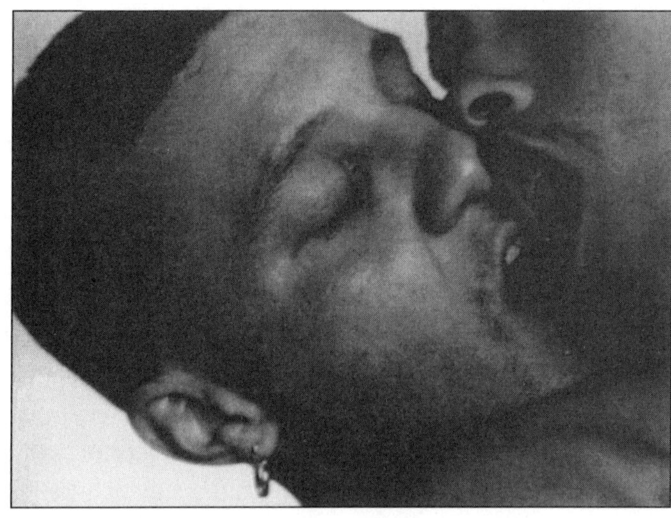

KISSING

Love and kisses is not just a cute close to a letter. Deep emotions, as well as delicious stimulation, are triggered by putting your mouth to another's, which is no doubt why men in some sexual situations won't do it at all. "After twenty-nine years, it still returns me to the nervous and excitable young man I was when I met my partner, and without it I'd die," says Raoul, age sixty-two. Others talk of "gasping with pleasure," "opening up completely," or "melting" with a kiss. Try it soft and yielding, deep and probing, with caressing hands, or just with heart.

SUCKING AND GETTING SUCKED

The soft head slides toward your throat and your lips close in an O of surprise. For me it is a surprise, always.

The gasps and murmurs in the back of his throat are like replies to what your mouth says without words.

Especially if it's someone you really like, his dick is no longer "it" but him. You have him in your mouth, his whole body balanced on your tongue.

"Cocksucker" may be a schoolyard insult, but in gay man's land it can be the highest compliment. Sucking someone's penis, or being sucked, is one of the great gay pleasures, and the most common form of sexual expression between men. How we get from schoolboys to gay men, as you know, is a complicated story, but the journey often takes us to at least two destinations: fellatio, where you move your head up and down, and irrumptio, where he does the moving. Sucking each other's penises at the same time—sixty-nine (or, for sophisticates, *soixante-neuf*)—lets you work for mutual pleasure.

The Risks

KISSING

Kissing's risky for transmitting emotion, but not for HIV. You can catch herpes or mono from a kiss, and if you've never had hepatitis B, there's some debate about whether deep, intense tongue twining might pass it along. There's also one single solitary reported case of AIDS in America from a man-to-woman kiss, but many HIV specialists are skeptical about this report. There have been, it should be pointed out, millions of wonderful kisses.

SUCKING

In GMHC workshops, the single most asked question is: How safe is it to suck? The short answer is that study after study has shown that oral sex comes with a drastically lower risk for HIV than anal sex. One study of more than a thousand gay men in Chicago, Los Angeles,

Pittsburgh, and Baltimore concluded that the risk was "statistically insignificant," meaning that if everyone had oral sex but anal sex stopped, the epidemic might slowly die out. A smaller study in San Francisco found that 8 out of 122 HIV-infected gay men reported getting HIV from oral sex. Whichever you prefer to believe, oral sex is not 100 percent safe, and you may not want to be one of those unlucky few who were statistical exceptions and got HIV from sucking someone.

A small number of HIV infections through oral sex (less than a hundred) have been well documented in professional journals. There have been many more individual reports of people who say they got infected from sucking. Scientists have found HIV in pre-cum, though it's unlikely that there's enough virus in it to result in infection. It is also definitely possible to get STDs from sucking, including syphilis, gonorrhea of the throat, herpes, and—if his uncovered penis has been up someone else's ass recently—hepatitis and parasites. And no, gargling with mouthwash afterward does not take care of the problem.

Certain things are thought to make oral sex more risky for HIV, such as if you have cuts or sores in your mouth, have just flossed or had dental work, or have an STD in your throat. If he has an STD, that might also make him more likely to give you HIV, too (see "Riskier Business," page 68). There's no evidence that how deep you take someone's penis in your mouth changes the risk. If you're into having someone stick it to you for hours, or like it really rough, or are drunk or high enough not to notice pain or tearing in your throat, that may make sucking riskier.

AIDS organizations in America have been telling gay men to use condoms for oral sex for years, and most gay men never have. Lots of gay men worry about it, though. One small study of gay men in Atlanta in 1997 found that even those men who get fucked without condoms—the easiest way to get AIDS during sex—worry more about getting HIV from oral sex. Who said sex was rational?

Some of us are willing to live with more risk than others. Think not only about how you feel about sucking a particular dick, but about how you're going to feel about it the next day. If you want to be absolutely certain you won't get HIV, don't suck someone who might be positive without a condom, or don't put your mouth over the head of his penis.

GETTING SUCKED

Read "Sucking," above. And then relax further, since getting sucked without a condom comes with an even lower risk for HIV than sucking. You can get gonorrhea, herpes, or other kinds of sexually transmitted infections from being sucked, and his teeth may pose the greater danger here. The central vein of your penis may become irritated enough for you to have to give it a rest. And if you do get a bite that breaks the skin, seek immediate medical attention. "The mouth is a lot dirtier than we imagine," says New York City urologist Franklin C. Lowe, MD.

ANAL SEX

The Pleasures

If God had meant men to have sex, jokes Craig Nelson in his *Finding True Love in a Man-Eat-Man World* (Dell, 1996), he would have put a little hole between our legs. If you're not laughing, relax: Grade-school jokes and preconceptions aside, anal sex is not a God-given gay requirement. If you're half smiling, relax: Anal pleasure doesn't mean only taking a penis the size of a small animal inside you. And for those of you smiling broadly, you probably are already relaxed, or know that the anus is a many-splendored thing, and the more you relax and get to know it, the more you'll love it.

Relax how? you ask. The "Seven Solo Steps Toward Anal Awareness," on page 25, offer some suggestions for finding anal pleasure on your own terms. If you haven't read them yet, turn back. If you're ready for work with a partner, there are other pleasures besides penetration: having him lightly stroke around your butthole with a fingertip and then gently tug the hairs there, for example. Dr. Morin's *Anal Health and Pleasure* (Down There Press, 1998) has a great series of exercises for anal explorers journeying together.

ANAL INTERCOURSE

I am totally receptive. Some guys are afraid to say it, or act all masculine to make it look like something else, but in my house it was nothing to be ashamed of. My mother and my aunts were in control, and I got it from them. What's wrong with sleeping with a big, strong man who makes me feel good in bed?

I like to watch my partner's face as I fuck him, to kiss him, to touch him, to cradle his body and touch his nipples, to activate as many pleasure receptors as possible. Eye contact can be incredibly important at these moments as the most direct path to the emotions. I love to fuck and then get fucked. That gets everything going.

It's all about attitude. You better make me believe that I'm going to feel it from my head to my toes, that it's going to be hot, sweaty, noisy, and intense, with no complex negotiations about equality of who could fuck who, or anything other than sex and feeling good and getting off. In a relationship, where there are romantic feelings, it's a whole different ball of wax. Then the person I want to fuck me is the person I care about, and I'm not as concerned about how wild the ride is.

My partner's knowing me and what I like makes it wonderful. I don't have to say anything. I do like it when he works my hole over with his finger or tongue first to loosen me up. Then I like to be on my stomach so that he can hold me while he fucks me. We love to do it with a candle lit and some great tunes on.

It's taken me a while. When I first heard it I just couldn't believe it. I mean, a dick in the ass, ouch. I just thought about shitting and how dirty and painful it must be. Then I thought, shitting feels good, so why not try it? There's a preconceived notion that it's feminine, but to me it's the ultimate expression of masculinity. I'm equal, not bottom.

"Passive" or "active" anal intercourse are the technical terms, though often both of you are active and it's the intercourse—the exchange of physical and mental energy between you—that can be more to the point. Whether the active partner is serving the needs of the passive partner or whether it's the bottom who's serving the top is one of those questions that runs into itself like a staircase in an M. C. Escher drawing, though it's certainly the case that the man who's doing the inserting is occupying the more traditionally defined place of power. In a number of cultures, past and present, it's only the man who gets fucked who's considered gay or somehow different from a "regular" man. Echoes of that thinking are still heard in those charming questions like "Which one's the woman?" that some gay couples are forced to field

FROM THE BOTTOMS TO THE TOPS, TOPS TO THE BOTTOMS

Besides your basic entrance tip—breathe and push your anus out slightly as he's putting his penis in—what makes anal intercourse better? Since everyone likes it different, there's no one rule or way to work. Virtually all studies of gay men's sex have found that most of us are versatile, changing back and forth from top to bottom. But here's what a few men who like to play one role offered to those who play another, with commentary from "sexpert" educators or medical professionals.

from our heterosexual fans. If you're interested in anal sex, though, you might ask yourself a more penetrating question: What do *you* think it means for you to put your penis inside another man, or to have him do it to you? How does either role affect how you see yourself as a man? As cared about? As a powerful force in the world?

Men and women, and men and men, have debated these issues for years. Shere Hite, a sex researcher in the 1970s, went as far as to suggest intercourse without thrusting as one form of power-balanced sex; feminist (and antiporn crusader) Andrea Dworkin, in a later model doomed to failure, proposed that the politically evolved would have no penetrative intercourse at all. A few exceptionally limber, creative, and persistent gay men have found ways to explode the top-bottom distinction by fucking each other simultaneously, though the position leaves you looking like a two-headed crab largely incapable of movement (one man lies on his back with his legs spread; the other one sits down on the dick of the first, facing away from him, leans forward, and then slides his own semisoft penis around and into his partner's ass—don't try this at home). Many more of us find it's not what we do but how we feel about who we do—is he younger, older, hot, not, a trick, a lover, sensitive, rough?—that most changes the dynamics of anal intercourse.

Questions of power—and what is masculine or feminine—exist in all our bedrooms and in all our imaginations. As often as not, writes Dr. Jack Morin, it's discomfort or tension with a situation—rather than something purely physical—that takes the pleasure away from anal intercourse. Big-bodied men can feel as though they're boxed into being tops, while small or slender men may get sick of being expected to submit. Racial stereotypes—the submissive Asian, or the Black or Latino stud—can also stunt our sexual expression. Condoms (see "Toys and Tools," in this chapter) can make a hard-on soft. If any of these is the case, then consider ways to work out those feelings with your pants still on. It might be as simple as airing your concerns with a sexual partner, suggests Dr. Morin, or as complicated as examining how you really feel about femininity in the first place. Butt sex is just one of many places where feelings about sexuality and gender and power come to the surface, and exploring those feelings outside of sex can free both mind and anal sphincter.

I don't remember him really asking. He just said, "I have some lube. . . ." I said, "Great," thinking I was going to do it to him like usual. Instead, he just shoved it inside me. I think it didn't hurt because I was so drunk, and then it started to feel good. Really good. I felt for the first time that I had really become a gay man, and felt what it was like to have someone inside me, my body causing another man's body to writhe and shake with passion. It was so great. I think if I wasn't so conservative, I would have stuck anything up my ass to get that feeling again.

Men Being Fucked Say:		Sexperts Add:
Play me.	"I like it when he spends an hour just warming me up, stroking me, sucking me. I usually lose my erection when he gets inside me, but I do get it back. If he helps."	Don't squeeze his penis at the moment you're inserting your penis. It causes the anal sphincter to contract.
Go slow.	"If it hurts, I need time to adjust."	The internal sphincter stays clenched for around thirty to sixty seconds and then relaxes. Also, the rectum takes a turn a few inches in (see Chap. 1). If you seem to hit a wall, don't ram; pull back, reposition, and be patient (see pages 32–33).
Grease is the word.	"I need a lot of lubricant. Start with a finger or a dildo, and be patient."	If you think you're using enough lube, use a little more. Avoid oil-based lubes, since they eat away at latex condoms and clog glands in his rectum.
Kiss.	"There's something about having his mouth on mine that just makes me melt."	Mmm-hmmm.
Stay tuned.	"I don't like it when he gets in and then just starts pumping like a piston. We're men, not machines." "He knows it's painful, so he does it lovingly, carefully. It's like I'm relaxing into him, saying, 'This is it, you can have me.'"	**COMMUNICATION**
Men Fucking Say:		**IS**
Let me know it.	"I don't know what's happening if you're just lying there. I know some guys don't like an active bottom, but everyone needs some feedback. Do you feel me? Is it pleasant? Let me know." "I'm guess I'm a fuzzy top (even though I'm hairless). I'm not one of those guys who just comes in and is all about topping. I want to do it with you, not to you, so if there's something you want, please work with me."	**CRUCIAL**
Squeaky-clean sex machine.	"What can I say? Cleanliness is appreciated." "It's so much hotter if I don't have to feel like I'm stuffing stuff back inside you."	Douching's fine, but not just before sex: It irritates the mucous membranes, and water may gush out unexpectedly. Also, if you do douche, make sure he's wearing a condom (for more info, see box on page 30)
Dirty does it.	"The nastier the better. I like to literally bang the shit out of you."	As long as it doesn't get in your mouth.
Squeeze play.	"I love it when he grasps my dick with his ass, when I can feel him milking it."	It's Kegel time (see page 41).

And just maybe, if things are right, you'll carry on the great gay tradition of finding something liberating and transformational in anal intercourse. We don't brag about it as much, but gay men are the real tits-and-ass men, daring to open both body parts up for exploration and challenging the whole idea of what real men do in sex in the first place. Plenty of us love the feeling of opening someone up during anal intercourse. Plenty more of us love the feeling of being taken over, overwhelmed by a seemingly irresistible force. "You know what *versatile* means on AOL chat rooms," jokes Sandy, a thirty-six-year-old AIDS activist from Atlanta. "You fuck me first, then I'll climb on top for five minutes until I lose my hard-on." Actually, men on both top and bottom have known the pleasure of changing roles in a night or over a lifetime, overturning old taboos and preconceptions. Remember those proclamations from gay newspapers in the 1970s? Fucking is an act of revolution.

FINGERING/BEING FINGERED

We were doing a standard sixty-nine, but not on our sides: I was on top, and he was on the bottom. Sometimes the rhythm isn't always the same with the other person, but this was one of those times when our rhythm was exactly alike. With one hand each of us was doing the cock and with the other the asshole. At the point that we came, our fingers were in each other's asses. The intensity was kind of mind-boggling.

Fingering is among the least discussed, and most practiced, of anal pleasures. "I always rewind porn videos to the few moments of fingering scenes and replay them over and over," says Wally, thirty-two, lamenting the little attention given to this kind of hand job. Neither too mild to ignore nor too intense to tolerate, fingering is the crowd pleaser of anal pleasure. Work his penis with your other hand (or your mouth), and it's easy to create that all-fronts-at-once assault that'll make him beg for mercy. Probe for his prostate (see page 32) as things get hot, and he may groan, grunt, or spurt a little faster.

On patience (yes) and poking (no): An unlubed finger goes in hard, can be stiffer than a penis, and can hurt. And if he comes while you're inside him, don't pull out abruptly. Ejaculation causes the sphincter to contract, as you'll feel, and the draining of blood from the area makes things suddenly more sensitive.

RIMMING

Not wishing the cock alone to have its role
My mouth too has joined often with that hole
My tongue, sopping, tried to devour the flower
Blooming in brown damp. The chute, unmanned
It's a sublime sugar bowl, a Promised Land
Aflow with other milk and honey, heavenly bower!

FROM "SONNET TO THE ASSHOLE"
ARTHUR RIMBAUD AND PAUL VERLAINE

To the uninitiated, the meeting of tongue and anus is mysterious, embarrassing, or even repugnant. To the rimming enthusiast, it's poetry. "If I could have a guy's tongue up my ass all day and still work and go to the gym, I would," gushes Evan, age twenty-four. Adds thirty-eight-year-old David, "It's that whole idea of someone using their tongue and mouth in an area that you think of for much more private functions that makes it so exciting."

ASSUME THE POSITION

How you position yourself for anal sex can make the difference between discomfort and delight. Here are only a few of the possibilities, described from the perspective of the man receiving:

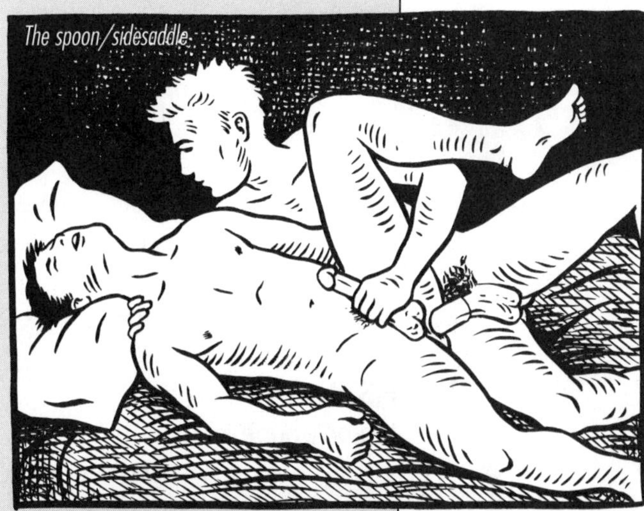
The spoon/sidesaddle

• *The straddle.* He lies or sits, while you lower yourself slowly onto his hard penis. Recommended by baby bottoms, those of us who don't have a lot of experience. "I like it because I control how deep he goes, and because I can put my hand down to make sure the condom hasn't slipped off, which I always worry about," says José.

• *The spoon/sidesaddle.* You both lie on your sides, your back to his front—a familiar position for snuggling, except this time you move your top leg forward to let him slide into you easily. A tender position, and another that gives you some control. He can easily masturbate you, and if it's too rough, you can stop or pull away. If you like it rougher, you can roll into either of the next two.

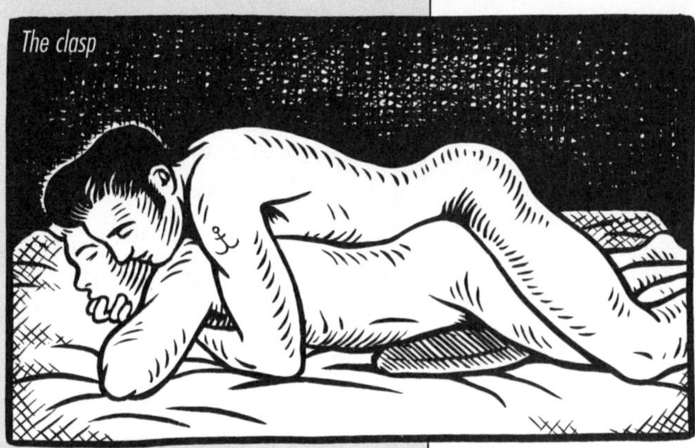
The clasp

• *The doggie.* You're on your hands and knees, and he's gripping your hips or laying his stomach and chest over your back while he sticks it to you. If you rest your weight on a single arm, you can play with your penis; if he leans forward, he can do it for you. Looks great in a mirror.

• *The clasp.* You lie on your stomach, with a pillow under you to raise your ass higher. He straddles your legs with his own, pumping in and out, while clasping your chest with a forearm. Deep penetration time.

• *The classic.* Face-to-face, where you can see each other's reactions. You lie, with a pillow underneath you, legs apart, and he slides in. Great for watching the effect your tight ass is having on him. He can see you, too, every shudder and moan. And you can kiss.

• *The classic plus.* Swing one leg onto his shoulder, with the other wrapped around his thigh. Or put both onto his shoulders, if that's comfortable. Deep and intense penetration.

• *The liftoff.* You sit on his lap (and on his dick). He holds your ass in his hands and moves you gently up and down. Again, good for kissing and feeling cradled.

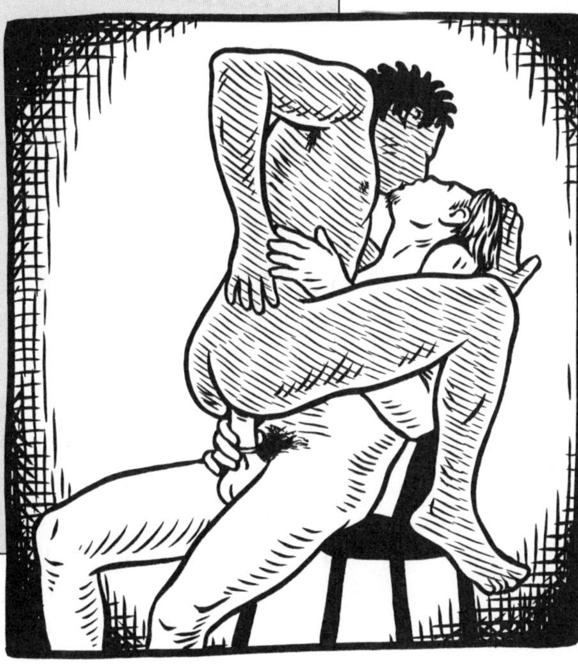
The liftoff

Rimmers, as well as rimmees, sing the praises of an act that they describe as "more intimate than fucking," "the single most important sex act, if I had to choose one," "the most intimate act, something saved for my long-term relationship," and "the end to a romantic evening." A well-placed wet tongue can dissolve the top/bottom divide, melting the recipient into openness, whatever his penetration preferences. Among rimmers' favored positions: with a freshly showered man squatting over their faces, or with his arms clasping his knees and his butt spread. "I have a big nose," says George, who claims to use it to great effect. "They've usually never had that done before, and it drives them crazy: back and forth, tongue, nose, tongue, nose." Risks more common than driving him crazy with pleasure are discussed below.

More of the men GMHC talked to in our totally unscientific, totally unrandom survey preferred to get rimmed rather than to rim. But bringing science to bear would probably be like those studies proving that tickling causes laughter or that caffeine is addictive: We knew that.

FISTING

I've only done it as a top, and I'm always shocked by the incredible sense of connection and intimacy. There's something so gentle about it. My image of fist fucking was that it was this incredibly violent act, like a kind of rape, something so physically traumatic and violent. I had instruction from a couple of other guys who were experienced, and they taught me that to do it well you have to be very in tune, sensitive.

French theorist and sex historian Michel Foucault said that fisting—the insertion of a greased hand into the rectum and lower colon—was an invention of the twentieth century, though no one's ever found his footnote. It's certainly true that few sexual acts have been more often debated—and perhaps as little practiced—in this century, though there is a small but committed corps of experts. Handballers have been known to develop an attentiveness to arms and hands that most people save for genitals, making a rush-hour bus ride in summertime as charged for them as changing in a locker room.

Fisters and fisted both talk of an incredible intimacy that can come from such deep penetration. "I know it's an illusion, but it's like I'm holding his heart in my hand," says one. Those getting fisted talk of a great sense of accomplishment during the act, and of an incredible relaxation and tranquillity afterward. Again, risks are discussed below.

The Risks

RECEPTIVE ANAL INTERCOURSE (GETTING FUCKED)

Listen to men talk about how they got infected with HIV if it happened recently, and it's often portrayed as a fluke: "The condom broke," "We had oral sex," "He put it in for a second," "I got it from pre-cum." But most gay men with HIV, whether we got infected last week or last decade, got infected through unprotected receptive anal intercourse (getting fucked) by someone positive. Except for sharing needles, which gay men have also been known to do, letting someone with HIV fuck you without a condom is the most efficient way to get yourself infected. Unprotected anal sex also exposes you to gonorrhea, syphilis, and other STDs.

Even with a condom, anal sex comes with risks. The least serious, and most common, is a little aggravation to your system—maybe some gas, or cramping, or runny bowel movements. If those don't go away shortly, or if you have a discharge of mucus, you may have an aggravated anus or a more serious infection or inflammation. Condoms help but don't completely protect you from warts or herpes, which can range from a pain in the ass to a serious and ongoing medical problem.

Oh, and one last thing. Lately, more gay men have been experimenting with a "just a li'l bit" approach, that is, putting your penis in (or letting him put it in) just for a little while without a condom. It sounds good, and it may feel great, but in safety terms it's a gamble. Remember high-school health class and how the withdrawal method doesn't prevent pregnancy? Having him pull out before he comes doesn't mean no cum or pre-cum gets inside you. And if you've ever tried to hold your orgasm back but still passed the point of no return, you'll know it's also a risk to assume that he won't pass that point, too. If you're on the bottom, no matter how well you think you know the pump of his hips or the tone of his moan, you can't necessarily feel it coming.

ACTIVE ANAL INTERCOURSE (FUCKING)

Yes, tops do get HIV, though being the one to put it in puts you at lower risk than getting fucked. It's unclear how much lower the risk is, so most AIDS educators across the world leave unprotected anal sex in the "high-risk" category. See the next page for some of the factors that might increase your risk as a top.

As for STDs, you can get most of them—herpes, warts, gonorrhea, syphilis, and others—from unprotected anal sex. A condom helps but does not fully protect you from warts and herpes.

ORAL/ANAL SEX (RIMMING)

In terms of HIV, rimming is more of a theoretical risk than a real one: Most studies haven't looked at eating ass as a sex act, and those that did haven't found evidence of HIV transmission. It's conceivable, though unlikely, that he'd have blood in his shit or his anus that would get in your mouth. For some of the more serious STDs, however, most notably parasites and hepatitis, rimming is definitely high-risk behavior. And sorry—while keeping clean down there is folk wisdom among gay men, doctor after doctor says it's impossible for cleanliness alone to wash away all the tiny eggs that transmit parasites (see page 154). Using plastic wrap with a dab of lubricant on the side that touches his hole can give you protection but still let you both feel the heat, says New York City doctor Dan William, MD, as will cutting a condom lengthwise to form a barrier. If what you're looking for is the pleasure of getting inside, or putting your mouth where it "oughtn't be," then you may choose to skip the plastic and turn your tongue loose on someone you know is STD-free. That kind of knowledge, though, usually comes only with long acquaintance and honest conversation (see Chapter 4).

Being rimmed does not put you at risk for HIV. You could get herpes or warts.

FINGERING

Fingering is safe in regard to HIV so long as you don't have cuts or cum on your fingers. The hyperhygienic use gloves, or little latex covers called finger cots, but keeping unwashed fingers away from your own ass, your mouth, or any body part your mouth will be touching should protect against parasites and hepatitis. Being fingered is safe, too, if his fingernails are smooth and short, and his finger hasn't been in his own or someone else's cum or ass. You can get

RISKIER BUSINESS

HIV is a lot less easily transmitted than viruses such as hepatitis B. As a consequence, getting a positive man's cum inside you doesn't always mean turning HIV-positive. Though the science is weak, guesstimates about the risk of getting HIV from unprotected sex with someone who is HIV-positive range wildly, from 3 in 10 to 1 in 1,600.

Whether or not you get infected depends on three things:

1. *The amount of HIV that gets in* (it's not just how much someone comes—people have more virus in their cum or blood at different times).
2. *How strong the HIV is and what fluid it's in.* Some strains of HIV seem to be more infectious, and unless you have an STD in your penis, blood usually carries higher concentrations of HIV than semen.
3. *The ease with which that fluid can get to the bloodstream.* The membranes of the rectum, say, pass the virus into the bloodstream more easily than the membranes of the mouth.

Researchers call this "Q, Q, R"—quantity, quality, and route of entry. Unless you're having sex in a lab, or with a lot of broken skin, only the last—the route of entry—is easy to control. But researchers do suspect that having oral or anal intercourse without condoms is more likely to transmit HIV if:

- *One of you has recently turned positive.* HIV production is highest in the early stages, leaving newly infected people more likely to infect others.
- *One of you has an open sore or other broken skin on the parts of the body you use for sex.* Getting semen on an open sore will let HIV into your bloodstream. If you have HIV and an STD, virus is often found in the liquid that comes from such sores.
- *One of you has a sexually transmitted disease in your penis, rectum, or throat.* If you're HIV-positive, having an STD that irritates the urethra makes you shed more HIV into your cum, pre-cum, or the discharge caused by the STD. If you're HIV-negative, having an STD in your penis, throat, or rectum weakens your defenses and draws cells to that location that can in turn be infected with HIV more easily.

Last, a word for positive men: A number of men who are on anti-HIV medications and tracking their virus load are getting word that their virus is "undetectable" (see box on page 407). This does not mean that they have no virus in their bodies, but rather that their blood tests aren't showing HIV. Active HIV has been found in the semen of more than one man with "undetectable" virus in his blood. And remember, warns Ken Mayer, MD, director of Brown University's AIDS program, that virus levels can change from the time someone got their last test results. "We simply don't know enough to say that very low viral loads mean no danger of transmission," says Mayer. Finally, the fact that you're positive does not mean you no longer have to worry about whether you get more HIV in your body—see the box on page 73.

herpes and warts from touch as well as penile probing. If you're HIV-positive, you may want to be especially careful about what goes inside you.

FISTING

Fisting, or the insertion of any large object in the rectum, is not risky for HIV, but it can be seriously dangerous. The inner walls of the lower colon, often described as having the consistency of wet paper towels, are soft and easily torn. The lower colon is also called the sigmoid (S-shaped) colon because of its several curves, including a sharp one about eight inches in. A jagged fingernail, an overly aggressive or ignorant approach, or a bottom who's high or tired or timid enough not to know or say when he's in pain can all lead to a break in the colon wall.

SAFER FISTING

If you are going to practice something as risky as fisting, experienced handballers offer the following advice:

- Use latex gloves, or even double gloves if you need to. Even a callus on your hand can be uncomfortable for the bottom. Keep spare gloves handy in case you need to change.
- Use Crisco or oil-based lube. Even though oil-based lube is usually not the best choice for anal play, in this case you need more lube, and wetter lube, than most water-based products can provide. The thicker latex of gloves is less easily worn away than condoms, so they are not likely to break during fisting.
- Don't let yourself be fisted by someone inexperienced.
- Clean out beforehand. Many men who get fisted go on special diets for several days before, and douche.
- Bring a series of dildos of graduated sizes, and make sure he uses them. It's not about getting there all at once.
- Reserve the right to stop.
- Be careful about being too high or drunk to know or say when you're in pain.
- If you have any follow-up pain, fever, or bleeding, seek medical attention immediately.

Internal bleeding isn't obvious from the outside, and peritonitis (poisoning of the system) is a real possibility. If you experience sharp pain, fever, weakness, or bleeding after fisting or anal penetration with a big dildo or large penis, go to an emergency room immediately, and take someone with you.

Even without these emergencies, opening the sphincter wide enough to take an arm or large dildo can cause the sphincter muscles to lose their tone, and make it harder for you to tell whether you're passing gas or fecal matter. The stories about older fistees in diapers are exaggerated, says Dr. Stephen Goldstone of New York City, but they're not pure fiction.

SEX WITH WOMEN

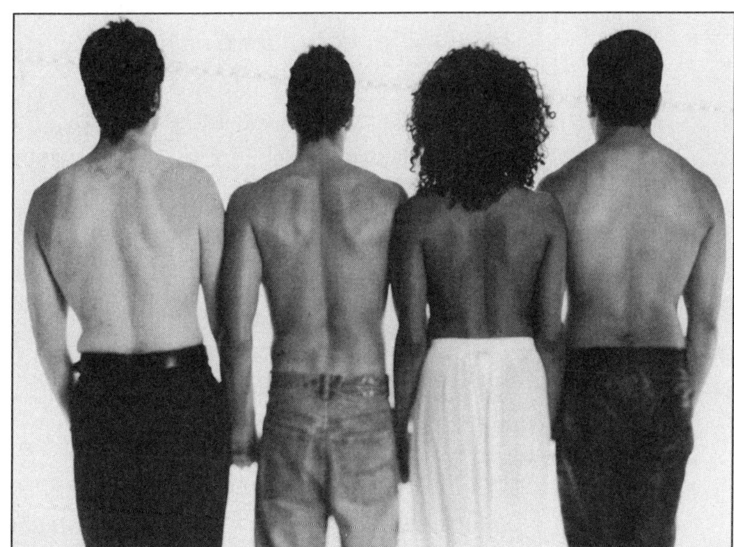

The Pleasures

The answer to the first question is yes, many of "us" enjoy those pleasures. Life isn't as tidy as our categories, people are more powerful than labels, and men who sleep with men may also find themselves in bed with a woman. Sometimes (can you believe it?) she might even be a lesbian. "When a lesbian and a gay man get it on, it opens up so many possibilities," says New York city sex activist Eva Pendleton, with the voice of experience. "You might fuck her, she might fuck you, or you can just play around and get to know each other's strange and exotic body parts." Sex with women usually involves many of the different acts already listed on these pages. But knowing a few things about how to make love to a woman can mean the difference between getting lost in space and frolicking in the Garden of Eden.

HINTS FROM THE HOMO SUTRA: *SEX WITH WOMEN*

LUBRICANT IS LUSCIOUS

"What is it with men and the dry fuck?" laments sex educator and masturbation maven Betty Dodson, Ph.D. Just because the vagina moistens itself doesn't mean she couldn't use a little extra lubrication. The wetter the better.

TRY HAND TO MOUTH

Don't just be a dick. Engage different parts of your body in stimulating hers. Feel your way around and get to know what kinds of touching, licking, and nibbling she likes. If you don't know what clitoral orgasm means, let her show you. "Men can learn a lot about sex from women," says Pendleton. "You can't just grab a woman's crotch and rub it like a dick. You need to use more nuanced kinds of touch to turn a woman on and get her off."

DRAW FROM EXPERIENCE

"Men and women have more in common than we're aware of," says Dr. Dodson. "The clitoral glans is a lot like the penile glans, for example." Just because she doesn't have a penis or a prostate doesn't mean you have no idea how she might like to be kissed or stroked. Anal pleasure is also not yours alone.

PLAY BALL

Why so serious? Some men get with women and immediately start defending against marriage plans, or feel as though their naughtiest natures are for men only. The sexual revolution includes all five genders (see Appendix B), not all of whom are out to domesticate you—especially if she knows you like men. So lighten up and enjoy. You may learn something.

The Risks

Unprotected vaginal and anal intercourse puts the woman at greater risk for HIV than the man. But much as with being the top in anal intercourse (with anyone), there's still a risk for HIV. Oral sex (going down on her, eating her out) on a woman is thought to be low-risk, not no-risk. As with rimming, some people cut open a condom, use plastic wrap, or choose a square of latex called a dental dam to protect themselves and their partners. Again, many find this changes the experience beyond recognition and so prefer other risk-reduction strategies (see "Beyond Condoms," page 85).

WATER SPORTS

The Pleasures

Four or five years ago I saw a flyer about a water sports party. I'd heard about it but I tried not to think about it, maybe the way a lot of people who aren't out yet try not to think about being gay. But I went and just watched. Part of me was disgusted and part of me was fascinated. It was years later that I let myself follow through on my fantasy. I was with this guy in a movie theater I felt really free with, and after he came I just asked him, did he want to pee on me? He said okay. I don't know if he had done it before. It was a feeling not of submission but of surrendering. I just lay back and felt the sensual feeling of liquid and warmth washing over me. It was like lying in the sun.

GOLDEN SHOWERS

Whether a relaxing surrender to warmth, a more formal humiliation, or somewhere in between, golden showers—the splashing of pee onto the body or into the mouth—can be a great pleasure. As with cum, some men are careful to distinguish between "on me" and "in me," though the distinctions here may have more to do with psyche than safety. "There's nothing like it when our eyes meet and lock," says forty-five-year-old Charles, a visual artist, who's a big fan of "in me." "I can see the physical relief created by his need to empty his bladder mingling with the power surge created by his need to dominate me. He understands my need for nourishment and lets me have it."

ENEMAS

Enemas, too, involve water, surrender, and release. They can be part of an S/M scene, an eroticized way of ensuring cleanliness before fucking, a replay of a charged childhood memory, or part of a bigger love for those areas where medical and sexual practices intersect. Enema enthusiasts, however, minister far more lovingly and deeply than most doctors or nurses, with everything from the insertion of the nozzle to the kneading of his lower abdomen to make sure everything's gotten in (and comes out) all right as part of the thrill. Or maybe you let him use the enema as a way of getting you to beg for release and watch you explode, in a reworking of the more common orgasmic theme.

The Risks

GOLDEN SHOWERS

Getting urine on your skin, so long as you don't have open cuts or sores, cannot give you HIV or other STDs. Drinking it poses a theoretical risk for HIV and other sexually transmitted diseases, since viruses such as CMV or herpes are shed in urine and could conceivably infect you if you got them in your mouth.

ENEMAS

Enemas pose no risk for HIV or other STDs, or (in moderation) for anything else. Do them a lot and you can deplete potassium and other electrolyte levels in your body, says New York City doctor Howard Grossman, MD, as well as build a dependence that will keep your bowels from moving on their own. If your immune system is seriously weak, use boiled water—cooled to room temperature, of course. Make sure to leave ample time not only for administration but for expulsion. Rush it at your own peril: You or your partner may find yourself greeting a brown geyser that arrives, without warning, in the middle of sex (or your dinner party).

Enema enthusiasts have special recipes: milk and honey, aromatic oils, even air. Some people use enemas for medicinal purposes. If you, or he, are one of those who like to use liquids other than water, be careful with anything but the most seriously diluted mixtures unless you really know what you're doing. The same mucous membranes in the colon and rectum that absorb fluid from your bowel movements absorb other things—alcohol, astringents, and so on—with equal readiness; this can be extremely dangerous. Also, enemas can cause tiny abrasions, so make sure to use a condom (and see the box on page 30) if you're planning on pairing them with anal intercourse.

SCAT

The Pleasures

Bottoms either get it or they don't. A few are grossed out and then they say, "Do it again." One called me from a Hawaiian vacation every time his lover left the room, and asked me to fart into the phone while he jacked off.

Scat is short for *scatological,* meaning concerned with the load produced not by the penis but by the bowels. Whether you're talking feces or farts, some men get a great charge from delivering them to a partner or receiving their delivery. There's also a fan mag, *Poohzine,* that features pictures—and rapturous descriptions—of various people's daily produce. (That's why they call it the information revolution.)

The Risks

Like rimming (see page 67) but more so. While there is a theoretical and unproven risk for HIV, handling someone else's shit puts you at high risk for parasites, bacteria, and hepatitis if your hands get anywhere near your mouth or your food. Eating someone's feces almost guarantees you'll get those organisms, unless you can be certain he's not infected.

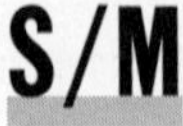

S/M

The Pleasures

Part of what's interesting to me is that orgasm is knocked off its pedestal. The physical sensation of struggle against the ropes, trying to reach that particular point where I can go so far and no farther, that's pleasurable.

S/M, or sadomasochism, is not really a specific sex act, or even a series of them. In many ways it's more of a mode of communication (see "S/M: Special Channel #1," page 107) that two or more men use as a way of exploring issues of power and pain, desire and domination. Much to the dissatisfaction of practitioners of specific disciplines, who may or may not see themselves as having anything in common, there are a bunch of acts that fall under the S/M umbrella—spanking and bondage, piercing and pissing, enemas and tickling and flogging and fisting and force-feeding and much, much more. Oh, and fashion. The pleasure of that part of S/M has been readily accepted by mainstream members of all sexual orientations who, their sunny interiors notwithstanding, sport jackboots and motorcycle jackets of dark leather. Lest you dismiss deeper involvement with S/M as the specialty of people more committed than yourself, consider all the following hazy areas of pleasure.

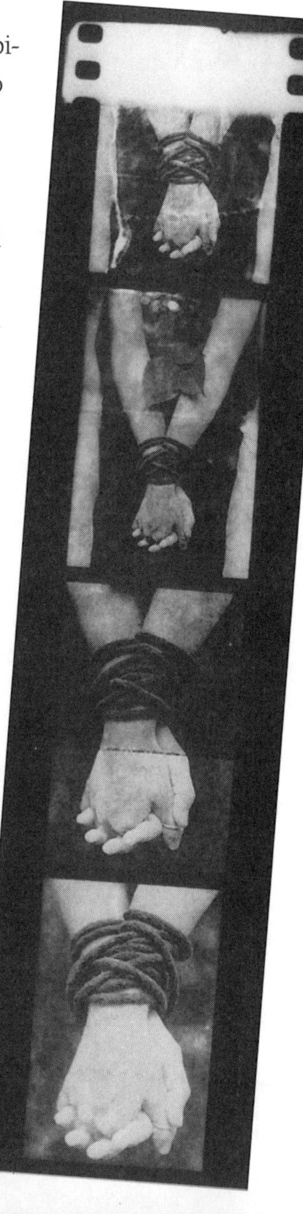

BONDAGE

This can range from the old bathrobe belt to a full-fledged, incapacitating, deliciously immobilizing concoction of ropes a scoutmaster wouldn't be able to undo. He wants you to worship his body? You'd better obey (your hands are tied).

SPANKING

You've been bad. Very bad. And now you're going to take down your pants and be punished with a series of slaps or hits on your buns—perhaps, if you close your eyes, by that coach you lusted after in high school. Or maybe your partner will want you to see his raised hand as it descends to slap, or soothe, your reddening cheeks.

TIT, COCK, OR BALL TORTURE

Is *torture* too strong a word? Think of anything from the pleasure/pain of an unshaven cheek against your nipple to the hard pinch of fingers all the way to clamps and needles. Working someone's equipment can benefit from gadgets available at your local sex shop, like a cock ring or ball spreader (see "Toys and Tools," page 75), but you can also make do with focus and hand work. "I like to stretch the sac tight and then spank it softly," says Seamus, thirty, a social worker, of his ball play. Another man suggests a gentler approach: grasping scrotum between thumb and middle finger, and then tantalizing the taut surface of the scrotum gently with your nails.

The Risks

Whether you're talking about bondage, spanking, tit torture, or cock and ball play, no blood should ever be drawn, or skin broken, without taking careful precautions. If you're using equipment, know its limits, and your own. A number of books, including the *Leatherman's Handbook* (Masquerade Books, 1997) and *The Safe Edge* (Alternate Sources, 1993), can help. Since S/M is so much about communication, lack of it is one of the most serious risks. See page 107.

HIV RISK IN THE NEW MILLENNIUM

IT AIN'T OVER YET

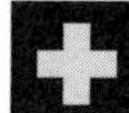

To HIV-Positive Men: Reinfection Realities?

Why bother with safer sex at this point? Plenty of guys dispense with condoms, particularly if they know (or think) their partner is positive, or if he doesn't say. Sure, anal sex without a condom may be a little risky for getting something, but it's not like getting HIV again. You already have it, right? Well, no. Not quite. More, says recent research, like wrong.

To HIV-Negative Men: A PEP Talk?

Why bother with safer sex at this point? Plenty of guys are thinking that even unprotected anal sex isn't that big a deal, that the new AIDS drugs make having HIV less of a trauma. There's even what some men are calling a "morning-after" treatment—PEP, or postexposure prophylaxis—where you take a month-long course of anti-HIV drugs right after you think you might have been

To HIV-Positive Men: Reinfection Realities? (cont.)

There isn't one virus—there are different strains and subtypes. And when someone else's virus gets in your body, it may combine with yours and make a new type. As of this writing, no one's sure whether having one of these recombinations means that you'll get sick faster or die sooner. But researchers are increasingly convinced that it's possible, and that new strains could be harder to treat, particularly now that so many people are on different combinations of AIDS drugs. If you get virus inside you from someone whose drugs have failed to work, the drugs he took may be useless for you, too. Some worry that mixing different strains of HIV will create a "super-virus" that is resistant to all AIDS drugs, and though there is no hard evidence of that yet, there *are* documented cases of positive men passing multiple drug-resistant strains to their HIV-negative partners. A 1999 study of recently infected gay men in New York found that 16 percent had a strain of HIV resistant to one or more drugs.

Fucking without a condom also means giving up a chance to protect yourself from other STDs. People talk less than they should about the ways that STDs are more dangerous for people with HIV (see Chap. 4). Think warts coming out of your anus, herpes sores that might stay for months, or liver damage just when you need your liver most.

Finally, there's him. Even if you don't care about STDs or getting more HIV, you're still at risk for infecting someone else. Just because he doesn't say, it doesn't mean he's positive. And even if he is infected, the same holds true for him as for you, and you could be exposing him to a disease, or new virus, that may seriously harm his health, or take his life.

There's gambling, having unprotected anal sex that potentially exposes him and you to disease and strains of the virus that could make your HIV much more serious. And then there's safer sex.

For ways to think about condom use and risk reduction, see the final sections of this chapter, starting on page 79. For more information on how resistance develops to AIDS drugs, see Chap. 9. For more

To HIV-Negative Men: A PEP Talk? (cont.)

exposed to prevent infection. "It's like abortion," says Jack, age forty-two, a lighting designer. "You don't want to use it, but it's good to know it's there." Unlike abortion, says New York city doctor Howard Grossman, MD, "you have to use it within forty-eight hours of the sex in question, and even then we aren't sure whether it works."

What do we really know about PEP? It's based on studies done in hospitals, where workers who got stuck with needles took AIDS drugs to reduce the risk of turning HIV-positive. The theory is that if you stop the virus from reproducing immediately, it never gets strong enough to turn you positive. And, at least with hospital workers in the studies, it seemed to reduce infection by an estimated 81 percent. But those people got their treatment right there in the hospital, literally hours after potential exposure, rather than the morning or two mornings afterward. Even in that best-case scenario, some health-care workers became infected. The studies have not included a control group of people who didn't take the drugs, so we don't know how many of them would have stayed negative anyway. Though increasing numbers of doctors are prescribing PEP, many insurers won't pay for it, deeming it unproven.

We do know what taking protease inhibitors and the other new AIDS drugs is like. Ask the thousands of gay men who are on them. They can tell you about how strange it is to have pills that are supposed to make you feel better make you feel sick, about the diarrhea and diabetes and nausea the drugs cause, about having to take up to twenty pills a day with different eating requirements and storage requirements, and about trying to make sure you have the insurance or the money to pay for them. With recent reports showing that hopes of completely eradicating HIV from the body were premature, anti-HIV drugs are a lifetime proposition. If you do gamble on unsafe fucking with someone of unknown serostatus, you may "win" dependence on a $15,000-a-year course of treatment for life—if the drugs work for you.

Finally, there's him. Not using a condom for anal sex not only may expose yourself to harm, but may expose him to STDs. If you think you know your HIV

To HIV-Positive Men: Reinfection Realities? (cont.)

information on sexually transmitted diseases and their effect on people with HIV, see Chap. 4.

To HIV-Negative Men: A PEP Talk? (cont.)

status but aren't really sure, you may give him HIV. Even if you're on the bottom in anal sex, you could be giving him a disease that may seriously harm his health, or take his life.

For ways to think through condom use and risk reduction, see the final sections of this chapter, starting on page 79. For information on the effects and side effects of new AIDS drugs, and paying for them, see Chap. 9. For more information on sexually transmitted diseases, see Chap. 4.

Location, Location, Location? HIV, Bathrooms, Back Rooms, and Bedrooms

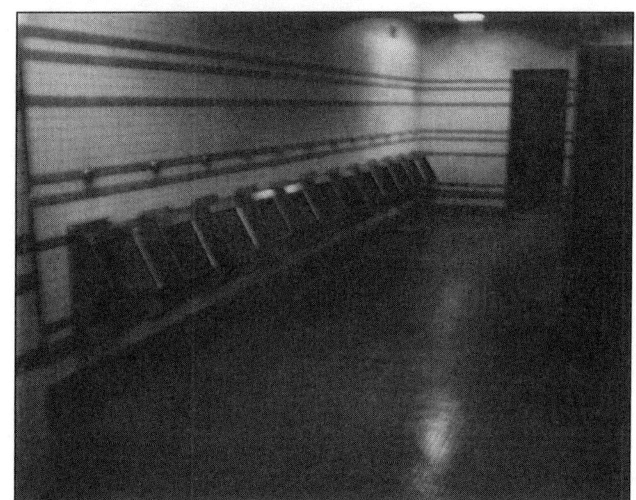

Yes, it's the sex you have, not where you have it, that determines risk for HIV. In broad terms, though, where you have sex is worth watching. Whether it's because we feel more intimate or simply have more space to lie down and relax, gay men are more likely to have anal sex at home than in public places. Public sex, on the other hand, tends toward the silent, which means more partners whose HIV status you don't know (see "Talking HIV," in Chapter 3). Before you slip into something more comfortable (including him) at home, ask yourself if love or comfort levels may be moving you toward risky sex that you're not ready for. Consider, before you step into that stall and bare your butt, if you would do the same things if you knew him to be positive. Finally, remember that sex in some places, particularly public parks and bathrooms, comes with other risks: entrapment or arrest (see box on next page).

Toys and Tools: Eleven that Can Please Your Body and Open Your Mind

Buy, Buy

Yes, maybe you *can* use that cucumber meant for last week's salad. But where and how you purchase a sex toy may have a lot to do with how much you come to understand and enjoy it. Many large- and medium-sized cities have at least one sex-toy shop or erotic boutique. The best, often gay- and/or woman-owned, have friendly, knowledgeable people behind the counter. Beware of the "dirty-bookstore" with the wall of shrink-wrapped products and the surly staffer.

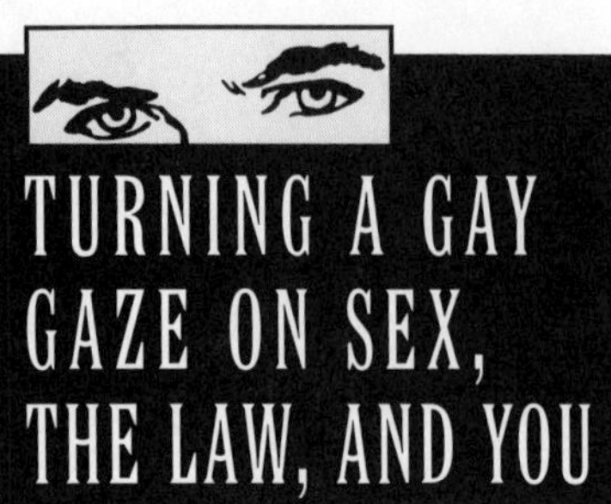

TURNING A GAY GAZE ON SEX, THE LAW, AND YOU

Laws make things normal by threatening punishment for those who don't follow them. Which makes it especially ugly that sodomy—meaning any kind of oral or anal sex between men, among other things—is illegal in sixteen states. Even the privacy of your home is no guarantee of safety. In 1986, with the *Bowers v. Hardwick* decision, the highest court in the land decided that sodomy laws—including the one used to arrest Bowers in his bedroom—were constitutional.

If you're having sex outside a home, though, then other laws come into play. "Lewd conduct," "criminal opportuning," and "lascivious conduct" are a few of the pretexts used to arrest or harass gay men who are having sex, asking someone to have sex, or even lingering where men have sex in public. Never mind that "public" in this case may mean a deserted park or bathroom stall. Never mind that most gay men are arrested not because some other citizen was inconvenienced but because a police officer staked out the cruising area, waiting there for hours or leading men to believe that he wanted to join in. Never mind that straight people make out all the time in cars, in parks, and on beaches and are more likely to be cheered on than given a warning. The laws against public lewdness are usually aimed at gay men and other "sex offenders." Cruising outdoors is also subject to the law of the jungle—some straight men go to cruising areas to bash, beat, or rob gay men.

If you are in legal trouble because you are accused of having public sex, get a good local lawyer. In the meanwhile, advises Evan Wolfson of the Lambda Legal Defense and Education Fund, say as little as possible. "You have the right to remain silent, and in almost all cases you should," says Wolfson, coauthor of "The Little Black Book," Lambda's excellent pamphlet on the subject of public sex arrests. In addition, Wolfson suggests, you should write down as much as you can remember about the circumstances of your arrest, make sure you know the legal charges and what happens if you plead guilty or innocent, and consider contacting a local antiviolence group or gay legal organization. Police sometimes engage in "fairy shaking," demanding money or threatening to out you as gay or HIV-positive in order to get a bribe or a guilty plea. You're not the first one to have faced that, and you don't have to face it alone.

For a free copy of "The Little Black Book," referrals to local legal organizations, or to help fight a pattern of prosecution across the nation, contact the Lambda Legal Defense and Education Fund. The American Civil Liberties Union can also help. Addresses for both are found in Appendix A.

It's perfectly okay to browse. Take the opportunity to listen to the staff: If they're serving up more attitude than advice, shop elsewhere. Don't be shy with your questions; clerks in sex shops have heard it all. "The only irritating customers are those that aren't really customers at all, the people who come in to see who else is in there buying what," says Eric, assistant manager of New York's Pleasure Chest. "But if you're asking questions because you want to find something to use and enjoy—even if that means going home and thinking about it for a while—we're happy to advise." If there is no decent shop within your immediate traveling range, try mail order or the World Wide Web. The following are a few of the most popular playthings.

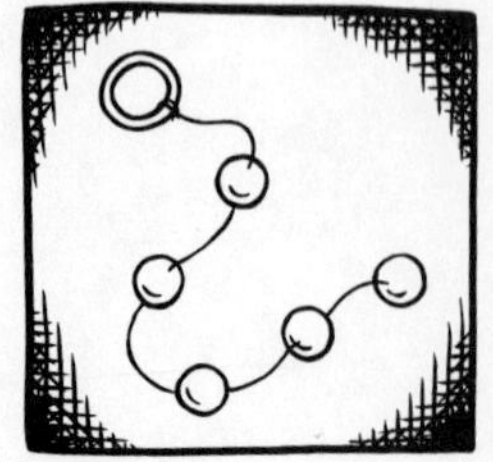
Anal beads

ANAL BEADS

Not your average string of pearls, anal beads usually come about five to a strand. They range in size, resembling marbles at one end of the spectrum and baseballs at the other. The plastic ones often have seams in need of filing, so skip right to the silicone or rubber varieties. One touted technique: Insert them slowly, one by one, as you are getting excited, then pull the string out as you come.

BALL SPREADERS

If your testicles can't rise up toward your body, you can't ejaculate. Which is what makes ball spreaders a tantalizing treat, allowing for increased scrotal sensitivity and prolonged pleasuring. Common models come in leather, denim, or nylon.

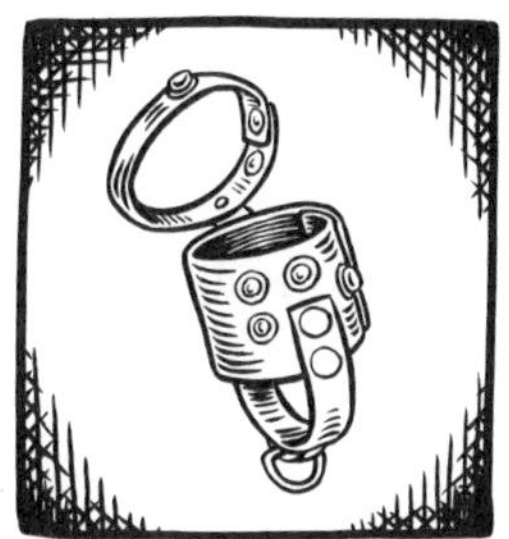

Ball spreader

BUTT PLUGS

These range from a slim, finger-sized model all the way up to something you might be tempted to string a set of lights on at the holidays. The key to butt plugs is that they're flared at the base to prevent them from slipping inside you. Some plugs are rippled to give added stimulation, while others provide one modest bulge for your rectum to grab. Beginners beware: The battery-operated vibrating plugs make the Energizer bunny look low-energy.

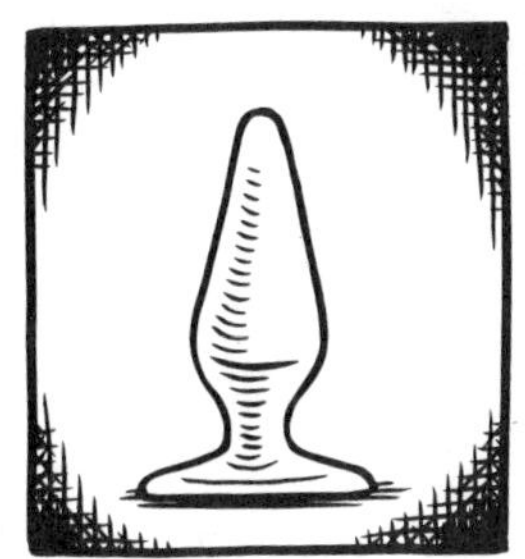

Butt plug

COCK RINGS

These squeeze the veins that carry blood into the penis, leaving you bigger and harder, longer. And when you do finally come, the increased intensity will be well worth the wait. There are metal rings, black rubber rings, simple rawhide ties, and adjustable leather rings with snaps. Most go around both cock and balls. Solid rings need careful sizing. Make sure to put your balls in first, and watch out for any ring so tight that circulation is cut off. Adjustables are best for beginners, and no one, no matter how advanced, should leave a cock ring on if there's any swelling, pain, or feeling of coldness in the genitals. Two more caveats: Never use rubber bands, and always take off a cock ring before you fall asleep.

DILDOS

Though available in materials from leather to Lucite and in a full range of colors, the dildo is the sex-toy equivalent of basic black. Whether you choose a "lifelike" model or a nonrepresentational one, the right instrument can provide years of faithful service. Silicone dildos, which have more warmth and give than most, are a good start. For beginners, the rule is start small; going big will probably only send you back to the store next week, and they're neither cheap nor returnable. Dildos with balls, a flared base, or a suction cup make for easier control and less fear of losing it inside your rectum. Some dildos are double-headed, making for two (or is that four?) buns of fun when used with a partner.

Having a real friend to insert your new inanimate one can add some spice to the soup. In this one instance, Mother was wrong: Don't share your toys, at least not without using condoms and changing them in between, or washing a dildo thoroughly with soap and hot water (and wiping it down with Betadine) to ensure you don't transmit HIV or other STDs.

NIPPLE TOYS

If the homemaker inside you says that clothespins will do, you're right. They're not adjustable, however. For more careful control, pick up a set of clamps from a sex-toy store. They come tweezer-style, or with screws that allow you to start easy, then increase the squeeze. Go easy, since the sudden return of blood to your nipples when clamps are removed is often more painful than putting them on. For pressure without a lot of pain, try the little suction cups that come in snakebite kits you can get at army-navy stores, or their higher priced erotic-boutique cousins. Overuse of these can cause blistering or even open sores. And the kits are suspected, though not proven, to cause CNS—Chelsea Nipple Syndrome, which is what gives certain boys in New York inch-long flesh plugs where you just know tiny tits ought to be.

PUMPS

For some, this is more than a toy—it's a medical device or a lifestyle choice (see "Big Talk," page 14). The casual user can find pumps—vacuum tubes that draw blood and fluid into the penis, leaving you temporarily bigger than you've been before—in either battery-operated or manual models. Having him pump you up physically can do the same emotionally, and leave you both raring to go. Manufacturers advise you not to pump for more than fifteen minutes, and don't be surprised if your bigger erection is also bluer and a little soggy-seeming. Bruising or pinpoint-size blood blisters on the head of the penis are also common. As noted in Chapter 1, overuse may cause structural damage to the tissue of your penis.

RESTRAINTS

For times when you want to give up (or take) control, employ the proper restraints. That old silk scarf can easily become too tight, and your nylon clothesline can burn. Handcuffs are widely available at sex shops and army-navy stores, but make sure to leave room to avoid cutting off circulation (the width of a finger is good). If you feel any coldness or numbness in a bound body part, have your partner loosen it immediately. If you're using handcuffs, keep a spare key nearby—they're easy to lose, and having to call local police for help may add a little too much realness to the fantasy. Leather restraints come in two sizes, designed to fit either wrists or ankles. They are often available with fleece lining if you prefer a gentler touch, although these can cost nearly twice as much as the unlined variety.

Don't use restraints around the neck, either alone or when playing with someone else. Teenage boys and grown men both have died because someone said you could get an extra orgasmic boost by choking yourself. Breath control, autoasphyxiation—whatever you call it, it's highly dangerous.

VIBRATORS

There is a world of electrically assisted toys beyond the vibrating butt plug and the old, yellowing plastic torpedo with the twist-on base. Plug-in models offer pleasures often unexplored by men; put a washcloth between you and it if the sensations are too intense. Wand-style vibrators have a wide surface that glides easily along the underside of your shaft; coil-operated vibrators resemble handheld mixers (one is even made by Sunbeam!) and give more concentrated, focused stimulation. Both kinds feature attachments for anal play, variable speeds, and "cum cups" that fit loosely over the head of your penis for a one-way ticket to ecstasy.

LUBRICANTS

Modern technology offers a passel of potions designed to keep you wetter and wilder. Yes, a few men will complain it's not spontaneous, or that they don't like the mess, or that they crave the extra friction of dry rubbing. But the heightened pleasures of slippery surfaces, the way lube can enhance the touch of a hand or the brush of a fingertip, can far outweigh the drawbacks. If you haven't found a lubricant that sets you slipping toward ecstasy, try a couple; there are many variations on the following three basic themes.

Oil-Based Lubricants

Best for jerking off, these great and greasy lubes include gay-targeted brands such as Mens Cream (no apostrophe, since *mens* means "wisdom" in Greek) and Elbow Grease, as well as old-style pharmacy favorites like Albolene Creme. Any kind of mineral or vegetable oil can also do the trick (now that's Wessonality!). A plastic bottle of peanut oil (twenty-four cents an ounce) is a simple pleasure. Heat it for ten seconds in the microwave, and it will quickly return the investment in electricity. One warning: For anal penetration, don't use oil-based lube. The oil plugs glands in the rectum, and all oil-based lubes (including baby oil, mineral oil, hand lotions, and petroleum jelly, better known as Vaseline) make latex condoms fall apart. Unless you're equipped with polyurethane protection (see "Five Steps to Condom Comfort," next page), stick to another lubricant.

Water-Based Lubricants

These, too, come in many varieties, from the expensive but exquisite Astroglide, the practical and pleasant Probe, and the new and improved KY Liquid to a host of cheaper, gloppier flavored affairs. The anally involved favor a pump or nozzle-style dispenser, so as not to dip a nasty hand in the tub (think peanut butter in the jelly), while the stain-conscious look at the list of ingredients on the back (the higher the water content, the safer those Ralph Lauren sheets). Different water-based lubes dry out at different speeds. Some men keep a spray bottle or mister by the bed. Elegant, no, but effective.

Those wanting an extra layer of HIV or STD protection have been known to seek out another common ingredient, the spermicide nonoxynol-9. Though nonoxynol-9 kills HIV in the test tube, it's rarely sufficiently concentrated in lubes to do that in your body, and it's never enough to use nonoxynol-9 by itself without a condom. Some recent studies have suggested that nonoxynol-9 is actually bad for HIV prevention, causing irritation that may increase your risk for STDs, including anal herpes and HIV.

Silicone-Based Lubricants

These are the new kids on the block but are fast becoming the homecoming queens in the lube pageant. Eros, a European import, now has a few local competitors, including Wet Platinum and Millennium. While the Food and Drug Administration will neither test lubes with condoms nor allow them to claim latex compatibility without tests, reports from Europe show silicone-based lubes to be condom-compatible. And since they don't dry out the way water-based lubes usually do, a dab'll do you for a good long while. Cleanup may be harder—but so, probably, will you.

CONDOMS

Scientists are working on a rectal microbicide—a gel that you can put inside you that would kill HIV without blasting the soft, sensitive tissues of your anus. There are plans for a liquid condom, a super-thin, fast-drying product you can squirt inside you to form a protective, invisible shield. But until those things move from research to reality—or unless you know your partner is HIV-negative—then using condoms for anal sex remains the best way around to protect him and you from HIV and a host of other sexually transmitted infections.

FIVE STEPS TO CONDOM COMFORT

1. *Go it alone.* Get comfortable with condoms before you find him gazing up expectantly at you with butt raised and legs spread. Take one out, lube it up, and masturbate with it. Experiment with stretching it and seeing if you can make it break. Condoms come in different sizes (see #3), though most stretch to fit over a fist. That should be big enough.

2. *Keep them handy.* Nothing breaks the mood like getting up and rummaging through your bathroom medicine cabinet while he's getting chilly and soft on the bed. Any dark, cool place—such as your bedside table drawer—within arm's reach will do.

3. *Find a favorite.* All latex condoms sold in the United States block HIV, but not all are created equal. There's flared for the big at the base among us, contoured for the heavy-headed penis, smaller for the small penis, bigger for the wider penis, and thinner for the heat-seeking missile. Don't use lambskin condoms, which are so thin they don't block all viruses. There's prelubricated and unlubricated latex, textured for more sensation or untextured for the quick-to-come, condoms with different colors and smells. There are even polyurethane condoms, marketed under the name Avanti, which transmit heat much better and allow you to use oil-based lube. Proceed with caution: As of this writing, poly condoms are FDA-approved only for those allergic to latex, and have broken more than latex condoms in a number of tests.

4. *Make it part of the play.* You don't have to know how to do it all. Get him to show you how to put it on. With his mouth, maybe. You or he can also put a cock ring over the condom if it helps keep it on (and you hard).

5. *Communicate.* This can be verbal or without words. Some men find it easier to do before he or you gets hard. Maybe you make it a point to say, before you go home with him, "I like to use condoms. Is that okay with you?" Maybe you've been home with him for years already, in which case you can say, "I love you, but I'm not ready to do this without condoms yet." Or maybe you just hand him a condom as you're going at it; he'll get the message.

I know it sounds crazy, but for me the sound of a condom packet opening is arousing. I hear it—wheet!—and I know something good is coming.

For me, it's talking about it that's the problem. Once I've said it, "I have safer sex. Is that cool with you?" then I can feel more relaxed about handing him the condom.

I want to get carried away. So if I have to use a condom, I'd rather skip the whole thing.

Condoms are a tool, not a total answer. They remind some of us of things we'd like to forget, like who's on top or the possibility of AIDS. They're a barrier—not only a latex or polyurethane barrier, but a psychological one—to intimacy that we may want to share with a loved one, to spontaneity and carefree caresses. But lost in the condom complaints or the jokes about "taking a shower with a raincoat on" is the fact that *not* using a condom with someone may also rain cold water on our efforts to be intimate and sexual. The fantasy that HIV is ignorable—sometimes appealing for the moment—is rarely a sturdy one, replaced quickly by anxiety over infection or infecting, ambivalence about how we should care for each other's safety, or the bitterness that comes from being with someone who does not seem to care (see "Talking HIV," in Chapter 3). Taking care of each other through condom use is a gay male specialty. Thousands of us have worked to find ways to make condoms easier, hotter, and safer. And condoms have worked for us, preventing HIV and saving lives. They do take time and effort, but compared to what: the six hours it took to pick him up, or the fifteen phone conversations you might have afterward about why you didn't use one? Think of it as a loving act for him, and a way to protect yourself.

How to Put On a Condom

1. Push the condom away from the edge of the foil package before you tear it open. Watch the sharp edges of the wrapper, and your nails. It's not a grenade. Don't open it with your teeth.

2. Before unrolling it, place a drop of water-based lubricant inside the tip of the condom to increase sensation.

3. Pinch the tip of the condom, squeezing the air out and leaving between a quarter inch and a half inch of space at the end for the cum.

4. Proceed to roll it down to cover the erect penis. Note the word erect: If it's not hard yet, a condom won't go on well. Hand-over-hand is the easiest method, though some favor the A-okay approach, ringing thumb and middle finger in the okay symbol and moving the ring down the penis. If you're uncircumcised, pull your foreskin down before you put on the condom to avoid "bunching."

5. Lube up the outside (and his inside) with water-based lubricant for easy entry. Add more as needed.

6. Enjoy. Many men withdraw before ejaculation for extra safety. If you do come inside him, hold the condom by the base as you pull out to prevent semen from spilling or seeping.

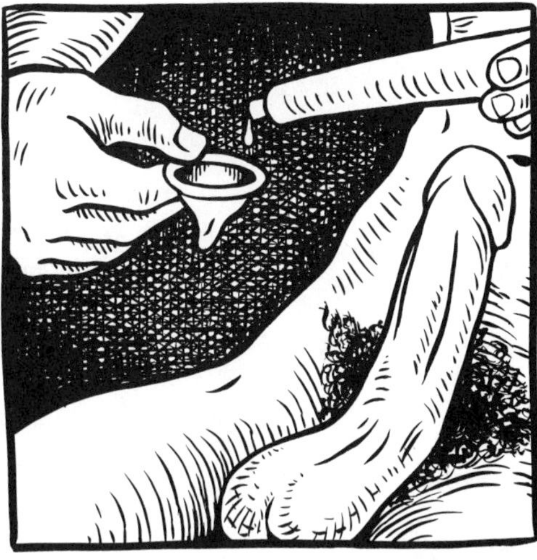

2. Before unrolling it, place a drop of water-based lubricant inside the tip of the condom to increase sensation.

Condom Complaints and Solutions

1. *They burn.* It might be the nonoxynol-9 in the lubricant, the powder that comes on unlubricated condoms, or the latex itself. Latex allergies have increased sharply since AIDS started, jumping an estimated 800 percent over the last two decades. Most allergies start mild, though if you have immediate or serious stinging after putting on a condom, get to an emergency room. To find out if you're allergic—or to test his claim that he is, and so can't be bothered—rub a condom against the skin on the inner arm; an allergic man will have a rash the next day. If you are latex-intolerant, investigate a polyurethane product such as Avanti, the "female" condom (see next page), and www.latex-allergy.org, the Web site for a latex allergy support network. And though it sounds like a bad gay joke, don't eat bananas or nuts. They're among the foods, along with papaya and avocado, that can make a latex allergy worse.

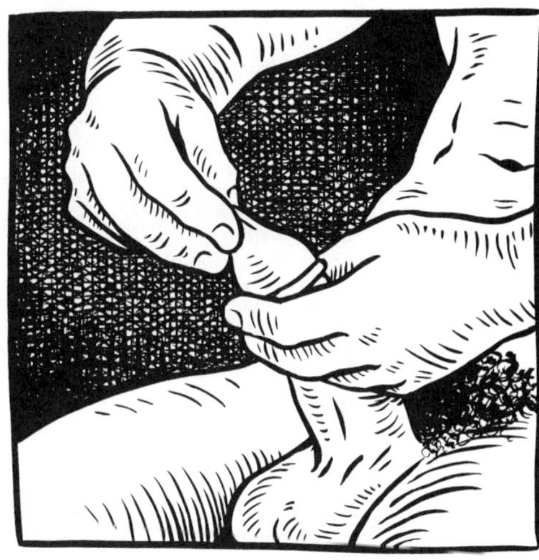

3. Pinch the tip of the condom, squeezing the air out and leave a quarter to a half inch of space at the end for cum.

2. *They're too small.* Condoms in this country usually stretch up to two feet, so it may be a matter of width. Try more lube inside, and if your penis is wide at the base, consider flared condoms, which help you feel more by gripping you less. A number of manufacturers make special condoms for bigger penises: Carter Wallace has Magnum, Trojan makes Trojan XLL, and Mayer Labs makes Maxx. Mayer also sells a polyurethane baggy condom, EZON, in Europe, which they say is not only roomier but the only condom that rolls down without a problem, even if you put it on "wrong side up"! As of this writing, the FDA has yet to approve it for sale in the U.S.

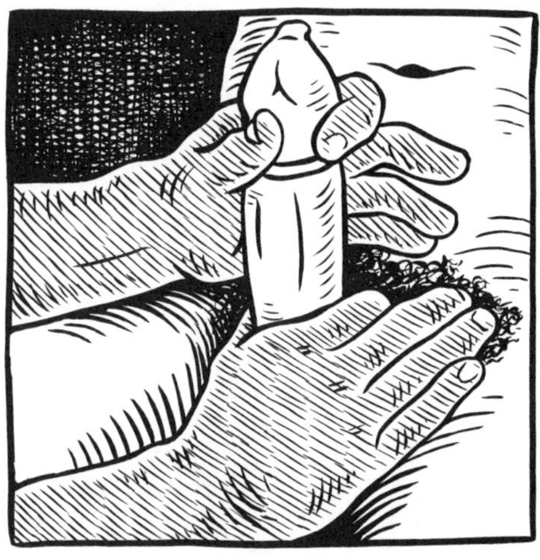

4. Proceed to roll it down over the erect penis.

REALITY?

Defenders say this is the best thing to happen to anal sex in decades. Critics call it as appealing as a plastic bag, and its use as appetizing as screwing an ass with a plastic bag hanging out of it. It's Reality, the "female" condom being tried by increasing numbers of gay men for anal pleasures. It's big, it's expensive ($4 a go), it takes some getting used to, and—unless you use a lot of lube—it squeaks. Still, defenders say its virtues—the ability to use oil-based lube, to stop and start anal sex (and avoid the now-that-the-condom's-on-let's-race-to-the-finish pattern), and to feel heat through polyurethane—make Reality more like a fantasy, at least for the man doing the fucking.

Designed in part to give women more control in contraception, Reality is used by the receptive partner in intercourse. It's more like a closed plastic funnel than a conventional condom, with a ring at the narrow end and another at the wider opening to hold it in place. Men insert the sheath into the anus and rectum, leaving an inch of polyurethane and the outer ring sticking out. It can technically be inserted up to four hours before use, though men who've used it say the insertion is best saved for the bedroom. Some men, complaining of the inner ring, have started removing that ring, and using a dildo or their partner's penis to get the sheath in place. No matter how you do it, it takes some getting used to, and a practice run—without anal intercourse immediately after—is in order.

A word of warning: Reality, with or without the inner ring, hasn't been tested or approved for use in anal sex. Neither, apparently, has any condom—it seems the fact that anal sex is still illegal in many states has the FDA squeamish. Still, a number of men have decided that if it's good enough to protect against HIV in women's vaginas, they'll try their luck. A survey of eleven gay couples by Chicago's Howard Brown Clinic found that Reality didn't tear during sex, though men did complain about feeling the seam (which runs the length of the condom) and the inner ring. Among a hundred men surveyed by the Stop AIDS project in San Francisco, the complaints included bunching up of the condom, slippage, and, most notably, difficulty getting the inner ring past the sphincter. Still, 84 percent said they'd be willing to try Reality again, and just over half said they preferred it to conventional condoms. The survey didn't distinguish between tops and bottoms, leading one to wonder whether it was the top half that felt most enthusiastic.

3. *They slip off.* The opposite of the advice in number 2: Beware the flare and avoid overlubing. If you're small, there are a number of special condoms for you, Barnett's Bikini, Ansell's Lifestyles Form-Fitting, and Safetex's Slims among them. Different brands have different amounts of stretchiness. Use only a dime-sized drop of lube inside—too much and your condom can ride up or slide off.

4. *They make you lose your hard-on.* Many men—in some studies, even the majority—report losing their erections while putting on a condom. Practicing the five steps to condom comfort on page 80 can help. So can knowing it's not just you.

5. *They break.* Every batch of American condoms has to be tested for leakage; Japanese condoms are tested even more rigorously, one by one. The most common causes of condom breakage are incorrect storage and mistakes in use. Heat, sunlight, and humidity all eat away at latex, and if your condom's past its expiration date, it's no good no matter how long you've left it in the dark. Human error with condoms takes many forms, including using oil-based lubricants (Crisco, Vaseline, hand lotion, olive oil, and the like) that cause latex to fall away. A less common cause involves the marathon-man syndrome. "After spending ten minutes with one man going through every condom breakage possibility I could think of, I finally asked, 'How long does it take?'" recalls Daniel Bao, director of the Condom Resource Center in Oakland, California. "He answered, 'About two to three hours.'" If you're in him for the long haul, change condoms every hour.

USING THE "FEMALE" CONDOM

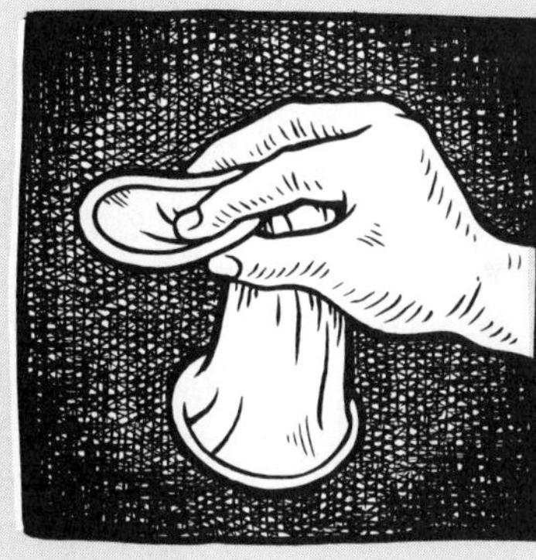

1. Hold the pouch with the open end hanging down and squeeze the ring at the closed end with your fingers.

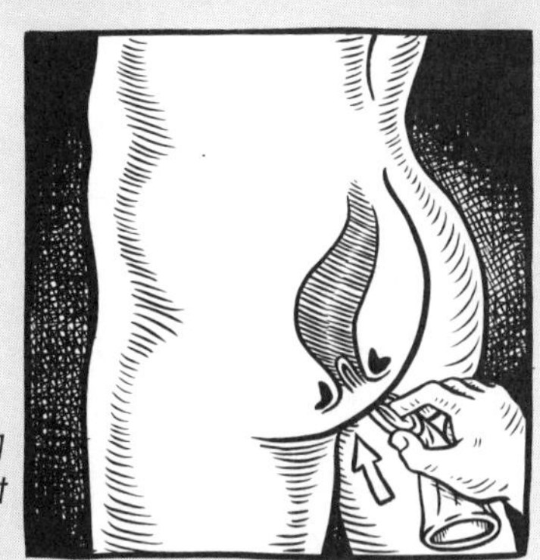

2. Still squeezing the ring, insert the condom.

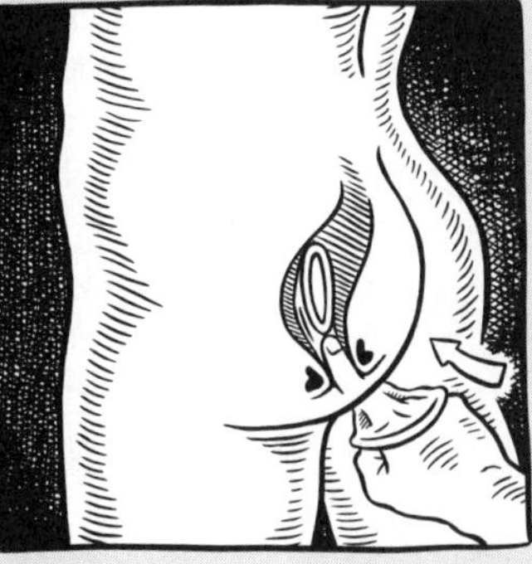

3. For maximum protection, the inner ring needs to go up inside you, past the sphincter muscle.

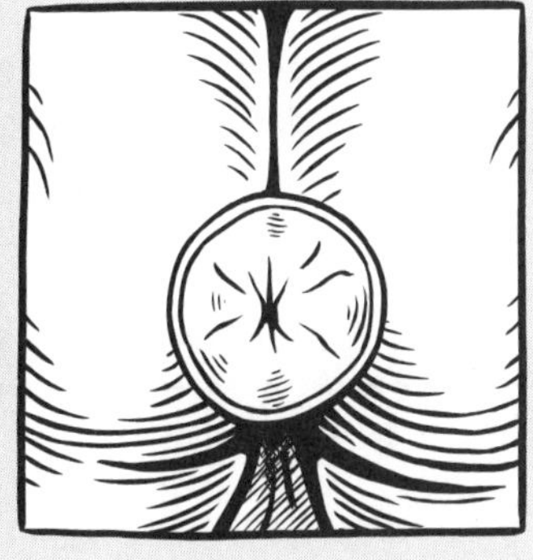

4. The wide opening of the pouch should stay outside, even after he puts his penis in.

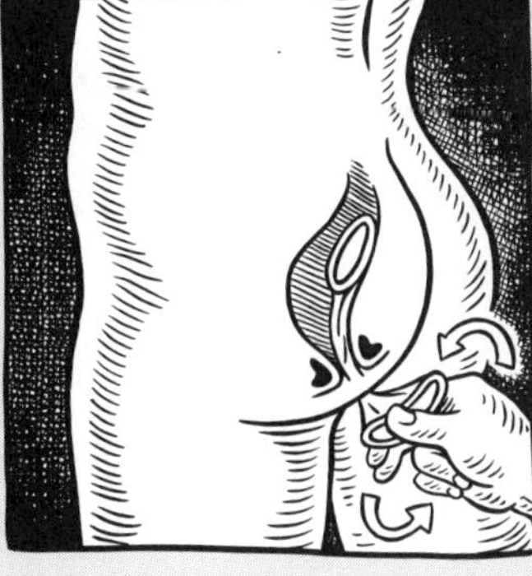

5. To remove, twist the outer part to trap the cum, pull it out gently and discard.

A little movement, from side to side or up and down, is common once his penis is in the sheath. If you or your partner notices that the outer ring is being pushed inside you, stop, pull it out, and add more lubricant. If he slips under or beside the sheath to get inside you, stop and have him put it in the sheath.

Condom slippage or breakage is more common than we like to admit. A number of studies of gay men estimate that as many as 17 to 25 percent of us have experienced it. The good news? Practice may not make perfect, but it sure does help. Among gay men in New York, one study found that those who used condoms for anal intercourse more than forty times a year had a breakage rate of only 0.4 percent, compared to the 15 percent breakage rate experienced by those who had anal sex with a condom only once a year.

If a condom does break on you (or in you), stop, wipe up, and get another. If it's at the time of or after ejaculation and you're on the bottom, stay calm—and don't douche. That will likely drive some of the semen farther inside you and abrade your rectum, says Bao.

TAKE A SHOT? HIV VACCINES AND YOU

If you live in New York, San Francisco, or forty or so other places around the country where gay men gather, you may have seen ads recruiting men at risk to test the efficacy of an HIV preventive vaccine. For gay men, researchers' definition of at risk usually starts with anyone who's HIV-negative, between the ages of 18–60, has had anal sex in the last year. The question is, do you want to take a shot?

The preventive HIV vaccines now being tested hope to work like other preventive vaccines, which inject a little bit of a harmful virus or bacterium into the body, and activates your body's defenses. Having learned to recognize and conquer a small amount of the virus, your body is ready to neutralize the invader even if a large amount gets inside you. At least that's the fantasy. The reality is that it will be many years before an effective vaccine is on the market. The vaccines being tested as we enter the new millennium are only a few of some 35 different vaccines now in some stage of testing, though they're the first to be tested for efficacy in humans.

Should you do it? If you're hoping to throw away the condoms, no. Any of the vaccines being tested for efficacy is not likely to give you HIV—they use only a piece of HIV or killed virus, rather than the live, whole kind, and have all been tested for safety first, in animals and people. Still, as of this writing there is no evidence that any vaccine will help protect you. Some could conceivably make it more easy for you to get infected if you were exposed to HIV. Similarly, if you're looking to get your name in the paper or be the subject of the television movie about the finding of THE VACCINE, sit it out. Many researchers, including those most optimistic about these current vaccines, think it will take many more than the studies now being done before we've found a vaccine powerful enough to stop the spread of AIDS.

If, on the other hand, you recognize that history is made up of small steps, that gay men have always led the way in HIV prevention and AIDS drug research, and that helping science in the long run helps many of the people most at risk, you should consider it. If we don't act in the short term to test possible vaccines, there won't be any long-term success. And experts are pretty unified in believing that a vaccine is the best shot we have at stopping the spread of HIV.

Though trials differ somewhat from vaccine to vaccine, there are a few things to think about if you are a volunteer on the verge.

FOUR POSSIBLE COSTS OF BEING PART OF VACCINE TRIALS:

- **You won't get HIV, but you may test positive for HIV on standard HIV tests.** With one vaccine, as many as 1/5 of participants may look as though they're positive on a standard test. Current vaccine trials advise participants to test only at the trial site to avoid confusion.
- **You may not get the vaccine at all.** Some participants get a "placebo," harmless injections. Neither you nor the staff at the trial site know whether you're getting the real thing.
- **You may suffer side effects, even serious ones, they don't know about yet.** Researchers have studied the effects of the vaccines in the short-term, and found them safe. Vaccines could have long-term side effects that are unknown.
- **You may get fooled into thinking you can take more risks sexually**. In some studies, people in HIV vaccine trials started taking more risks once they went into the trial. There is no evidence that vaccines offer enough protection to do without condoms. In fact, it's possible that the vaccine may even make it more likely that you'll get infected with HIV if you are exposed.

FOUR POSSIBLE BENEFITS OF BEING PART OF VACCINE TRIALS:

- **You get free, regular HIV testing**. Many trial sites offer you regular, routine HIV tests as often as every four to six months, as well as tests any other time you want, for as long as three years.
- **You get free, regular counseling on HIV prevention.** The staff at the trial site don't just inject you, they offer support.
- **You get a little cash**. It's an "incentive" to participate, not a way to pay the rent. Still, every little bit helps.
- **You help the world.** Without trials like these, and people willing to be in them, we'll never learn what we need to know to stop the spread of AIDS.

Finally, a few big-picture reminders. A vaccine is not a cure: even if it did work, many people with HIV would still get sick. And though vaccines are an incredibly powerful idea—the government and private industry are not the only ones drawn to the idea of being able to throw away the condoms and stop talking about embarrassing things like drug use or sex—technology, even if effective, is not enough. Don't let attention to the future promise of vaccines reduce our national—or your personal—investment in awareness of what you're doing here and now, and the consciousness-raising that is our real best shot at HIV prevention.

For more information about the issues surrounding vaccines and your participation, check out the Web site of the AIDS Vaccine Advocacy Coalition (AVAC), at www.avac.org.

HIV is not transmitted every time you have unprotected sex, though that may not be enough to relieve your anxiety. Various kinds of HIV tests (see Chapter 7) can tell you what's up, but you'll have to wait at least a few weeks or longer if you use the most common.

Another possibility now under evaluation for condom breakage situations is PEP, postexposure prophylaxis, a month-long course of anti-HIV drugs administered to HIV-negative men after condom breakage. It's also known as PET, postexposure treatment, though PEG—postexposure gamble—might be more appropriate (see "It Ain't Over Yet: A PEP Talk," page 73). If you think you may have been infected and want to consult your doctor about taking drugs, do so as soon as possible. Though standards have not yet been set up about when PEP is appropriate, after what kind of sex, for whom, or even whether it helps, experts suspect you have to do it within forty-eight hours for it to have any effect at all.

Beyond Condoms: Risk Reduction and You

I use a kind of Arabian strategy: left hand for things to do with the ass, and right hand for playing with everything else. And I keep track, like if I touch his nipple with that left hand, then I don't put it in my mouth.

I hook up with people online, and I search their profiles, right up front, for the words HIV-negative. And then we use a condom. Sure, it could break, but I'm more willing to play Russian roulette if all the shots are blanks.

First, I only eat out a butt that I know has been freshly showered. Clean as a whistle. Second, it may be fun to proceed from butt-licking to penetration with fingers, sex toys, or a cock. But once there has been any penetration, I don't go back to licking butt. Slipping a finger or anything else in the can will drag out traces of fecal matter you don't want to have in your mouth. Eating out is never a risk-free proposition. However, I've gotten food poisoning at least three times dining at restaurants, and I've never gotten sick from eating butt.

I only want to be with other guys who are positive. I don't want to deal with a negative guy's drama about sex, and I feel more relaxed.

I just don't have anal sex. I think that's why I survived. It was never that important to me anyway.

With every pleasure, risk. It's a concept we accept every day in our nonsexual lives. On one hand, with more than forty-one thousand fatal auto accidents each year, you have a chance of being crushed to death by two tons of metal each time you jump in the car. On the other, driving has tremendous benefits, getting you to work, home, to see friends or a movie. Some of us even enjoy it. The same can be said for living in cities or drinking alcohol, both of which have their own peculiar pleasures and dangers. The level of risk we find acceptable for an activity tends to depend on how useful it seems, how much we feel comfortable denying, and what we think we can get away with without hurting ourselves. It's why some of us cross against the traffic light, smoke, ski the advanced slope, or stick the Q-Tip all the way inside our ear even though the instructions tell us not to.

Sex—even if the instructions we've received are that we should never have it, or never have it if it carries the slightest risk of HIV—is a similar though more powerful proposition. Heterosexuals have made their peace with it: No one would ever suggest, for example, that women not have sex because of the risk of dying in childbirth. Gay men, too, even before AIDS, have had long practice weighing the importance of sex against its risks: risk of arrest, risk of going home with someone who may turn violent, risk of getting kicked out of your job, getting bashed in the park, or contracting a sexually transmitted disease. AIDS complicated the calculation terribly, not only because we could get sick and die from sex but because we could make other people sick. And gay men responded amazingly, going from a time when most of us had never even seen a condom unwrapped to a time when, according to recent studies, two-thirds of us use them most or all of the time for anal sex. It is a behavior change that health officials describe with words such as *unprecedented* and *historic*.

And yet sex and love and the ways they combine have proved powerful enough so that some of us—increasing numbers of us—have had occasions when we went ahead with sex without a condom. Some of us looked at the use-a-condom-every-time approach as a short-term solution, a detour; two decades later, we are trying to find our way back to a latex-free life the same way that people in Sarajevo or Beirut got used to the snipers and started going about their daily business. Often our strategies are long-term—deciding, for example, that we'll skip anal sex but risk oral sex with no cum, or that we'll trust a partner who's also HIV-negative to stay safe outside the relationship and fuck without condoms inside (see "Negotiated Safety," page 113). Other times the calculations are more off-the-cuff, with each man juggling a series of questions—"How much do I want sex tonight?" "How healthy does he look?" "Am I inserting or receiving?" "How will he react if I talk about condoms?" "What do we plan to do together?" "How should I respond now that things are going a little differently than I expected?"—with the focus of a mathematician solving a multivariable equation. Even when we don't know each other's HIV status, most of us manage to get home safely, stay out of jail, stay sexual with a lover, and have no virus pass between us. But too many of us miscalculate, or overload, and wind up infected or infecting others.

And he just turned around and backed onto my bare dick. It felt great for a moment, and then I thought about it and lost my erection. "What's wrong?" he said. I didn't know what to say, so I just started making him the center of attention.

Among young gay men, or men in gay urban centers, as many as half of men surveyed say they've had anal sex without a condom at least once in the past year. Look a little more closely—as GMHC did in a 1999 study of more than 7,000 gay and bisexual men in New York City—and it appears that much of that condomless sex occurs when men believe their partner's HIV status to be the same as their own. GMHC's study did find that 11 percent of gay and bi men reported having anal sex without condoms and with someone of unknown or different status in the past year. Why would men risk it? For every study or bar-stool psychologist who says unsafe sex is caused by self-destructiveness or lack of caring, there is another who claims it's about intimacy, love, or the desire to get past barriers. That may be less gay than it is human; research among heterosexual couples where one partner is infected, for example, shows that an estimated 80 percent don't always use condoms. Among gay men, studies say we don't use condoms because we're feeling optimistic, or because we're feeling low and need a lift. We do it to show our love and trust with a long-term partner, or because we're seeking new sensations with a new man. We do it because we mistakenly assume we have the same HIV status as the man with whom we're having sex, because we believe that on top means out of danger, or because we, just for right now, really don't want to have to think about it. We do it because we're already positive and feel like we have nothing to lose, because we've lived so long around AIDS that staying uninfected in the future doesn't seem important, or because we're so young that we can't really imagine a future. We do it because we're drunk or high and aren't thinking—or because we thought about it, decided that tonight we wanted to have no-holds-barred, special sex, and got drunk or high to help.

Different studies produce different general principles: that men are more likely to have unsafe sex when they've just gotten out of or into a relationship, for example, or that young men are more likely to have unsafe sex when they're feeling bad before the sex, whereas older men are more likely to do it when they're feeling good. If you're among the men who are struggling with safer sex, these rules may not work any better to keep you safe than the general principle that tells you to use a condom every time. What can work is looking honestly at the sex you're having, looking at the risks and the pleasures, and trying to come up with an increased consciousness of choices you didn't know you had.

Thinking Through Arousal

French photographer Henri Cartier-Bresson would study situations looking for what he called "the decisive moment." Sex can be made up of many such moments, though often things happen so silently, and so fast, that it's easy to feel as though you're watching the movie rather than acting a main part. "Too often, when men talk about unsafe sex, they say, 'It just happened,'" says GMHC's HIV prevention director, Richard Elovich. "Yes, it happened, but how?" Sexual arousal is a kind of altered state: Men at GMHC workshops often talk of feeling like what they do when they're turned on is almost outside of their ordinary selves (see box on next page). Researchers on other mind-altering behaviors, such as alcohol use, talk of what they call "SUDs"—seemingly unimportant decisions. You drive home alone from the party, for example, and decide to stop in for a drink at the bar, talk to a guy who's cute, have a few more, and somehow, the next thing you know, it's the next day and you're calling your best friend and freaking out because you swallowed someone's cum or let him put it in you for a few minutes.

I remember praying as I waited for my test results that if I could just be HIV-negative, then I'd never take those risks with Bob again. And then sure enough, a year later, I found myself waiting at the same clinic with the same prayer. It's like I live my life in yearlong cycles: test, pray, promise, hold out, fail, test, pray, promise, hold out, fail.

I fell in an AOL hole again last weekend—not even hooking up with people, but just flirting, answering messages, trying to line people up. It's like I'm a lab rat, pressing the bar over and over again, except that instead of a food pellet I only get the shock, some kind of jolt of electricity about the possibility that the next guy is going to be even more to my liking. By the end of the weekend, I felt wasted.

THE MIND/BODY PROBLEM?

My mind said I was going home, but my body was walking to the sex club.

I had seen his pill bottles in his medicine cabinet in the bathroom. I don't know why, but when I went back out, I still found myself lowering my mouth over his dick without a condom. Even as I was doing it, I was kind of thinking I didn't want to be doing it, but I did it anyway.

I let him do it, initially, and it was this new feeling of fucking and having no condom on. And then, afterward in my mind, it became about something else. Like, by doing it, am I influencing him to do this with other people? I'm negative, but does he know that? We talked about it a little afterward, and I said, "You know, you should never do that." "I know," he said, "and I have condoms. But you aren't positive, are you?" I said, "That's a stupid question to ask now. You should never, ever do that." A few days later, in the heat of things, we did it again.

It's an old Yiddish expression: When the prick gets hard, the mind goes soft. Some research has even suggested that brain function during certain kinds of sex, as in other intensely emotional or powerful moments, is actually physically distinct from other thought, using the most primitive, "reptilian" part of the brain (didn't you just know men were snakes?). Though biological processes are not sufficient to explain it, many gay men know the experience of doing things while turned on that they might not "want" to do when less aroused. "It's like there's the smart Bill and the dumb Bill, and the smart Bill is just watching the dumb Bill go at it without a condom," says one man.

Center for AIDS Prevention Studies researcher Rafael Diaz, Ph.D., cautions that in this case biology is not destiny, and that accepting the mind-penis split means giving up a whole range of options to protect yourself or your partner. In detailed interviews with a small group of men in San Francisco, Diaz identified that split between sex and the rest of one's feelings and thoughts as a powerful predictor of risky sexual behavior. He suggests a number of signals for what he calls the "trip to fantasy island" that is unsafe sex: feeling intense or painful emotions prior to the sexual encounter, use of drugs or alcohol to ease discomfort about the sexual behavior and facilitate the split, seeing your partner as more of a fantasy object than a man, and feeling nonetheless as though you yourself have little control over the sexual situation. Australian researcher Ron Gold, Ph.D., investigating what he calls the split between "on-line, off-line cognitions," has worked to explore the way our thinking about risk is different when we're caught up in the heat of the moment than when we're talking in the cold light of day. Giving men questionnaires or asking them to fill out sexual diary entries, he looked at the list of justifications they used to explain what their thinking "looked like" at the moment they decided not to use condoms: everything from "This guy seems so clean" to "This guy seems intelligent, so I'm sure he's been careful." Identifying the specific justifications, says Gold, may be less important than becoming aware of their existence, recognizing the thinking that may be operating when we decide to have unsafe sex.

Stewing in sexual anxiety, or swearing you won't do what caused it again—until you do—is a more common pattern than most of us like to admit. An alternative, if the never-again approach doesn't seem to be working, is to start with smaller changes. Begin by looking at what you're doing—not to judge it, rationalize it, or "get to the bottom" of how you could have done it, but to be more conscious of the seemingly unimportant decisions that lead up to the result. Spare yourself the "How could I be such a slut?" "Why did I believe love was worth this?" or the "Why am I so weak?" kinds of questions. Instead, take some time to see where you feel good about your sexual behavior and where you don't.

Try This at Home

Compare two different sexual interactions: one where you felt good about the sex, and one that felt risky or worried you. (If you're never worried, great—just think about the good experiences.) In each instance, try to go back to the experience and lead yourself—or better yet, someone else—through the details. "It sounds contrived, but telling it to a friend can help you hear it in a way that's hard to do by yourself," says GMHC's Elovich. Find someone to listen, he suggests, "who isn't going to reassure you, or judge you, or try to 'fix' the situation. You want them just to help you get through the story, the way someone would spot you while lifting weights at the gym." If you don't have anyone you feel comfortable with, see if a local AIDS organization offers any kind of HIV-prevention support groups. If you can't or aren't comfortable doing that, write yourself a detailed diary entry.

START WITH THE POSITIVE

In both instances—including the one that didn't work out great—start with the positive. Focus on what you wanted that day or night. What you were looking for? Bring yourself back, not just to the moment, but to the lead-up. What was attractive about the situation? Whom was it with? What drew you to him or them?

Play with yourself—not literally, but in the telling. It can be vivid, not just dreary. What was the sex like? What were you thinking or feeling as it progressed? Avoid the generalities—"It was hot," "It felt so good"—in favor of vivid specifics. And it's not vivid enough to say "I loved sucking him." What exactly did you like so much about it? The feeling of making him come? Feeling as though you "had him"? Feeling romantically merged? Taken over?

Bernie Zilbergeld, Ph.D., whose *New Male Sexuality* (Bantam Doubleday Dell, 1999) is often cited as one of the most comprehensive guides to the male psyche, sex, and the intersection of the two, writes of what he calls "conditions" for good sex. In his work with straight men—his book, though excellent, is not quite "new" enough to include gay men—these range from not being too drunk or tired to more detailed emotional states such as feeling safe or feeling as though your partner is not going to make fun of you. Some of these—not being too tired, for example—may seem universal, though any of us who's ever found himself going home with someone five hours and seven drinks too late has certainly ignored it. Others are highly personal: a voice, a feeling. Try to figure out what your "conditions" for good sex are. How do they relate to your fantasies? Your feelings about the other person?

TRY TO SPELL OUT THE RISKS

These may be less evident in the situation that you felt good about, though next to the risky or worrisome situation, the comparison may be revealing. What was it that made you worried? Was it related to the sex itself or to something else: the time and energy or money it took to get it, for example, or what it revealed about your relationship? Were you worried from the start, did you become concerned only afterward, or was there some point in between where things went from comfortable to not? Would it have changed if you had known the other person's HIV status? Or was the issue that you knew it? Did your discomfort have to do with what was going on inside your head, or the feelings of your body?

HOW MIGHT YOU HOLD ON TO THE POSITIVE FEELINGS AND CUT DOWN ON THE RISKS?

Return once more to the progression of events. If you had stayed on the phone sex line for half an hour instead of four hours, would that have worked better? If you had felt less used, more like he knew you better, would that have helped? If it was a risky encounter for HIV, how might you have held on to the pleasure and reduced the risks? If, for example, you loved sucking him but freaked out when he came in your mouth, could you have said, "Pull out before you come, okay?" as you started? If you were afraid that stopping for a condom would make you lose your hard-on, might you have asked him to put one on you? If you like to be with "straight" guys but worry that they'll pull off the condom, could you have only oral sex with them until you know if you can trust them to watch out for you?

Those changes may sound small. But small steps can still be steps toward sex that keeps you safer or more satisfied. Even talking about the sex you have in front of someone else can be a step. "It's about bringing things to consciousness," says Elovich, "making the internal external and then allowing yourself to internalize it again."

Risk in Context

Sex isn't like flying in an airplane, where everyone on board has basically the same risk of survival. In sex, risks are contextual, not categorical, depending upon who you are, where you are, whom you're with, and what you think of as a problem. If you're not out at work, being seen by someone you know at a rest stop may be more serious than if everyone already knows you're gay. If you're supposed to be monogamous, getting an STD from someone you played around with may be a lot more serious than if you're a man about town. If you're both HIV-negative, there aren't really any sex acts risky for HIV. Rules about risk are personal: Some positive men, for example, in spite of the risk of reinfection, decide that they'll take the chance of cum in their mouths but not in their asses. Others go further, or less far, with "harm reduction": choosing to be on top without condoms during anal sex but not on the bottom, sharply limiting the number of partners with whom they don't use condoms, or deciding they'll allow someone to put his penis inside them so long as he doesn't come. The same is true for men without HIV, who choose different levels of risk according to their comfort level. Risk elimination—deciding not to do something at all—is easiest when the thing you're giving up is not important to you.

A growing number of media stories have focused on "bugchasers" or "barebackers," men who go as far as to claim that they consciously choose to fuck without condoms and don't care about preventing infections in themselves or others. There may be a few men who fuck indiscriminately without regard to getting infected or infecting, though research suggests they may be rarer in reality than in magazine stories. Only 2 percent of the more than 7,000 men in GMHC's 1999 study were positive and had anal intercourse with someone of unknown or different HIV status at all in the course of a year. Far fewer still did that with multiple partners. In GMHC workshops, men who begin by saying they "don't care whether they get infected," or that "it's the other guy's problem if he doesn't protect himself," often find their confidence in those statements eroding once they get deeper than the sound bite.

Many more of us are conflicted, at once wanting to have a good time free from HIV and feeling bound by a deep sense—by turns clear or cloudy—of caring for ourselves and others. It's something less talked about than how to put on a condom: how many of us want an opportunity to forget about the virus, and how we have to balance that over and over against the need to protect ourselves and others from infection.

Most important of all sex acts and facts is that most sex happens with another person. Whatever pledges you take or resolutions you make about your sex and safety, they will be tested—and confounded or confirmed—by the communication between your body and another. For more on that, read the next chapter.

Free at Last? Fourteen Random Places You Can Go to Find Your Way Toward Sexual Liberation

For the Bisexual at Heart
Anything that Moves
Mark Silver
2404 California Street #24
San Francisco, CA 94115
(415) 703-7977x2
qswitch@igc.apc.org

For the Disabled, and the People Who Love Them
The Disability Rag
PO Box 145
Louisville, KY 40201
(502) 894-9492

Come on In, the Water's Fine
Fraternity of Enema Buddies
Frank Ball
2421 West Pratt Boulevard, #1116
Chicago, IL 60645
(312) 561-7188

For Trannies and Their Admirers
The Transsexual News Telegraph
41 Sutter Street #1124
San Francisco, CA 94104

For Daddies, Boys, and Other Pain Pigs
Gay Male S/M Activists
332 Bleecker Street, #D23
New York, NY 10014
212-727-9878
www.gmsma.org

For the Nonmonogamist in Us All
Abundant Love Institute (ALI)
Deborah Anapol
PO Box 4322-BB
San Rafael, CA 94913
(415) 507-2739
pad@well.com

For Those Who Love with Body and Soul
EroSpirit Research Institute
PO Box 3893
Oakland, CA 94609
(510) 428-9063
www.erospirit.org

For Long-Hair Lovers
BROS (Brotherhood of Long-haired Men)
PO Box 17931
Rochester, NY 14617

Needles and Syringes and Scalpels, Oh My!
Epidermal Intrusions
Carla Love
PO Box 6430
Phoenix, AZ 85005-6430
(602) 272-1483

If Toes Make You Tipsy
National Foot Network
John or Tim
PO Box 150790
Brooklyn, NY 11215-0790
(718) 832-3952

For the Tiny-Tooled and Small in Stature
Small Etc.
J. Meisler
PO Box 610294
Bayside, NY 11361

Fisting Anyone?
Red Hankies of San Diego
Bill Freyer
PO Box 3988
San Diego, CA 92163
(619) 688-8668

For Older Men and Their Admirers
Prime Timers International
Woody Baldwin
PO Box 436
Manchaca, TX 78652-0436
(512) 282-2861

For Cigar Lovers
Hot Ash
Tony Shenton
PO Box 20147, London Terrace Station
New York, NY 10011-0002
(718) 789-6147

FURTHER READING

Condom Resource Center. (1994) "Condom Educator's Guide" (pamphlet). Oakland, CA: Condom Resource Center. Every detail of condom variety and application.

Dodson, Betty. (1996) *Sex for One: The Joy of Self-Loving*. New York: Crown Publishers. Masturbatory hints from a seasoned sexpert.

Michael, Robert T., et al. (1994) *Sex in America: A Definitive Survey*. New York: Warner Books. Among the most scientifically rigorous and carefully constructed of American sex surveys, though the authors themselves admit they didn't get a lot of good gay data.

Rotello, Gabriel, and Evan Wolfson. (1993) "The Little Black Book" (pamphlet). New York: Lambda Legal Defense and Education Fund. A short, smart guide to legal issues for any man who's ever been arrested for public sex or worried about the possibility.

Rubin, Gayle. (1989) "Thinking Sex." In Carol Vance (ed.), *Pleasure and Danger*. London: Pandora Books, pp. 267–320. Perhaps *the* essay to read about sex, ethics, pleasure, and society.

Sanderson, Terry. (1994) *A to Z of Gay Sex: An Erotic Alphabet*. London: Other Way Press. Like the title says.

Silverstein, Charles, and Felice Picano. (1992) *The New Joy of Gay Sex*. New York: HarperPerennial. The groundbreaking encyclopedic guide to gay sex, from "anus" to "wrestling."

Spencer, Colin. (1996) *The Gay Kama Sutra*. New York: St. Martin's Press. A beautifully illustrated, modern gay reworking of the Indian classic, offering hints on how to help him (and yourself) find ecstasy.

CHAPTER 3

Two to Tango: Cruising, Coupling, and Communication

Open Wide and Say "Uh . . ." • Hallmarks of Arousal • Pillow Talk • Saying No Nice • When No Means No: Rape • Special Channels of Communication • S/M • Tao and Tantra • Negotiated Safety • Talking HIV • Boyfriend Basics • Sex Life Versus the Rest of Your Life? • Sex and a Long-Term Partner • Monogamy?

Gay men talk a lot about sex, but what *don't* we say? While we may ogle the waiter or boast about how that gorgeous man did us three ways to Wednesday, when it comes to our emotions—the rush of thoughts we get just before we're about to kiss for the first time, the feelings we get when someone sidles up next to us (or slides up inside us), or how it was that we let him do that without a condom—we get quieter. Often gay sex talk can sound like sports reports: full of great details about how high or how hard or how big or how fast or how many times. Less racy declarations about the sexual mysteries—Why do I find it easier to have sex in the park than with my lover? Why do I lose my hard-on when I put on a condom? Why am I so excited to be going home with this man whose partner I know?—we tend to keep to ourselves.

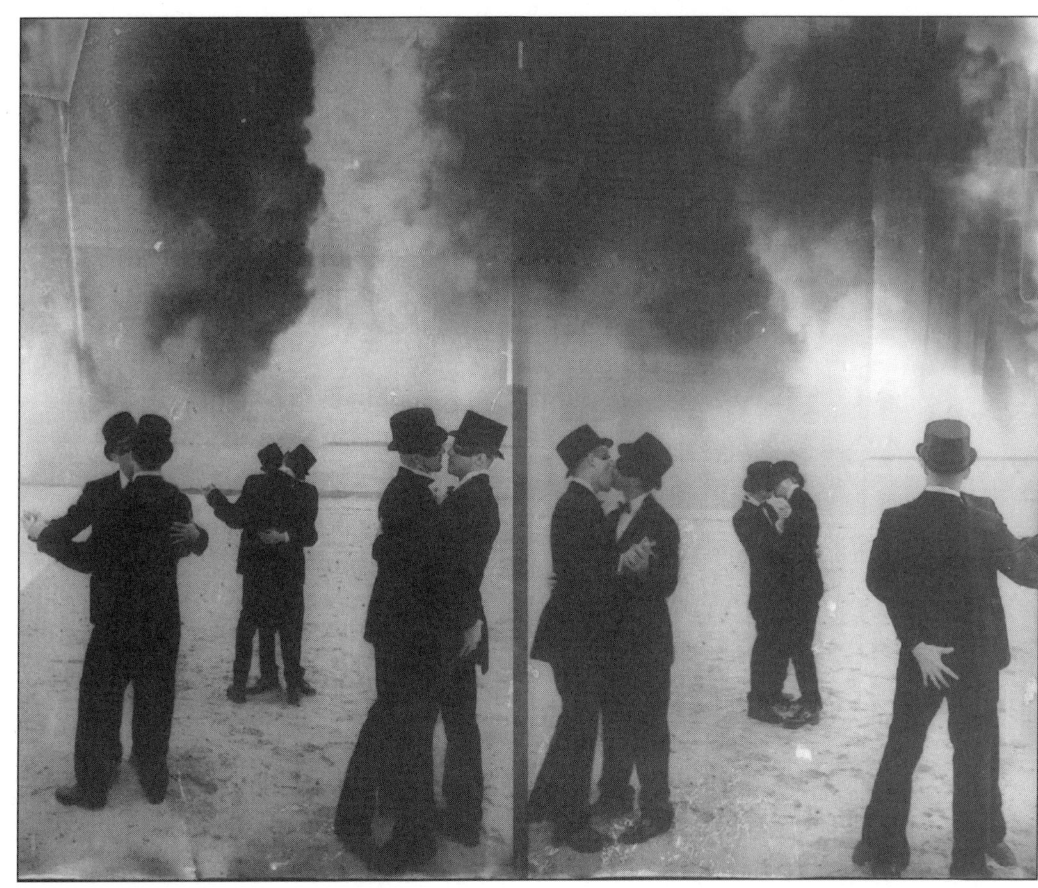

Sex can be about athleticism, or recreation, or total number of orgasms logged. Sex can also be about love, an antidote to hatred, indifference, or isolation. It can be about great adventures—

the way we get lost in each other's eyes or sweep into each other's lives—and great escapes. It can be about reaffirming our commitments and connection, getting attention or affection, or expressing things we don't have other ways of voicing. "When I'm having sex, it's like a different part of myself is singing," says Roy, forty-five, a performer from New Jersey. Even when we work to avoid the emotional content—when we turn away from each other in bed, or turn ourselves (or him) into a hungry hole—there are plenty of emotions present. Because no matter how (or where) you put it, no matter how much it may seem like going to the gym or cracking your knuckles, sex involves one or more other people, human beings with different needs and wants and ways of trying to meet them.

Project SIGMA, an English group doing extensive research on gay sexuality and HIV prevention, has suggested that researchers, and the rest of us, might do well to reframe our approach to sex. Instead of focusing on what the individual does, propose Peter Davies and his coauthors in *Sex, Gay Men and AIDS* (Falmer Press, 1993), think of sex as a conversation. Like conversations, sex changes according to whom you're having it with, where you're having it, and how you're feeling. Some sex, like some conversation, is forceful, some mild; some is cold and some is warm; some is pleasant, some exuberant. Some is conflicted—unsafe sex you have even as you're worrying about why you shouldn't, for example, might in Project SIGMA's formulation be thought of as an argument. Just as there are suckers for argument, or people who are argumentative, there are some who may find themselves actively engaged in sex that's full of that kind of conflict. Others of us find ourselves drawn in almost by accident, or manage in the course of the exchange to find ways to defuse or avoid the argument.

Unlike conversations, though, most sexual communication is nonverbal. Long-term lovers may work their way through discussions about sex, and a few exceptionally gifted dirty talkers may find ways of articulating their true desires amid the stream of common commands. Virtual sex—phone and cyber—relies heavily on the spoken or written word, at least for the parts that precede meeting in more tangible forms. Once you're there in the flesh, however, sexual expression is more often achieved by pulls and pushes, moans, looks, and the intersection of private, half-conscious fantasies.

Therein lie the complications, since even the most expressive groan can leave things open to interpretation. There's chemistry, the lucky moments when everything fits and clicks and he and you both seem magically to understand what pleasure means. In the long run, though, and often in the shortest of them, most of us need communication. "There's absolutely no way that anyone else is going to know what stroke or tickle you need," says *New Joy of Gay Sex* author Charles Silverstein, Ph.D., "unless you find some way to tell them."

Open Wide and Say "Uh . . ."

Gordon is from the school that says you shouldn't need to express it. But I need an "ahhh" or an "ohhh" or something. Sex doesn't follow the golden rule that what you like is what he likes.

I went home with somebody who was into underarms. I'm sixty-two years old, I've had a lot of sex, and I've never paid attention to my underarm. He was a master at it; he knew what he wanted. And it worked for me. If that gentleman sleeps with me again, you can be sure I'll take his head and guide it to my armpit.

I try to give as much positive affirmation as I can. I say, "Remember when you did that? I loved that." He doesn't say anything right away, because he doesn't want to let on that he's taking advice. And he's too clever to do it again right away. But a few weeks later, I notice that he's heard me.

Sometimes I can't stop talking, especially if I'm feeling uncomfortable. But after I've gotten to know a person, I might just get up on the bed in a frog stand, upside down, with my greedy butt spread.

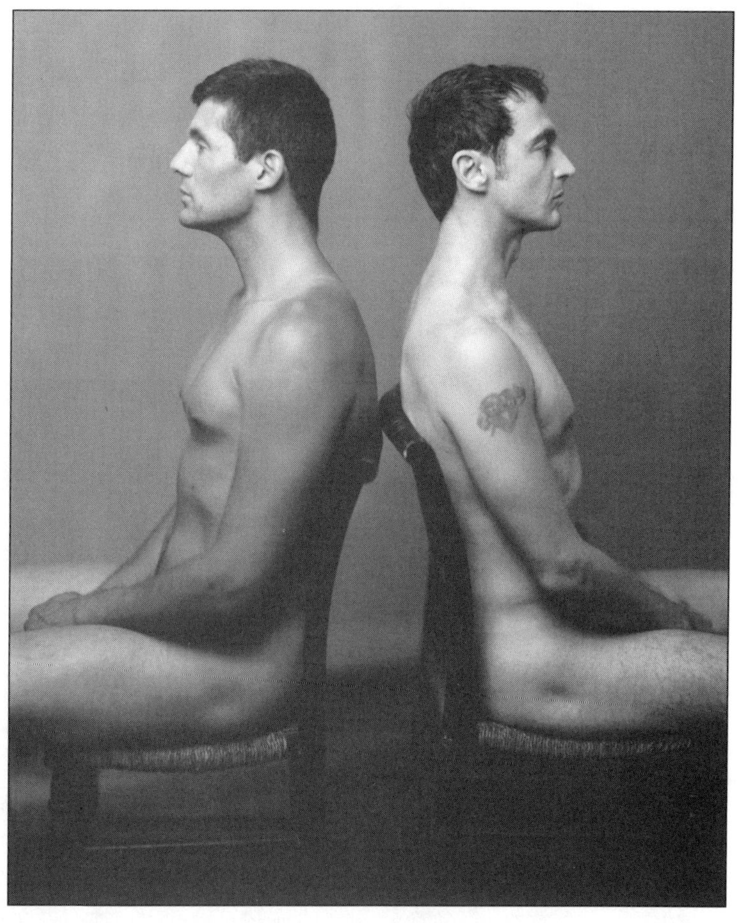

I think people asking for what they want is attractive—to say "I need to be tied up tonight" or "I will not fuck you without a condom, forget it" is hot because it's willful, not passive.

The eye contact–smile–let's screw scenario doesn't give me time to get comfortable with another person, no matter how good-looking he is. I think it comes down to trust. I need to trust a sexual partner at some level, and that doesn't happen without conversation. It might be minimal, but it's almost always there.

Even if the acts themselves are all the same, what we want in sex often depends on whom we want it from. What do you imagine doing with that drop-dead-handsome man who's the center of attention at the bar and pays you little mind himself? How about with your long-term boyfriend, who may know both your favorite pleasure points and all the weak points in your character? Think back on the different "moods" of sex you've had throughout your life: the sex after a first date, after a fight, before you leave for work, or in a drunken haze late at night. How has your mood changed the "conversation" between your body and someone else's? Where have you found the line between raw heat and something painful? Between comforting and completely boring? Are you listening to his body or tuning out the feedback that might let you know the way to something deeper or new?

Often fear of upsetting that apple cart may keep us from communicating anything at all. "The message I get is that good gay men know what they're doing in sex already," says Jim, sixty-eight, a Utah native now exploring sex with men after forty-five years of marriage to a woman. "If you have to ask, you need more practice." Ruben, forty-five, has been with his partner for twenty years, but says he too stays silent: "After so many years of having sex the same way, John would see it as an attack." Others say they wish their sex partners worried more about offending. "I was with a guy—actually inside him—when he answered his cordless phone and asked somebody else to come over and have sex with him," recalls Lawrence, thirty-seven, a New Jersey photographer. "Of course I couldn't help but stay around to see who it was. Later I regretted the whole thing."

Hallmarks of Arousal: What Turns You On?

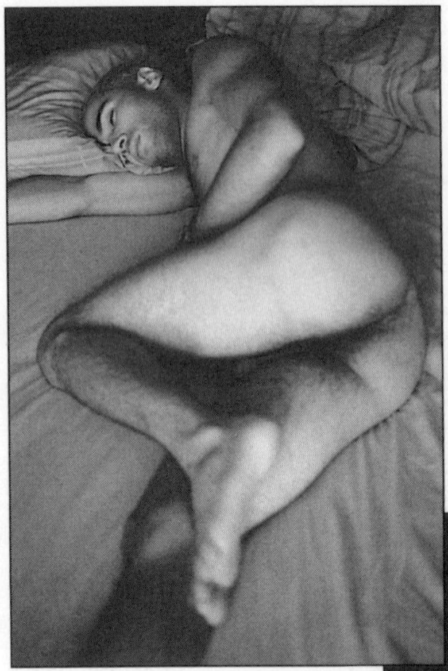

One thing that makes sex special, says Jack Morin, Ph.D., is that pleasure and displeasure are so closely linked. While many sex therapists go for a neat and tidy approach to sex, trying to find ways to eliminate anxiety or guilt, Dr. Morin has worked to tease apart the ways in which conflict—in the right doses—plays a role in sexual satisfaction. His book *The Erotic Mind* (HarperPerennial, 1996) discusses his survey of hundreds of people, including many gay and bisexual men, about their peak erotic experiences and central erotic themes. While widely varying, says Dr. Morin, these suggest what he calls the "four cornerstones of eroticism."

Longing and Anticipation

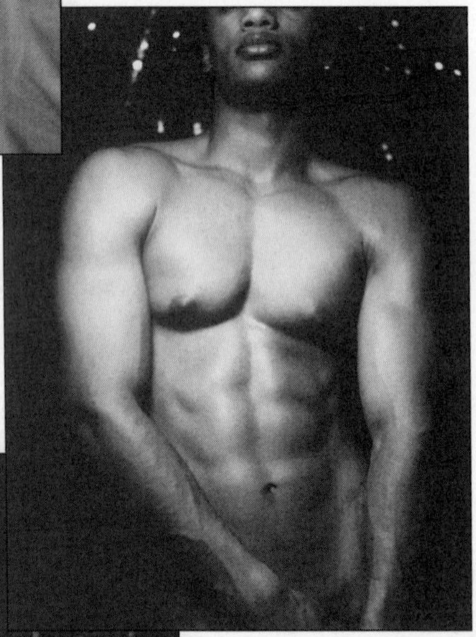

Think of the boy you lusted passionately over but never quite found a way to touch in high school. Or the way your lover's two-week trip makes you miss him in ways that don't happen ordinarily. Longing can be immediate, such as the frenzy you feel building up inside you as someone teases you and then stops short of your orgasm, or part of the thrill that comes as you pursue someone you aren't sure you can ever have. It can even be the way that our memory of being without a boyfriend years ago makes us grateful to receive the affections of our long-term lover today.

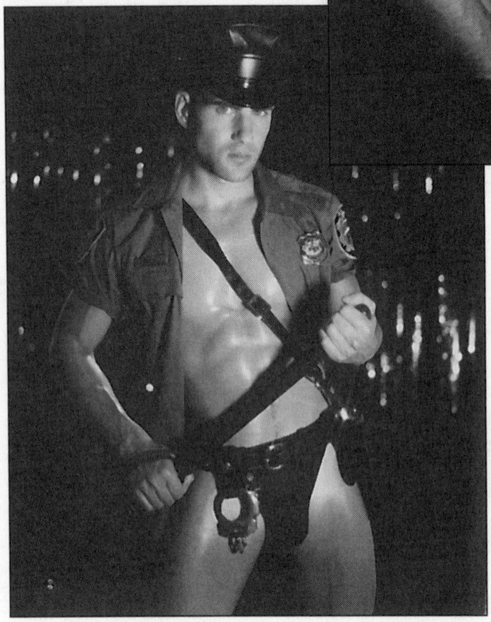

Violating Prohibitions

This is one reason why it may feel naughty and nice to steal a kiss from someone else's boyfriend or have quick sex in the steam room while a gym manager or unsuspecting straight men linger outside. Or why, in some cases, going without a condom, even when you know about safer sex, can seem like an act of erotic affirmation.

Searching for Power

It's not just about S/M fantasies or experiences, though those would fall into this category. Power—and the desire to give it up—are present in everyone's sexual experiences. Is the top serving the bottom's need for pleasure, or is it the other way around? Is the young, hot man serving the older, richer, less physically stunning one? How can you tell?

Overcoming Ambivalence

It's an old story: You're attracted to someone even as something about him seems repellent. He takes you home, the sex is every bit as brutish as you'd imagined, and you leave feeling both turned on and repulsed. Later, though, recalling the scene, it seems erotic, and you can't wait to see him again. Or perhaps it's another scenario of ambivalence undone: your long-term partner asking you to rim him after years of resistance, or appearing, naked under his coat, at your office.

Boiled down like this, these individual cornerstones may seem deceptively simple. Dr. Morin's book goes into greater depth, identifying the way that several of these themes can work together. But the basic principle—that the same things that turn you off can, in smaller doses, help turn you on—is important to understanding how complicated sexual dynamics often are. Entwined around each of Morin's cornerstones are what might be called the anti-aphrodisiacs: anxiety (that you won't get what you want, or that he'll make you sick), guilt (that you've been "bad"), and anger (that you have to fight for power). It's the process of both experiencing and overcoming those feelings, Morin suggests, that gives a sexual interaction its erotic force. Lose them by feeling too safe (or too sure you're wanted, or too powerful), and you lose some of the charge.

Pillow Talk: Ten Ways to Hear Him (and Yourself) in Bed

Just as with conversation, styles differ. But if you want to work toward mutual sexual understanding, there are ways to do it nicely. Below find suggestions for sexual etiquette from gay therapists and an amateur Mr. Manners or two.

Five Beyond Words

1. *Be there.* Otherwise known as dance with the one who brung you. Whether you're at dinner with a date or under the covers with your long-term partner, try to be present. "Cruising is a fact of life," says Shelby, thirty-two, a Jacksonville arts administrator, "but when your date starts looking into his butter knife to see who's behind him, something's wrong." In sex, being present means listening to your body rather than the inner voices saying how late it is or that you could have gone home with someone hotter or how he forgot to pick up the dry cleaning. If it's early in your relationship—even if it's going to be a one-night-long relationship—see how it goes before deciding it's right or wrong or that you'll never be married. If you are married, or close, you may be thinking about how he bullied you at dinner or how you really need to re-grout the bathtub. Let that go. Focus on sensations.

2. *Hold the phone.* And the beeper. And the cell phone. This is really a subset of #1. No matter who you are or how long you've been together, you really should think before you answer the phone during sex. And turn down the answering machine. Listening to your best

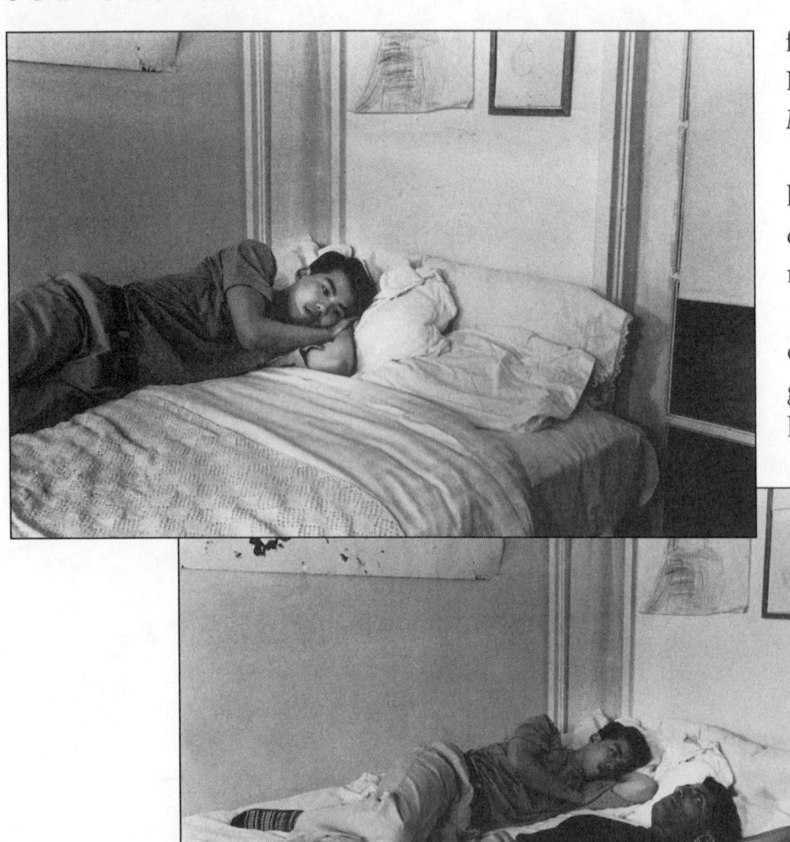

friend go on about how much she and Orville Redenbacher enjoyed that late-night rerun of *Mahogany* never did much for a sexy moment.

3. *Actions can speak louder.* Moving his hand gently up or down, adjusting your hips, or spreading your lips can sometimes say more than a mouthful of words.

4. *Moan—but mean it.* A gasp or moan can tell a lot about the right touch (or a caress gone wrong). If he's making you feel good, let him know it. If he's wearing the last shred of skin off your penis, let him know that, too. Mock moans and pseudo-sighs confuse the situation, particularly when he repeats the same touch or tickle over and over thinking you like it.

5. *Come and gone?* No matter how long you've been married or how much you know you don't want to be, it's not over after your orgasm. He may be fine with sleep instead of orgasm, or with a service-only arrangement. But have you checked?

Five Talking Points

Everyone feels vulnerable about sexual techniques and performance. If you're going to open your mouth—for whatever sexual purpose—do it with care.

1. *Be direct but not accusing.* If you know you want something, ask for it as simply and clearly as you can. "'I've told you a hundred times' may be meaningless if you've been ambiguous," advises Dr. Silverstein. "And no matter how you're feeling, avoid accusations, harsh criticisms, or guilt trips. They're more likely to make him defensive than responsive."

2. *Stay flexible.* "If it's not endangering your safety, or his, why not try it?" says Silverstein. "Deciding in advance what you don't want cuts out a lot of pleasure."

3. *Feedback.* If something feels good, make sure he knows it. If you're trying to give him pleasure, find a comfortable way for him to let you know what feels good. "Touching him in a couple of different ways and asking which feels best will tell you more than vague questions like 'What turns you on?'" says Dr. Morin.

4. *Talk about the bad and the good.* Rather than driving him crazy—in a bad way—with your special tongue flick, or silently suffering through his body odor, leave yourselves room to talk about how things could be better. Choose the right time. In the middle of sex may not be the best moment for criticism, says New York City therapist Michael Shernoff, MSW, since people feel vulnerable already.

5. *Patience and moderation.* In general, showering commands on someone—faster, harder,

stop, start, softer, wetter, softer, harder, stop—is not sharing, it's stifling. Ask, say many couples, and you shall receive—but not necessarily right now. "I find that talking with my partner introduces a temporary awkwardness," says fifty-year-old Craig, a writer. "It may take a while before you get back to working by instinct again."

Saying No Nice

Dogs 2 Men

Sometimes Don will say, "Do you mind if I just hold you while you jerk off tonight?" I appreciate that. There's a world of difference between that and just pushing me away or falling asleep.

I went into this cubicle with this man who I just knew would never talk to me if it wasn't for sex. I mean, we're talking White, perfect body, all that. And he said, "Sorry, I'm not into it." So I said, "Oh, I'm sorry." And he said, "What are you sorry about? I just don't want to have sex with you." I really appreciated that. I learned something from him about how I like to be treated, and about how other people can be treated, that stayed with me.

You know that moment when you find out the guy on the other end of the phone line is a bottom, too? When he says, "Good luck, guy," as he moves on to the next? I value that instant of politeness.

Strategies to bow out when sex isn't working can be as varied as those to get into it in the first place. But many a man has found himself traumatized when someone unceremoniously zips up, walks out, rolls over, or rings off. Acting civilized, on the other hand, lets you leave, and leave him, feeling good.

Are you a dog who doesn't want a bone, or a man with a heart? The golden rule—treat others as you'd like to be treated—may not work for having sex, but it should for skipping it. Below, what makes the difference between the animal and the human.

Phone or Cyber Sex

Bottom line: Quick turnover is par for the course. That's why technology has offered us anonymity, the option to press the pound sign to move on and the ability to "instant-message" ten people at once.

Bad dog #1: Beep off without a word when the man is midfantasy, describing what he'd like to do with you. Is it your problem he believed you when you said you were a six-foot-two hairless top with ten inches?

Bad dog #2: Don't tell him when you recognize him from his picture or screen name—just tell all your mutual friends.

Human minimum: Muster at least a cursory "Sorry, I've got to go" to anyone you've spent more than a minute or one instant message on. And if you don't tell him you know him, don't tell others, either.

Postscript: The supply of men in virtual sex, and the hope that you'll make one more, hotter connection, is inexhaustible. You are not. Stop when you start getting tired, or mean.

Hooking Up After Phone, Online, or Personal Ad Introduction

Bottom line: In person is worth a thousand words and quite a few digital pictures, so often it doesn't fly. You don't need to fake a cramp in your foot or a long story about how you locked your cat in the closet. It'll only make it more awkward when you see each other online ten minutes later.

Bad dog #1: You walk in, decline to sit down, and say, "Swimmer's body? I don't think so."

Bad dog #2: You walk by the coffee shop, see your man waiting, as agreed, and keep on walking.

Human minimum: Spend a minute in conversation. If it's not happening, explain politely that you're sorry it's not going to work and excuse yourself.

Postscript: If you're going to meet in person, the truth, or something very close, will out. Describing yourself unrealistically, or leaving out a major detail of your physical appearance, is a setup for both of you.

In a Sex Club or Bathhouse

Bottom line: Lots of men and little time make Jack—and John and Jeff and Jerome—fickle boys. But we're still human. Gently removing a hand is different from flinging it off your body and scowling. Once things are started, if you want out . . .

Bad dog #1: Drop his dick, turn on your heel, and walk off in search of greener pastures.

Bad dog #2: Stare in silence at the wall, ignoring the man at the door of your cubicle looking interested.

Human minimum: Decline aloud. "I need to take a rest" or "I need to take a break" seem to get high marks.

Postscript: If you've had one great experience in a visit, it's okay to stop. Really.

With a "New Friend" at Home

Bottom line: Home is where the heart is. If he's invited you inside, show a little tact.

Bad dog #1: You stand up, say "Actually, I'm tired," and exit.

Bad dog #2: You make up a long story about how you haven't done this so much before and you're really nervous and you don't think you can go through with it after all. (This is "good dog" behavior. You'll both still feel bad later.)

Human minimum: You say, "I'm sorry, I'm pretty tired, would it be okay if we didn't have sex tonight?" Then you stand up. Or say, if you mean it, "I'm sorry, I'm feeling really tired, can we just sleep?" Or you hold or kiss him while he brings himself to orgasm, and say sweetly, "I'm sorry, I'm really tired." Or . . . you get the picture.

Postscript: Afterward, don't ask for his number if you don't intend to call. "I don't mind if it's not going anywhere," says George, thirty-six, a magazine editor. "But I feel embarrassed later if he acts all enthusiastic and then I never hear from him again."

With a Long-Term Partner, at Home

Bottom line: Sex isn't as fresh for him as it was in those early days, either. Be merciful.

Bad dog #1: You say "Don't!" and press the volume button on the remote.

Bad dog #2: You lie there limply, waiting for it to be over.

Human minimum: You say, "I'm not feeling so sexy tonight," and snuggle up to him. Or see "With a 'New Friend' at Home," above.

Postscript: If the same thing happens ten times in a row, or if you both simply stop asking, see "Relight My Fire," page 130.

When No Means No: Rape

After he left I took a long shower, standing under the water and crying. The smell of him was on my body, his semen was between my legs and I washed with soap over and over, lathering and rinsing continuously. . . . I did not seek counseling or formal support, nor did I confide in any of my friends for several years. I was ashamed and embarrassed by what had happened, identifying the experience as a form of bad, regretted sex.

Those are the words of Michael Scarce, rape survivor and author of the book *Male on Male Rape* (Insight Books, 1997). They, or something uncomfortably like them, could be the words of many more of us. Though rarely discussed beyond the occasional prison joke or frat fantasy, male-male rape—penetration of a man's mouth or anus, with a penis or any other object, against his will—is a silent reality. A full 5 to 10 percent of assaults reported at rape crisis centers are male-male. A number of studies of gay men have found that a staggering 29 to 40 percent of us report being forced into sex at some point in our lifetime.

Where bad sex turns into rape can be a cloudy issue, particularly for the many of us

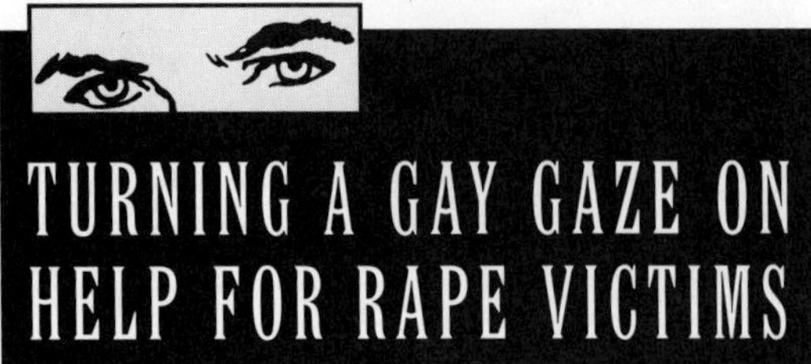

TURNING A GAY GAZE ON HELP FOR RAPE VICTIMS

When it comes to the law, gay rape victims' reluctance to seek help has just cause. Laws on male-male rape are inconsistent, varying from state to state. Some states fail to distinguish male-male rape from sodomy between consenting adults. In Idaho, consenting gay sex carries a minimum penalty of five years, while male rape gets only one. "The modern legal protections for female rape victims—such as rape shield statutes that prevent a survivor from being questioned about past sexual history—often do not apply to male victims of sexual assaults," says Bill Rubenstein, J.D., a law professor at the University of California, Los Angeles. "And the fact that sodomy laws are on the books in some sixteen states means some gay rape survivors face not only the fear of being disbelieved, but the possibility of being charged with a crime themselves once they are."

If you have been raped, though, seek help. Among the places to turn:

- ***The emergency room.*** If possible, find a hospital with a rape advocacy center that pairs survivors of sexual assaults with advocates who can lead you through the process of being examined or treated. "As much as you'll want to take a shower to get rid of the smell, taste, and memory of your attacker," says Scarce, "it's best not to brush your teeth, eat, drink, shower, pee, move your bowels, or change your clothes before your exam." Saliva, hair, and semen can all help identify your attacker. Bring an extra set of clothes—they may take yours as evidence, and the replacements they have on hand are sometimes available only in women's sizes and styles. If your assailant has ejaculated inside your mouth or anus, make sure the hospital takes samples of semen from those places. In addition, they usually offer you treatment to prevent STDs like gonorrhea and syphilis, and may also suggest PEP, postexposure prophylaxis for HIV (see chart on page 73), if you are HIV-negative. Finally, suggests Scarce, they should perform a colposcopy to look for trauma to the anus and rectum. The illumination and magnification provided by the colposcope can provide better and more detailed evidence of rectal trauma than the anoscope usually used for anal exams. This will provide crucial evidence if you decide to press charges.
- ***The police.*** It is up to you and the local district attorney whether you decide to try to prosecute; the police get the name of every sexual assault victim who receives treatment at a hospital, but no further information. Even if you know you don't want to prosecute, filing a police report may be necessary to get state help in paying for medical treatment or follow-up counseling. Most hospitals should put you in a private area for treatment and questioning, and give you a choice of a man or a woman to talk to. If you don't have the privacy you need, if authorities seem to suggest that you in any way "asked for it," or even if you're just feeling overwhelmed, ask if you can come down to the station or talk to a detective at your home the following day.
- ***A rape crisis center.*** Don't be put off by an unfriendly voice on the other end—since most men calling such centers do so to harass or ridicule the staff, counselors are often suspicious. Scarce, who coordinated a rape crisis center at Ohio State University, says many are getting better at dealing with male survivors, but that inexperienced counselors remain. Steed, a forty-five-year-old survivor from Wisconsin, agrees. "The first place I called asked me if I was a rapist, or if I was masturbating on the other end of the phone. It took me years before I sought help again."

who've gotten high or drunk and found ourselves under a man who's pounding into us so hard it hurts. The roughness gay men use with us when we are younger, especially, can leave us feeling both flattered and violated. "An older neighbor banged the shit out of my sixteen-year-old ass while I screamed with pain," says Juan, a dancer from Miami. "It's not that it wasn't exciting; it was. I talked him up, I drank his beers, I even went with him again. But each time, afterward, I felt so bad." Realizing that someone hurting you in sex has more to do with who *he* is than who you are is work that gay men—whether we've been raped or just pushed into something we don't feel good about—often find difficult.

Forceful, coercive sex—involving weapons, violence, or sex by force even after you've said no clearly—are much more likely to be acts of control by straight men than anything gay, though that too remains cloudy in the minds of most rape survivors. Clearer, says Scarce, is the fact that openly gay men, in what little documentation has been done among male rape survivors, are raped more frequently than our heterosexual male counterparts. Black men seem to be raped more frequently than White men. The experience, in virtually all cases, includes forced unprotected anal intercourse. And whether it is assault by someone unknown to us, rape in a college dorm or other all-male setting, "acquaintance rape" of the kind experienced by Scarce, or part of ongoing domestic violence between men in a couple, it is likely to go unreported.

Why don't we hear more about this? Mike Lew, a Brookline, Massachusetts, expert on sexual abuse of male children and author of *Victims No Longer* (HarperCollins, 1990), traces one cause of silence to rigid notions of masculinity. "Our culture provides no room for a man as a victim," says Lew. "Rather than 'Who did this?' men are subjected instead—or subject ourselves—to the question 'Why did you let this happen?'" If the survivor happens to be adult and gay, says Michael Scarce, he gets a double dose of suspicion, facing both "the accusation that he was too unmanly to prevent it and the stereotype of gay men as hypersexual beings unable to control our own bumping and grinding."

"I honestly thought that my attraction to men meant being with this kind of man," says Jason, thirty-five, who was raped when he was twenty and just coming out of the closet. "I didn't realize until much later that the man who raped me was not part of the gay community, and that he was looking for someone else who didn't have connections, who wouldn't tell his family or friends. He knew to use my closet as a cloak." The confusion is one factor that leaves gay men—perhaps even more than women survivors—reluctant to turn to medical authorities or the legal system.

Show Some Emotion?

Even revealing your emotions about being raped to those known to you may take years. "I didn't tell my lover for ten years," says Jason. "I think he was shocked and hurt, but I felt unclean and didn't want him to think he'd gotten less of a person than when we first got together." Patrick, who was raped, burned with a cigarette, and alternately beaten up and tenderly embraced by his attacker until 6 A.M., showed up for work at 8. "I wanted to get control of what had gotten control of me," he says. "Two days later I was in Seattle on a business trip, surrounded by a bunch of people I didn't know, and I looked down at my burns and bruises and wondered what had happened." Scarce says reactions to being raped can be varied, though he names those below as some of the most common.

SHAME, GUILT, OR CONFUSION ABOUT YOUR ROLE

Rapists will often close their act of violence, or follow it up, with statements like "I love you," "I need you," or "I loved being with you," that make it sound as though you wanted it. Date rape is probably the most common, and confusing, experience of sexual assault. But going home with someone, or lying still until he finishes, is not the same as consent. Nor is there any connection between having a rape fantasy, which lots of men have, and having the actual experience. Involuntary erection or ejaculation during rape are also common. None of these things mean you chose to be raped or that it was okay for him to do that to you.

CHANGES IN SEX

In many cases, having sex after you've been raped means asking your partner to understand certain requirements—talking more before sex, going slowly for particular acts, even using a mirror to see his face during anal sex. One man interviewed by Scarce recalled the aftermath of an assault in which he was struck repeatedly in the face. "I remember talking to people before I had sex," he recalled. "I said, 'Don't touch my face. It freaks me out too much.'"

FEAR AND VULNERABILITY

Many rape survivors find themselves scared to go out, or imagine that they see their assailant in many places. Gay men may feel that they were singled out because of their sexual orientation, and feel more afraid to reveal it. "Having my first sexual experience be one that was violent, painful, and required hospitalization shoved me back in the closet for five years," says one survivor. Male survivors fear that they themselves will become perpetrators of abuse or rape, making counseling especially important so that you can explore and defuse that preoccupation.

DEPRESSION, SELF-DESTRUCTIVENESS, OR RISK TAKING

Sexual violence can leave many men feeling lost, suicidal, depressed, or numb. Studies of gay men forced to have sex with other men have also found them significantly more likely to have unprotected receptive anal sex later on in life.

If you have been assaulted and don't know where to go for help, call the Rape, Abuse and Incest National Network (RAINN) hot line at (800) 656-HOPE and give them your zip code. They'll patch you through, toll-free, to the rape crisis hot line nearest you. Michael Scarce's book contains an extensive bibliography on male-male rape, as well as a number of organizations that can connect you with sexual assault survivor services in your area.

Special Channels of Communication

Tips on Scripts

If sex is a dialogue, certain conversations can seem scripted. Long-term lovers narrate their roles with equal parts of humor and weariness: "I take care of him, and lay back, and he takes care of me, and he reaches for the blue towel we keep under the bed to the left and wipes his stomach first. . . ." Those not coupled find solace in scripts, too, using them in the search for sex and in the acts themselves. "I went through a period where I was dating three times a week, and every date was the same—dinner, back to my place to look at photos of my exotic travels, Bulgarian women on the stereo, candlelight, make out on the purple beanbag chair, maybe sex or maybe not," says David, thirty-nine years old. Then there's phone sex, whose opening lines—"Hey, how you doin'?" "Pretty horny, how about you?"— occur with the regularity of a television theme song no matter what the ensuing episode. The next question, "What are you into?" is rarely answered with "Reading Victorian novels" or "Following the latest constitutional crisis on C-SPAN." "What do I say? 'Just hangin' out, looking for some hot buddies to party with,' of course," intones John, a thirty-nine-year-old English professor, dropping his voice a half octave in demonstration.

The nuances vary, even in a seemingly rigid medium. "How I introduce race is a delicate thing," explains Shelby, thirty-two, of his phone-sex cruising. "Always mention it, but not right away, and never in response to 'What do you look like?' It's later, after there's been some interest. I say, 'How do you feel about Black men?'" Breaking from the formulas comes with its own risks and rewards. "Say something too real and people stop and say, 'Oh, maybe we should actually have coffee and get to know each other better,' except it rarely happens," says Shelby. Sullivan, thirty-three, an AIDS educator from Toronto, says his cruising formula is "one part humor, two parts daring. When someone asks me in that super-serious voice what I get into, I say, 'Kittens and raindrops.'" Lawrence and David, lovers who met at a Berkeley, California, bathhouse, kept the daring but left the humor. The sex was good, they say, but it was each man's willingness to talk about his spirituality, and his confusion about it, that made them take each other seriously.

Sex changes depending on whom it's with, but favorite motions or moves often get repeated. "Like novelists or dramatists, few of us wander far from the formulas of their most predictable successes," offers John Gagnon, Ph.D., who with coauthor William Simon has written extensive analyses of the scripts they claim lie at the heart of everyone's sexual behavior. For Gagnon, sex is a "little like jazz, full of improvisation and nuance, but also returning to certain familiar melody lines and patterns."

There's also Muzak sex, the gay-porn-robot mode that may be the lowest common denominator of gay sexual communication. Sure, it works in a pinch. Use at the risk of boring him, or yourself (see below).

HOW TO BE A GAY PORN ROBOT

1. Say "Oh, yeah" a lot. And deep, like it's coming from your abdomen: "Yeaaaah."

2. Refer to all body parts as if they, or you, were across the room. "Suck that dick." "Give me that ass." "Use that mouth."

3. Tell, don't ask, when soliciting feedback—as in "You like that, don't you."

4. Use *hot* and *shit* as often as possible, though never "hot shit" (too country). Best in combination with #1 and #2, as in, "Oh, yeaaaah, that dick is hot. You are so hot. Shit, that's hot." Or even, "Shit, it's getting kind of hot in here. Mind if I take off my shirt? Oh, yeaaaah."

S/M: Special Channel #1

People who don't have experience with S/M imagine that the pain is like the pain you experience when you go to the dentist. The Little Shop of Horrors image of the sadistic dentist is what most people think of. We need to invent a new term. Pain doesn't describe the sensation that's involved. Some people use the term pain/pleasure. Pain is this horrible, bad thing that nobody wants to experience, and the sensation in S/M is something other than that. It's pain transfigured.

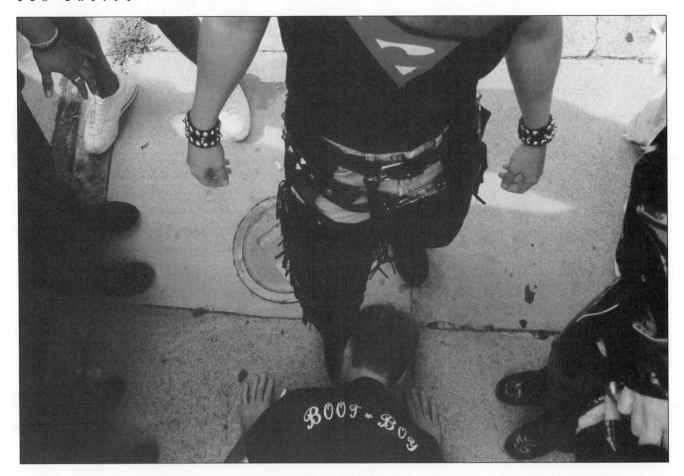

Perhaps no sex is more highly structured, more scripted, than S/M, a formal language two or more men use to explore desire and domination, pain and control. In some sense, of course, all sex uses that vocabulary. Who hasn't felt the struggle between comfort and discomfort in sex, the tension between pleasure and the pain of its delay? What sex doesn't involve some element of power or submission, or attention to certain roles or body parts? S/M intensifies the focus, isolating certain details and highlighting them until they expand into an entire erotic landscape. In vanilla sex, for example, your balls might be something he sucks on for five minutes before returning to your penis. In an S/M scene, they may well be the central point of pleasure, the object of four or five hours of work in which they're shaved, bound, teased with hot or cold, stretched, weighted, twisted, and caressed. A feeling in sex—the giving in, for example, that is a piece of settling back for a blow job—can in an S/M scene become drawn out until it *becomes* the sex, a prolonged act of submission that renders oral sex itself unnecessary. Even time—which stands still in orgasm—becomes more generally extended in S/M, lengthening and pulling away from sex as arousal increases. Vanilla sex lasts an hour or two. An S/M scene, and the variety of activities it involves, can often go for five hours, eight, or a weekend.

Where exactly, does vanilla end and S/M begin? Is giving someone a hickey, and the accompanying blend of pleasure and pain, an S/M act? How about ordering him to his knees and watching as he sucks you off? What if the man whose neck you're biting, or who's sucking you, is blindfolded? If he's tied with the sash of your bathrobe, is that S/M? If you trade the bathrobe sash for handcuffs, is that S/M? Like most sexual acts, S/M is more a matter of intention than equipment, a way of making explicit the give-and-take of power that often goes unspoken.

How and when that happens—and what is true S/M or not—means many things to many people. "There is a cornucopia of options," says John Weis, chairman of Gay Male S/M Activists (GMSMA) in New York City. "For some, unless you blindfold them, they don't respond. For others, spanking is the only thing that gets them going. The level of play or its intensity is less important than your mind-set going into it." Some S/M players focus on body parts—hairy bellies, armpits, cock and balls. Others focus on practices: bondage, flogging, piercing, or mummification. Still others take on roles: daddy and boy, master and slave.

The intensely specific nature of these desires may seem limiting or liberating, depending on how well you like them. "I started going to the Spike—a leatherish bar—when I turned forty-five, because it was the only gay bar where I felt welcomed or saw anybody who looked like me," says David, fifty-four, an art history professor whose latest love—besides the boyfriend he met at an S/M bar—is nipple play. "It was the first time in twenty-five years that people had helped me learn how to think about sex, about what I was willing to try and where that might take me." For many, finding their way to S/M is like a second coming out. "As a gay man, I knew that society's attitude toward gay men was the problem, not gay men," says Dorian, thirty-two. "But it took me much longer to feel comfortable with my interest in bondage. I used to walk by those bars in Boston and wonder, could I ever go behind those doors? What would I learn there?"

I was tied up and I could see that he was placing these candles on the floor, and I thought, "I wonder if there's going to be hot wax dripped on my body," and I've never done that before and wonder if it's going to be painful and awful. He picked one of the candles up and he could see that I was tensing up. And he continuously whispered in my ear: "Relax, breathe." And he gave me some breathing exercises and explained what he was going to do and how good it was going to feel, giving me confidence. And he took me someplace I'd never been before.

The pleasure of learning and instruction finds echoes throughout S/M culture. S/M organizations offer workshops and seminars, frequently in contexts that are not sexual. Inexperience in vanilla sex may feel like something to hide, but S/M personal ads often advertise for novices. "Never lie about your level of expertise," says John Weis. "If you want to learn, there's someone to teach you."

Cracking the codes of S/M desire—red hanky on the left means fister, one on the right, fistee—is the stuff of gay T-shirt shops. Serious S/M players know that the color of your handkerchief or what side your keys fall on is only the beginning. "It's all about what you tell and when, what hidden or forbidden things you can get the other person to enact," says Jeff, forty, a self-proclaimed "little bottom boy" who delights in training new tops. "Words are the most important S/M instrument. You use them to coax out the selfish part of someone, the part they didn't even know wanted to be served."

For all the instruction manuals and workshops, the most important S/M skills—building trust and setting limits—are found in the context of personal exchanges. Going places you thought you couldn't reach is part of S/M's appeal—but so is finding the right person to go there with. Good tops often started as bottoms. Good bottoms know that if he doesn't seem in control of himself, you don't want him in control of you. "Usually the tops I play with will take a long time to talk to me beforehand, laying out their ground rules: how they play, how they keep you safe, how they feel about safe words," says Dorian. "During a scene, they can drive you up the wall, asking if you're all right every five minutes." In a bar, it's common practice for a top to introduce a bottom to a few people to show he's known and reliable. And no matter what, says Weis, trust your instincts. Does he smile? Does he meet your eye? Does he seem like he knows other people, or is he a dark figure in the shadows who, while alluring, seems untrustworthy? There's an S/M expression: A little pain never hurt anyone. "Bad judgment certainly does," says Weis.

If the "safe word" (see box below) is a hallmark of trust, "safe, sane, and consensual" is the overarching framework. Many S/M players recite it like a mantra to spell out the difference between healthy S/M sex and the kind that might be coercive, sick, or self-destructive. Gil Kessler, a past president of GMSMA, defines the terms as follows:

> ***Safe*** is being knowledgeable about what you're doing. This means knowing your equipment and how to use it, and knowing your partner and how to keep him healthy both physically and psychologically.
>
> ***Sane*** is knowing the difference between fantasy and reality, and observing that difference. You may know how to do something, and even get consent for it, but it may be best left for one-handed reading.
>
> ***Consensual*** is respecting the limits imposed by each participant. Consent is an ongoing right, and can be withdrawn at any time. You cannot consent to give up the right of consent! Nor can the content of any master/slave contract negate that right. "You can do anything you want to me, even if I really want you to stop" is a statement that only an irresponsible top would take seriously.

No matter how neat the definition of consent, of course, S/M is also about what Michael, a thirty-six-year-old writer, calls "the tensions between two seemingly contradictory impulses: respecting limits and pushing boundaries." In other words, when does no really mean no? When do you ignore what the bottom says to take him just a little bit further? For all the scary potential of that kind of judgment call, many men find it a relief to walk that hazy line, particularly given the clarity that also comes with S/M's explicit recognition of the power of limit

SAFE WORDS

Most good tops will be able to sense your limits and push you right to them. One way to make sure a scene doesn't go farther than you want it to—and to relax as you approach your edge—is a safe word.

"Safe word" is the term for a word chosen for the scene that, once said aloud, means it's time to stop. *No, don't,* and *stop* are no good, since those are things you might moan even when you want him to continue. Some men use *halt,* or references to a traffic light: *yellow* means "slow down," *red* means "stop immediately." If you're gagged or bound, you agree on a safe gesture, a hand signal that means "let me out of this."

Good tops check in regularly with the bottom, seeing how things are going. The safe word keeps them from going too far. If you can't trust someone to respect the boundaries of a safe word, then play with someone else.

setting. "I'm much more comfortable bringing up my HIV status in an S/M context, and I always do," says Dorian. "He'll say, 'I want to tie you up and hang you upside down and then fuck you for hours,' and I'll say, 'I'm HIV-positive, and I'm pretty tight so I can't get fucked easily, but the first part sounds good.' Talking about things like how to meet medication schedules and what practices you like to do most is easier when there's a tradition of that kind of discussion." The skills and thrills of seeing where boundaries are respected, and where you're pushed past them, can also take you well beyond the crude modes of genital pleasure and risk of HIV transmission. "There was a period in my life when my sex focused on my genitals," says Dorian. "Suddenly I've discovered that I have a whole body, a whole range of sexual sensations."

Tao and Tantra: Special Channel #2

Semen and HIV may be contained by walls of latex. Energy—the transformative, healing energy released by sexual arousal—is not. So say modern practitioners of Taoism (pronounced "dow-ism" and meaning "the way"), an ancient Asian philosophy that, though encompassing far more than sex, is now uniting increasing numbers of modern couples in orgasmic bliss. You may be more familiar with Tao's South Asian cousin, Tantra (Sanskrit for "to weave" or "web"), whose practices of sexual and spiritual delights are based on Indian texts, including the mother of all sex manuals, the *Kama Sutra*. The terms differ between Taoism and Tantra, but both share certain beliefs and practices, including the idea that sex is an experience of the soul and your partner is a stand-in for God or the universe.

Freeing the flow of *chi* (pronounced "chee"), the bioelectric or life force inside each of us, is a staple of Eastern medicine (see "Acupuncture," page 314). Tao seeks to circulate one of the most powerful energies—*ching chi*, or sexual energy—throughout the body. What we call getting hot or horny, Taoists call an accumulation of *ching chi* (which certainly sounds classier). But whereas most Western orgasm involves blocking off this energy below the chest until you force it all out your penis through ejaculation, Taoist practitioners seek to retain and recirculate, turning orgasm into an affair of the head, heart, and spirit.

A spiritual connection to your partner—and attentiveness to the details of his experience—is a necessary starting point. Sexual techniques include slow and varied movements during intercourse or mutual masturbation, breathing in sync, long, locked gazes, and an internal process Taoists call the Draw, in which partners bring their sexual energy away from their genitals and up into the rest of the body. The key moment is just before ejaculation, when "you are totally at a peak and full of sexual energy," says B. J. Santerre, a gay Taoist instructor in Miami, Florida. "That's when you transform the energy, drawing it up out of the perineum [see page 23], up the spine to the crown of the head, touching your tongue to the roof of your mouth to complete the circuit and channeling it back down the front of the body, from eyes to heart to belly button. Now you've done a full loop."

Obviously this takes a little practice, in a workshop, with a book, or (perhaps best) with someone already versed in the Draw. Most instructors agree that the key lies in a mastery of breathing and meditation, practiced outside of sex as well as during it. "I know lots of people who can raise their energy just by breathing deeply after they've been training for a while," says Collin Brown, director of Body Electric, the touch-based healing arts school centered in

THE MALE MULTIPLE ORGASM

When we were kids, our house had a slanted roof, and we used to throw a tennis ball up and see how high we could get it and still have it roll down. It's like that: You bring yourself right to the brink, but not so far over that you have to wait while you walk around and get the ball and start all over. I can come five or six times.

Sisterhood is powerful, and the spontaneous multiple orgasm remains one of women's special privileges. Male students of sexual and spiritual energy, however, as well as a relatively small number of naturally lucky men, have found that a little work and practice can also give them repeated waves of pleasure that include the heart-pounding, mind-stopping pleasure of orgasm—without ejaculation.

The road to male multiple orgasm begins like the one-shot deal, with you aroused and erect. It's right before you hit the point of no return that the two roads diverge—one leading to ejaculation, the other toward multiple orgasm. Pay close attention to the signs of increasing arousal: the climb of your heartbeat, the change in your breathing, and the series of prostate contractions that mark the start of ejaculation by pumping fluid into the urethra. Once the fluid's there, two small muscles close the urethra above and below, creating a pressure buildup and the feeling that blastoff is "coming." The trick with multiple orgasm is to stop stimulation as soon as you feel that initial fluttering in the prostate and pelvic floor. Then wait twenty seconds or so, and resume stimulation. With practice, you'll start to feel waves of pleasure each time your prostate contracts, growing more and more intense as you repeat the process.

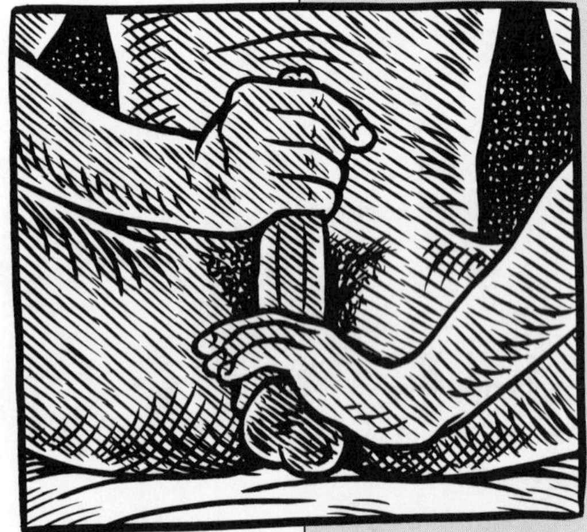
The scrotal tug

How do you put on the brakes? Doing Kegels (see page 41), keeping your breathing deep, and consciously uncurling your toes and relaxing your thighs can all help. Other interventions include squeezing the head of the penis firmly (see the squeeze technique on page 177) or gentle but firm tugging of your testicles away from the penis (the "scrotal tug") to delay orgasm.

Mantak Chia and Doug Arava, authors of *The Multi-Orgasmic Man (HarperSanFrancisco, 1996),* also suggest pressing your finger to the first joint into what they call the "million-dollar point," a spot on your perineum just below your prostate. "However you do it," suggests Collin Brown of Body Electric, "take yourself to the edge and then back away. Relax into the erotic charge."

With a little practice, you may start experiencing multiple orgasms within a few weeks. Not masturbating the regular way, devoting yourself instead to this new approach, will get you there sooner. The Tao preaches that the highest state of health and energy is achieved by conserving your semen and not ejaculating "at all." Does anyone in the Western world have *that* much self-discipline?

Oakland, California. "Others focus more on the feelings at the root chakra [energy portal] just above the anus, and consciously pump energy up their spine." Learn how to work with your energy, says Brown, and your body can become a "total erotic zone."

The result of ongoing Taoist practice? In addition to a kind of meditative awareness and a greater sensitivity to your and your partner's experience, think of honey flowing, fireworks, or whatever other images are provoked by the idea of wave after wave of orgasm (see box above). Since this is orgasm without ejaculation, says Santerre, your body—no longer depleted by wasting the vital life force of semen—will feel refreshed and energized after sex, rather than exhausted. "If you take all the honey from the honeycomb, the bees have to get busy making new honey," explains Santerre, detailing why so many of us feel shot after we shoot.

The Taoist approach to orgasm works for solo flights, but its greatest benefit—even as you perfect it—can be to taking couples to new heights of sexual and emotional connectedness. "Moving beyond orgasm to the study of energy frees men up to let go of the erotic machismo," says Collin Brown, "replacing it with an ability to experiment, to be playful, and to make mutual consideration and pleasure an explicit value." Joseph Kramer, the founder of the Body Electric School and currently the director of Erospirit Research Institute, agrees: "It's about communion, melting together. I've known many couples who found that Eastern approaches to sex involving touch were just as, if not more, fulfilling than insertive sex. It's true intimacy, two becoming one."

If some of Santerre's claims for Taoist practice—a boosted immune system and total sexual satisfaction—seem grand, that is in keeping with a long tradition. "If a man has intercourse without spilling his seed, his vital essence is strengthened," advises the venerable *Discourse on the Highest Tao Under Heaven*. "If he does this twice, his hearing and vision are made clear. If three times, all his physical illness will disappear." By the seventh time, according to the *Discourse*, your thighs and buttocks are firm, and by the ninth your life span will have increased. That's enough to keep even the most impatient homosexual lingering a bit longer on his *lingam* (it means "wand of light" in Sanskrit).

Even if you're not ready to commit to full-fledged spiritual practice, you may find Taoist sex to be a great way to postpone ejaculation until you are ready to shoot a thundering geyser. Western medical practitioners suggest at least some ejaculation to avoid congestion of the prostate (see page 40), while Taoists recommend massage of perineum, testicles, and tailbone to relieve the pressure caused by holding back ejaculate.

A note of caution: Virtually all written texts on Taoism and Tantra focus exclusively on heterosexual models, and are sometimes decidedly homophobic (including early writings by Taoist master Mantak Chia). Chia's later book on multiple male orgasms (see box on previous page), however, includes a gay-specific chapter. Margo Anand, the Tantra instructor who has authored an introductory text on Tantra, *The Art of Sexual Ecstasy* (J. P. Tarcher, 1991), is also open to the notion of gay sex, though in the past she has not allowed people with HIV to take her advanced courses. Even if you're a beginner reading your way toward ecstasy, you'll have, once again, to translate the penis-into-vagina discussion, and the pronouns, into terms you find more meaningful.

Negotiated Safety: Special Channel #3

My boyfriend and I just stopped using condoms after ten years, and I have to say, it's wonderful. We did the whole thing: testing together, talking. I think I was scared to have the conversation, not because I didn't trust him, but because I didn't know if he should trust me. I have to admit, though, that I'd forgotten about how good it would feel.

We're both negative, we've been together a year and a half, we don't have sex with other people, and we still use condoms. "I'm old-fashioned, and condoms saved my life," Steve says, but he knows I've never experienced anal sex without condoms and would like to try.

He has started to let me get a little of his cum in my mouth—after, not during—oral sex. I see that as a step.

I think in some ways AIDS is one of the things that has kept us together. We've been together since before AIDS started, and we don't have sex with other people, so we've never used condoms.

If negotiated safety—the name Australian AIDS educators gave to an HIV-negative couple's decision to fuck without condoms—doesn't sound sexy, the practice itself is far more appealing. To the pleasure of condomless anal sex—the lack of fumbling with condoms, the ability to move easily back and forth between anal and other kinds of sex, and the warmth of skin-to-skin contact—is added a different kind of warmth: that of an exclusive bond between you and another man.

Lots of men, maybe even most of us, have experienced anal sex without condoms. Getting to condomless sex that comes from a formally articulated commitment to caring for each other—rather than deciding for the moment that you don't care, or that you care enough about the present to take some chances with the future—is less common. In many ways, reaching that point takes a "practice" as formal as Tantra or S/M, one that involves more outside steps and discussions. Negotiated safety is not just fucking without condoms, or assuming you're both the same HIV status and fucking without condoms, or even both testing negative and fucking without condoms. It's fucking in a framework, pledging to protect each other and your special relationship, and being honest if or when you can no longer honor that pledge. That can feel as freighted and important as trading rings at an altar. Given how many marriages, gay and straight, break up over misunderstandings or dishonesty about outside affairs, the negotiation part of negotiated safety may be harder than a simple "I do."

"Test, test, talk, trust" is the four-word summary that Australian AIDS researchers use to describe how you get from condoms to a place where you no longer need them. You both test for HIV, and if you're both negative, you wait a month (the time it usually takes for new infections to show up on the new, improved HIV antibody test—see Chapter 7) without having unprotected sex and test again. If you're both still negative, you talk about whether you're willing to swear off unprotected sex with anyone but each other. For some couples, that can mean no sex with anyone else, or just no sex with anyone else that involves risk for HIV. "Gordon and I weren't ready for the whole monogamy conversation," says Sam, forty, a Connecticut photographer, "but we don't use condoms. Our agreement is that if I or he should happen to be with someone while the other is out of town, then we can get sucked but not suck. And nothing goes inside us, not even a finger. We don't want to bring something home, and I want him around to be with me when I'm an old man."

Making sure you are both comfortable with the same idea of what safer sex means is one part of the conversation. Coming up with a mutually agreeable understanding about monogamy, or how to have safer sex outside, is a more complicated one (see "Boys on the Side," page 132). But the hardest, and an absolutely essential, part of negotiated safety is the commitment to be honest with your partner if at any point you find that you've strayed from the terms of the arrangement.

Some couples agree that either partner has the right to cancel the arrangement at any time, without explanation, though the idea that you could call the whole thing off without a conversation is unlikely. Any kind of agreement should be postponed if you feel like you're having trouble being direct or honest with each other, or if you have misgivings you don't know how to voice (see box below).

Some positive men, also, are opting for unprotected sex with each other. "The feeling of having someone inside of me—and coming inside me—is a pleasure like none other, and what I do to my body is my business," says Gerard, twenty-four. Unprotected sex between two positive men may not risk new HIV infection, but given the possibility of reinfection (see box on page 73), this is less negotiated safety than calculated risk. If you are positive and decide that the chance of getting more HIV doesn't seem scary enough to warrant condoms for anal sex, think about how else you might reduce your risks: not fucking with people who might have STDs, for example, or not letting him come inside you. Things that increase blood flow to your ass, or create tiny cuts inside it—poppers, douching, rough sex, prolonged sex—may all increase your risks.

NEGOTIATED SAFETY MEANS . . .

• *Taking two HIV tests to find out if you're both negative.* Assuming you are, or that he is, because that was true a year ago isn't good enough. Is testing something your relationship feels strong enough to survive? Is it a good time to test (see page 303)? Think and talk about what you would do if both of you tested positive, or if one of you did—*before* you go to have blood drawn.

• *Frank talk about sex and safety.* Is that kind of conversation something you have now? Can you really be honest about your current practices outside the relationship? About what you believe is safe? If you aren't sure, or are nervous or suspicious of his definition of safer sex, don't go to condomless fucking no matter what pressures you may feel.

• *Honesty about unanticipated "screwups."* Think about how you feel when one of you has done something "wrong" or broken an agreement in the past. It doesn't have to be sexual; it might be spending shared money, or forgetting to do an errand. Can you talk about it honestly with your partner? Have you been able to tell him the truth without fearing you're risking the relationship, or retaliation? Do you believe he tells you the truth? Negotiated safety isn't the time to try out a new resolve to be more open.

• *Choosing.* Just because it's possible doesn't mean it's necessary. If you're at all uncomfortable, "I'm not ready" is a response that he should understand.

• *Sex without condoms.* This is a wonderful benefit, well worth other stretches and sacrifices.

Talking HIV

It's a mood breaker, that's for sure. It's like saying "I'm Catholic" in the middle of sex. I mean, what's he supposed to do, say, "Ooh, that sounds hot? What's your favorite prayer?"

We went out to lunch, and then afterward he kind of walked me into a doorway and said, "I'm positive." He was so scared he was shaking. When we went to bed I still did the same things I'd done before. I cared for him too much to let him think that it had changed things between us, and we weren't having anal sex anyway. Actually, and this is my stuff, I think it drew me closer to him to think of him as positive, and needing to be cared for.

I had this guy really want to suck my dick. I kept pushing him away gently, turning, trying to do something else. "What's the matter, aren't you safe?" he murmured, fighting my hands away. I let him do it. I mean, I didn't want to get into an argument.

At the beginning I asked, casually, "How are you finding dating in the age of AIDS?" without telling him I was positive. He didn't say much, but for several dates I kept trying to get my tongue into his mouth and he wouldn't let me. "I have HIV and no T cells," he said finally, when I asked him to spend the night. "I'm sorry to hear that," I said, "but I'm also relieved." It was the first time we shared an open-mouthed kiss. We were together until he died.

Of all the conversations about sex, verbal and nonverbal, those that deal with HIV are among the most difficult. Thinking about infection—or infecting someone else—isn't sexy. Thinking about illness, loss, or the potential for both isn't sexy. Certainly in the midst of sex—when you most want to be swept away—talking about anything complicated and multilayered means a change in your experience, and the possibility that you'll get more information than can fit your fantasy. "Since my lover told me he's positive, I won't go down on him," admits Sammy, twenty-six. "But if I'm with a man whose status I don't know, I'll sometimes go ahead and suck." Not talking sometimes leaves us freer, though not necessarily free, of worry. "I know it doesn't make logical sense," says Sammy. "That's why talking about it freaks me out. I don't even want to think about it."

Think about it. AIDS broke the silence on gay sex, drawing thousands of men to safer-sex workshops, and moving discussion of anal sex from porn magazines to public health campaigns. Our fight against AIDS raised the profile of gay male caring, challenging the stereotype that our lives were solitary and selfish and soulless. But AIDS created silences even as it broke them, because at base—and beyond politics—the idea of getting or giving HIV has never lost its stigma. "Even as gay men were battling the idea that babies and hemophiliacs were the 'innocent victims,' we were creating our own guilty: those infected after we 'knew better,'" says Berkeley-based psychotherapist Walt Odets, Ph.D. Today, amid calls for greater responsibility for protecting each other and increasing numbers of laws making HIV transmission criminal, the specter of what you knew and when you knew it still haunts gay men's bedrooms and our decisions to disclose our HIV status. That's assuming that you're in a bedroom. Or that you're talking to the person with whom you're having sex. Or that you have tested recently enough to know your HIV status with any certainty.

With long-term partners of different serostatuses, the question is not usually whether to tell—the fact of being HIV-positive is too important to keep secret from your lover—but whether to test. With a casual partner, the question of disclosure—even if you know your status—depends on the relationship. "I'm not going to believe someone I've just met if he tells me he's negative," says Tim, a thirty-year-old New York City writer who thinks he's negative but hasn't tested in two years. "So what's the point of asking?"

Positive and negative men both say that how serious the relationship seems is the most important factor in determining what they'll say about HIV. "When I was husband hunting, I always told men I was positive," says Darryl, fifty-two, an administrative assistant from Maine. "If I know we're not going to do anything risky, then I figure there's no point in bringing it up." Deciding beforehand "how serious it is," or what will happen in sex, has obvious pitfalls. "Things went better than I thought, and on the third wonderful weekend together, all I could think of was how much I didn't want to scare him away," recalled Tom, a man in a GMHC workshop. "When he asked if I was positive, all I could come up with was, 'I don't know my HIV status, but I don't think it's in great shape.'"

Men of both HIV statuses say often that they just "assume everybody's positive," or that "he knows the score, and if he doesn't ask me to use condoms, that's his choice." But don't-ask-don't-tell policies also keep us from asking ourselves about the emotions attached to the fact that some of us have a potentially fatal virus and some of us don't. "When you're negative and ask his status, one of the things you're really asking him—at the level of feelings—is, 'Are you dangerous? Will you contaminate me?'" says Dr. Odets. Similarly, he says, a positive man's rationale that "he would have asked me to use condoms for anal sex if he wasn't positive himself" sounds clearer than it is. "Almost every positive guy knows that he may be doing damage to his partner in that situation," says Odets. "If he gets closer to his feelings, that's going to be experienced as guilt, anxiety, self-hatred, anger. Even if he's angry at having been infected himself, it's not going to help him feel any better."

Complicating the equation are the vastly different stakes negative and positive men have in telling. Saying you're negative is at worst a kind of challenge to your partner: "I'm negative, how about you?" Revealing that you're positive, says New York State Psychiatric Institute researcher Robert Remien, Ph.D., means "not only risking rejection, but giving up control of information with implications far outside the bedroom. It's an intensely personal piece of information many men feel should be shared only with someone they know, trust, and care about." Not all sexual partners meet those conditions.

Papering over these kinds of painful distinctions is one of the things that made the "condom code"—the advice to use a condom every time—so attractive, says Richard Elovich, GMHC's director of HIV prevention. Reckoning with those differences, on the other hand, is what is needed if we are going to avert another generation of gay men struggling with a lifetime of toxic medicines and new HIV infections. "The reality is that HIV is undesirable—in *all* our lives," says Elovich. "It's difficult to say, because for guys living with the virus there's a real struggle to keep a tenuous hold on feeling okay about being infected. But unless all of us can affirm that living with HIV should not be a normal way of life for the gay community, we might as well give up on HIV prevention."

Instead, though, we sometimes find it more comfortable to give in to fantasies that let us skip disclosure in favor of denial. Among HIV-negative men, one such fantasy is that silence equals safety—that if he doesn't mention anything or look sick, he must be free of HIV. Some positive men describe a parallel fantasy: that their infection is meaningless. "There are times when you want to think, 'What difference does it make if I have one of the zillion viruses living in the human body?'" says Gary, thirty-eight, a communications consultant from San Francisco. Ironically, even unmentioned, HIV can be an absent presence, making itself felt as you try to figure out what the sex you're having means about him. "It felt good to be inside him without a condom," says thirty-two-year-old John, an actor. "But then I kept thinking, why would he let me do this? What's wrong with him?"

Imagining the other side—what it would be like to be your sexual partner and get infected—is one of the things that motivates men both to use condoms and to talk about their status. "For all the talk of every gay man for himself," says David Nimmons, an HIV-prevention specialist for the Center for AIDS Prevention Studies at San Francisco (CAPS), "the majority of gay men are thinking of others already." Researching motives for sexual caretaking among gay men, CAPS interviewed positive and negative men in San Francisco and New York about what motivated them to stay safe or disclose their status. The overwhelming majority of positive men cited concern for their partner as one of the reasons they use condoms or tell their partners they're positive. "They didn't want someone else to have to go down this same road or do to someone else what somebody did to them," says Nimmons. More than half described disclosure and safer sex as an "ethical, moral, or spiritual commitment." Interestingly, positive men's concern about telling did not seem matched by their negative brothers: Only 10 percent of negative men said they regularly asked their partner's status or disclosed their own.

What Do You Know? Looking at What Keeps You Silent on HIV, or How You Talk About It

You may not have been tested, or not tested recently, for HIV. "Most people who say they're negative are basing it on a two-year-old test anyway," says Dr. Remien, one reason why he says he "doesn't believe that disclosure of a new partner's negative HIV status should be the sole basis for decisions about risk behavior." Whether or when you ask is almost never simple. It can help, though, to ask yourself some questions, and then use those answers to make decisions about safer sex.

HIV-Negative Men		**HIV-Positive + Men**	
What do you know?			
"There are a lot of things I won't do if he says he's negative, because I don't necessarily believe him. But if he says he's positive, there are a lot more things I won't do."	If you don't know his status, or don't know him well enough to trust him if he says he's negative, ask yourself: Would you really do the same thing if you knew he was positive?	*"He came over and as we were playing around some of my semen got in his eye. He didn't seem to mind—he was going on about how he loved my big load, about how many guys at the gym he had wanted to do but how glad he was to hook up with me. Later, when I told him I worked for an AIDS organization, he asked if I was positive. When I said yes, he panicked. I explained that semen in the eye was not a common route of transmission, that I had a low viral load, but he wasn't listening. He was no longer interested in me, my situation, my load—he was just worrying. He left totally upset, and I was, too. We were just masturbating. Should I have told him beforehand?"*	Silence doesn't mean his status is the same as yours, or that he shares your definition of risks worth taking. Are you making decisions for him by not telling?

HIV-Negative Men		HIV-Positive ✚ Men	
What are you waiting for?			
"It's a major buzz kill."	If you're wondering about his status, why not ask? Positive men have the most to lose by talking about it, yet the burden of the discussion seems to fall to them.	*"People talk about responsibility, but why is the responsibility always up to me as the positive man to bring it up? I am so relieved when people ask. I mean, this is year nineteen of the AIDS epidemic. Hello?"*	How to know if things are serious enough for you to tell is a common problem. But all the stories of lost erections and tense silences suggest it's better to talk about it before you take off your clothes.
What do you say?			
"Telling him I'm negative is a way of asking him about himself. It's also like a little string around my finger reminding me to stay that way."	Saying "You're negative, right?" or "You're clean, aren't you?" isn't really asking for an honest answer. Disclosing your own status is also gentler than just turning and saying, "Are you positive?"	*"It's my moral standard: freedom of choice. I would never have sex with someone before telling them. If they don't want to be with me, I want to know before. If they act like an asshole, that's not me, that's not my responsibility, and at least I've met mine."*	Even if you don't want to disclose, you should think about how you'll tell if asked. Hedging or hinting isn't the same as telling. Lying is never okay.
What aren't you saying?			
"He told me he was positive, and I told him I was negative, and he still kept asking to fuck me without a condom. This was not even someone I knew well. I thought, 'What kind of person do you think I am?' I care about myself."	Claiming "It doesn't make any difference" or "I assume everyone's positive" may accurately describe your condom use, but probably not your mental state. It's unlikely that something with as many implications as HIV makes no difference to how you feel.	*"Finding out he was positive was like a burden coming off my back."*	Same as for negative men. If it really makes no difference, then why is it such a relief to find out he's positive, too?
What do you do?			
"I always observe lines that I've laid down for myself, one of which is that oral sex without ejaculation is okay. But when he told me he was positive, my first reaction was just a wave of anger washing over me, like, 'How could you let me suck on you for twenty minutes and not tell me?' I'm sure he saw it on my face."	Learning he has a potentially fatal virus is not like finding out his zip code. Conflicted feelings—such as simultaneously feeling emotionally attracted and sexually nervous—are common. But turning on your heel and leaving without a word, or shifting immediately into "Why does this always happen to *me?*" are not responsible responses. Do unto others. . . .	*"It's like going home with someone and you say, 'Oh, by the way, before we start, I have a tiny little dick.' Tell them you have HIV and you watch them just transform from someone who was all over you to someone totally cold."*	Talking about something as complicated as HIV means giving up a lot about yourself. Worrying that he'll drop you like a hot potato, or feeling that the anxiety of it all makes negative men too much to deal with, is common.

HIV-Negative Men		HIV-Positive ✚ Men	
What are you afraid of?			
"He hadn't been tested, but I did what they always tell you to do: talk about your sexual history. He told me, 'I've been with about six hundred men.' And I thought, 'Okay, what now?'" *"After going through the death of two lovers and maybe ten friends, I'm gun-shy."*	Is it getting HIV? Is it being involved with someone who might depend on you or get sick and leave you? Knowing can help.	*"Telling is like planting the seed that says, 'Go away from me.'"* *"I called to tell him I was positive, and he just hung up on me. He was terrified of having to go home to his family, who were Jehovah's Witnesses, in Colorado. We didn't talk for six months."*	Fear of infecting someone else is one thing; fear of rejection is another. So is fear of having to face someone else's concern about your sickness. Separating the issues may help you face them.

HIV Disclosure in Public Sex

How do you tell someone when they're going down on you in a room where there are fifteen people around?

I like sex where we don't talk. It lets me get out of my head, out of my worries about what and who and how. I've never had unsafe sex that way. But I don't want to talk about HIV or much else, including what my responsibilities are. I see my responsibility as treating people decently, and that's about it.

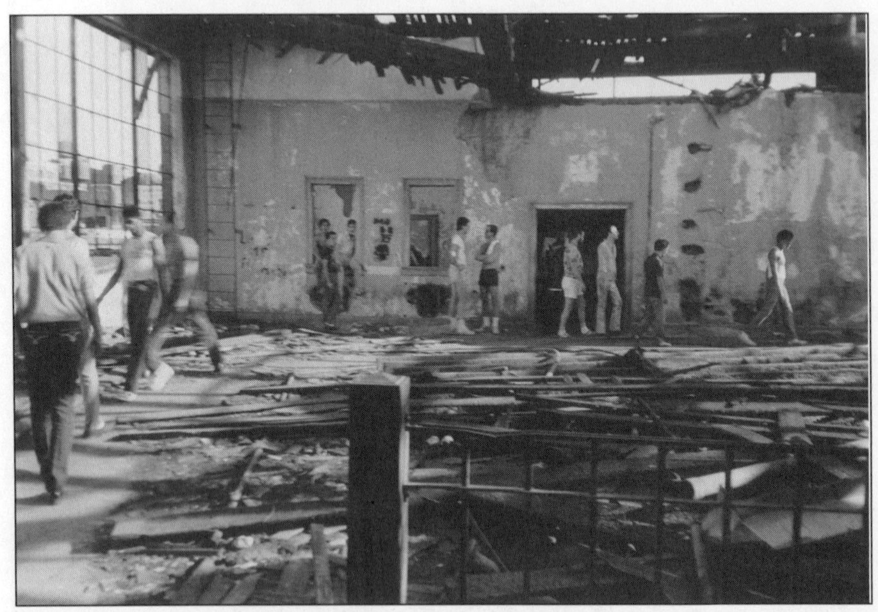

When speaking more than a few sentences is unlikely, then talking about HIV is *really* unlikely. That's one reason why public sex—in a park, in a gym, or in a bathroom—is attractive to some of us. It's also one reason why it can be risky. Be real about what that silence means. The way he looks can tell you a lot about his fashion sense, or about whether he's the kind of man you fantasize about, but it can't tell you much about his HIV status.

If you are going to have public sex in parks or rest stops, make sure you bring your favorite brand of condom along. If you're paying to go into a sex venue, it's still a good idea to bring condoms; you may not like the ones they have. If they don't have condoms, water-based lube, and safer-sex information available for free and in great quantity, ask why not. Any place that charges four dollars a drink or takes your ten dollars at the door can certainly afford the twenty cents a person it takes to give you a condom.

TURNING A GAY GAZE ON HIV DISCLOSURE LAWS

Giving someone HIV through sex is against the law in most states. Some states, such as Michigan, have made it a crime for people with HIV to have any penetrative sex, with or without a condom, without telling their partners they are positive. Other states have used public health statutes, or more general laws against attempted murder or manslaughter, to prosecute people accused of transmitting HIV through spitting, biting, or sex. If you know you are HIV-positive and knowingly set out to infect someone else, you can (and should) be held liable. You are also at legal risk in the much more common, much less clear-cut situations where you may not have set out to infect someone, but where you can still be seen as "reckless" or "negligent" since you didn't warn them about the danger.

The law, with its focus on what you intended to do when you took an action, isn't great at sorting through the ethics and emotions of something as complicated as sex. HIV transmission laws actually encourage people to avoid the knowledge that can save their life, since they punish those people who've taken the HIV test in the first place. As gay men in the middle of an epidemic, we deserve better. Responsibility for making sure that no virus passes between two people does not rest only on the one who's infected. HIV-negative men, those who don't know, and those who are positive can all ask questions and take actions. If you're not sure where to draw the line for safer sex, see Chapter 2.

Boyfriend Basics

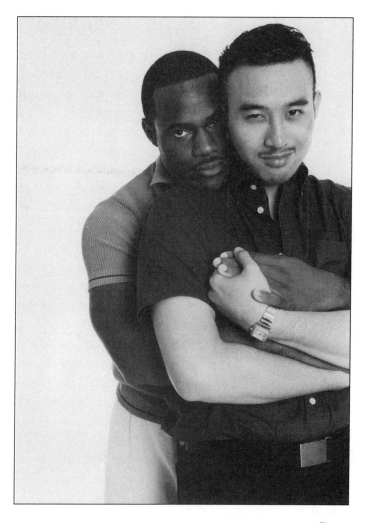

Listen closely and you'll hear it, rustling over the phone wires, echoing in the silence of the turned-off jukebox after last call, murmured on Gay Pride marches, confided to best friends over coffee, or lamented to ourselves as we turn to face the singles scene and find our stomachs turning in the process. Some therapists say it's the national call of the gay urban man with too many choices or the rural one with too few, a six-word soliloquy whispered wistfully and too often: "Why don't I have a boyfriend?"

Another question to ask is if you really need one. "Lots of gay men feel like they're doing it wrong because they've passed their late twenties and still haven't gotten into the Meaningful Relationship, the Big One," says New York City therapist Steve Ball, CSW. "And though it's been said a zillion times, I don't think most of us see more than two stages to personal development: coming out and getting settled." The storybook version of life has us all married by thirty, agrees Daniel Garces, a therapist at Houston's Montrose Counseling Center, and just because it's a heterosexual story doesn't mean it's not powerful. "We tend to go with what we know," says Garces. "If you want a traditional relationship—a 'heterosexual' homosexual relationship—you can definitely work for that. But it's also important to ask yourself why you want it. Is it to balance some sense of loss you feel from coming out that might be filled in another way? Is it something you were raised with? Is it your friend's idea of what you should be doing? Or is it a desire that's coming from within you?"

Having a partner is a beautiful thing, but it's beautiful for reasons. Some of those—intimacy and sexual companionship and social support—you can find with a boyfriend, in spite of him, or without having one at all. "Some people fall so much into a particular role in a relationship that they're not challenged," says Bruce Koff, LCSW, a Chicago therapist and former executive director of Horizons Community Services. "I don't believe in a hierarchy—lover, family, friends—so much as having ways to bring the different parts of your life and self together."

Would you be really be happier with a nice boyfriend, or manfriend, or transfriend, who understood your life and needs and sexual desires? If you find yourself complaining about the lack of Mr. Right, don't just repeat to yourself that you're doing something wrong. Instead, ask yourself a few questions about whether you're ready or how to proceed:

Are You Serious? Six Questions to Ask if You Think You're Ready for a Boyfriend

1. Are You Happy with Your Friends?

The need to feel connected to other people, to have a "watcher" in your life, is nearly universal. The need for those people to be your sexual partners is not. The real question is whether, as Bruce Koff puts it, you have somewhere in your life where you feel "fully known." What that means is a little like the famous judicial characterization of obscenity—you can't define it, but you know it when you see it. It doesn't mean bonding on the weekends or at the circuit party and then feeling isolated the rest of the week. It doesn't mean that there are some people who know the "work" you and others who know the "gay" you. It does mean having friends who appreciate both the "party" you and the needier you, people you can ask for help and for whom you don't have to put on a show. It does mean establishing relationships with people who interest you on a number of levels at once, who challenge you to do more and do better. Do you have people following your growth through life? Does anyone know both your family and your friends?

If you have deep friendships, feel good about that—instead of the "intimacy issues" everyone blames for lack of boyfriends, you may have the gay gift. A 1983 study of two hundred (presumably straight) men asked them to name their close friends; three-quarters could not name a single one. Gay men, by contrast, work to forge deep and lasting bonds. If you don't feel as though your friendships are deep or broad enough to include the different parts of your life, then focusing on those relationships may be a place to start your journey toward coupledom. Even if you found a partner, you might not know how to keep it deep. And no boyfriend can meet all a man's needs.

2. Are You Having Sex with Anyone You Know?

"Know" is open to interpretation. Start with more than name, place of employment, town or city of origin, penis size, and an hour's worth of conversation. No, you don't have to know people to have good sex with them. But one of the things that makes a boyfriend special is that he knows you—at least somewhat—*and* has sex with you. If hard-ons seem easy and emotional connections hard, suggests Michael Shernoff, one strategy may be to meet a few times before having sex and see how that feels. "Don't get me wrong—there's nothing wrong with casual sex," says Shernoff. "But sometimes it becomes an anesthetic for feelings of loneliness, boredom, or sadness. Experience those feelings, or their opposites, without sex, and you may be able to tell when an emotional connection with a man is addressing some of those other needs, or when you and he are going nowhere."

On the other hand, if you have good sex and good friends, the only thing you may be lacking is an attitude adjustment. What do you expect from a boyfriend that you're not getting already? How you answer that question—"a sense of permanence," "someone I can talk to about my interests," and so on—may determine where you start to look.

3. Are You Available?

Do you go to the movie you really want to see with Tom and Dave, your older married friends, leaving husband hunting for 11 P.M. and after? Are you so joined with the group of "sisters" you spend every Saturday night with that it would be too painful or intimidating for someone new to join you? Boyfriends sometimes find you, but only if you let them. And you have to make time for them to turn into boyfriends.

4. Are You Selling Your Short-Term Relationships Short?

Most of us have to flounder around a bit, though that doesn't mean we're not learning anything. "Relationships don't have to last for years to be opportunities for intimacy," says Garces. Rebound relationships, dates, and flings all "count."

The question is, are they all the same? "Is there the opportunity for conflict in that relationship, or do you jump out at the first sign of trouble?" asks Garces. Contrary to popular belief, boyfriend success rarely means finding someone with interests all the same as yours and with a better body. As important, in the end, is how you deal with difference.

5. Do You Have "Gay-D-D"?

That is, gay attention deficit disorder: obsessively scoping out every guy who comes within a block of you? "You know, like when you're in the local gay café, cruising guys in the pupil of the eye of the friend you're talking to," says Rob, twenty-nine.

6. Are You Your Harshest Critic?

"I counsel both straight and gay couples," says Steve Ball, "and both come in expecting that this kind of commitment is something we should know how to do without asking." If gathering all your friends and family together and proclaiming some version of "till death do us part" still ends in divorce for half or more of heterosexuals, even with all the legal perks that come with marriage, gay men certainly deserve some slack. "If a couple were buying a house, they'd know that it takes plenty of advice and helpers and brokers and technicians before they felt comfortable making and maintaining their home," says Ball. "What makes us think that having an ongoing love relationship would take less struggle or support to maintain?"

Sex Life Versus the Rest of Your Life?

I was twenty-six before I had sex in a bed.

What do you call someone you share everything with—companionship, a house, interests, holidays—except sex? A lover? We need a new word in the language.

I like the steam room. It's cloudy, dreamy, like a fantasy. I come easily there; you don't see the warts, the expectations or disappointments. It seems simpler.

Where does your sex life meet the rest of your life? That's a question that takes different forms throughout our lives and loves, changing with age and circumstance. If you're looking for a lover, or looking to keep one, you'll probably face the question of whether the place you find your sex is also where you find your friendship. Which is not to say that you'll never meet a boyfriend in a bathhouse, or that long-term partners necessarily give up on having satisfying sex together. In a world of so many sexual choices, though, trying to find the intersection between sex and love and daily life—or decide if you mind the lack of overlap—is a common cause of confusion.

Some men are sustained by slipping out of their ordinary lives for sex. Men describe public sex particularly—the randomness, the danger of discovery, and the joy of the hunt—as a special kind of thrill. Those into it talk of how it can intoxicate them into "an extrasensory sensitivity," of the way that waiting for sex in a rest room attunes you to "every footstep or door creak or water drop." In public sex spaces where men pay to hook up—bookstores, bathhouses, sex clubs, and cinemas—there's an additional charge: the electricity that comes when men dispense with ordinary politeness to get to raw sexuality. There are plenty of new rules to learn; public sex is often highly formalized. But the availability of so many interested men can create a kind of collective sexual arousal, the intoxication of knowing that hard dicks and hungry mouths are all around you and the hope that a stranger, by opening your pants or his own, may also be opening your soul. Cyber- and phone sex start with a verbal version, and the added excitement of never being able to see all the potential partners present.

The abundance that intoxicates can also make you sick. "When there are too many men to focus on, I become crazed," says Billy, twenty-three. "If his body's not hard enough, if he says the wrong thing, I'm on to the next." The same men who find a sex club stimulating one Saturday can find it lonely and alienating the next, or wonder if the pattern is a waste of time. "It's the same thing over and over: getting off and going nowhere," complains Jerry, twenty-eight, a security guard in Los Angeles. Animal arousal can seem brutal if you're looking for more human interaction. "People talk about sex clubs like they're all democratic, that anyone and everyone goes," says Tom, thirty-three, a Minnesota native whose five-foot-nine-inch frame carries more than two hundred pounds. "But even if you brave the fifteen or twenty rejections and find someone willing to give you the time of day, you walk out the door and feel just as alone, ignored, and shut out as you've always been."

OPEN UP IN THERE: HOW TO TELL THE DIFFERENCE BETWEEN HIM AND A PIZZA

"Fast-food sex," "quick-pick sex," "wham-bam-thank-you-Sam sex"—whatever you call it, there are times when the fast way to bust a nut can seem like it's the only way. "It's like ordering take-out," explains Neville, age thirty, matter-of-factly, "though not always as satisfying. You say what you're 'into,' deliver what's agreed upon, and that's the end of it." The fact is, he's not a pizza unless you want him to be. If you want more of the human element, go back to basics. Try demanding of yourself, the next time you have sex with someone, that you be able to answer four of the following five questions.

1. Who are this man's closest friends?
2. What's one of the most important things to him?
3. Is what he does for a living something he wants to be doing?
4. How does he spend his free time?
5. Does he have a boyfriend?

Then ask yourself a question: What are *you* like when you're with him? "Something common to many gay men is a learned habit of accommodation, of pleasing someone else," says Bruce Koff. "It's easy to focus on 'How does he feel about me?' and not ask 'How do I feel about him?'" Think in terms of not only shared values, but also whether or not you feel a little bit of a challenge with this man, suggests Koff. "Is this someone who connects you with a deeper sense of yourself? Does he make you feel bigger or smaller? More important or less important?"

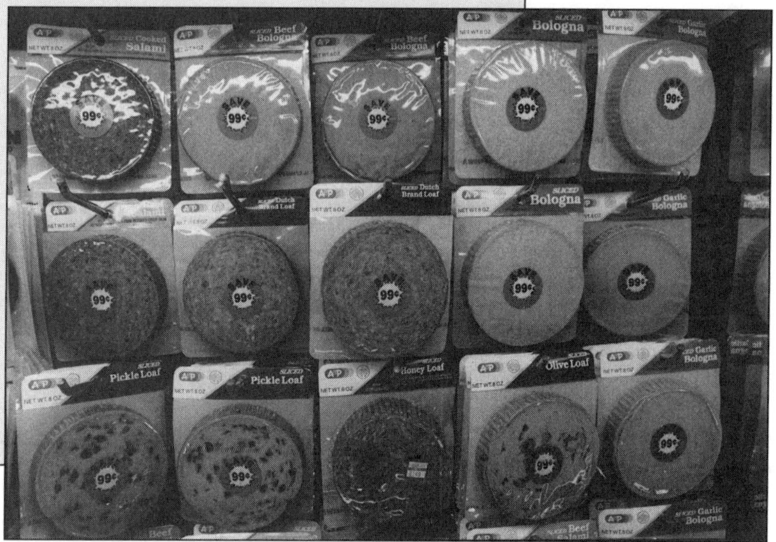

Cruising for What You Want

Many men are spending time searching for signs of more compassionate life in the gay universe. Wanting to be known for more than just your physical presence is one of the many factors that keep "Date Baits"—the get-togethers where gay men pay to gather, listen to each man speak for thirty seconds, and then rate each other as potential love interests—drawing sellout crowds in gay community centers and bookstores on both coasts. Wanting to be known is what swells gay publications with personal ads from men ISO (in search of) LTRs (long-term relationships) w/GMs of every age, race, serostatus, and sexual inclination. Ironically, wanting to be known on a deeper level is what keeps many gay men pumping iron and crunching their abdomens at gyms (see Chapter 5). "It's a purely marketplace decision," says forty-year-old Isay, a two-hour-a-day gym goer from Hawaii. "If you can't get them to look twice, then how will they ever look deeper?" Some of those who can't bear the market mentality, or the skin-deep judgments of that type of dating game, may turn to political organizations or potluck socials. The consumer within may prove harder to escape. "I can sit in a room and have opinions about every single guy there without even hearing him speak," says Ryan, twenty-six. "It took me years before I realized that if I didn't want to be alone for the rest of my life, I was going to have to ease up." Martin, forty-seven, confesses to "dumping one guy I was dating because I didn't like his wallet."

Focusing on what you want, rather than what you don't, is a step toward sexual and emotional satisfaction. Below find five variations on that theme: ways to make a kinder, gentler connection.

1. Cruise for What You Want, Not Just for What's Familiar

Think about what you want in a boyfriend, preferably in a moment when you're feeling calm or satisfied. Things get harder to sort out when you're horny, but you can still do the same. Again, it's about mindfulness. Pause before you go out or log on and ask yourself how you're feeling. How was your day? All things being equal, would you rather get off or get together with someone to talk?

If you do go out, imagine yourself as a scuba diver: Stop every hour or so, take a few deep breaths, and ask yourself how you're doing. It's 2 A.M.—are you getting what you came for? If stopping and thinking is precisely what you *don't* want to do, or if you have the feeling that what you're doing is happening in spite of you, that's also something to think about.

2. Right Place, Right Time?

The follow-up to #1, above. If you've been to the same bar thirty times and always felt as though everyone ignored you, then maybe there's another bar—or another type of gay meeting place—that would be better. If you're sick of superficial body culture, is that friend of a friend who always runs down other men's defects at the gym really your ideal date? Will phone sex after an exhausting day make you feel connected or numbed out? You don't always know—every interaction is what you make it, and it's the hope that the next one will be extra satisfying that keeps us all coming back—but notice if you're going to the same place and expecting different results. If you feel like you're completely off the gaydar screen, or can't find anyone whose interested in the things you are, go somewhere "nongay" where you share people's interests. As we so often say: We are everywhere.

3. Put It Out There

If you do have a romantic interest in someone or find him attractive, say it simply and without playing games. This runs counter to the best-selling "Rules" approach to romance (keep him waiting at least two days before calling back, never accept a date for Saturday unless he calls by Wednesday, et cetera), but the gay dating pool is already full of attitude. Delivering a compliment is not the same as a wedding proposal, and no expression of interest, no matter how much of a long shot, is *that* incomprehensible. Even if he's not interested, he's likely to be flattered. If you're the one being approached and you're not interested, make that clear, too, again as simply and unhurtfully as possible. Don't say "maybe" if you mean "no." He'll appreciate the clarity, and your ability to say what you want will attract other men like moths to a flame.

4. Quiet the Critic

So his shoes aren't perfect. So his chest is a little sunken. So he doesn't like Eryka Badu and thinks the Spice Girls are soulful. He's not you. "Learning to put up with loss is essential in order to have a successful relationship," says San Francisco therapist Michael Bettinger, CSW. "Foremost is the loss of the fantasy of the perfect person."

5. This Is Not the End

GMHC runs a periodic workshop called Love Stories, where gay men get together to write about moments of great intimacy. Often no sooner have men recalled a wonderful memory than they recall another feeling, too: the fear that there will be no more like it. Feeling as though we can't sustain something so good is one reason why gay men jump ship even when the sailing seems smooth (see "'Don't I Know You?'" in box on next page). But feelings aren't facts. And if you have broken it off with someone you'd hoped was forever, there is one rule worth remembering: There's hope for another relationship. We *are* everywhere.

SEX AND A LONG-TERM PARTNER

When I go to grab my lover now, he laughs and squirms away. "Stop," he says. "You're tickling."

It's harsh, but hard to argue. Study after study, therapist after therapist, and couple after couple, gay and straight, say the same thing: Stay with someone long enough, no matter how hot, and the flame flickers. Why the erotic edge is dulled by time together is often discussed, with theorists saying your growing sense of closeness makes sex seem like incest, that man desires most those things he's not sure he can have, or that no single story line can plot the rise and fall of many passions. Couples' responses to this challenge are communicated mostly by the roll of a gay eye when monogamy is mentioned, or the sideways humor in straight male jokes of the "Take my wife . . . please!" variety.

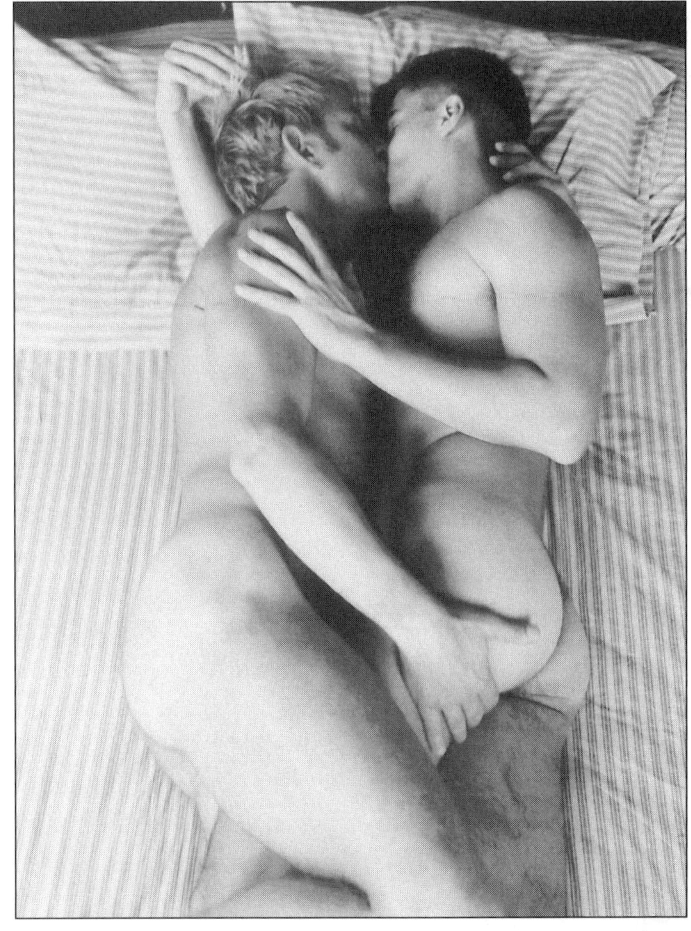

How much sexual activity declines in couples, or what that means, will vary. How sexual was your relationship to start? How much does each person depend on sex, or miss it if it doesn't happen? Factor in what else is going on between you and your partner. "In a couple, what happens in bed is not distinct from what happens outside the bedroom," says Bruce Koff. "Unless there's HIV or some other physiological issue, if someone says they're having sexual issues, I urge them to look at what's happening with their roles in the relationship, with money, or over the breakfast table." The better you know each other, the more sexual relations are relations, involving all of the same issues—power, competition, and dependency—that couples face throughout their life

"DON'T I KNOW YOU?": SPEAKING OUT ON GAY ROMANCE

Excerpted from remarks by Walt Odets, Ph.D., Berkeley psychotherapist, addressing the Gay and Lesbian Medical Association, August 1996

Gay men talk all the time about relationships. One reason for this is that we often feel hopeless about them. There are some obvious reasons that gay men might harbor such hopelessness: the traditional acculturation of men, which makes relationships for all men so difficult, is one. But gay men almost universally share another, even more pervasive experience. This is the experience of disappointing others simply by virtue of who one is.

In being gay, we are not who our parents expected us to be, and most of us thus "fail" in these two early, very important relationships. That failure is most often and most powerfully experienced as the failure of oneself—as "*I* am a disappointment." We may spend the rest of our lives trying to be particularly good and particularly accomplished—by becoming doctors, for instance—but in intimate relationships we fear being really known; the sense of being a disappointment persists tenaciously. The feeling of too many gay men attempting relationships is that a partner will eventually discover who we really are, and everything will be lost. Unfortunately, the fear of being disappointing to others is too easily experienced as the less painful disappointment in others and leaves us too ready to leap from a relationship before our partner finds out who we really are and leaps himself.

Unlike heterosexuals, we are not working on the problems in our relationship in a socially supportive environment. The gay marriage initiative—regardless of how one feels about the details of the issue—has made one thing very clear: American society does not support gay relationships. In fact, gay men have received more support over the last decade for getting sick and dying than for relationships with a recognized, respected social presence. In America, social values nearly prohibit two men on television from touching affectionately, much less kissing. But night after night we broadcast stories of men threatening each other, beating each other, and blowing each other's brains out with guns. We talk about whether this might be "hurting" our children. In truth, it is killing many of us.

We live in a deeply disturbed society that professes "decent family values" but demonstrates a clear preference for fear, hatred, and aggression over love between any two people who are able, against all odds, to muster it. But I have also seen that as gay people—men and women—we live not only with impediments, but with real opportunity to make something authentic, decent, humane, and loving of our lives. We must not let them—the self-hating and the hateful—make us in their image. We can and must seize our opportunities as gay people and make something better—something much better.

together. The tools you use to mend a sexual break also tend to be the same (see "Fighting Fair," in Chapter 12).

If you're at home and in a slow period of sex together, take heart. Couples reinvent themselves as often as Madonna, drawing closer and more distant even as we stay together. Sexually, it's nowhere near as simple as a long, slow fade. Researchers McWhirter and Mattison, surveying a hundred White gay couples in the 1980s, reported sexual rejuvenation—and nonexclusivity (see "Monogamy?" on page 129)—to be common between years five and ten. Men in the second decade, the study found, experienced a decline in frequency of sex together, but an increase in the quality of lovemaking. After twenty years came the renewal phase: greater affection, interest, tenderness, and, sometimes, sex (for more on stages of coupling, see page 503).

Monogamy?

Miles thought he asked my permission, and came back saying what a nice time he'd had with Tony. Somewhere between his mouth and my ears that turned into the sentence "I no longer want to be your lover." That turned into the conversation about what he really wanted from being together. And I realized if Miles was asking me to get a dog or move to Denver, I would entertain it, so why wouldn't I entertain this new way of being in order to give him something he wanted? The deal we made was a trial period and we each reserved—really reserved—the right to say, "I tried this, I can't live with it." Fast-forward to nine years later: I've been a little tramp and he's mostly been a nun. A few years ago I would have said it hasn't hurt our relationship, and now I would say it has actually helped. If I had hit midlife feeling like I still had some sexual oats to sow, I would have felt angry. It's been a way to demonstrate the difference between what we have and what's out there. He's the one I come home to, and coming home to him reminds me of how special he is to me.

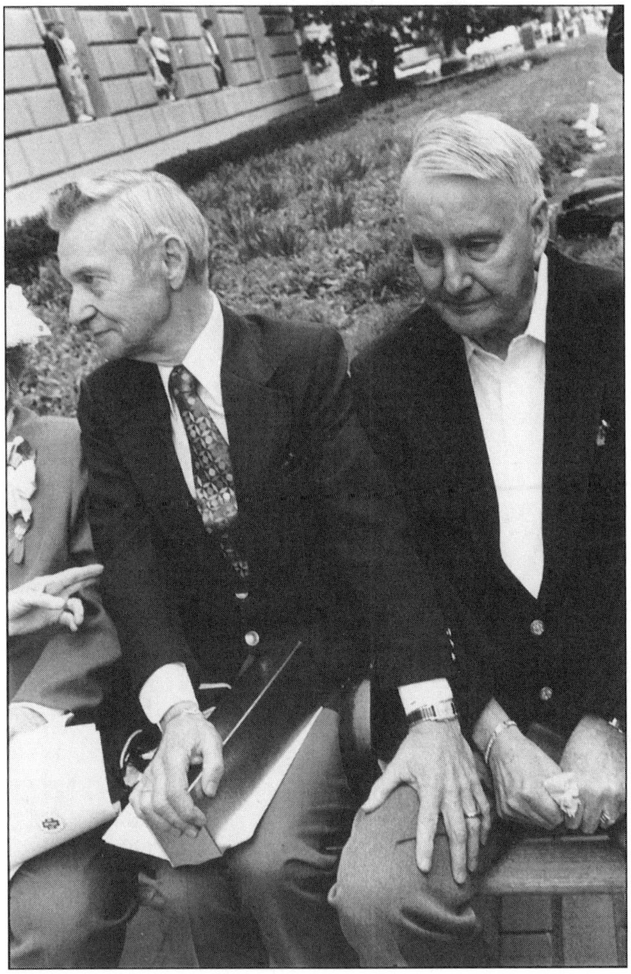

Sex what it used to be? What is? Robert and I are closer than ever, to each other's families, to each other, more able to work out conflicts and share our hopes and our bank account. Eight years later, being home together feels less like we're missing some dance party and more like settling down with a wonderful friend. I have terrible pangs—like "Why would I settle for that little sex?" "Am I really that old?"—but I never want it enough to go outside for it. It would feel like breaking something so private, so tender, that we have together.

We were always honest, but in some ways it was the beginning of the end. I'd go to see someone on Saturday; he'd stay home. I'd sleep in on Sunday, and he'd get up and prowl the beach. None of them were serious boyfriends, but we didn't plan for how much time they'd take away from what we did together. Eventually they edged us out. There wasn't time for all of us.

The "open" heterosexual relationship seems to have gone the way of the be-in and the VW bus, its structure as hazy and hard to grasp as a plume of smoke from a sandalwood incense stick. Married men and women still wander, but they don't talk about it much, and straight society continues to use a system of rewards and punishments to keep the married folks at home. Porn shops are barred from many residential neighborhoods, adultery is regarded as grounds for divorce and loss of child custody, and marriage—heterosexual marriage, that is—is shored up

RELIGHT MY FIRE: TEN SUGGESTIONS FOR LONG-TERM COUPLES

Even after twenty-five years, or especially after twenty-five years, there are some things I just don't feel like I can talk about. So we write each other notes.

Some couples don't mind their mellow sex lives: Once every three weeks may be fine, and they have other ways of bonding. Some keep it lively with frequent, high-pitched fights and "make-up" sex, though that doesn't make a great long-term strategy. If one of you wants more sex than the other, though, or if masturbation alone replaces all shared sexual activity, you may want to relight the fire. How is it done? "If I had a simple or effective answer, I'd be a millionaire sitting in an Italian villa surrounded by beautiful young men," says Dr. Silverstein from his Manhattan office, revealing both the difficulty of the problem and one possible solution: a rich fantasy life. Silverstein and other therapists working with gay men offer some additional suggestions.

1. ***Change the frame.*** "What that means is going to be different from relationship to relationship, but change the way you relate in sex," says Silverstein. "That's not simple. If you do everything the same and just add a sex toy, that's not going to do it. Experiment with ways to change the *structure* of how you interact: the roles you play, the tones of voice you use with each other, how you express your desires." Dr. Jack Morin's hallmarks of arousal (page 98) give you some themes to play with. So do some of the suggestions below.
2. ***Accept the awkwardness.*** "I hate the crap in pop literature: be closer, be adventurous, communicate, then everything will be great," says Dr. Morin of the struggle to stay sexual over the long haul. "If you want to explore this territory where sex and closeness intersect, then you've got to be able to talk about it, and to tolerate the resulting anxiety and awkwardness." Remember how it worked with coming out? Bind up anxieties, or try to pretend they're not there, and they grow powerful. Find ways to talk them through with people you trust—in this case, your partner—and you feel them and then get through them. For hints on how to get through conflict without destroying your relationship, see "Fighting Fair," in Chapter 12.
3. ***Review the sexual communication basics*** (see "Pillow Talk," page 99). Pay particular attention to two: staying flexible and avoiding accusations. Taking about sex can trigger all a couple's most powerful defensive mechanisms. One strategy some couples find helpful is the "trade fair" exercise: One of you talks for five minutes, while the other just listens without challenging or responding. If you're the one listening, really do so, rather than just gritting your teeth and watching the clock. Take him in. After five uninterrupted minutes, switch.
4. ***Share your fantasies.*** What you secretly think about can be a way to recharge your erotic battery, and can give both of you ideas about role playing or other new directions. If you don't have a fantasy, or don't feel comfortable sharing it, try buying a book that contains a number of different ones and reading a favorite aloud to one another. Some couples do the same by renting porn videos, each choosing one they find appealing, though make sure you're focused on sharing rather than getting sucked in by the television. And again, be kind; fantasies are intensely personal. "The one that turns you on like nothing else is probably the most personal one there is, and we're all afraid of being judged, so start with one you're not quite as attached to," suggests Morin.
5. ***Try touch without sex.*** Often, particularly after long periods of no sex, expectations can make everything seem too tense. Break the tension by experimenting with touch that leaves the genitals out of it. One of you agrees to be the "giver" and one the "receiver:" The receiver lies down, naked and newly showered, and the giver spends twenty minutes or so touching, kissing, licking, and rubbing every part of his front and back except ass, penis, and balls. This is a variation of sensate focus, used often to help overcome early ejaculation (see page 176).

6. ***Prioritize sex.*** "If he comes up behind you at the stove and presses himself suggestively into you, think before snapping, 'I'll burn the chicken,'" suggests Michael Shernoff. If you are doing the pursuing, don't be put off by the first flimsy excuse. Turn off the flame under the chicken, and turn up your own.

7. ***Break the routine.*** This is a cliché, but it's no accident that many waning sex lives pick up on vacation (if you're trying to heat it up, think twice about vacations apart). Rather than dinner at home and TV every night, try going out on a date or spending a Saturday night at a hotel. Or try "tricking," getting home from work and suggesting he get down on his knees ASAP. "Lots of us have to break through our own version of the madonna/whore syndrome, the gay equivalent of 'How can I ask the mother of my children to do that nasty thing for me?'" says Shernoff.

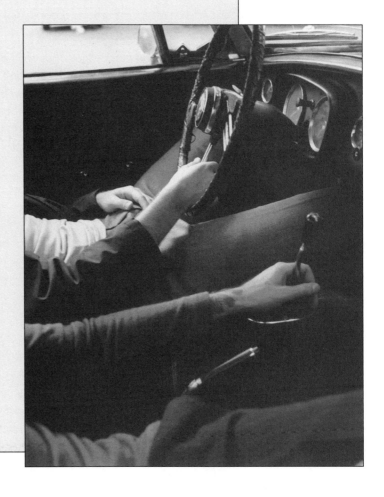

8. ***Invest.*** Diversifying is a good idea for husband hunting, above, but can distract you from your husband once you have one. If you are having sex with other men, or masturbating daily by yourself, save some of that for him. It's no wonder that your boyfriend can't compete with idealized porn images or a mysterious stranger.

9. ***Couples counseling.*** It's not only for people breaking up. If you can afford it, and will both agree to try it, this may help. Choose a therapist neither of you sees individually to keep things simple, and see "Dr. Love," in Chapter 4, for more advice on how to choose.

10. ***Appreciate the edginess.*** "Where you get stuck is often the edge of your growth, the most important thing to work on," says Steve Ball. "No conflict, no growth."

with cold cash: inheritance rights, disability benefits, and health insurance.

Gay men, left to our own devices and temptations, use them liberally, often choosing something besides a one-man strategy. Whether we're more honest about lust or whether our freedom's just another word for nothing left to lose depends on whom you talk to (and often on *his* last experience). Our choices change depending on where we are, what we value, or how easily we find outside opportunities. Some gay men are happily monogamous thirty years later; others say they really wouldn't want to be. How you decide to deal—whether you find fuck buddies fascinating or finally unacceptable, or think monogamy a moral or practical necessity—depends on you both, and how you talk about it.

"The issue isn't monogamy or nonmonogamy for me," says Lidell Jackson, a community activist whose work has included "safe-sex" parties for men of color and helping to found New York City's Lesbian and Gay People of Color Steering Committee. "The issue is whether you're able to examine the paradigm rather than stepping into a role and hoping that somehow you'll

BOYS ON THE SIDE

My partner thought we should go to an orgy. There were many handsome men, and my every orifice was filled. You know what I was doing in my mind? Balancing our checkbook.

I'm in a monogamous relationship now, but I couldn't have done it ten years ago. In my relationship with Jaime, the one before this, I wasn't ready. At the same time, without that earlier experience of slutting around, I don't think I could have settled down.

I was determined that neither of us should have outside sex. I demanded it. It was probably four months before he told me he couldn't keep his end of the bargain, and when he said it, I realized I was wrong: I wanted to be with him even if it wasn't exclusive. By then, though, he'd given up on me in some sense. I'd been out of town, and he'd taken a mutual friend back to my apartment—he had an apartment of his own, mind you—to sleep with him. I could adjust on monogamy. Not on trust.

What's in a name? Nonmonogamy means different things to almost every couple. What marks forbidden territory—what lines you or he cannot cross without the risk of explosion—may change from year to year, boyfriend to boyfriend, or conversation to conversation. Whatever you decide, say men who've tried, be clear, and don't break an agreement you've reached unless you're willing to risk terrible consequences. Renegotiation is okay, and many couples have rules of conduct as full of amendments as a constitution. Among the styles men have found acceptable:

- ***Alone together.*** "I think of it as a Pandora's box, full of issues I'd rather not get into. We don't go outside for sex, or invite others in."
- ***Don't ask, don't tell.*** "Do what you like. Just don't talk about it."
- ***Three's company, two's a problem.*** "As long as we do it together, it's fine."
- ***Anonymously yours.*** "No sex with friends or acquaintances, and no anal sex with anyone else ever. Keep it anonymous if at all."
- ***Hi-fi.*** "For Jack and me, it's fidelity that's important—meaning making sure we're faithful to each other emotionally. Anything that feels too serious outside has to end."
- ***Time travel.*** "No sex with anyone else as long as we're both in the same time zone."
- ***Home alone.*** "Our bedroom is ours alone. What he or I do outside is our business."
- ***Open your heart to me.*** "Our love for each other is top priority, but we do tell each other about outside experiences. The stories are like gifts we bring home for each other."
- ***Together apart.*** "We've been together for thirty years, don't have sex outside, and don't live together. As for flirting and time apart—you might call it emotional promiscuity—that's part of what has kept us alive and well for so long."

magically be satisfied." Examining the choices alone, by the way—as in "He's cute; should I or shouldn't I?"—doesn't mean you've really looked at them. Have you talked it through with your partner, or just left a silence you both interpret as you like? If his going outside would hurt you deeply, or vice versa, don't mistake the silence for agreement. Nor should you go along with it—whatever it is—just because he wants you to. Saying nothing out of fear of conflict rarely pays off in the end. You get the conflict anyway.

For years we did the open relationship thing, but when we moved to Florida, I thought, "No. I want to know that this is going to last forever." That became our priority: letting ourselves, and other people, know that this was it, that we were together, just the way our parents and their parents had been.

As with negotiated safety, whether you're ready to talk about monogamy depends on how honest you think you can be about your disagreements. Do you feel the need to conceal minor "screwups" from him out of fear of retaliation? Do you tell "white lies" about the friend you spent an evening with, what you ate, or the movie you saw? Putting off the monogamy discussion until you've worked on honesty in those other areas may be a healthy response. Sex is hard enough to talk about even when the channels of communication are clear.

Three's Company

David was a friend of George's first, and lived pretty close to us. He spent an evening with us, and we had a nice time; that turned into a summer. He had a car, we didn't; he was crazy about George and me, and we were crazy about him. We slept with one another, separately, together, however it worked out. It ended as warmly as it began, when he got a new boyfriend and moved in with him.

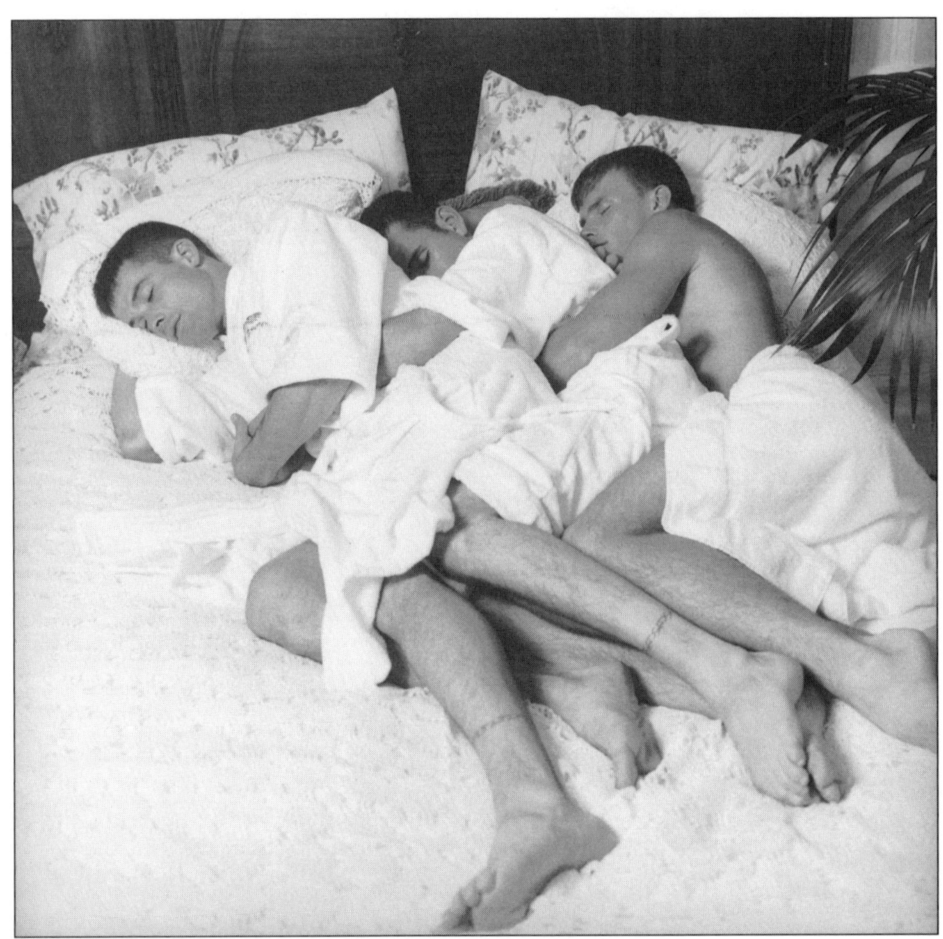

Bringing a third into your bed can add some heat, but don't get burned by poor communication. If you're looking for a threesome to get things going, think through some of the sticky issues beforehand.

• *Who chooses?* Whoever asks, both of you should agree that the time, and man, is right. It helps if he's enthusiastic about both of you as well. "Does that mean you both have to go over and interview him or look at his online profile?" says Carl, sixty-two, with an authority born of experience. "I would have to say yes."

• *Two's an insult.* Unless watching is part of the plan, abandoning your boyfriend for the newer man in bed is bad form. If you're together, be together. "Charles and I try to make eye contact throughout the threesome," says Juan, age thirty-four. "Not to make the other guy feel left out, but just to keep our sense of connection strong."

• *A kiss is just a kiss?* Discuss with your partner what is okay to do and what isn't. Doing something with the third that you refuse to do with your partner is asking for trouble, but other things may also push his pissy button. "Don't ask me why, but it's kissing that gets me most jealous," says Sam, twenty-five years old.

• *When in doubt, cancel.* Reserve the right to call it off at any time. It'll be no fun for anyone if you're just going through the motions. And if your partner's the one to cancel, make sure you support him.

• *HIV?* Will you disclose to your third what both of you already know? Few people enjoy being the only one in the dark.

• *Future shock.* Is it okay for one of you to see the third man by yourself? Even threesomes raise issues of monogamy.

Finally, don't look to adventure as a cure. Making an agreement about monogamy or threesomes doesn't mean one of you won't be wracked by jealousy. And it's no accident that *want* in English means both "to lack" and "to desire." To want what you don't have means you're alive, not that you are necessarily unhappy. No approach known to man—and no man, however wonderful—can fully conquer longing.

FURTHER READING

Berzon, Betty. (1988) *Permanent Partners: Building Gay and Lesbian Relationships That Last*. New York: NAL/Dutton. Clear advice from a seasoned couples counselor.

Chia, Mantak, and Douglas Abrams Arava. (1996) *The Multi-Orgasmic Man*. New York: HarperSanFrancisco. Even has a chapter on gay couples, unusual for a book on Taoist practices.

Davies, Peter M., et al. (1992) *Sex, Gay Men and AIDS*. London, New York, and Philadelphia: Falmer Press. Great thinking from some of Great Britain's leading researchers on gay male sex.

Jacques, Trevor. (1993) *On the Safe Edge: A Manual for SM Play*. Toronto: Whole SM Publishing. A Heloise's Helpful Hints and intellectual introduction for the would-be whipped (or whipper), the leather lads (and daddies), and the bondage-bound.

Lew, Mike. (1990) *Victims No Longer: Men Recovering from Incest and Other Sexual Child Abuse*.
nal testimonies and therapeutic advice.
's Guide: Finding a Man, Making a Home, Building a Life.
in clear, considered prose.
Unlocking the Inner Sources of Sexual Passion and
rennial. Much more than sexual how-to, this book looks
e, and suggests ways to better understand your own.
ve in a Man-Eat-Man World: The Intelligent Guide to Gay
ve. New York: Dell Publishing. Smart and sassy, full of

Rape. New York: Insight Books. Insight, information,
's experiences of rape.
man's Handbook II. New York: Carlyle Communications. A
sequel to the original classic.

CHAPTER 4

Sex Troubles

Sexually Transmitted Diseases (STDs) • Erection Troubles • Erection Solutions • Ejaculation Troubles • Sensate Focus and Other Solutions • Sexual Compulsivity • Dr. Love: Finding a Sex Therapist

Everybody has had the fear that they're not doing it right. But there are times when things seem sexually out of order enough—physically or emotionally—that some kind of help is needed. Often there's a physical alarm: the appearance of a sore or another symptom, or the failure of an erection or an orgasm to appear. Sometimes the warning sign is purely mental, expressed by persistent feelings of anxiety or unhappiness tied to sex, desire, or their lack.

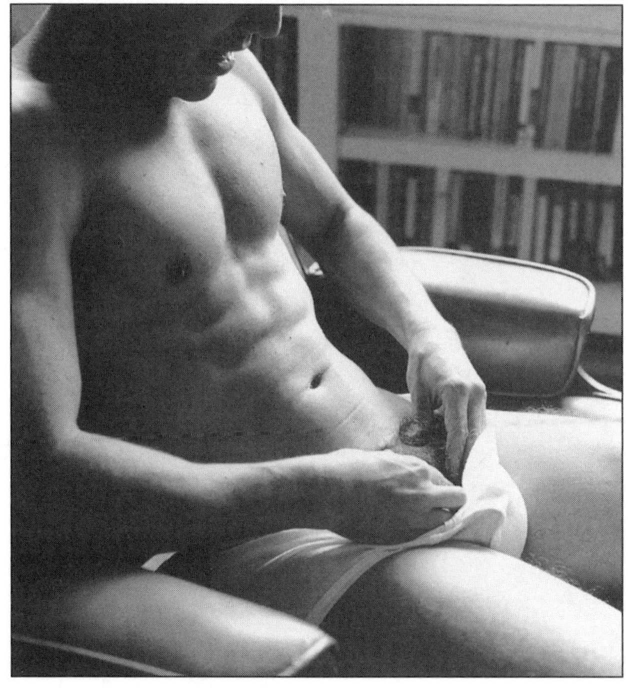

Sex, as the previous chapters have stressed, doesn't usually involve you alone. Neither do sexual problems or the strategies to resolve them. Though it's easy to fall into me-and-my-penis thinking—what am *I* going to do to make my penis harder, how can *I* be better in bed—sexual function is shaped by all kinds of forces, including the way you're relating to your work, your sexual identity, your health, and your particular sexual partners. If you have a problem, getting a reality check from a doctor is a good place to start. If you have a regular or long-term sexual partner, you should also talk to your doctor about how best to include him in the process, whether that's getting him treated for the same sexually transmitted disease (STD) you have or bringing him along for the next discussion of your problem getting a hard-on.

If you don't feel comfortable talking to your doctor, think in the short term about going to a gay health center or a public STD clinic. Page 571 contains a list of some gay health centers. The national STD hotline, reachable at (800) 227-8922, can refer you to public STD clinics that, while not gay-specific, offer lots of experience at little or no cost. Clinics tend to use more on-the-spot diagnoses and fewer expensive tests than private doctors, but they've seen it all and then some. And if your problem is not an STD, they should have referrals to doctors who can help. In the long run, if you can't talk to your doctor openly, think about changing doctors (see Chapter 7 for hints on finding one). What your primary-care physician doesn't know *can* hurt you, especially if it's because you don't dare tell him.

SEXUALLY TRANSMITTED DISEASES (STDs)

Remember herpes? It made the cover of *Newsweek* in the 1980s, and the top of the American sexual anxiety list, until HIV blew it and every other STD out of the water. For gay men especially, the devastation of the last twenty years has swept a whole range of sexual health concerns under the carpet of AIDS consciousness. Understandably so: HIV, with its fatal outcome, long incubation period, prolonged and expensive treatment, and ugly association with stigma and discrimination, is no ordinary STD. But gay men also wrestle regularly with other problems of sexual health, ranging from the inconvenient to the incapacitating. Even mild STDs may in fact be fueling the HIV epidemic that has obscured them (see sidebar).

Nobody, it seems safe to say, likes an STD. At best, as with something like crabs, they're disturbing proof of the primitive: reminders that we are animals with other organisms living on or inside us. At worst, they can land us in bed with acute illness, as with hepatitis, or leave us feeling tainted as we wrestle with a lifetime of flare-ups, as with herpes. They also mean a trip to the doctor for discussion of parts of our lives, or lives of our parts, that most of us would rather not have under the microscope. The idea that the same sex that can bring us excitement can also bring STDs may seem minor after nearly twenty years of AIDS, but it's still painful. "I don't even like to say the word *herpes* aloud in an exam room unless I'm sure, because people panic," says Scott McCallister, MD, former medical director of the Howard Brown Clinic and now a physician in private practice in Chicago.

The tension between health and sex is particularly awkward for gay men, whose sex has long been labeled sick. AIDS, you'll remember, was originally known as "gay-related immune deficiency," or GRID. Some doctors still refer to a cluster of STD-related anal, rectal, and intestinal disorders as "gay bowel syndrome," as if there were something about our sexual orientation that yielded the unpleasant result. It's true that gay men get STDs from one another—and that specific sex acts affect where STDs show up and which ones you get. Just as kids playing in the sandbox can pass along everything from the flu to chicken pox, you can easily pick up an STD from a guy you play with, whether he's your one true love or someone whose name you don't know. But contrary to the hype, there's nothing any more inherently gay about STD transmission than there is in little Bobby's getting a case of the sniffles. Some STDs are not much more of a health issue, either. "It's important to get beyond the oh-my-God-I-knew-gay-sex-was-dirty reaction to recognize that different STDs have different consequences," offers Dan William, MD, of New York City. "Hepatitis B can cause serious, lifetime liver damage. Crabs are nothing more than a venereal cold."

Dr. William is among the many, however, who believe the gay nation would do well to review the ABCs of STDs. A 1997 report from the Centers for Disease Control showed a 74 percent increase in the incidence of gonorrhea among some gay and bisexual men. Herpes rates among the American public, including gay men, are now 30 percent higher than they were in the late 1970s. Hepatitis A has been epidemic among gay communities from Seattle to New York over the last two decades, and rates of hepatitis B are sharply higher among people with multiple sexual partners, including gay men. "It would be nice to believe that we have learned the lessons of history," says Dr. William, who was among those in the early 1970s who started New York's Gay Men's Health Project to raise awareness of and testing for STDs among gay men. "Instead, we seem to be repeating them."

DOUBLE TROUBLE: STDS AND HIV

Think of it as a safer-sex fact that got lost: Certain STDs help fuel the spread of AIDS. If you're HIV-negative, STDs that inflame your rectum or urethra make unsafe sex with a positive man even riskier, because the same white blood cells that are drawn to the area to fight the STD are those that are most vulnerable to infection with HIV. If you have HIV, those same STD-related inflammations can boost the amount of virus in your semen, making you far more infectious. STD-related inflammations in the urethra, for example, may increase the amount of HIV in your cum by more than tenfold. HIV is also highly concentrated in the liquid that comes from sores caused by herpes or syphilis.

Whether certain STDs are cofactors for AIDS, speeding progression of the illness, has yet to be definitively proven. It's clear, though, that the combination of HIV and STDs means short-term increases in levels of HIV, as well as other medical complications. Warts can run out of control when you have HIV, and herpes don't respond as well to treatment. Even an easily cured STD such as scabies can turn into a chronic, highly contagious condition if your immune system is weak.

Among those ignored lessons is the fact that information and STD testing alone are not enough. The following section outlines some of the most common STDs that face gay men, but remember: You don't get STDs from sex, you get them from another person. As with HIV, one part of prevention is thinking about your partner, and that means more than "nice smile, good body." Would he be likely to tell you if he had an STD, or be in touch enough with his health to know? Do you know him well enough to say? Would you do things differently if you knew for sure that he had, say, herpes? Or, if you're the one with an STD, think about what it would take to protect him: a conversation, a condom, deciding to kiss and call it a night?

Some STDs are mild enough that you may write them off as a necessary hazard in the search for satisfaction. That's different from tuning out the information in the first place and freaking out later. Learning about STDs can go a long way toward helping you grapple with a delicate doctor's visit, a sex partner's panic, or your own anxiety (see box on page 140).

I've Got You, Babe: Telling Him You Have an STD

So I said it: "I've got herpes, and though I don't think I'm contagious, I want you to know." He said, "It's worth the risk," and kissed me. It was the beginning of a wonderful night.

You know those stories where a straight couple breaks up because she finds a long hair in the bed, and it's not hers? That's what crabs have been like in my life.

First, a crash course in artful dodging. You can get a parasite from mountain streams, not just mouthing ass. The viruses that cause warts and herpes can be inside you for years without showing themselves. Nongonococcal urethritis can flare up in only one member of a monogamous couple. Hepatitis A can come from seafood, salad, or a bad glass of water as well as oral-fecal contact. It's possible. Really.

Excuses aside, though, telling your sexual partner when you have an STD is important, and not only because it opens conversations about where else you may have wandered. Gonorrhea

WHAT AN STD, OR FEAR OF ONE, CAN TELL YOU ABOUT . . .

If you often find yourself wracked with worry, absolutely convinced that some organism has found its way onto your body or into your system, you're not alone. "I've seen a lot of 'worried well' at the clinic," says Scott McCallister, MD, "men who are afraid that they've caught something and just need to be reassured. Others, convinced that there's something 'in their penis,' may spend so much time tugging on it that the trauma alone will create a drip." While repeated checkups don't hurt—many STDs have no discernible symptoms in men—self-examination may be a more telling test. Ask yourself what an STD, or fear of one, can tell you about . . .

. . . YOUR CHOICES

Try to separate out your feelings about an STD from those you have about where you might have gotten it. Is it the idea of gonorrhea of the throat that's making you upset, or the idea that in retrospect he didn't seem worth getting it from? Are you freaking out about the fact of crabs, or about what having them might mean for your sense of self-respect or for your long-term relationship?

. . . YOUR LONG-TERM RELATIONSHIP

Often, say doctors at STD clinics, it's guilt about having strayed, rather than symptoms, that send men to the clinic for a checkup. Is it a communicable disease you're afraid of, or just communication? Waiting until you really do have an STD is probably not the best time to explain to your life partner that you're uncomfortable with your monogamy agreement (see "Monogamy?" in Chapter 3).

. . . YOUR HIV RISK

STD anxiety can often be a stand-in for its more powerful shadow, HIV anxiety. Some of that is well placed. If you find yourself with rectal gonorrhea, for example, it means you've also been at risk for serious infections such as hepatitis B and HIV. Getting tested for and vaccinated against hepatitis A and B, and taking an HIV test, are highly recommended (see Chapter 7). So is reading the next paragraph.

. . . YOUR PATTERNS

If you find yourself seeing doctors repeatedly for the same STD or fear of it, awareness may be as important to your health as antibiotics. Dr. William, for example, estimates that eight of ten men he treats for the parasites transmitted by rimming are men he's already treated for the same condition. Getting three STDs in as many months, or getting ones transmitted in the same way as HIV, should mean rethinking your sexual safety. Read the last part of Chapter 2 for ways to do that, which include using a condom, reducing the number of your sexual partners, or talking more to the partners you have.

and syphilis can be cured quickly, and without complications, if they're treated early. Vaccination can help prevent hepatitis A, even after exposure. Treating your long-term partner can break the ongoing back-and-forth cycle that keeps some STDs going for weeks longer than they should. Even if he was a one-night ticket to nothing special, letting him know is a way of helping him, and yourself, grapple with the fact that sex has consequences. Think of it as a step toward undoing the possibility of an unpleasant surprise, a way gay men can care for each other, or a simple application of "do for others what you'd like them to do for you."

STD BASICS: WAYS TO REDUCE RISK OF STDS AND THEIR COMPLICATIONS

SEEK PROMPT TREATMENT

If you have any common symptoms of STDs—discharge from your penis or anus, itching or burning of either body part, pain or stinging when you urinate, and sores, blisters, or rashes on your genitals or in your mouth—go right to the doctor. Some of these things can come from the ordinary wear and tear of sex, but over-the-counter creams and ointments, or long delays, can complicate diagnosis. "Lots of men come in and say, 'I had a sore here four or five days ago—what do you think it was?'" says Ken Mayer, MD, of Brown University. See a doctor while it's fresh on your skin, not in your mind.

THE MORE THE RISKIER

As with HIV, it's not technically how many men you have, it's what *they* have and what you do with them. Most STDs are a lot more easily transmitted than HIV, though, and the statistics are clear: The more partners you have, the less likely you are to be STD-free. It's no accident that STD rates among gay men are highest when we're younger and experimenting. Again, you may decide it's worth it. Still, when it comes to STD prevention, multiple partners means multiple risks.

GET VACCINATED FOR HEPATITIS A AND B

You'll see this repeatedly throughout this book, because it bears repeating. If you haven't had hepatitis A or B, and you're sexually active, go get vaccinated (see page 298). The process, completed over the course of six months, can be costly—but not compared to the weeks of lost work, serious liver damage, and worse that may be the alternative.

DON'T FORGET CONDOMS

Short of STD-free monogamy, condoms during anal sex remain one of the best ways to protect yourself from a number of STDs. Using latex and other risk-reduction strategies for sucking and rimming (see Chapter 2) can further enhance protection.

The following are some real-life suggestions of what to say from men who've done it. Take one or make up your own.

- "I didn't mean for this to be your problem, but I just found out that I have warts, and you should probably get tested, too."
- "I just got an outbreak of herpes, and I know it's awkward, but I figured if I was in your situation I'd rather know than not know. If you begin feeling tingly or like you have the flu, that could be what it is, and there's medicine to help control it."
- "I just found out that I have hepatitis A. I'm not sure how I got it, but it can be sexually transmitted, and my doctor suggested that you might want to go in for a shot to protect yourself."

Some states have programs to force the issue, requiring doctors to give your name to the health department if you have gonorrhea, syphilis, or certain other infectious diseases. The state health department in turn asks you for the names and numbers of recent sexual partners

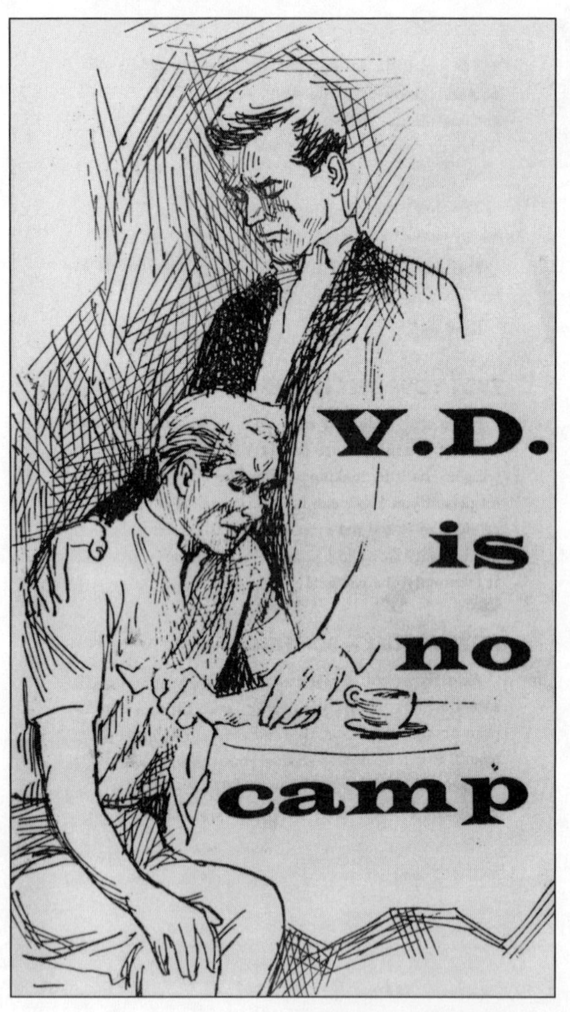

so that they can call them and let them know—without naming you—that they may have been exposed. Other states have voluntary versions of the same partner notification process, where they call partners for you if you ask them to do so. Make sure in either case that you ask them how long a backlog they are working with: Some health departments are running months behind, making it a better idea for you to do the work of disclosure yourself.

Local STD clinics, or your local health department, can advise you about laws in your area. They are sometimes less than iron-clad in practice: Many private doctors find themselves "too busy" to pass your name along to the health department, and some STD clinics will see you anonymously, or allow you to give any name you want at the desk. "Even if you are contacted by the health department, you're unlikely to be arrested or fined if, for instance, you can't remember the names of your contacts," says Bill Rubenstein, a professor of law at the University of California, Los Angeles. Think seriously, though, about how helpful it can be to find out about an STD, and how much *you'd* rather hear it from someone you slept with than from some scary-sounding public health official.

The full spectrum of sexually transmitted diseases can fill volumes. The following—grouped roughly by mode of transmission, and then in descending order of seriousness—are among the most common that confront gay men.

Skin Surfers: Herpes, Genital Warts, Molluscum, Crabs, and Scabies

Condoms definitely help with herpes and warts, but these invaders aren't always covered by latex barriers. Crabs, scabies, and molluscum aren't contained by condoms at all. Here's where you need mutual communication and consideration, as well as regular condom use.

HERPES

Description

Herpes is from the Greek word meaning "to creep," because herpesviruses—and often their unpleasant effects—seem to keep creeping back. Some herpesviruses—such as Epstein-Barr virus (better known as EBV) or cytomegalovirus (CMV)—are so easily passed that the vast majority of gay men have been exposed to them in childhood and suffer no ill effects as long as their immune systems remain intact. Others, such as genital herpes, you get from sex.

Most people who talk about herpes are referring to herpes simplex virus (HSV), the most well known of herpesviruses. HSV comes in two types: HSV I, which generally causes the cold sores that appear in or around your mouth or nose, and HSV II, which usually causes similar sores on the anus or genitals. Though people refer to them as oral and genital herpes, both viruses can and do cause sores above and below the waist.

The Centers for Disease Control estimates that forty-five million Americans, one in five of us over age twelve, is infected with HSV. Among Black Americans, the estimate is a staggering 46 percent. Another statistic is simultaneously soothing and scary: Fewer than 10 percent of those infected report experiencing symptoms, and the overwhelming majority do not know that they have HSV. If you do get herpes, you won't necessarily be covered in sores. If you do get sores, it doesn't necessarily mean he knew and was hiding something.

Incubation Period

Usually from two to twenty days, though you can carry around the virus for years before showing symptoms.

Symptoms

A few days (or even just hours) before any lesions appear, you may feel an itching or tingling sensation around the penis, anus, or mouth. Sores—from tiny red pimples to large raw blisters—tend to erupt shortly thereafter, appearing wherever you made contact with the virus: penis, anus, rectum, throat, on or around lips and nostrils. Touching sores can spread them to other parts of your body, including, rarely, your eyes. Herpes can also cause systemic effects, such as fever, muscle aches, and other flulike symptoms. Sores last anywhere from two to seven weeks, with the pain usually peaking at week two.

Subsequent outbreaks, if you have them, are usually milder. "You may have outbreaks every month or two at first, then go to once or twice a year, or they may never come back again," says Peter Hawley, MD, medical director of the Whitman-Walker Clinic in Washington, DC. Often, prodromal symptoms—itching or burning at the site of the infection, or feeling as though you're getting the flu—will warn you of an impending outbreak.

How Doctors Diagnose It

If you haven't fiddled with them much or waited long, visual diagnosis is usually enough. Herpes can also be diagnosed by scraping, by culture, or by blood test.

Treatment

There's no cure for herpes, but three antiviral medications—acyclovir (brand name Zovirax, but also generic), famciclovir (brand name Famvir), and valacyclovir (brand name Valtrex)—can all help lessen symptoms, severity of the outbreak, and contagiousness. All are available in pill form, though serious cases may require intravenous administration.

Those drugs can also be used to help prevent or lessen future episodes. Some men have had success taking them as soon as they feel the itching or burning that warns of an outbreak, while others take them daily. Since they aren't cheap (or always covered by insurance), check with your doctor and weigh the costs and benefits. "If you're only having small outbreaks once a year," says Dr. Hawley, "there's no sense in taking antivirals all year, every day. If you're getting monthly outbreaks with dozens of sores and terrible pain, it might be worthwhile to try to suppress them."

How You Get It

Usually from contact with sores, or with a hand that's had contact with sores. The mucous membranes of your anus and mouth are especially vulnerable to infection. With people who are chronically infected, doctors suspect that asymptomatic viral shedding, perhaps from sores too small to see, may be responsible for transmission when no other symptoms are visible.

How You Keep from Getting or Giving It

If you see (or have) sores, call sex off: Condoms work if they cover all sores, but they may miss some. For that matter, don't have sex if you have the itching or burning that precedes an outbreak, since that's when you are most likely to be contagious. Taking antivirals may make you less infectious. If you're chronically infected—even if your skin looks clear—condoms for anal and oral sex are advisable.

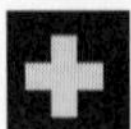 **HIV Connection?**

People with HIV frequently get bigger, longer-lasting herpes sores, and have more of them. HIV is also highly concentrated in the sores. If your immune system is weak, HSV can spread through the bloodstream, with lesions appearing in the esophagus, colon, lungs, brain, or elsewhere. Internal herpes lesions are diagnosed through biopsy and are often serious enough to require intravenous treatment and hospitalization. Herpes resistant to acyclovir can be treated with foscarnet (brand name Foscavir). If you're HIV-positive and have severe lesions that won't go away after treatment, herpes is considered an AIDS-defining event. If you are HIV positive, check with a doctor about taking medication to prevent such outbreaks.

OTHER HERPES VIRUSES

These other viruses in the herpes family are particularly important to know about if you are over age sixty-five or HIV-positive.

***Varicella zoster* Virus**

This herpesvirus, which causes shingles and chicken pox, is not transmitted primarily through sex; most of us get it in childhood. The virus stays for years in the spinal nerves, and when reactivated travels along those pathways to erupt into sores or a rash on one side of the body. Other symptoms include sharp pain, fever, headaches, and fatigue for the two to three weeks that sores remain. About 15 percent of people continue to experience pain even after the sores have disappeared. Treatment with HSV medications (see page 143) can relieve symptoms, reduce the length of an outbreak, and cut down on pain. Once you have shingles, they're contagious until the sores have cleared.

If you're HIV-negative and have never had chicken pox, a vaccination can protect you. If you're HIV-positive, as of this writing, the vaccine's not safe. A shot with *Varicella zoster* immunoglobulin may reduce your risk of infection if you get it within ninety-six hours of exposure. Shingles are most common in older people and in those with immune suppression. If you are under sixty-five, don't know your HIV status, and get shingles, consider an HIV test (see page 302).

Cytomegalovirus (CMV)

As many as 90 percent of gay adults are thought to have been exposed to this herpesvirus, which is passed through unprotected oral or anal sex when one person is newly

COLD (SORE) COMFORT: SELF-HELP FOR HERPES OUTBREAKS

The pain and itching from a herpes episode can be pretty intense. Don't use over-the-counter anti-itch medications with hydrocortisone, which could make the sores worse. Sores will heal faster if you take warm baths with baking soda three to five times a day and keep them clean and dry. Try a blow dryer on the lowest setting after you get out of the tub and sprinkle a little cornstarch or baking soda on the sores once you've dried off. For sores on your genitals, wear loose-fitting cotton boxers. Topical application of licorice root extract may also help—check with your doctor or herbalist.

Stress, cold wind, and sunburn are among the factors thought to trigger recurrences of herpes, and reducing your exposure to them can help keep you outbreak-free. Nutritionists also advise against foods that contain the amino acid arginine (cereals, chocolates, grains, and nuts, among others) as well as vegetables in the nightshade family, such as tomatoes, peppers, and eggplants. Foods containing lysine (including beans, chicken, eggs, and fish) are said to prevent outbreaks, and some people have also had good experiences preventing or treating herpes by taking lysine pills. Check with your doctor. Finally, there are many support groups for sufferers of herpes. Check the STD hot line, (800) 227-8922, or search online for one near you.

infected. While it is suspected in some cases of chronic-fatigue-like syndrome, CMV causes few or no symptoms in most healthy adults. Its complications in people with HIV can range from blindness to pneumonia to inflammation of the brain or ulcers in the intestine. As with HIV, there are different strains of CMV, so even if you already have it, it's a good idea to use condoms to prevent reinfection.

Epstein-Barr Virus (EBV)

Infection with the Epstein-Barr virus is better known as mononucleosis, or the "kissing disease," since kissing is one way to get it. Again, 90 percent of us have been exposed to it by the time we reach adulthood, though far fewer manifest symptoms. EBV is thought to be the cause of a mouth infection, oral hairy leukoplakia, in people with HIV, and is associated with, though not known definitively to cause, HIV-related non-Hodgkin's lymphoma. It can also cause fatigue, swollen glands, and other symptoms in both HIV-negative and HIV-positive adults.

Human Herpesvirus 8

Also known as KSHV, this virus, recently discovered, is a herpesvirus suspected to be a sexually transmitted cause of Kaposi's sarcoma (KS). KS is a cancer that appears most frequently in older men of Mediterranean extraction as well as those with compromised immune systems. If you have HIV, getting KS is an AIDS-defining event (see Chapter 9). Studies in 1999 showed as many as 15 to 20 percent of gay men to be infected with HHV-8. Popper use, a history of other STDs, and higher numbers of sexual partners were all associated with infection.

GENITAL WARTS

Description

Genital warts are caused by a virus known as the human papilloma virus, or HPV. Like genital herpes, they usually appear below the waist, but can also develop in the mouth and on the lips and face. They're even more common than herpes, and like herpes, they often recur. Since HPV remains in your body even after a wart goes away, your first outbreak is unfortunately unlikely to be your last.

Genital warts grow easily in many places: on the shaft of the penis or under the foreskin, around the anus or inside the anal canal, on the skin underneath your pubic hair, or on your inner thighs.

Incubation Period

Warts have an incubation period ranging anywhere from several weeks to several years.

Symptoms

External warts on your penis are the ones most easily seen and felt. They're not usually painful or itchy, and often look like small, flesh-colored bumps on white skin, or especially dark bumps on skin that's darker. Though it's harder to see warts on your own anus, you may feel them at the outside of the hole or on your perineum: clusters of small, rough, cauliflower-like growths called condyloma acuminata, or in old English medical books, "figs" (clearly the English could see the poetic in anything).

Internal warts are usually not visible to the one who has them. Nor can you always feel them, though you may well notice their effects: pain, itching, or bleeding after bowel movements or sex.

How Doctors Diagnose It

Visual diagnosis, sometimes with the help of a little vinegar, which turns the warts white, confirms their presence. If you have external warts, always make sure to have the doctor look inside to see if there are internal anal warts as well—otherwise you may be "reseeding" yourself with every bowel movement, and have to face the doctor's office and a sore rectum for months. "I've seen men who, six months and twenty thousand dollars later, never got rid of their warts because their dermatologist didn't use an anoscope," says Lester Gottesman, MD, a colon and rectal surgeon at St. Luke's–Roosevelt Hospital in New York City. If warts are internal and you're HIV-positive, a doctor may biopsy the warts to see if the virus causing them is among the varieties associated with anal cancer (see box on next page).

Treatment

Genital warts can only be treated under a doctor's supervision. Do not use over-the-counter wart medications on your delicate penis or ass! If the warts are external, small, and easily accessible, you have a couple of doctor-supplied, home-applied alternatives. Most common is a cream called podofilox (brand name Condylox) that burns the wart away (along with any other skin it touches, so be careful). Applying zinc oxide or Vaseline on surrounding skin before you put on Podofilox can cut down on burning. Another cream, imiquimod (brand name Aldara), enhances immune function, so warts may slowly disappear over the course of sixteen weeks. Neither cream works well for large warts, or for ones inside your anus, rectum, or mouth. For those, you need a series of doctor's visits.

Doctors get rid of warts in a variety of ways: by burning them with trichloroacetic acid

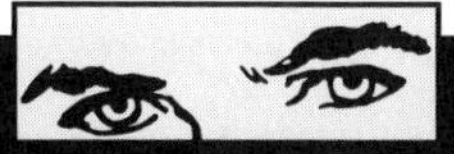

TURNING A GAY GAZE ON PAP SMEARS

Certain strains of HPV, the cause of anal warts, have also been linked to anal cancer. Exceedingly rare as that disease is (at last estimate it affects only about thirty-five of every hundred thousand gay men), a number of experts are seeing growths in the gay male anus that they suspect may signal a rise in the disease. "Anal cancer is already more common among gay men than cervical cancer was among women before routine screening and examination," says Joel Palefsky, MD, whose studies of HPV and the anal health of hundreds of men in San Francisco puts him in the vanguard of the gay rear end. In addition, says Palefsky, an associate professor in the Department of Laboratory Medicine at the University of California, San Francisco, careful examination and follow-up show that many men have precancerous cells in the anus that follow stages made familiar—and ominous—through the study of cervical cancer. HIV-positive men, in particular, have proved five times more likely to have the "high-grade" cellular growth (dysplasia) that may be associated with an increased risk of cancer.

Palefsky and a handful of other specialists are recommending to men with HIV procedures similar to the ones that have helped lower cervical cancer rates among women: Pap smears (a quick and painless swab of the anus); visual examination; biopsies of warts to see if there is also high-grade dysplasia mixed in; and, if necessary, surgery to remove abnormal tissue. Even as he makes the suggestion, Palefsky adds a warning: Most places in America have neither doctors trained in anal Pap smear administration and interpretation nor surgeons skilled at removing precancerous tissue. Having an unskilled surgeon could leave you with a narrowing of the anal canal and serious postoperative discomfort, not to mention a bill some insurers may refuse to cover.

A number of other experienced doctors and surgeons raise a bigger question: whether the slim odds of getting anal cancer really justify the pain and expense of having precancerous cells cut or burned away. As with the prostate-specific antigen test (see page 351) and a number of other diagnostic tests, the ability to measure something doesn't mean people agree on when it's useful to do so or on what to do if you receive an abnormal result. "Among my patients, removing all precancerous tissue would in some cases mean removing unjustifiably large portions of the rectum," says Dr. Gottesman, who favors "watchful waiting" to detect actual cancer over surgical intervention for dysplasia. "Very few men I've seen in ten years of practice have developed anal cancer. The quantity of the damage isn't worth the theoretical risk." Dan William, whose practice has included gay men for most of the last two decades, tends to agree. "In twenty years of practice, I've seen only three cases of anal cancer, all operable," says William. "I'm not sure that warrants Pap smears and preventive surgery for everyone."

All doctors concerned acknowledge that we don't yet have studies showing whether anal cancer is on the rise now that men with HIV are living longer, or whether removal of dysplasia will help. Palefsky, now collaborating on one such study, points in the meanwhile to the example set by our sisters in women's health: Cervical cancer rates, never much higher than those of anal cancer in gay men, have dropped more than fourfold as a result of the adoption of annual Pap smears as a national standard. New York City surgeon Stephen Goldstone, MD, offers a simpler analysis: "If I had something that might become malignant inside me," he says, "I'd want it out."

(TCA), podophyllin (brand name Podocon-25), electrocauterization, or laser therapy; by freezing them off with liquid nitrogen (known as cryotherapy); or by surgically removing them with a blade. An experienced eye and hand can make a big difference, so make sure to ask your doctor about his or her previous experience, as well as whatever help with pain—such as application of a local anesthetic—he or she can provide. "With use of anesthetic, there's no reason for removal of anal warts to be excruciating," says Karl Beutner, MD, an associate clinical professor of dermatology at the University of California at San Francisco, though many gay men's experience says otherwise.

The frequency with which anal warts recur (as often as 30 percent of the time, even after surgery), makes their removal an ordeal for nearly everyone who has experienced them. Persistent warts may be helped by injection of interferon into the base of the lesion after the wart has been removed by conventional means. The treatment is expensive, may make you feel depressed or as though you have the flu, and tends to be less effective for people with CD4-cell counts under 200. In the self-help—and clinically untested—arena, some men have reported success with vitamin E oil, squeezed from capsules and applied daily to external warts for a few weeks.

Even STD doctors tend to use only one method of removal, so if you haven't seen results in three to six visits, says Beutner, see an experienced surgeon or dermatologist. Whoever the practitioner, it's best to make follow-up visits as often as once every week or two until the warts are gone, and to go back for frequent checkups, including internal examination, to make sure they stay gone. If you have large warts removed, it may take several weeks or longer for the wounds left by the surgery to heal. Make sure your doctor gives you the pain medication you need.

How You Get It

Skin-to-skin contact with the warts of another, the fluid they produce, or conceivably with a towel or other surface that has recently touched a wart can transmit HPV. The wart-causing virus can be carried inside you by any penetration, not necessarily just by intercourse; a finger or dildo can also do it.

How You Keep from Getting or Giving It

As with herpes, what you see is what you don't want to get. If someone has visible warts, pass on unprotected sex involving that body part. Also as with herpes, condoms are a definite help but not a fail-safe method: There may be lesions condoms don't cover, and HPV can be carried in fluid or by the touch of a finger. If you're playing with someone's ass, be sure to wash your hands before touching your own, and vice versa.

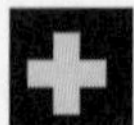

HIV Connection?

HIV often worsens a range of skin problems, warts among them. HIV-positive people are more likely to develop more genital warts, more frequent recurrences of warts, and larger and faster-growing warts. If your immune system is weak, warts can also appear anywhere on the body, including on your hands or inside your mouth. Recent studies are also raising the possibility that people with both HIV and HPV are at significantly higher risk for anal cancer (see page 147).

MOLLUSCUM CONTAGIOSUM

Description

Caused by a virus like herpesvirus or HPV, molluscum usually appears on the thighs, lower abdomen, or buttocks, though it can also show up on the face, anus, genitals, or anywhere else.

Incubation Period

Growths appear anywhere from one week to six months after exposure.

Symptoms

Molluscum lesions are smooth, waxy bumps, about three to five millimeters in diameter (a bit smaller than the head of a tack). They are often flesh-colored or whitish, but can be gray-white, yellow, or pink. They are usually painless, do not itch or ooze, and usually have a dent or crater in the center.

How Doctors Diagnose It

Visual inspection or biopsy usually suffices for a diagnosis.

Treatment

Trying to pop or scrape off molluscum yourself can make it worse. Doctors remove the lesions through cryotherapy (freezing with liquid nitrogen), electrocauterization (burning with electric current), or surgical scraping. "Liquid freezing tends to leave discolored spots, particularly on dark skin," says New York City dermatologist Jeffrey Roth, who favors surgical scraping as the most effective method. "Scraping's painful, but the scabs heal within a week, and tend to leave less of a trace."

Topical treatments similar to those used for small genital warts can sometimes be effective for small growths. Some people also report success with the prescription antiacne liquid tretinoin (brand name Retin-A), the anti-CMV medication cidofovir (brand name Vistide), and injections of interferon. As with warts, keep going back until the lesions are gone, since it's easy for them to recur and multiply.

How You Get It

Molluscum is caught through skin-to-skin contact. Children pass molluscum to each other while playing, as do adults. You can also spread molluscum by scratching yourself, or, when it's on your face, through nicking the bumps while shaving.

How You Keep from Getting or Giving It

Avoiding contact with the lesions will prevent you from getting or giving it.

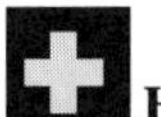 **HIV Connection?**

Men without HIV may get as many as ten or twenty molluscum lesions; people with weak immune systems can get dozens or hundreds. "I've gone to the dermatologist every two to three weeks for the past four years," says one positive man who has tried liquid freezing, scraping, and burning.

Anti-HIV medications that reduce viral levels in the blood can sometimes help to clear molluscum. As with warts, seeing a dermatologist with HIV experience is advisable for persistent cases: Specialists can offer a range of treatment options, as well as diagnosis of more serious infections such as histoplasmosis or pneumocystis, which are sometimes mistaken for molluscum by less experienced practitioners.

CRABS (PUBIC LICE, *PEDICULOSIS PUBIS*)

I'll never forget it: I went to spend the night at my grandmother's, and a few days later I realized I had crabs. And I just kept thinking, "Oh, my God, what if I gave them to her from the towel?" But I just couldn't bring myself to call her up and say, "Granny, there's something I think you ought to know. . . ."

Description

Crabs are gray, flat, and about a millimeter long, which means that they are visible to the naked eye. They live off your blood, so when they've eaten they change from their normal pale gray color to a dark red. They look like tiny crabs, of course, and nestle in warm, hairy areas such as your groin or armpits, barely moving once they get settled. It is easier to see their eggs, waxy white specks attached to the base of individual pubic hairs. These are called nits, and they are usually so well cemented that they often need to be removed with a very fine comb or between two fingernails (hence the term *nit-picking*). Take the time to do a thorough job, as missing a few eggs can cause reinfestation.

Incubation Period

Usually five days after you've been bitten. But if someone you've slept with in the last few days tells you he's got crabs, start looking for them anyway. The sooner you get to them, the easier they are to get rid of.

Symptoms

Itching, itching, and more itching, though some people are more allergic to the bites than others. Itching is generally concentrated in warm, hairy places: your crotch, your ass, and maybe your thighs and/or lower abdomen. Pubic lice have claws uniquely suited to grab pubic and underarm hair, though not the finer hair on your head. The exception is facial hair: Crabs can nest in eyelashes, eyebrows, and beards, crawling up your body or taking the shorter route from his pubes to your beard or mustache if the conditions are right.

How Doctors Diagnose It

Doctors use visual inspection to diagnose crabs.

Treatment

Over-the-counter shampoos with permethrin, such as Nix or RID, may kill crabs, with two applications spaced a week apart. There's also the prescription favorite, lindane (the lotion formerly known as Kwell). You can't use shampoo or lotion around your eyes, though—in the case of a colony on your brows or eyelashes, coat them with Vaseline and they'll suffocate. You'll also have to wash your clothes, sheets, towels, and everything else that touches your body in hot water, or put them in sealed plastic bags and let them sit for ten days (to allow any stray eggs to hatch and die). Perhaps most important, if you share a bed or toweling with another, treat your partner. Passing critters back and forth is a common cause of recurrence. And unless you're a yogi, he can get down there and look for eggs far better than you.

A word on after-crab syndrome: Crabs are so creepy, literally, that it's common to imagine the tiny things crawling on you for weeks afterward. That in turn causes overdousing for delousing, with the harsh shampoos causing dry skin, flaking, and itching in your groin that makes you think you're still infested. Most recurrences are the result of not covering all your body, or your boyfriend's, in the first week. If you do that and can't find any eggs or any crabs, they're probably gone.

How You Get It

Both crabs and scabies can be transmitted through everything from toilet seats and towels to a quick romp with Mr. Right Now, though the romantic impulse to stay the night might be the best way to guarantee an extended visit from some new "friends."

How You Keep from Getting or Giving It

There's no real way to keep from getting crabs, aside from never rubbing your naked body over someone else's, never sharing a towel, and never having a slumber party.

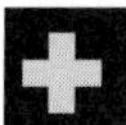 **HIV Connection?**

Crabs don't pass HIV from one person to another, and they like your blood just fine whether it has HIV in it or not.

SCABIES

Description

If you're itching like mad but can't see any sign of crabs, and especially if the itching is concentrated in your hands or groin, then you may have scabies. Known as the "itch mite," its discovery in the seventeenth century made scabies the first disease to be linked to a known cause.

Mites are much smaller than crabs, measuring about the size of the period at the end of this sentence. Instead of attaching to the surface of the skin the way crabs do, scabies burrow underneath to lay their eggs. The paths traveled by burrowing mites appear as short, wavy lines, usually limited to the webbed skin between the fingers or on the wrists, elbows, or penis.

Incubation Period

If you've never had them before, it takes about ten days for your skin to develop an allergic reaction to the presence of the mites. If it's your second time around, or more, then you'll itch faster.

Symptoms

Small bumps or blisters often come along with burrows. Unlike crabs, *everyone* who has scabies has some degree of itching, which tends to be most intense at night or after a hot bath. If left untreated, scabies will become a chronic condition, which is why they got the nickname "seven-year itch."

How Doctors Diagnose It

The skin problems caused by scabies are easily mistaken for many other conditions, from eczema to a rash to insect bites. A scraping can detect their actual presence, and an experienced doctor can often provide a visual diagnosis.

Treatment

Scabies are treatable with lotion available only by prescription. The more recently developed permethrin (brand name Nix or Elimite) is now used often in place of lindane, which used to be the sole standard treatment, and to which a few varieties of scabies are now resistant. Other alternative treatments include sulfur ointment and the newest, still experimental, ivermectin (brand names Mectizan and Stromectol).

To rid your body of mites, rub the lotion thoroughly into every inch of skin, from the soles of your feet all the way up to (but not including) your head. You should also wash all clothes, sheets, and towels and anything else that comes in contact with your body in hot water. As bad as the itching may be, avoid hydrocortisone cream, says Dr. McCallister. If you must have relief, he says, try oral antihistamines such as diphenhydramine (brand name Benadryl) and hydroxyzine (brand name Atarax).

A word on after-scabies syndrome: The itching from the mites lasts after they've been killed, since their skeletons and fecal matter continue to irritate your skin. Don't panic, and read the information about after-crab syndrome, on page 151.

How You Get It

Like crabs, you catch scabies from any touch or from sheets, towels, or even a toilet seat.

How to Keep from Getting or Giving It

Complete abstinence from touch of any kind. So don't worry too much; just deal if you need to.

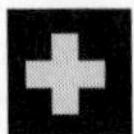

HIV Connection?

You can't get HIV from scabies, but people with weak immune systems can get an acute condition known as Norwegian or crusted scabies, which causes the skin to erupt into scaly, highly contagious patches. Whereas an ordinary case of scabies involves about seven to ten mites total, crusted scabies can involve millions. Regular lotions, rigorously applied, should take care of the problem, and some physicians have used the experimental medicine ivermectin with success.

Fecal Foes: Bacteria, Parasites, and Hepatitis A

There's a story some STD doctors tell about an experiment done in 1978. Scientists put two gay men in a laboratory, painted the asshole of each with dye that showed purple under a black light, and asked them to have sex. After the two men came, the researchers switched on the black light. Both men glowed purple from head to toe.

Whether or not the story's real, you get the point. Shit happens, and it happens to get around in more ways than we expect when having sex. Unfortunately, so do the bacteria and parasites it contains, which—if they find their way from his ass to your mouth—can make you sick.

BACTERIA AND PARASITES

Description

Four common bacteria found in feces can cause severe gastrointestinal problems: *E. coli*, shigella, campylobacter, and salmonella. While all of these may sound familiar from recent reports of chicken and beef contamination (see "Food Safety," in Chapter 6), they can get to you through human waste as well. There are also several common parasites passed through oral-fecal contact. The most common of these are amebas *(Entamoeba histolytica)* and giardia *(Giardia lamblia)*. Infection with *E. histolytica* is also known as amebiasis or amebic dysentery.

Incubation Period

Symptoms can begin within twenty-four to thirty-six hours of infection.

Symptoms

Symptoms of most bacterial and parasitic infections are similar, ranging from no symptoms at all to watery diarrhea, cramping and gassiness, smelly or bloody diarrhea, or abdominal pain. In some cases, more systemic effects such as fever, nausea, vomiting, and/or headache occur.

How Doctors Diagnose It

Effective testing for intestinal invaders usually means as many as three "purged stool" samples, each a day or more apart. "Purged stool" is the medical name for pretty runny fecal matter from pretty high up in your bowel, forced out by drinking a superlaxative. Often you go to the lab yourself for hot-on-the-spot delivery of the sample—if you don't, your sample shouldn't sit for more than an hour or two before it's sent.

An experienced doctor and lab are recommended, since detection can be difficult. You can also get false negative results if you're taking milk of magnesia, Mylanta, Maalox, Pepto-Bismol, Kaopectate, or any of a number of other common laxatives, antacids, or diarrhea medications, or if you've had an enema in the past few weeks. If symptoms persist, even after a negative test, colonoscopy—examination of the lower colon with a flexible instrument—and biopsy can help to detect the cause.

Treatment

Bacteria are often treated with antibiotics, with ciprofloxacin (brand name Cipro) a common treatment for shigella and salmonella, and erythromycin used for campylobacter. Metronidazole (brand name Flagyl), alone or combined with other drugs, is often prescribed as a first defense against giardia and some amebas. Using metronidazole leaves a metallic taste in your mouth and means taking nine pills per day. Contact with the tiniest bit of alcohol—including the amount in mouthwash, or in some cases hair gel—can increase the nausea that is among its side effects, and taking it with either alcohol or disulfiram (brand name Antabuse) will make you seriously nauseated. Tinidazole (brand name Fasigyn) is commonly used outside the United States for treating parasites, with treatment ranging from a single day for giardia to six days for amebas.

Parasites can be resistant to treatment, and may require a number of combinations of medicines. The longer they linger, the harder they are to get rid of, so it's best to get at least one purged stool sample after treatment to make sure they're gone. Symptoms may continue for up to a few weeks even after they're cured. For tips on relieving diarrhea, see "On the Runs," page 256.

How You Get It

You don't have to touch mouth to ass directly to get a tiny particle of shit in your mouth. A hand that touches an ass can rest on a shoulder, which is kissed; perspiration can carry a little bit of something down to someone's balls, which are licked, and so on.

Again, while cleanliness does reduce the risk of fecal foes, virtually every doctor interviewed for this book stresses that no amount of washing can eliminate every microorganism. "It's like throwing Clorox in the ocean," says Dr. William. "Looking clean doesn't mean you don't have microscopic eggs," warns Dr. McCallister. "You only need ten or so shigella bacteria to feel the effects," sighs Dr. Mayer.

How You Keep from Getting or Giving It

No oral-fecal contact (meaning an awareness of what hand's been where, no rimming, and no sucking after anal intercourse, among other things) is the best way to avoid parasites and bacteria. "Ass open, mouth closed," offers Dr. William cheerfully. Careful eating out of other kinds is also important, since bacteria are found in undercooked meat, and parasites are found in mountain streams (see "Food Safety," in Chapter 6). Finally, some men use condoms, dental dams, or Handi-Wrap to eat ass more safely (see Chapter 2), though many say they'd rather skip it.

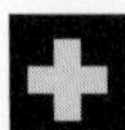

HIV Connection?

With factors from HIV itself to anti-HIV medications causing diarrhea, both diagnosis and treatment of parasites can be harder in men with HIV. In addition, many men with weak immune systems experience chronic problems, wasting, or, rarely, death from other ordinarily self-limiting parasites such as *Isospora belli* or cryptosporidium. Some immunologists argue that there is a link between the presence of amebiasis or giardia and faster progression to HIV illness, although a cause-and-effect relationship has not yet been definitively established.

HEPATITIS A (HAV)

Description

Hepatitis is the term used to describe liver inflammation caused by any variety of causes, including viruses, alcohol, medications, and bacteria. Of the many varieties of viral hepatitis—now identified as hepatitis A, B, C, D, E, G, and counting—only A and E are fecal foes, transmitted by getting microscopic particles of infected shit in your mouth. Hepatitis E is almost unknown, but nearly half a million Americans a year get hepatitis A.

Incubation Period

If you notice symptoms, you're likely to do so two to six weeks after exposure.

Symptoms

Severe flulike symptoms, vomiting, fatigue, achiness, pale feces, and dark urine are among the symptoms of acute hepatitis A, though many men don't have any symptoms at all. In addition, some people get jaundice (yellowing of the skin and eyes), abdominal pain, and itchiness over all or part of their body. In rare cases liver enzymes climb to critical or fatal levels.

How Doctors Diagnose It

A blood test will show elevated liver enzymes and the presence of antibodies to the hepatitis A virus.

Treatment

Lots of rest, no drugs or alcohol, and a simple, low-fat diet is the basic treatment for hepatitis A. Check with your doctor before taking any kind of oral medication: Almost all are a bad idea, and the ordinary pain reliever acetaminophen (Tylenol) can be especially dangerous. Liver-cleansing substances include dandelion root, milk thistle, and schizandra, as well as the dietary supplement alpha-lipoic acid (ALA), though you should check with your doctor before using any of them. If you're vomiting constantly, suppositories of prochlorperazine (brand name Compazine) or other drugs can help slow the flow. While symptoms usually begin to subside after several weeks, continued rest is important, since you can easily get a relapse of symptoms during the first six months.

How You Get It

While most HAV cases result from contaminated food and water, the viral ailment—along with its blood- and semen-borne cousin, HBV (see "The Condom Containables," page 156)—also passes between gay men through sex where any oral-fecal contact is involved.

How You Keep from Getting or Giving It

Ideally, by getting vaccinated (see page 298). Otherwise, as with parasites, avoiding oral-fecal contact is key. If you're ill with HAV, don't share dishes or glasses with anyone without washing them with soap and hot water, and make sure to wash your hands thoroughly after going to the bathroom. Virus continues to be found in your shit up to three weeks after you become ill, so it's best to avoid all kinds of anal sex during that time. Once you've had HAV, you can't get it again.

Hepatitis A is at its most contagious one to two weeks before symptoms appear. If you think you may have been exposed within the last few weeks, check with your doctor about getting an injection of immune globulin (also called gamma globulin) to help fight infection. Immune globulin has been shown to provide protection against recent HAV exposure approximately 75 percent of the time, and it is safe for people with HIV.

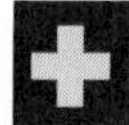 **HIV Connection?**

None, though getting HAV may mean having to stop all AIDS drugs or putting increased strain on your already medication-strained liver. HAV may also cause a spike in the amount of HIV in your blood.

The Condom Containables: Hepatitis B and C, Syphilis, Gonorrhea, Nongonococcal Urethritis (Chlamydia, Mycoplasma)

Latex condoms can block the transmission of these STDs, which are passed from person to person through bodily fluids, including semen, blood, vaginal fluid, and penile discharge. In the case of syphilis, the sores and rashes caused by the infection also transmit the disease.

HEPATITIS B (HBV)

Description

Another of the viruses that causes inflammation of the liver (see hepatitis A, page 154). This one can sometimes cause ongoing damage to the liver.

Incubation Period

Anywhere from a month and a half to six months after infection. The average incubation period is about three or four months.

Symptoms

About one-third of people infected with HBV have no symptoms at all and don't realize they're infected. Symptoms, when they occur, are similar to those of hepatitis A: nausea, fever, vomiting, achiness, jaundice, yellow eyes, dark urine, and pale stools. In 90 to 95 percent of cases, symptoms of acute illness usually pass in several weeks, leaving you without lasting liver damage and protected against getting HBV in the future.

About 5 to 10 percent of those with HBV, however, become chronic carriers. Blood tests are the only way to know if you are among this group, since symptoms can vary from acute, life-threatening liver failure to nothing at all. Even without symptoms, chronic carriers are at increased risk of cirrhosis and liver cancer, and can pass HBV to their sexual partners.

How Doctors Diagnose It

Blood tests can detect two different types of antigens and antibodies to HBV, which mean either that you have HBV now or had it in the past. If you have one of these, known as a surface antigen (HBsAg), it means you have an active HBV infection; if HBsAg remains in your blood for more than six months, it means you are a chronic carrier. Those with chronic HBV should have regular blood tests, and in some cases liver biopsies and other regular monitoring, to see how the virus is affecting the liver. Viral load tests similar to those used for HIV (see Chapter 9) can also be useful to track progress of HBV infection and help determine appropriate treatment. Finally, get vaccinated for hepatitis A if you haven't had the illness, or the vaccine, already: HAV can seriously complicate chronic HBV infection.

If a blood bank informs you that you "tested positive" for HBV, ask which tests they did. Generally, more tests are needed to find out if you had HBV in the past and are now immune, if you have it now, or if the whole thing is a false alarm.

Treatment

As with HAV, lots of rest and no medications, no alcohol, and a low-fat diet are recommended for those with initial HBV illness (see treatment for hepatitis A, page 155). Again, acetaminophen (Tylenol) may cause you special problems. Symptoms usually begin to pass in several weeks.

For chronic carriers with high levels of virus and elevated liver enzymes, standard treatment is to inject yourself with interferon, either daily or three times a week, for four months. Typical side effects include fatigue, fever and chills, diarrhea, nausea, achiness, and intense depression or anxiety, leaving researchers looking for a better solution. The anti-HIV drug lamivudine (brand name Epivir, also known as 3TC) was approved for use against HBV in late 1998, though make sure you have an HIV test before using Epivir as a hepatitis medication and test periodically for HIV throughout the course of your treatment. Epivir for HBV is prescribed at half the dose used to fight HIV. If you're positive, you don't want the HIV in your bloodstream to develop resistance to one of the most powerful anti-HIV drugs available (see Chapter 9 for more on resistance and HIV treatments). As with HIV, more and more research is suggesting that combination therapy may be more effective against HBV than taking only one medication. As with hepatitis A, herbal or complementary treatments for HBV include dandelion root, schizandra, milk thistle, and alpha-lipoic acid. Again, check with your doctor.

How You Get It

HBV is transmitted in the same way as HIV, through infected blood or semen, though it is an estimated hundred times more easily transmitted.

How You Keep from Getting or Giving It

Getting vaccinated against HBV is the best protection (see page 298). Shared needles, razors, toothbrushes, nonsterile tattoo needles or piercing equipment, and unprotected anal intercourse are all risky for HBV. Since HBV is found in saliva and semen, sucking and being sucked are both potentially risky, too. Sharing plates, silverware, or food is not thought to spread the virus, though some researchers suspect that deep kissing can pose a risk. If you think you've been exposed within the last few weeks, a shot of hepatitis B immune globulin may help fight infection.

TIPS FOR CHRONIC CARRIERS OF HEPATITIS B

HBV, like HIV, is carried in blood and semen, but it's so much more contagious that it takes even more care to prevent infection. The following recommendations are adapted from the Hepatitis B Coalition in St. Paul, Minnesota:

- Contact with your blood can get someone sick. Cover all cuts and sores with Band-Aids or bandages, and tell your physician or dentist about your condition. Don't share needles, razors, or toothbrushes.
- If you haven't had hepatitis A, get vaccinated against it.
- Avoid alcohol, and check with your physician before taking any drugs or medications: underground, over-the-counter, alternative, or prescribed.
- Check your liver enzymes at least once yearly, and get an annual screening for liver cancer.
- Sorry, aphrodisiac lovers, no raw oysters—they carry both hepatitis A and a bacterium, *Vibrio vulnificus,* that can cause serious or fatal illness for those with liver disease.
- Protect your sex partner. If you don't know whether he's been vaccinated or is immune to hepatitis B, advise him to get tested and vaccinated. In the meantime, use latex condoms for anal sex, and know that HBV—found in saliva and semen—may make sucking or being sucked, or even deep kissing, high-risk.

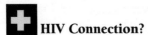

HIV Connection?

HBV often produces more severe symptoms in people with HIV. People with HIV are also more than twice as likely to become chronic carriers of HBV. Those using Epivir as an anti-HIV medication and then switching to another drug may experience flare-ups of HBV after stopping the Epivir. More generally, since many AIDS medications are hard on your liver, having HBV may also mean fewer HIV treatment options. The excellent Web site hivandhepatitis.com offers people with both HIV and hepatitis the latest information on "coinfection."

HEPATITIS C (HCV)

Description

This type of hepatitis was formerly known as non-A, non-B hepatitis. Rates of chronic HCV are very high, with around 80 percent of those with HCV becoming chronic carriers, and one out of five developing cirrhosis of the liver. Primarily transmitted through blood or shared needles—an estimated 3.9 million Americans are infected—HCV is the most common reason for liver transplants. HCV-related liver illness may take as long as twenty years to manifest itself.

Incubation Period

Same as for hepatitis B.

Symptoms

See information for hepatitis B, page 156.

How Doctors Diagnose It

Health care personnel diagnose HCV the same way as HBV, through blood tests looking for antibodies and elevated liver enzymes. A "home test" for HCV was also approved in 1999—as with the HIV test done at home, you prick your own finger at home, send your blood in to a lab, and call in for the results (and, if necessary, for medical referrals). As with HIV, antibodies can take as long as six weeks to show up after infection. If you do test positive, get a viral load (PCR) test to see how much virus is in your blood.

Treatment

Injections of interferon, three times a week for six to twelve months, has been standard treatment for HCV, though fewer than 20 percent of patients get sustained results. A combination of ribavirin (Virazole) with interferon, approved by the FDA in 1998 and marketed under the name Rebetron, works better, though in addition to the depression and flulike side effects of interferon you get the possibility of anemia. Sold together, the combination is expensive, though some pharmacies now compound ribavirin specially, and will sell it at a greatly reduced price. Trials have also shown promise for the flu medication amantadine (brand name Symmetrel), alone or in combination with other HCV medications, and a new, once-a-week interferon regimen is on the verge of approval as of this writing. Complementary treatments recommended by herbalists and others include schizandra, milk thistle, dandelion root, and alpha-lipoic acid. Again, check with your doctor. And make sure you get vaccinated for hepatitis A if you haven't had the illness or the vaccination. Getting HAV can be seriously dangerous for those with chronic hepatitis C infection.

How You Get It

Hepatitis C is transmitted through blood. Recent reports, complete with scary magazine covers featuring a big red *C*, have hailed it as the next major epidemic, playing up stories of people getting it from even the tiny amounts of blood on coke straws (that's cocaine, not the soda). Sexual transmission of HCV is suspected, though data about whether semen transmits HCV remains inconclusive.

How You Keep from Getting or Giving It

No shared needles, piercing equipment, razors, toothbrushes, S/M equipment, or rough sex.

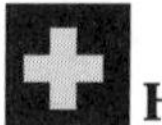

HIV Connection?

In some studies, 40 percent of people with HIV are coinfected with HCV. As with HBV (see page 156), liver damage may decrease your tolerance for HIV medications and accelerate the progression of both HIV and HCV.

SYPHILIS

Description

Syphilis was incurable until penicillin was discovered in 1943, leaving history full of references to "diseased minds," "tainted blood," and "moral weakness" that sound familiar in the age of AIDS. "Diseased minds" was a physical as well as moral description in the case of syphilis, which can cause damage to the brain and central nervous system. Healthy minds, and the education, testing, and treatment they produced, have now brought syphilis levels to their lowest point in years. Still, its seriousness—and outbreaks among gay men in Chicago, Seattle, and other cities in 1999—make it a disease worth watching.

Incubation Period and Symptoms

Syphilis has three stages, with different symptoms and incubation periods for each.

STAGE	INCUBATION PERIOD	SYMPTOMS
Primary syphilis	Anywhere from a week to three months after contact.	One or more red sores, called chancres, on the genitals, rectum, or mouth. Chancres are usually painless, are not always visible in the rectum, and go away by themselves in two to six weeks.
Middle-stage syphilis	Usually begins about six to eight weeks after the sores have healed, though this stage can appear while a sore is still present or up to six months afterward. This stage usually lasts two to six weeks.	Rash on the body, including palms of hands and soles of feet. Other symptoms include sore throat, achy muscles and joints, headaches, lymph node swelling, fever, hair loss, loss of appetite, skin growths (condyloma lata) on moist body folds, and mucus patches (silvery gray on light-skinned people, or a gray/blue on people who are darker-skinned) on mouth and genitals.
Late-stage syphilis	Ten to twenty-five years.	Variety of problems in central nervous system, in cardiovascular system, and, more rarely, in liver and eyes. Symptoms include meningitis, stroke, dementia, paralysis, and spinal cord degeneration. Among HIV-positive men, these occur more often and more quickly (see "HIV Connection?" below).

How Doctors Diagnose It

A blood test identifies the bacteria in the primary and secondary stages of the disease, though false negatives and false positives are both possible. For neurosyphilis and other late-stage syphilis, a lumbar puncture (spinal tap) may be required.

Treatment

Treatment for the early stages of syphilis is with an intramuscular injection of penicillin. Doses may vary depending on stage of disease and doctor. Rapid progression to neurosyphilis among men with HIV has led many doctors to treat syphilis in gay men aggressively with megadoses of antibiotics from the start. Neurosyphilis is treated with ten days or more of intravenous penicillin.

How You Get It

Syphilis is transmitted by blood and semen, as well as by contact with a sore, rash, or skin growth on the body of someone in the primary or secondary stage. If you have unprotected anal or oral sex with someone in one of these stages, you have an estimated 50 percent chance of being infected.

How You Keep from Getting or Giving It

Using condoms for anal and oral sex, and avoiding contact with any sores or rashes, will prevent transmission.

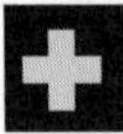

HIV Connection?

As many as half of people with HIV may develop neurosyphilis, even if the syphilis is in an early stage or has been treated with a standard dose of antibiotics. All men with HIV should have a syphilis test, even if they have no symptoms, and all who test positive and are treated should have regular follow-up blood tests to ensure that treatment was effective. If you have had neurosyphilis, follow-up may require spinal taps every six months.

BURN, BABY, BURN: GONORRHEA AND NONGONOCOCCAL URETHRITIS

Rectal inflammation. Prostate inflammation. Inflammation of the urethra, the throat, or the epididymis, the tube at the top of your testicles. All of these—known respectively as proctitis, prostatitis, urethritis, pharyngitis, and epididymitis—are symptoms of some of the most common condom-containable STDs. Often inflammations caused by these infections are matched with a milky discharge, which is how gonorrhea—Greek for "flow of seed"—got its euphonious name. Though among the most easily treated, these STDs—particularly when located in the urethra of the penetrator or the anus of the penetrated—are the ones most responsible for boosting HIV infection during unprotected sex. Urethritis increases the amount of HIV in your semen if you are HIV-positive, and proctitis draws easily infected CD4 cells to your rectum. Even if you have no burning or inflammation, you may have an STD—in many men, symptoms are nonexistent, or are so mild as to go unnoticed.

GONORRHEA

Description

With the discovery of penicillin and the subsequent fifty years of talk about how gonorrhea is easier to cure than the common cold, you'd expect "gone-orrhea" to be this bacterial infection's new name. But seriously, ladies and germs, this one's on its way back up, with gonococcal urethritis among the most common STDs reported at gay clinics. This is partly because gay men are having more unprotected oral and anal sex, and partly because gonorrhea has become increasingly resistant to common antibiotics. In addition to inflaming your urethra, you can also get gonorrhea in your rectum and, less commonly, in the throat. Often gonorrhea is accompanied by chlamydia or mycoplasma (see next page), transmitted the same way and frequently causing the same symptoms.

Incubation Period

Often as short as two to five days, although symptoms can take as long as two weeks to appear.

Symptoms

Swelling, inflammation, and discharge are among the symptoms. At least 10 percent of men don't have any symptoms with urethral gonorrhea, and more are asymptomatic when it's in the rectum or throat. Thick, mucous discharge and burning on urination are the usual signs of urethritis, along with some reddening of the little lips at the opening of the urethra. When rectal gonorrhea is symptomatic, which it is only about a third of the time, the symptoms range from mild anal itching to discharge, blood or mucus in the stool, pain during bowel movements, or a false urge to have them. Symptomatic gonorrhea of the throat usually feels a lot like a sore throat, though not as severe as a strep throat. Sorry—antibiotics for a regular sore throat won't take care of gonorrhea.

Symptoms of gonorrhea go away, but the organism itself does not. Left untreated, gonorrhea can travel deeper into the body, causing prostatitis (swelling of the prostate, pain, fever, and so on—see page 39) as well as the scrotal swelling, soreness, and even sterility associated with epididymitis (see page 23). In rare cases, advanced gonorrhea can cause arthritislike symptoms, or bloodstream and heart valve infections.

How Doctors Diagnose It

Techniques for diagnosis of gonorrhea include swabbing of the throat, rectum, or urethra for examination under a microscope; culture; DNA test; or urine test. Swabbing is the most common, and for a brief moment (they don't call it the "white light" test for nothing) the most painful.

Treatment

So many gonorrhea microbes are penicillin-resistant that the old injection has been replaced by newer oral antibiotics such as cefuroxime (brand names Ceftin, Kefurox, and Zinacef) or ceftriaxone (brand name Rocephin). You take the former for a week and the latter for a month. You also want a course of antibiotics active against chlamydia (see next page).

How You Get It

Unprotected anal or oral sex. Gonorrhea can travel from or to a penis during sex, though it's more easily passed from penis to throat or rectum than the other way around. Since the bacteria are present in discharge, someone need not come in your mouth or ass to infect you. Pre-cum can be infectious.

How You Keep from Getting or Giving It

Using condoms for anal and oral sex prevents the spread of gonorrhea. Urinating immediately after sex may help flush out bacteria from the urethra, although there is not much hard evidence to support this folk remedy.

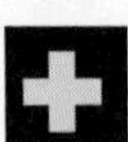

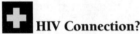

HIV Connection?

As mentioned, gonorrhea can make you more infectious if you're positive, and more likely to get infected if you're not.

NONGONOCOCCAL URETHRITIS AND PROCTITIS (CHLAMYDIA AND MYCOPLASMA)

Though caused by several different strains of bacteria, these STDs have the same symptoms, route of transmission, method of diagnosis, and long-term complications as gonorrhea (above). Chlamydia is the most common STD in the United States, though more of gay men's urethritis tends to come from similar bacteria known as mycoplasma. Both nongonococcal ailments can be treated the same way—a one-dose oral regimen of azithromycin (Zithromax), or a week-long course of antibiotics in the tetracycline family. They so often occur at the same time as gonorrhea that many doctors will combine this prescription with gonorrhea treatment as a matter of course.

As many as 40 percent of chlamydia infections are asymptomatic in men, though you're still infectious even if you have no symptoms. Have your partner treated, too, or you may never get rid of it.

ERECTION TROUBLES

Having no sexual desire at all is usually a sign of something amiss: depression, stress, testosterone imbalances, or a bad reaction to medication. In certain circumstances, though, the problem isn't desire, exactly, but delivering. The psychic reasons for erection problems can be as entwined and complicated as arousal itself, ranging from how we feel about our partners to all the things—power, control, intimacy, you name it—that we associate with sex. These dovetail with physical causes, too—an estimated 80 percent of erectile dysfunction, for example, is thought to have a root cause in the body, not the mind. Healing sexual dysfunction, whatever its cause, means considering both.

Among gay men, even being a bottom, there's all this emphasis on getting hard, and on the cock. So when you don't fit that profile, you get a sense of inadequacy. I don't talk about it with my sexual partners beforehand; I just wait to see whether or not it happens. Of course, it's worse with people I don't know because I feel ill at ease.

My boyfriend insisted that I not use a condom. I'd tell him I wasn't ready, that I wasn't comfortable, and he just kept insisting that I was negative and should go ahead and fuck him. I was negative, but for two years I couldn't get hard for anal sex.

It's not an all-or-nothing thing. I can get an erection about 80 percent of the time, but with great effort and persistence: using fantasies and manual stimulation. I still feel pleasure when it doesn't get hard, though it's not as fulfilling.

Every man at some point is likely to experience some trouble getting or maintaining an erection. For between ten and thirty million American men—one in every four—the National Institutes of Health says that trouble is consistent, and called impotence. With its connotation of complete powerlessness—which hard-on trouble is most certainly not—a number of men have come to prefer the term ED, or erectile dysfunction.

Erectile dysfunction has many causes, though it gets more common with age. At age forty, according to the National Institutes of Health, about 5 percent of men have experienced "a consistent inability to sustain an erection sufficient for sexual intercourse"; by age sixty-five, as many as 25 percent of us have had the experience. What that means for you, however, is a good deal less talked about or understood. Is it a serious sexual problem? That depends on what you and your sexual partner want. Not every man has intercourse as the center of his sexual life. Not every penis that's too soft to stick in an ass is too soft for other pleasures. Nor is everyone's idea of a satisfying sex life dependent on full erections. One famous set of interviews, published in the *New England Journal of Medicine* in 1978 and still cited more than twenty years later, interviewed a hundred self-described "normal" (and straight) couples, and found that the majority of them had some form of "problem" with sexual arousal or orgasm but considered themselves satisfied nevertheless. A 1999 University of Chicago study found that 31 percent of men and 41 percent of women had various forms of sexual problems, including low sexual desire, premature ejaculation, or inability to reach orgasm. How that correlated with their happiness—and whether they'd have been happier if experts and high-school health classes had told us all years ago that perfect and constant sexual "function" is closer to a myth than a norm—has yet to be explored.

The urologist told me there were a number of different oral and physical therapies. When I mentioned this to the psychiatrist, he became very defensive and said, "Oh, well, if all you're interested in is function . . ." I wanted to shout, "Of course I want function! Why are you minimizing function? It's been over twenty-five years since I had my last erection, and it's the primary cause for my depression and the physical, mental, and social state I find myself in now, you idiot." But I didn't. I simply decided that I wanted "function" now . . . and then I'd work on the psychological.

The doctor tested out injection therapy in his office to see if it would work for me, but I didn't feel comfortable about it. There was something so unerotic about it, so mechanical. I'm taking arginine and ginkgo biloba now, pills that I get at the health food store, and they seem to be helping.

Yes, I got Viagra. But I wanted to know: Why wasn't my doctor concerned that this is a symptom of something else rather than a condition of its own?

Treatments for erectile dysfunction come in two approaches, roughly speaking: You can address the cause, or you can work on the soft penis that is the symptom. Eliminating the cause of ED, when that's an option, most often involves working on your life—seeing a therapist, reducing stress, stopping smoking, or changing your diet, whom you're having sex with, or what you expect from it. The symptom-centered approach usually involves pills or some more mechanical intervention: shooting the penis full of substances, pumping it up, or strengthening it with rods, rings, or hidden inflatable mechanisms.

Given the stereotypes about tools and mechanics and preferring action over introspection, you can guess what most men choose. We are aided in this regard by the rapid growth in the past decade and a half of the field of impotence technology, the growing reluctance of HMOs and other insurers to cover psychological or nutritional approaches to anything, and an increase in the number of urologists in America who tend to have more training in plumbing the tubes and vessels of the penis than the complexities of the mind.

The rush to fix the symptom, however, does not mean it's okay to ignore the cause. "Erectile dysfunction can be a highly important warning sign for other, much more serious health issues," says Mark Litwin, MD, an assistant professor of urology at the University of California, Los Angeles. Research studies underscore his point, finding that as many as 25 percent of men with impotence suffer a stroke or heart attack within five years of the condition's onset. Even if your hard-on problems are not caused by arteriosclerosis or diabetes, fixing your part should not be mistaken for addressing your health as a whole. "In the nineties, we can give just about every man an erection," says Dr. Kenneth Goldberg, director of the Male Health Institute in Irving, Texas, and author of *How Men Can Live as Long as Women* (The Summit Group, 1993). "Effective treatment means thinking of the entire man: diet and exercise, physiological problems, relationships with his partner, and his ability to communicate."

Less likely than women to seek medical support in general, men tend to find a visit to a urologist—and the sexual discussion that goes along with it—especially daunting. "It's not unusual for men to wait a couple of years, suffering quietly, before they seek help," says Stephen Manley, Ph.D., a psychologist at the Male Health Institute. With openly gay urologists a relative rarity and sexually explicit conversations a must for the treatment of erectile dysfunction, gay men may have to look even harder for a doctor with whom they can be frank (see Chapter 7), though if you have a local gay clinic, that's a good place to start. The local Yellow Pages, too, may work in a pinch. Urological practices with expertise in erectile difficulties are often listed as "male health centers," offering yet another reminder—as if you needed one—of the odd ways that our penises are seen as the center of all things male. Asking how much experience a clinic has with gay patients before you go there is perfectly acceptable.

Erectile Dysfunction: The Mental

An array of simple tests at a doctor's office can help determine the cause of your erectile dysfunction. The first of these, however, you should administer to yourself: asking whether you can be honest with your health care provider about the details of your sex, work, financial, and emotional life. Questions about these are the usual starting point for an investigation whose first aim is most often to ascertain whether your erection difficulties are emotional or physical in origin.

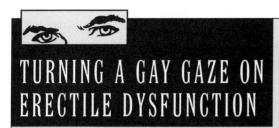

TURNING A GAY GAZE ON ERECTILE DYSFUNCTION

If you are consulting any of the vast amount of literature about impotence, get your language skills ready: Virtually all of the huge numbers of brochures and scientific studies have to be translated from the original heterosexual. Effectiveness studies and satisfaction surveys of men who use impotence treatments have all involved "stable, monogamous," and—you guessed it—heterosexual couples.

In addition to getting beyond the repeated references to your female sexual partner in the literature, this means several things for gay men.

1. ***Approved treatments yield erections of varying hardness.*** What works for unprotected vaginal intercourse may not be enough for anal intercourse with a condom, so if that's a goal of yours, make sure to discuss that with your doctor.

2. ***It's a couple's world; you just live in it.*** If you're single, ask about how that might affect your options. A vacuum pump that gets high marks from couples that have been together for thirty-five years may not be the most romantic sex toy to whip out of your backpack after you've gone home with that hunk from the bar. Or maybe he'll be into it.

3. ***Another negative of being positive?*** The idea that sex is a healthy part of all our lives seems sick to some of those who claim they're here to help. Urologists convened a special session at their 1997 conference to discuss the "ethics" of helping men with HIV get erections; a year later, an Alabama legislator proposed outlawing Viagra prescriptions for any man with HIV. Low-income gay men with HIV are in double trouble, since some states—for the first time in history—are also proposing banning Medicaid coverage of that erection inducer.

WHAT'S ON YOUR MIND?

Since every doctor treating erectile dysfunction should ask you about your frame of mind, you might prepare by asking yourself. Dr. Manley says he prefers to talk with patients rather than interrogate them, but in the course of the conversation he looks to answer some of the following questions:

- Was there any time in the last few years when you were successful in getting an erection? What were the circumstances?
- Do you get hard with one partner and not with another?
- Do you get hard during masturbation, but not during sex with someone else?
- Do you go limp during or before a particular sex act, or when a condom is involved?
- Did your erection difficulties begin during a period of increased stress or after receiving unexpected or bad news?
- Do you feel yourself in conflict with your sexual partner?
- Are you experiencing other signs of depression?

If the answer to any of these questions is yes, your erection difficulties may have a primarily psychological cause: deeper issues about your life or sex partner, or anxiety about performance. If that's the case, then some work with your partner, a counselor, or a sex therapist, perhaps bolstered by Viagra or one of the other ED treatments, should be able to reverse it. Insurance, though—even those plans that cover erectile dysfunction treatment—may not pay. Many cover only "medically necessary" treatment for "impotence with a physical cause."

Though that distinction sounds neat enough, the division between mental and physical causes of erectile dysfunction is not so simple. Particularly in sexual matters, the mind and body are never neatly segmented; each influences the other in a constant exchange of information and sensation. Erectile problems feed into a kind of vicious cycle that makes it hard to know which came first, the problem or the anxiety about the problem. You know: You don't get hard, you worry about it, you feel increased pressure for the next time, you don't get hard, you feel even more pressure. After a while, most men can't tell the difference between a physical inability to get hard and an emotional one. One way of getting some clarity may be to look to the dream world, and the "stamp test."

THE STAMP TEST: BECAUSE THE NIGHT . . .

Since night is a time when even the most stressed-out among us get erections, doctors treating erectile dysfunction often look for what they call NPT, or nocturnal penile tumescence—that is, whether you are getting hard in your sleep. It's normal to get between two and four nighttime erections, each lasting up to half an hour; the famed "piss hard" you may experience in the morning is simply the last of them (and has nothing to do with a full bladder or peeing). Some doctors may ask you to sleep in a hospital for observation, or will more likely send you home with a snap gauge or a Rigiscan, two different mechanisms that go around your penis and monitor whether and how much it swells during the night. The snap gauge uses threads that are broken by erections of different firmness, while the Rigiscan actually transmits data to a graphing device that charts your ups and downs for later examination. A cheaper, homier approach is the stamp test. Wrap a strip of postage stamps (the cheapest are fine, and avoid the self-adhesive kind) around the base of your limp penis, sticking one end to the other. If the stamps are separated along the perforated line when you wake up in the morning, you're getting stiff at night, and the problem is unlikely to be physical.

Even if you determine that your hard-on problems are primarily physical in nature, you should consider getting some kind of mental support. "While not 100 percent of men's impotence is caused by psychological problems, 100 percent of men are affected psychologically," says Dr. Goldberg. If you have a regular sexual partner, erectile dysfunction is very much a couple's problem, not an individual one, and you should try to include your partner in doctor's visits. "It's crucial for each of you to be able to imagine what the other's going through," says Goldberg. "Not getting an erection is a threat to your masculinity, but it's also a threat to your partner's sense of attractiveness." Communication, adds Dr. Manley, may relieve some of the pressure and anxiety that is causing the problem to repeat itself. While you're desperately trying to pump and grind yourself into a hard state, he may be wishing you could just relax and cuddle. While you may have discovered that your problem is caused by your ulcer medication, he may think you're having an affair with someone else.

In some locations, Impotence Anonymous and I-Anon groups offer men and their partners a way to discuss their situations. "It's a little like coming out of the closet," says Yaacov Gershoni, an openly gay therapist who facilitates the New York City groups. "Men come and say, 'What a relief! I can finally talk about this.'" Based on Alcoholics Anonymous in their volunteer-run, confidential approach—though without a "twelve-step" orientation—the groups are not always listed in the phone book, but can often be found through the urology departments of large hospitals. The Impotence Institute of America, which has a national directory of physicians, counselors, and support groups (though no gay-specific information), also keeps a master list. Their toll-free number and their address—in evocatively named Maryville, Tennessee—can be found on page 577.

Having an erection is not the same as having a desire for sex, fixing up relations with a partner, or resolving ambivalence about sex. If it has been a while since you had sex with a hard-on, then regaining your erections may also mean revisiting feelings about sex and experimenting with what makes you and your partner feel comfortable.

Erectile Dysfunction: The Physical

Since erections involve a complex interaction between nervous system and blood flow, anything that interferes with either of these can be a physical cause of erectile difficulty. Hard partiers know about "crystal dick," an unwelcome limpness experienced as a side effect of using methamphetamine, as well as the failure to engorge that comes from chronic alcohol and cocaine use. Medications prescribed for high blood pressure and other conditions, including ulcers and depression, can all keep you softer than you want to be (see box on next page). Prostate problems, low testosterone levels as a result of age or HIV infection, and surgery or accidents that affect your neurological system are all potential causes. Perhaps most important, an estimated 70 percent of ED is caused by diabetes, high cholesterol, or high blood pressure—three serious medical conditions particularly common among men over fifty. "Everyone talks about heart attacks, but people aren't used to thinking of a penis attack," says E. Douglas Whitehead, MD, director of the Association for Male Sexual Dysfunction in New York City. "The most common cause of impotence is for the penis to be starved of blood."

Getting help with a physical cause of erectile dysfunction may mean a process of elimination—taking a number of tests to rule out different causes. The first of these is a review of medications or other drugs that you're on, to see if one of them may have an undesired side effect. Though your doctor may not have mentioned it, changing from one brand of medication to another—or stopping alcohol consumption—may do the trick. Having ruled out medicines or psychological causes, the doctor will usually follow up with three more basic questions designed to help.

WHAT'S IN YOUR HEART?

Or, more exactly, in your entire circulatory system, and the blood that flows through it. Testing your blood pressure and your blood is probably the most important step in determining what physical cause, if any, is contributing to your impotence. These tests can look for evidence of diabetes, high cholesterol, and hardening of the arteries, among other things. Though hormonal imbalance usually affects desire rather than erections, your doctor should also test your testosterone levels. HIV-positive men in particular can have low hormone levels and may benefit from treatment (see box on page 348). Even intense bicycle riding can affect penile blood supply, so skip the racing saddle in favor of the cushy seat that spreads your buns, and the pressure, more widely.

Other, more sophisticated tests measure blood flow directly into and out of the penis, injecting dye and following it to see where and how long it takes to leak out. These tests have long names (cavernosography, duplex ultrasonography, arteriography) and high costs, and are generally necessary only to refine treatment options or when surgical solutions are proposed.

WHAT'S ON YOUR NERVES?

Neurological problems—the result of an accident, surgery, or diseases such as diabetes, Parkinson's disease, or multiple sclerosis—can all be a cause of ED. Tests can be simple: stroking the inner thigh and seeing if the scrotum on that side retracts (it's a natural reflex), or squeezing the head of the penis and timing how long it takes for the muscles around the anus to contract (that's natural, too). Others, such as biothesiometry (where an electrical tuning fork is laid on your penis to see what level of vibrations you feel) or BLCB testing (where the head of your penis is electronically stimulated, and a needle measures how long it takes for your anal muscles to contract), are more involved.

WHAT'S WITH YOUR PROSTATE?

What some people hail as a magic button of bliss may also be the cause of erection problems, particularly when the gland gets enlarged or infected. A prostate exam (see page 352) should be a part of any evaluation for erectile problems.

CURING ME SOFTLY

More than two hundred commonly prescribed medications have been known to have side effects that can decrease a man's ability to get or maintain an erection. This can create a catch-22: Your lack of erections makes you anxious, and your antianxiety medications hamper your ability to get an erection. It is never advisable to change your medications without consulting a medical professional, and walking in and demanding a different brand may be neither appropriate nor effective; most blood pressure and heart medications, for example, inhibit erections. If you suspect, however, that a medication may be responsible for your ED, ask. Cimetidine (Tagamet), for example, may help your ulcer but hinder your hard-on; ranitidine (Zantac) may not. Many antidepressants also delay your orgasm (for more on that, see "Ejaculation Troubles," page 175).

These are but a small sample of the drugs that may keep you softer than you want to be:

- Antianxiety drugs, including buspirone hydrochloride (BuSpar), diazepam (Valium), and alprazolam (Xanax)
- Antidepressants, including fluoxetine (Prozac) and sertraline (Zoloft)
- High blood pressure and heart medications, including propranolol (Inderal) and metoprolol (Lopressor)
- Party drugs, including methamphetamine (crystal), MDMA (Ecstasy), marijuana, and alcohol
- Drugs to treat addictions, including methadone and disulfiram (Antabuse)
- Ulcer medications, including cimetidine (Tagamet)
- Antifungal medications, including metronidazole (Flagyl), fluconazole (Diflucan), and ketoconazole (Nizoral)

Erection Solutions

The approval of sildenafil, aka Viagra, in March of 1998 made erectile dysfunction and the little blue diamond-shaped pill that could help cure it the talk of the town in America. Within weeks, doctors were reporting cramps in their hands from writing so many prescriptions—an estimated one hundred thousand a week in the first month alone. Black markets for daddy's little helper sprang up worldwide, including in the United States, with peddlers hawking it (and imitations with names like Vaegra and Viagro) on the Internet and on the street. The fact that the drug's manufacturer was careful to stress that it enhanced erectile ability but not desire was lost to the many who obviously fervently desired a boost in bed. Within two weeks, Viagra accounted for 79.2 percent of new prescriptions written for erectile dysfunction. A month after its release, the market for sexual disorder treatments had jumped more than 500 percent. Six months after Viagra's approval, more than 4.8 million prescriptions—and every conceivable joke, off-color reference, and exploration of the pill's apparent effects—had been written, making it among the most successful drug releases in pharmaceutical history. The figures were all the more remarkable given the backlash from the insurance industry. Afraid of breaking the bank by bolstering boners, they balked, with half of the insurance companies in America either refusing to pay for the treatment or sharply limiting how many of the $10-a-pop pills they would cover. Many restrict coverage to three pills a month, the amount of intercourse the *Sex in America* survey (see box on page 49) reported as average for a heterosexual married couple.

If Viagra is the best and biggest example of erection fever, it's not the first. Upon the creation of erection injection therapy in 1983, the urologist presenting it at the conference of the American Urological Association appeared onstage in a pair of gym shorts. The presentation began with the doctor ascending the podium to discuss the breakthrough, and ended, some half an hour later, when he dropped his shorts and paraded his splendidly firm penis in front of the admiring attendees. Perhaps not surprisingly, the field took off, with tens of thousands of men using erection-inducing drugs without Food and Drug Administration approval throughout the 1980s. In 1995 the FDA approved one of these, prostaglandin E1, for use as an erection inducer. Three years later Viagra popped out of the pipeline, and the rest was history.

Except, of course, that history marches onward. New treatments, including several rumored to boost desire as well as your erection, are slated for release. Injections and vacuum pumps remain useful for some who don't respond to pills. For those with serious physical obstacles to erections, implants can be helpful, too. Viagra's prescription rate has slowed somewhat, due in part to reports of more than seventy deaths associated with the drug, most caused by people having heart attacks during the sex they were no longer used to having (see "Systemic Solutions," on next page, for further details). Men with erectile problems due to prostate surgery, nerve damage, or the desire for a more permanent solution often opt for the more effective (and more invasive) options detailed below. In guidelines on erectile dysfunction issued pre-Viagra, but which stand the test of time, the National Institutes of Health suggests what could well be termed a basic rule for making hard choices for hard-on help: Try the least invasive procedure first.

Systemic Solutions: Pills

SILDENAFIL (VIAGRA)

Viagra is so successful in part because it is the least mechanistic of the many erectile dysfunction solutions. Other treatments give you an erection, like it or not: with Viagra, taken anywhere from half an hour to four hours before sex, you get a lift only when you're feeling aroused. Though it comes in varying doses (all at the same price, leading some men, against medical advice, to buy the bigger-dose pills and cut them in half), taking more than you should makes you neither harder nor hornier. Overdosing does increase the chance of side effects, including headaches, seeing blue, and upset stomach.

Viagra causes a potentially fatal drop in blood pressure when combined with nitrites, which include both the nitroglycerin that some men use for heart disease or anal fissures and the poppers they use for pleasure. Even if you're not using nitroglycerin, suffer a heart attack on Viagra and the ambulance crew might. "We've had reports of several patients who had heart attacks during sex and were given nitroglycerin by EMS," says Marshall Forstein, MD, medical director of Mental Health Services at Fenway Community Health Center. "They died." There's not yet a cheap and chic Viagra-alert bracelet ("I'm on Viagra . . . can we talk?"), though there is a high-end silver chain with a single, mysterious-looking Viagra tablet cast in gold. Check with your cardiologist about the wisdom of using Viagra if you have any heart problems, since the exertion of sex (heart attack risk rises for as much as two and a half hours afterward) is what seems to be a major cause of fatalities.

Viagra stays in your body for at least twenty-four hours (and, depending on your protease inhibitors or other drugs, as long as forty-eight), so even taking a Viagra on Saturday night and using poppers at a Sunday tea dance can be deadly. "Don't combine the two, period," says New York City doctor Howard Grossman, MD. "Even if *he's* using the poppers and you're using Viagra, being in the same room could conceivably provoke a bad reaction, because the poppers are in the atmosphere and could be inhaled." HIV-positive men, particularly those on protease inhibitors, should be aware that Viagra is metabolized by some of the same liver enzymes as Norvir, Crixivan, Rescriptor, and even antibiotics such as erythromycin. While Viagra is unlikely to decrease levels of protease in the blood, it may well stay in the body longer if you're on these anti-HIV drugs, or give you side effects even at a low dose. Check with a doctor before combining Viagra and protease inhibitors.

TRAZADONE (DESERYL)

Trazadone is an antidepressant whose side effects can sometimes include erection enhancement. Especially when taken with yohimbine (see sidebar), trazadone has yielded some positive results, though it may send you to the emergency room with an erection that won't go down (see "Too Hard Too Long," page 172). Work closely with a doctor to determine if it's worth trying, since it may not react well with other antidepressants (or your mind, for that matter).

Local, Nonsurgical Solutions

Don't try these at home, at least not before you practice with someone who knows what he's doing. Any kind of treatment that involves the penis also takes practice. "I use the teach-

HERBALLY HARD

Yohimbine, made from the bark of an African tree, is sold by prescription in some states, and over the counter in others, as an erection enhancer. Some OTC brand names include Yohimbe, Yocon, Yohimex, and Aphrodyne, though buyers beware: It's not much cheaper over the counter, dosages of yohimbine vary widely by brand or even by package, and you won't get reimbursed for OTC preparations by insurance. Doctors who believe in yohimbine suggest you try it for a month—it takes at least two weeks to begin to work—while critics blast it as no more effective than a sugar pill. "I tell most of the men who come to see me for impotence to try a month's supply," says Franklin C. Lowe, MD, of New York's St. Luke's–Roosevelt Hospital. Whether placebo or natural cure, yohimbine's effect can be sweet: More than a third of men who used it in a number of clinical trials got partial or full sexual function back. It works best for those whose problems are not related to serious circulatory or nerve damage, and its side effects can include dizziness, jumpiness, sweating, and anxiety. If you have diabetes, kidney problems, or high blood pressure, you should avoid it.

Ginkgo biloba, made from the venerable ginkgo tree (whose life span can exceed two thousand years and which supposedly was one of the few species to survive the bombing of Hiroshima), is another of the herbal hardeners. Popular also as an "herbaceutical" remedy for memory loss and Alzheimer's prevention, ginkgo is thought to boost circulation in the brain as well as the penis. See page 309 for a discussion of some of the pros and cons of herbal medicine in the Western world.

one, do-one, see-one method," says Dr. Lowe. "I go first, we work together on the second, and I observe the third." Three doctor's visits may sound like a pain, but not compared to the botched results of the unpracticed.

VACUUM PUMPS

As with yohimbine, there's an over-the-counter version (you may remember the Acu-Jack ads in men's magazines). As doctors tend to do, urologists come out strongly in favor of using a medically prescribed product; some can even give you a loaner to try out. Buying a pump through a doctor is more expensive, though you often do get the option of the instruction, as well as an organized way to order replacement parts and, in some cases, insurance reimbursement.

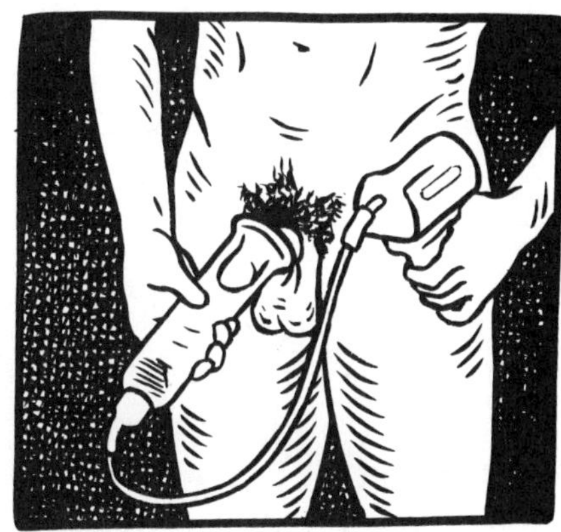

1. Slide a plastic sleeve over the penis

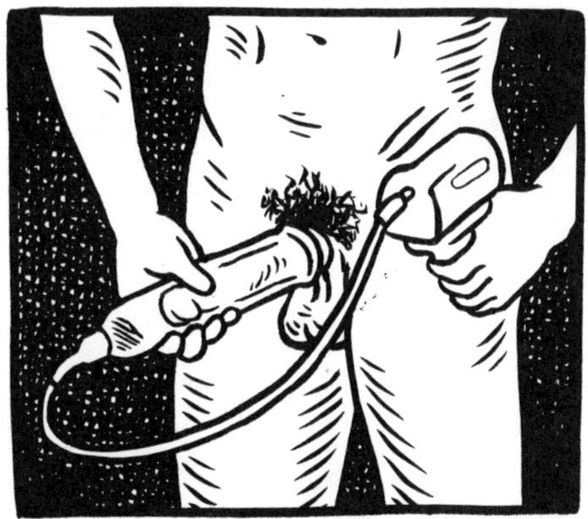

2. Suction air from the sleeve

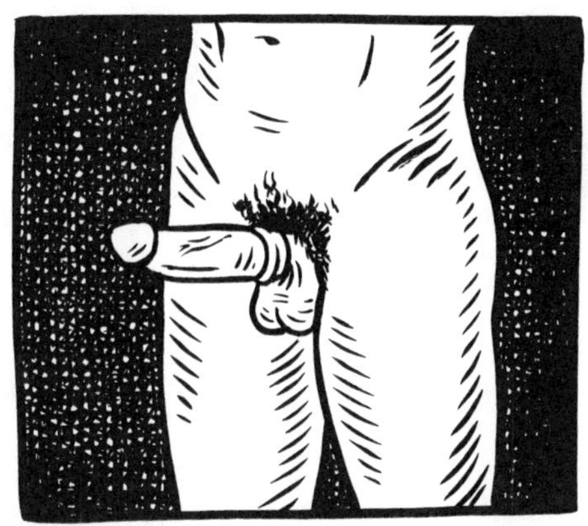

3. Slide the sleeve off and slip the tight plastic ring down over the base of your penis.

Wherever you purchase a vacuum pump, its use for erectile dysfunction is the same. You slide a plastic sleeve over your limp penis and plant it firmly against a lubricated (and, for best results, shaved) patch of skin at the base. Then, using either a manually operated or battery-powered pump, you suction out the air from the sleeve, creating a vacuum and drawing blood into your penis in the process. Slide the sleeve off, slip a tight plastic ring down over the base of your penis, and you should have an erection.

The upside of vacuum devices are that they require no surgery, are relatively cheap (around $500 for a top-of-the-line model, plus an additional $50 or so for an annual supply of lubricant and plastic rings), and can be used often. The battery-operated models require less dexterity—for the others, you need both hands (and for beginners, a low table on which to rest your plastic sleeve). Practice is recommended before you try it out, since bruising, petechiae (patches of tiny red dots), and a little pain are not unknown. Obvious problems are those of spontaneity and the fact that the erection you get with it is slightly floppy and bluish, colder than normal, and lasts only about twenty minutes. It's also virtually impossible to ejaculate with a plastic ring squeezing the base of your dick (though you still need condoms), so the satisfaction of spurting all over someone's chest is lost. It's later, when you remove the ring, that cum comes trickling out.

ERECTION INJECTIONS

Administered about a third of the way up the penis shaft, with a hypodermic needle about the width of a human hair, these work by relaxing the smooth muscle of the penis and allowing blood to rush in. The injections are minimally painful—"like a pinch," one man said—and with the proper dose erections last about two hours and continue even after you ejaculate. Get the dose wrong and you may find yourself with penile pain or priapism (see box). The most popular product is marketed as alprostadil (brand name Caverject). Users of erection injections should definitely consult with a physician to get the dose correct, going for several trial runs.

TOO HARD TOO LONG: PRIAPISM

Use of some erection enhancers raises the risk of priapism, an erection that won't go away for hours. That may sound great, but in fact it is both unpleasant and unhealthy, threatening to permanently damage the tissue of the penis. If you are having problems coming down, applying an ice pack to each inner thigh (hot, huh?) may help. "Though technically priapism begins after about five or six hours, if you don't go soft after about two or three, I advise an emergency-room visit," says UCLA's Dr. Litwin.

The biggest downside with injections, obviously, is the idea of jabbing yourself in a sensitive area. "I've had dozens of patients say they could never stick a needle into their penises, but you'd be surprised what you're willing to learn once the mood takes over," observes Dr. Lowe. To avoid priapism, small nodules of scarring, and the Peyronie's disease (see page 21) such scarring may cause, urologists advise patients not to use the needles more than two or three times a week, and to vary injection spots. Still, dislike of the needle and its consequences are among the main reasons that half or more of those who use injections stop within a year. Another disincentive may come from insurance policies—including Medicare—that don't cover such injections. At as much as $22 a shot, that could provoke serious pain.

SUPPOSITORIES

In your penis, that is. In 1997 the Food and Drug Administration approved a way to get a prostaglandin-induced erection without the needle. Instead, you plant a medicated pellet about an inch into your urethra, using a handy plastic applicator with a push-button release. Ten minutes after administration of the product, sold under the brand name MUSE, you have a stiff penis that will last for another couple of hours, come what or who may. Absorption of the drug via the urethra is less efficient than with direct injection, which means higher doses of prostaglandin, a higher failure rate than the injections, and erections that are less likely to be diamond-hard. There's also mild to moderate penile pain, which occurs (though not every time) in about a third of users. Peeing before you insert the pellet lubricates the urethra, helping it to work better and hurt less. At $22 each, and available only in boxes of six, some also find the price of the drug hard to take. On the other hand, there are no needles, no scarring, and less priapism, meaning fewer embarrassing ER episodes unsuitable for television broadcast.

Surgical Solutions

IMPLANTS

Known as the Cadillac of impotence treatments in the seventies, these should still be known as the Cadillac of treatments: that is, big, expensive, slightly old-fashioned, and not for everyone. Getting a penile implant requires significant expense—around $10,000 to $20,000, depending on the model and installation procedures—and also means irreversible structural changes. While you can urinate or ejaculate in the same way after the operation as you could before it happened, you will never go back to having normal, unaided erections.

Implants come in two basic varieties: solid and inflatable. *Solid implants* can be installed in an outpatient procedure, though you need to wait four to six weeks before actually putting them to use. The simplest consists of two rods that are slipped into the penis, leaving you with what looks like a kind of adjustable but permanent hard-on. You either push it down between your legs when not in active use or snap it up for action. Men who want a more discreet implant may opt for the more expensive kind, which consists of a series of small plastic blocks strung along a cable. A spring pulls the whole unit tight when you want an erection, and allows it to hang loose when you don't.

Inflatable implants also come in several varieties. One is a single-piece, semirigid device that swells further when a pump behind the head of the penis is squeezed. The easiest of the inflatable implants to install, this is also the least natural, since it—like its solid counterpart—remains semirigid at all times. While that might not be bad in the locker room, the skin of the penis occasionally stretches, leading over a couple of years to a floppy erection and the need for another operation.

More natural-looking, and more expensive, is the two- or three-piece inflatable model. A reservoir full of fluid is implanted in the abdomen and connected via tubing to inflatable cylinders in the penis and a pump in the scrotum. Squeeze the pump, and the penis fills with fluid. Squeeze it again, and it drains. One design even expands as it inflates, making it the only implant that affects penis width as well as length. If you are unable to have abdominal surgery, there is a two-piece option, with fluid and pump both in the scrotum.

Because they are more complicated, inflatable models fail more often—for a three-piece model, the American Urological Association puts the failure rate at about one in ten, twice as high as for the semirigid implants. Make sure to ask your surgeon for his experience and success rate, since these implants don't always give you a really hard erection, and incorrectly installed models can wear through the skin and have to be redone.

SURGICAL RESTORATION

In cases where physical trauma has damaged veins and arteries that supply blood to the penis, surgical repair is sometimes possible. Even the best candidates for these surgeries—nonsmokers between the ages of eighteen and fifty—experience failure rates of 40 percent, reversal of the effects of surgery after a year or so, and a host of complications, from shortening to scarring. Even if you are among the few who might be eligible for such surgery, it should not be attempted without complete testing by a doctor of ebb and flow in blood vessels of the penis.

Future Treatments

If erection injections warranted a firsthand display of the goods and Viagra boosted stocks and sticks worldwide, one can only imagine what delights will be planned for the launch of no fewer than three other new and yet-to-be-approved oral treatments. But as pharmaceutical companies rush to produce new medicines for erectile dysfunction, a few students of sexuality suggest men may do well with a dose of a different kind of medicine: attitude adjustment. "An enormous amount of anxiety about our hard-ons can be relieved if we get beyond the idea that the only good cock is a hard cock and the only real sex is penetration," says Collin Brown of the Body Electric School. A different but related appeal for perspective has been made by certain professionals within the fields of urology and sexology, who caution that a relentless focus on the function of our penises can blind us to deeper issues of what we're doing with them. Preoccupation with technological evaluation and "the authority of objective fact," writes Leonore Tiefer, a former associate professor of urology at Albert Einstein College of Medicine, can lead doctors to forget to ask the people involved how they feel about their own functioning. Tiefer's book, *Sex Is Not a Natural Act* (Westview Press, 1995), describes the scene at one urology conference, where a urologist in the audience insisted that the sixty-five- to seventy-four-year-old patients being discussed did not have rigid erections at night and were therefore dysfunctional. The presenter disagreed, noting that both the men and their wives reported happy sex lives, but the urologist persisted. Since seventy-four-year-olds can have rigid erections, the urologist argued, the fact that this group wasn't having nocturnal erections meant something was wrong with them, no matter what they or their wives said.

Keith, age forty, offers a different insight on the problem. "I tell my friends who are dick-crazy to open their minds," he says. "What I'm really into is balls. That all-meat-and-no-potatoes diet is just not healthy."

Ejaculation Troubles

Anxiety about length is not just a question of penis size. Plenty of men are concerned that they come too fast, too slow, or in certain situations not at all. While there are some physical causes for these problems—antidepressants, for example, can delay or prevent orgasm—many instances are compounded by some version of performance anxiety: fear of how we're measuring up to some mythical standard.

Premature Ejaculation

Worries about premature ejaculation, more sensitively known as "early ejaculation," should immediately raise the question: compared to what? Kinsey's early research found that 75 percent of married, heterosexual men lasted two minutes or less from the beginning of sex until orgasm. Young men often come faster than older ones; many men come faster in one form of sex than other, and the pleasure you experience during orgasm usually depends on many things, not just how long you take to get there.

As with erectile dysfunction, there are both medical and psychological steps to take if you'd like to last longer. Following in the wake of advances in antidepressants and erection enhancers, the pharmaceutical industry seems poised on the brink of great strides in treatment of premature ejaculation. Existing treatments, in fact, include low doses of antidepressants, since one man's unwanted side effect is another man's treatment. Fluoxetine (Prozac) or another of the selective serotonin reuptake inhibitors (see page 489) are among the most commonly prescribed.

Increasing awareness of the arc of your arousal is another route to treatment, says Charles Moser, MD, professor of sexology at the Institute for Advanced Study of Human Sexuality in San Francisco. It's a similar principle to that of the Taoist approach to multiple orgasm (see page 112). When masturbating by yourself, or with a partner, pay close attention to all phases of the approach to orgasm, no matter how short. Just before reaching that point of no return, stop (or have him stop) stimulation. Then begin again, doing it three or four times before you come. The more you get to know your arousal, the more likely you are to be able to control it.

Bernie Zilbergeld, Ph.D., describing this stop-start technique in his *The New Male Sexuality* (Bantam, 1999), suggests rating your arousal on a scale of 1 to 10 and stopping somewhere near 4 or 5. If you're working with a partner, agree on a verbal signal for stopping (a wild shake of the head may just look like you're having fun), and wait up to a minute before he begins again. You can talk while you wait, or just relax. Experiment with Kegel exercises (see page 41) to help avoid blastoff, and notice how your leg and foot muscles tighten as you approach orgasm. Relaxing them and breathing deeply can often do wonders. So can the squeeze technique, which can be done by you or your partner (see "Sensate Focus and Other Solutions," next page).

Delayed Ejaculation

I don't know if it's that I don't want to or I can't, but if I'm with someone who's expecting me to be my image—big, butch, needing to be satisfied—something just switches off.

I can't come. It's embarrassing, but it can also be a blessing, because if he doesn't call me back because of that, I think, well, in the long run, I'm probably better off.

If I don't know him, I'm fine. But I'm telling you, once somebody I like starts huffing and puffing and blowing and kissing down there, the pressure is too much, and I just freeze up.

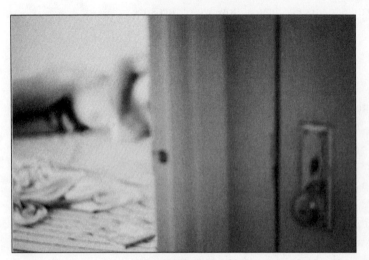

Hardly talked or written about in the pre-Prozac straight world, delayed ejaculation—also known as "retarded" ejaculation—has been a subject of gay concern for some time. Therapists interviewed for this book repeatedly cited difficulty in coming to be an ongoing complaint among their gay male clients. Dr. Charles Silverstein chalks some of it up to the "control queen" factor—not wanting to release in front of another man—while New York City therapist Steven Ball wonders if "it's an unconscious way to say you're something more than the sex machine the other guy may think he's gone home with." AIDS, and the idea that semen is nasty and infectious, can't have helped, notes Ball, though pre-AIDS surveys of gay men also found delayed ejaculation to be an issue. The rise of antidepressants, and the fall in both sexual desire and speed of orgasm that is an unfortunate but common side effect, has made the problem more pronounced.

Whatever the cause—and there are many—a common symptom once you start to worry about coming is what sex therapists refer to as "spectatoring": a feeling that you're somehow outside the sex you're having, watching it and judging it. In certain instances, medications—among them pseudoephedrine and phenylpropanolamine, found in common cold medications—can help stimulate the physical process of ejaculation, so check with your doctor about using them to help. As with early ejaculation, exercises that help disrupt the usual expectations and patterns of sex and replace them with something more relaxed can also be of use. "If you had a broken arm, you'd adjust your usual routine to help it mend," says Dr. Moser. "Sexual dysfunction is no different—something's not working, and you need to change, rather than repeat, your usual way of doing things." If you're in a couple, one way is to work toward change slowly, with exercises where orgasm is not expected.

Sensate Focus and Other Solutions

One of the most useful and commonly proposed sex therapy exercises for erectile dysfunction, early ejaculation, or inability to ejaculate is called sensate focus. It involves plenty of touch and a simple ground rule: For the first few sessions, leave the genitals out of it. The idea, as the name implies, is to focus on sensation rather than erection or orgasm, on pleasure without the need to produce.

To try, make sure you and your partner have talked it through and are both willing. Decide who will "give" and who will "receive." Though one of you may have "the problem," both of you should be willing to play both roles. "With sexual function issues, the couple is the patient," says Moser. 'Tis often harder to receive than to give, especially if you're a perpetual pleaser type.

Then, in a comfortable, relaxed setting, get naked, and let the giver touch and massage the receiver for an agreed-upon time—ten or twenty minutes. Experiment with different kinds of touch over the front and back of the body, but leave the genitals alone. If one of you gets a hard-on—even if the failure to get one has been an issue—ignore it. This may take some self-control from both of you—remember that you're each likely to be anxious to move beyond the problem. It's probably best for the receiver to keep his eyes closed, says Dr. Moser, so that he can relax into the sensations. No verbal response is necessary; just relax into the pleasure of touching and being touched. Afterward, spend a few minutes talking about what felt best and what was least comfortable.

After a few sessions of this, if they want to, couples can move to the next steps: genital stimulation without orgasm, and then, perhaps, to orgasm. "There's no recipe or cookbook approach," says Moser, who suggests that couples consult with a sex therapist if things seem stuck, and use variations on the theme depending on the problem at hand. A few of the standard suggestions are found below.

For Erectile Dysfunction

The "giver" should provide stimulation with an aim toward producing pleasurable sensations rather than an erection. Again, leave the genitals out of it, and if an erection appears, ignore it. If no erection appears, don't worry—there's always medical help (see "Erection Solutions," page 169). The point is to focus on what feels good, and to recognize that hard-ons can come and go. Often, breaking the anxiety that you won't get hard can be enough to let you do so in the future.

For Delayed Ejaculation

If you can come by yourself but not in front of another person, says Dr. Moser, most sex therapists will use what's called a "bridge technique." What the giver gives here is permission for his partner to relax and experience arousal in his presence, but without any expectations. Once the receiver is comfortable getting a hard-on, he masturbates himself to orgasm, with the "giver" in the next room or somewhere nearby but out of sight. Gradually, as each step is achieved successfully, the giver gradually moves closer, entering the room but not focusing on the receiver, then moving to nonsexual touching, sensual stroking, and eventually genital stimulation.

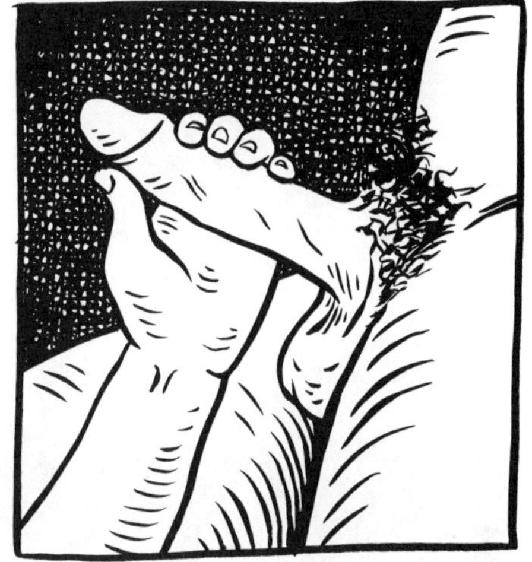

The squeeze technique

For Premature Ejaculation

If the "stop-start" technique described on page 175 isn't working, try the "squeeze technique." When your partner gives the signal, grasp the head of his penis firmly, with your thumb underneath and first and second fingers pressing just below the ridge at the top of the head. Squeeze gently but firmly, and his urge to come tends to vanish painlessly. Repeat a few times. Obviously, a few false starts—or rather, finishes—are likely as you experiment. Start without lubricant, then move to masturbation with lube. Once you have the hang of that, practice other forms of stopping and starting, such as placing his penis in your mouth or ass with no motion for a few moments. Work gradually.

An exercise you can do on your own is what Dr. Zilbergeld calls "getting your mind on your side." In *The New Male Sexuality,* Zilbergeld suggests what is a form of sexual creative visualization. Take five minutes every day to imagine yourself performing sexually the way you'd like to—lasting longer, being harder, whatever. If you have recurring negative thoughts about your sexual performance ("I come too fast," "I'll never get hard"), Zilbergeld suggests replacing them with an analysis of the facts, and credible positive statements that counteract them. Think "I don't get hard in anal intercourse, but I do stay hard for oral sex," or "I come quickly in intercourse, but I'm working on that. And I give a great blow job." If you feel comfortable—but only if you do, Zilbergeld cautions—go as far as "I will be a great lover" or "I know I can overcome this problem."

If you are dating, there's one other tool that can be incredibly useful for defusing the tension: talking. Imagine what would happen if you said as you were on your way home with someone new, "I'm really glad to be doing this, but I get nervous on the first date and can't come." "Rejection is a possibility," says Dr. Silverstein, "but it always is." And open conversation before sex may do more for your future together than the same conversation after an awkward ten minutes in the bedroom.

SEXUAL COMPULSIVITY

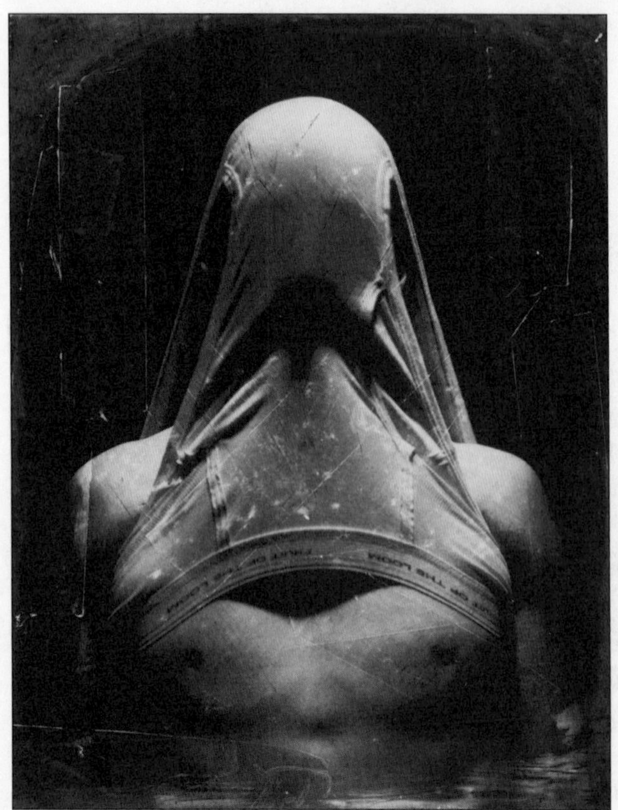

The night Terry's mother called me to tell me that he had died, I spent the rest of the night having sex in the basement of a porn theater. I never cried, but I went back every night for three weeks.

I was a mess. I was in the parks until all hours of the night. I almost got arrested in the bathroom at the local university. I narrowly escaped. I went back and the guard recognized me—it turned out I was trying to go in when it was spring break. I went in again the next week and he recognized me again. The last straw was when I had been in the park until the middle of the night. The next day I was sick, dragged myself to work late, and on the way home stopped in the park again. When I started always being late for work, or getting to the Greenmarket too late to buy the pretzels I love, those were real warning signs for me.

People have always used sex as a way to escape their solitude, forge connections, and gain a sense of power or pleasure. Gay men in particular have found that exploration of sex together—lots of it—is a means of healing homophobia, an affirmation of gay pride, a way to feel a sense of God, or just plain good. Well, most of the time.

Sometimes, having lots of sex—or looking to have it—doesn't feel so good. "Sexual compulsivity" is a term used to describe patterns where sex feels powerful without being pleasant, something you repeat over and over with less and less reward or sense of control. Examples of this can range from repeated attempts to act out sexually with people who have not consented—flashing your genitals, say, or fondling strangers on the mall escalator—to the more common and murkier pattern of unsatisfying sex sought out when you want to numb some other intense emotion. Feeling as if you're losing your ability to choose when and how to be sexual, having lots of sex with people whom you find abusive or unattractive, or seeing your sexual partners as objects to be used rather than people to connect with are all cited as symptoms of sexual compulsivity. Describing a common cycle—feeling driven to use sex to try to reach some magical altered state, and then experiencing a deeply depressing letdown afterward—some men talk about the problem with a different phrase: "sexual addiction."

Addiction and *compulsion* are controversial terms when it comes to sex, with battles over the implications of each. Addiction makes sex sound too much like a poison better given up, like alcohol, say some, when in fact there is no physiologically addictive component to sex, and having it is a sign of health. Compulsion ignores the incredible powerful social role of sex, counter others, and reduces sexual behavior to another symptom, like washing your hands too much or not stepping on cracks. Some students of gay history worry about both approaches, remembering the way that diagnoses of disease have long been used to cast a cloud of shame over any sex that does not fit the majority's idea of "normal." Some critics of gay society worry in the opposite direction, alarmed that the call for sexual freedom is silencing discussion of how many men have lots of sex without nearly so much satisfaction.

In practice, though, the differences between the terms *addiction* and *compulsion* (used interchangeably in the rest of this section) seem less important than the common themes expressed by men who find them meaningful. "I don't know whether I was addicted or compulsive, but I know that I would sit on my bed and cry if I didn't pick up someone every night after work," says Sam, age thirty-five. "One time I picked up three people on my block, one right after the other, and arrived late for an extremely important appointment." Other common stories include seeking sex immediately after important emotional events like the death of a parent or a friend; alternating sexual binges with periods of depression and total aversion to sex; and risking illness, arrest, or financial ruin in the pursuit of unsatisfying sex. A general feeling of numbness or dissociation during sex (the word *trance* comes up a lot) is also common to people struggling with these issues. Some of the men who describe themselves as sexual addicts report a childhood history of physical or sexual abuse, or emotional neglect. Many more report another addiction or behavior disorder—alcoholism, eating disorders, gambling, and the like.

If complaints about numbing or overpowering sex sound suspiciously like an effort to tidy messy realities into some unthreatening fifties fantasy of what sex "should be," talk of sexual compulsivity can carry that danger. People throughout history have certainly gambled, and lost a great deal, in the pursuit of sexual excitement, including excitement whose charge comes precisely because it's naughty or illegal or inappropriate or objectifying. Virtually everyone has had the experience of sex for reasons—mastery, a sense of power, an escape from worry—that may be more about changing a feeling inside ourselves than about experiencing one with someone

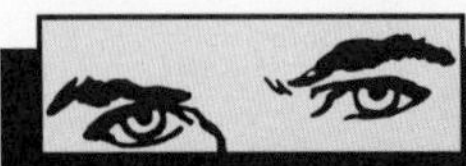

TURNING A GAY GAZE ON SEXUAL ADDICTION

SHAME ON WHOM?

Shame about sex, and keeping it secret, are red flags for sexual addiction in much of the psychological and addiction literature. But having grown up experiencing your desire for other men as something not valued or appreciated—something to be acted out apart from your family and friends—it's natural that many gay men would keep their sexual lives secret or split off. Coming out doesn't magically heal that split, or the shame and ambivalence it helps create. Trying to separate out the confusion about sex that society instills in us from the guilt and shame that fuel a psychological compulsion is a delicate proposition at best. "I've had men come in to me and say, 'You have to help me, I'm addicted, I masturbate every day,'" says New York City therapist Michael Shernoff, MSW. "And I have to ask, 'Well, why do you think that's sexually compulsive?' If you leave important meetings and go do it in the middle of the men's room, that's one thing. If you do it by yourself, in a stall, that's another. If you're doing it at home because you can't get to sleep unless you have an orgasm, that's yet another. There's no such thing as a pure motive in sex. It all has to be differentiated."

STRAIGHT TALKING

Gay culture—partly because we don't usually meet sex partners at work or through family, and partly because of the belief that there are models other than the monogamous child-rearing couple—has created some ways of being sexual that don't show up on the ordinary radar screens of the straight world. Some of those things—such as anonymous sex, cruising for sex, or having "fuck buddies"—may well show up on your local therapist's sexual addiction assessment, however.

One of the original self-help groups for sex addicts, Sexaholics Anonymous, goes as far as targeting "sex outside of heterosexual marriage" as a warning sign. Clearly, we're all diagnosable.

STRANGER THINGS HAVE HAPPENED

Consider gay realities as well as straight ones. "Just because you have sex with a stranger doesn't make you a sex addict, or mean you're not one," says John Sealy, MD, director of a treatment center for sexual disorders at Del Amo Hospital in California and a board member of the National Association of Sexual Addiction and Compulsivity. "It's not what you're eating, it's what's eating you." Similarly, it's tempting to want to split your sexual self into parts: the "bad" part, which feels drawn to the dangerous thrill of sex in the park, say, and the "good" part, which is monogamous and loving, brings home flowers, and gives your boyfriend soulful looks that would make Betty Crocker proud. "The reality of sexual life is more complex," says therapist Stephen McFadden. "Evaluating those complexities means looking at what you're getting or not getting from various kinds of sex, not just wishing lust away or dismissing gay culture."

ARE WE ALONE?

Most discussion of addiction, whether a physical addiction, such as alcoholism, or a compulsion, such as an eating disorder—uses a disease model, looking at the problem as something that an individual works to heal within himself. "That gets complicated," warns GMHC director of HIV prevention, Richard Elovich, "because most sex happens between two people, not just you. It's not something you 'have a case of.'" Treating sexual compulsivity as your problem alone can reinforce the isolation many gay men feel about their sexuality in the first place.

BEWARE ABSTINENCE ABSOLUTISM

Many men who feel there's some compulsive element to their sex jump at an I'll-never-do-that-again approach. While abstinence, freely chosen, can be helpful, says Jack Morin, Ph.D., author of *The Erotic Mind,* going to battle against sexual behavior can sometimes be the worst thing to do. "Struggle fuels compulsion," says Morin. "The solution is not for one side to win, but to integrate the warring selves by looking at what you are actually feeling while you're being compulsive. Conscious self-examination can disrupt some of the intensity, and much of the confusion."

else. And of course gay people feel shame about sex—straight people teach us to. Deciding where that shame comes from or what it means is a tricky business (see sidebar).

All of that makes it essential for gay men to cut themselves some slack during assessment of sexual "addiction," but not to rule out the exercise entirely. "The goal is be able to integrate your sex life with other things you want—feelings of freedom, self-esteem, intimacy, whatever—in such a way that you can be at relative peace with the sexual part of yourself, " says New York City therapist Stephen McFadden. "What that means has to be an individual definition."

"Treating" Sexual Compulsivity

STEP 1: AWARENESS

If you're not risking your life, courting arrest, or violating the rights of others through compulsive behavior, struggling with sexual compulsion usually begins with the same medicine prescribed for those seeking better sex or safer sex: mindfulness (see "Beyond Condoms," in Chapter 2). The same exercise that works for sex in general—asking yourself about what you do and how you feel, before, during, and after sex—can help you to grow conscious about your feelings of compulsion. Don't limit your thinking to direct contact with others; include phone sex, masturbation, and online cruising if you do them.

People grappling with sexual compulsion—as with eating disorders, alcoholism, or other powerful forms of behavior—talk of "triggers," the people, places, or things that activate intense cravings or behavior that feels out of control. For alcoholics, that trigger might be a bar where they used to drink; for someone who feels sexually compulsive, it could be a beach, a college bathroom, or an adult bookstore. Emotional "spots" you're in can also trigger compulsive behavior, as is captured in the oft-quoted acronym HALT—meaning feeling vulnerable when you're hungry, angry, lonely, or tired. Is it that you're horny or that you're alone on Saturday night and can't stand being in your apartment? Do you want sex or some way to escape the fact that you just got home from a difficult visit with your family? "I tell people, forget about monogamous, nonmonogamous, you have sex this way, you don't have sex that way," says therapist Michael Shernoff. "If you say you're on the way to the university bathroom to have sex, ask yourself: Is sex what you want, or just something you know how to get? I've spent months with people trying to help them figure out what it means to be horny, as opposed to anxious or bored or depressed or tired."

Other triggers for compulsive sex are found in the intersection of addictions, such as when you start drinking after a period of being sober, or start binge eating after not doing so for months. "Shame in general is a big trigger," says Joe Amico, M.Div., executive director of Minnesota's gay and lesbian chemical addiction center, the Pride Institute, "particularly when folks feel like what they're doing now stirs up bad memories of past experiences. For someone with a history of sexual abuse, for example, sex can trigger intrusive feelings of guilt about who you are and what happened to you. It feeds itself: More sex is a way of escaping the pain."

STEP 2: TALK ABOUT IT WITH SOMEONE

Not everyone needs ongoing therapy or to go to group meetings to deal with sexual addiction. A few counseling sessions or conversations with a close friend or pastoral counselor can be enough for some people to begin to feel aware. And unlike physical addictions to substances

DIAGNOSING SEXUAL ADDICTION

Sex, like food, is something that everyone needs—the question is how nourishing you're finding it. Rather than rushing to judgment, or treatment, of your sexual practices, take a look at them. "Most of us don't understand our sexual life—we have rules or methods for how we get off, but we don't necessarily sort out those rules or the mystery about them," says GMHC's Richard Elovich. "There is such a thing as sexual compulsion, but there's also natural confusion that may fit the diagnosis." Dr. Sealy agrees. "If you answer yes to fifteen out of twenty questions on an assessment test, that *may* or may not indicate addiction," he says. "The real question is whether you're selling out your integrity and tromping on your sense of spirituality and self. Can you sustain a sense of sexual satisfaction, or is there only dread?"

With those warnings in mind, below are some of the questions designed to try to gauge sexual compulsivity. They're a tool for inquiry, not an acid test.

- Do you think of yourself as overly preoccupied or obsessed with sex?
- Do you feel driven to have sex in response to the effects of stress, anxiety, depression, or other intense emotions?
- Have serious problems developed as a result of your sexual behavior (for example, injuries, illnesses, or loss of a job, or fiscal stability)?
- Do you find yourself constantly cruising or scanning the environment for a potential sexual partner, even when you don't feel it's appropriate?
- Do you often find yourself preoccupied by the idea of making sexual contact with a particular man you've seen or heard about, even if you don't know him?
- Have you repeatedly tried to stop or reduce certain sexual behaviors and been unable to do so?
- Have you missed important events in the lives of your family, friends, or life partner because of the time you spend pursuing sex?
- Do you feel yourself violating your own ethical standards or principles in sex?
- Do you worry about turning HIV-positive, yet regularly have risky sex anyway?

And here are a few questions that need to be balanced against the realities of being gay in a largely straight world, but are still worth thinking about.

- Do you keep the extent or nature of your sexual activities hidden from friends and/or partners?
- Do your sexual encounters place you in danger of arrest for lewd conduct or public indecency?
- Do you often have sex with men because you're feeling aroused and later regret it?
- Has your involvement with pornography, phone sex, or online sex kept you from other kinds of intimate contact with romantic partners?
- When you have sex, do you feel depressed, guilty, or ashamed afterward?
- Has the money you have spent on sex-related activities seriously strained your financial resources?

Adapted from Sexual Compulsives Anonymous's "Twenty Questions" and materials from the Del Amo Hospital in California

such as alcohol or heroin, sexual compulsivity is often not a lifelong struggle. "For the first two years I was in Sexual Compulsives Anonymous, I cried and whined and screamed, and people rolled their eyes at me and had compassion for me and got me through," says Charles, a thirty-seven-year-old public relations executive from Pennsylvania. "Now I can trick occasionally and go to the local porn theater for forty-five minutes, and not for five hours, and not for five hours every day for three weeks." Amico says that many people "go to meetings and treatment for a couple of years and then drop out of the scene." For others, issues are so strong it may mean a lifetime of investigation.

STEP 3: MAKE A PLAN

If you do seek therapy or peer support, don't have it be all talk and no action. Try to implement a plan, a way of finding what McFadden calls "a combination of understanding what contributes to the problem and a strategy about how to change it." That may just be returning to step one, above, or writing out a "contract" of the kind made by members of Sexual Compulsives Anonymous.

Self-Help: Finding a Twelve-Step Meeting

I was so relieved when I went to my first meeting, I just sat there, crying with relief that I wasn't alone.

There are at least half a dozen organizations nationwide that provide free fellowship and support for sexual compulsives. Each of these groups has its own traditions, approach, and familiarity with gay sexuality, though all are modeled on the twelve-step fellowship approach pioneered by Alcoholics Anonymous (AA; see page 277). In addition, there are support groups (S-Anon, Codependents of Sex Addicts, and Co-Sex & Love Addicts Anonymous) for sexual partners of sex addicts. "God makes us and we find each other," jokes Paul, a forty-three-year-old actor from Los Angeles. Actually, depending on where you live, what you find in terms of self-help programs can range from a gay-specific meeting for sexually addicted survivors of

SELF-HELP FELLOWSHIPS

SCA, SA, SAA, SLAA: If you thought sex was confusing, try the array of acronyms for sexual recovery programs. That there are so many different groups speaks in part to the complicated facts of sex, and to the many different opinions of how they can best be approached. Below is a list of a few of the more popular fellowships.

Group Name	Operating Principles
Sexual Compulsives Anonymous (SCA)	Founded by gay men, and still gay-friendly. Asks members to design their own written recovery plan and encourages them to change it as they change themselves.
Sexaholics Anonymous (SA)	Homophobic—it urges no masturbation or sex outside of "established heterosexual marriage." Gay men are welcome, but only if they're willing to be celibate.
Sex Addicts Anonymous (SAA)	Urges abstinence from "compulsive, destructive behavior" and "out-of-bounds" sex, which you define. Includes gay-specific information in literature and conferences.
Sex and Love Addicts Anonymous (SLAA)	Often straighter and with more women than SCA, but also welcomes gay men. Deals with romantic obsessions as well as sexual ones. "No bottom-line behavior" is their bottom line, and you define what that behavior is for you.

Further contact information is listed on page 580.

childhood abuse to no meetings at all. If you have access to the Internet, there are a number of online support groups as well.

As with AA, participants in sexual recovery programs work to support each other in maintaining their "sobriety," though what sobriety means differs from program to program (see box on page 183). Many participants are also in another twelve-step program.

Professional Help

Finding therapy for sexual compulsivity, or a place to talk it through, involves many of the same kinds of decisions as finding help for other sexual problems (see "Dr. Love," below). The exercises and homework of the "sex therapist" proper are likely to be less useful than finding a counselor or therapist willing to address broader issues of desire, anxiety, and motivation. Treatment can be a few counseling sessions or ongoing individual or group therapy, including medication or without it. Certain kinds of compulsive thoughts or urges, including some compulsive sexual behavior, have been minimized by use of antidepressants, particularly by some of the selective serotonin reuptake inhibitors (see page 489). And for cases where chemical dependency or compulsive behavior is putting you or others in danger, at least six hospitals around the country offer inpatient programs and treatment. The National Council on Sexual Addiction and Compulsivity (see page 580) maintains a list of these programs, and gay members of their board may be able to offer a referral to a therapist or gay-friendly program in your area.

DR. LOVE: FINDING A SEX THERAPIST

I have a good therapist, cool, relaxed. But when I talk about sex, I can't get over the nagging feeling that he doesn't know what I'm talking about.

How can I talk to my therapist about these things? I don't know how to talk about them myself.

Largely gone are the days of gay "sexual surrogates," when therapists routinely hired sex workers to help patients work out the details of their sexual difficulties in a controlled setting. "The threat of lawsuits was too high, and the training too erratic," says Dr. Silverstein. Ironically, the latter part of the criticism—lack of training—is the same one that Silverstein and the handful of others with extensive experience working with gay men would level at many therapists of today whose methods are more orthodox. For the difficult business of good sex, finding good therapy is also difficult.

The problem is not exactly lack of choice: If you're experiencing problems with desire, arousal, or sexual performance, there's an array of professionals out there willing to help.

Therapists and sexuality counselors, from social workers to psychoanalysts, all work with individuals on issues that often lie at the heart of sexual difficulties: self-image, exploration of conscious and unconscious urges, compulsions, and desires. These professionals may also provide education—a little bit of a reality check to let you know if you're operating under some misconceptions about what other people do and don't do in sex.

Family or couples counselors are therapists with experience helping people work on the dynamics of family life, including maintaining (or finding a healthy way to end) a committed romantic relationship. Issues like monogamy and decreased desire are among their specialties. And since the 1970s, when headlines claimed Masters and Johnson could reverse 90 percent of problems with sexual function, a new class of professionals, called *sex therapists,* have been working with couples on specific ways of addressing sexual problems. Sex therapists often tend to skip the deep psychological analysis, working instead with specific exercises and "homework" designed to alter a couple's response to problems such as delayed ejaculation, premature ejaculation, or failure to get a hard-on. Good therapists often see results, says Dr. Moser, though sustaining those results in the long term can prove more difficult.

In all these fields, gay men may find it hard to find professionals whose thinking about the complexities of desire and sexual expression have moved beyond safer-sex platitudes and a basic knowledge of a few Masters and Johnson–era exercises (see "Sensate Focus," on page 176). "In California, psychologists are required to have a mandatory ten hours of training, and people say, 'Okay, that's it, I know all about sex,'" says Dr. Jack Morin. There is no formal license for sex therapy in any state, says Dr. Silverstein, and many therapists have "no knowledge of the data, and only a little more curiosity."

Whether you want a gay therapist is up to you, but gauging a therapist's comfort level with gay sex is essential. "Ask what he or she thinks are some of the most pressing sexual issues," suggests Michael Shernoff, "and see how they respond to your questions. Do they welcome them, or do they seem defensive? If he or she acts like the great white doctor—'How dare you ask? Don't you see my certificates on the wall?'—then that tells you something." Actually, so may the certificates on the wall: two different societies, the American Association of Sex Educators, Counselors, and Therapists (AASECT) and the American Board of Sexology, offer ongoing training and certification for their members. AASECT will send you a regional members list upon request, though they don't separate out therapists who are gay or especially practiced in gay issues.

While grilling someone on the ins and outs of anal sex is probably beyond the call of duty, it is appropriate, no matter how embarrassing or awkward, to ask a few questions (see box below). If the therapist tries to set you "straight," cancel the whole affair and get a referral from someone else, says Silverstein. "That's one network you don't want to be a part of."

TALKING SEX: QUESTIONS TO ASK A POTENTIAL SEX THERAPIST

- Do you think homosexuality is an illness?
- Are you certified as a sex therapist?
- What do you do to keep current on sexual thinking?
- Do you read any journals or attend any meetings about sexual research?
- Where would you go for information if we encountered sexual issues you were not familiar with?
- How many gay men with issues similar to those I'm describing have you treated?
- Are you still in supervision with a more experienced colleague? (Yes is a good answer, not a bad one, here.)

FURTHER READING

Goldstone, Steven. (1999) *The Ins and Outs of Gay Sex.* New York: Dell. A gay surgeon's account of, and tips on, gay men's sexual ailments and their care.

Holmes, King K., et al. (1999) *Sexually Transmitted Diseases*. New York: McGraw Hill. A highly technical, completely comprehensive guide to the subject.

Penn, Robert E. (1997) *The Gay Men's Guide to Wellness: The National Gay and Lesbian Health Association's Complete Book of Physical, Emotional, and Mental Health and Well-being for Every Gay Male*. New York: Henry Holt and Company. Like this book, an overview of many gay male health concerns, including sexual health.

Tiefer, Leonore. (1995) *Sex Is Not a Natural Act and Other Essays*. Boulder, CO: Westview Press. Pre-Viagra, but extremely insightful on the thoughts behind and beyond erectile dysfunction treatment, including some not found in namby-pamby impotence literature.

Whitehead, E. Douglas, and Terry Malloy. (1998) *Viagra: The Wonder Drug for Peak Performance.* One of a dozen books published within a year of Viagra's release. Contains basic info on erectile dysfunction as well as on the "wonder drug."

Zilbergeld, Bernie. (1999) *The New Male Sexuality*. New York: Bantam Books. Not new enough to include gay men, but full of interesting exercises and suggestions about sexual function, communication, and the intersection of the two.

PART 2

BODY BASICS

CHAPTER 5

Skin Deep?

Exercise Basics • Aerobic Exercise • Strength Training Basics • The Gym • Hurts So Good? • Chemical Catalysts: Steroids and Supplements • Exercise Control? • Mind and Body • Skin Care Basics • Plastic and Beautiful? • Hair Care, Hair Loss, and Hair Removal • Balding Basics • Watch Your Mouth

A popular game in classrooms across America finds schoolchildren staring at a willing but unsuspecting playmate. "Look at your fingernails," comes the first command. "Now stand up, drop your pencil on the ground, and pick it up. Carry a notebook two steps across the room. Look at the sky. Sit down and cross your legs." When the participant is done, the other schoolchildren—their delight increasing with the amount of trouble in Genderville—render the verdict. "Boys" look at their nails by turning their palms up and folding their nails toward the heel of the hand. "Girls" stretch their fingers out away from them, contemplating the back of the hand. Boys pick up their pencils by bending at the waist; girls, by lowering their knees toward their heels. Male-style book carrying is with hand by side; female, with book clutched to chest. Boys lift their chin skyward, craning their necks, while girls throw their eyes to the sky. Finally, boys rest the ankle of one leg on the knee of the other, avoiding the feminine placement of one knee on top of the other, or the even more girly hooking of the toe of the top leg under the calf of the bottom leg. Take this test and *voilà!* You, penis or no, may be revealed as three-, four-, or even five-fifths—100 percent—woman.

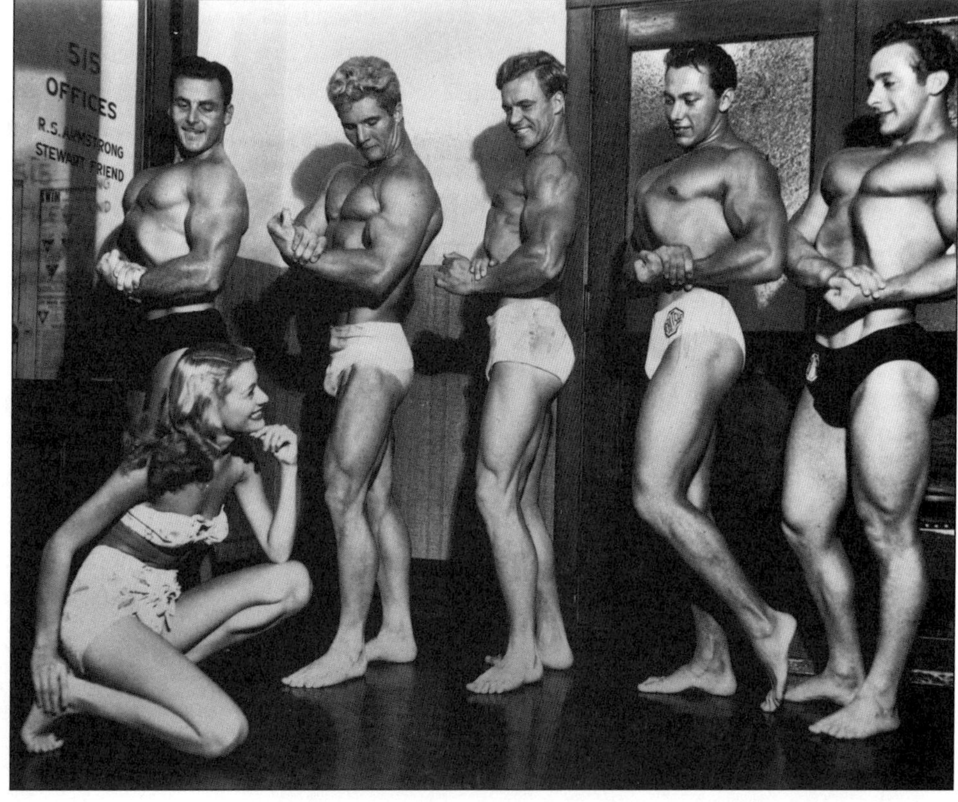

From the mouths of babes. It's a lesson little homosexuals, sensitive straight boys, tomboys, and young trannies-in-training learn over and over again: It's not just what your body looks like but what you do with it that counts. It's why some of us deepen our voice when asking for change at the gas station or firm up our handshake at the business meeting. It's part of why we work out at the gym, making sure that our arms, even if clutching books to our chests, are rippling with muscles. It's why switching and swishing, rolling alternate buttocks, or strutting sway-backed and seductive may get you a date, an appreciative laugh from your friends, or a fist in the mouth. French feminist Simone de Beauvoir summed it up simply: "The body," she wrote, "is a situation."

I remember dangling at the end of the rope for the obstacle course, completely unable to climb it, and completely unwilling to try. I just hung there limply, waiting for the coach to blow the whistle in disgust.

When I'm dancing—just swaying with my friends, all of us moving together—I get filled with this joy, this pride in what we can do. I love our movement! I love our style! We are so alive at that moment, I just close my eyes and sway and want it to go on forever.

He just said one word. He called my skin "caramel." If anyone ever says that, he has a special place in my heart. And because it was in Europe, it was that much more exciting.

Grade school may be over, but the tests and triumphs are not. Feeling comfortable with your body and where you put it is a challenge that continues in all ages and stages of gay life. HIV—the fear of looking like you have it, and coping when you do—has been one of the most painful forms of bodily struggle for gay men in the last two decades. For men of certain generations, those of us with the half-empty address books, the wasting of AIDS has probably done more to get us to the gym than any health bulletin, sending us in search of a look—backward baseball caps, hairless chests—that recalls a time when we were all younger and uninfected. Some see the piercing trend as another way to mark an expression of bodily innocence lost in the age of AIDS, a literal version of the pain of an on-me-not-in-me era. But it doesn't necessarily take direct experience of HIV or a Prince Albert through the penis to feel as though your body is something you're stuck with, a physical manifestation of your difference from the rest of the world. "When I come into Chicago and the gay scene, I feel myself vanishing," says Paul, twenty-four. "I mean, you say hello to someone on the street and they look through you, like, 'How dare you even talk to me when you don't have a body?' And as much as I hate it, I turn around and do it to someone else, not looking at someone so much as rating him." Men in their forties and fifties—including fit, well-muscled men—often talk not of feeling bodily changes so much as feeling as though their bodies have ceased to exist. "You get used to seeing yourself in terms of the heads that turn toward you, the glances you catch," says Vincent, forty-five years old, his body toned from daily yoga and biking, "and then you realize that it no longer happens, that you've crossed over some line into the land of the invisible." (See "Off the Gaydar?" page 341, in Chapter 8.)

These are not just gay thoughts; alienation from the body, the single person's search for connection, and a sense of fragmentation haunt the experience of most people, especially city dwellers. Gay ghosts, though, may rise up in different places. Step into all-male domains, especially—gyms, hardware stores, some gay bars and cruising areas—and body consciousness can return with all the force of schoolboy jitters. That's not always true; there *are* gay men who feel at home on a construction site or swing weights around the gym with the cool assurance of bartenders mixing cocktails, just as not all gay men played with dolls or were scared of sports as kids. But go to a party sometime and ask how many men (including the big hunky ones) were picked last for teams at school. When put on an all-male team, most of us learned to masquerade or melt into the background, confused by the difference between what attracted us—men—and all the little tests and comments that suggested we weren't one of them.

The difference between what you want and who you are remains confusing, and arousing. You see that ambivalence in the gay personal ads from men looking for straight-acting partners, or in the guys who say they like to sleep with straight men best. You hear it in men's complaints about the superficial, hard-body-obsessed gay magazines we don't like but nonetheless can't seem to put down. Men talk about it in workshops at GMHC, acknowledging the importance of their inner selves at the same time they detail the ways they imagine a different body would give them a different life. "If I had a gym body . . ." "If I weren't Asian . . ." "If my head were smaller . . ." "If I were Latino . . ."

It's true that there are places in the gay community where the size of your basket is more important than the size of your brain, or where pecs count for more than personality. It's true that good-looking people often get better jobs, and that people who are overweight are treated worse. It's true that we live in a free-market society whose efforts to sell you something—clothes, cologne, sexual services, a masculine mythology—are fueled by images of a just-out-of-reach ideal that keep us buying and trying. Women have talked about it for years: the pitfalls of trying to live up to a picture-perfect image, and the way the straight white men in power benefit from keeping us more concerned with bathroom scales than pay scales, more worried about how we look than how we're treated. It's also true that the times are changing, with men and women, gay and straight, increasingly buying into the idea that young and fit is where it's at. In 1986 few had heard of personal trainers; by 1996 twenty-three thousand such trainers had been certified by the American College of Exercise. Americans now spend $4 billion annually to look young, and more than $33 billion on diet programs, pills, videos, books, and "thinning" surgery.

But there's no absolute center to the world, gay or otherwise. Widen your focus and you may see a different picture. Hot go-go boys are on the covers of some gay magazines, but by no means all. In *Bulk Male,* a magazine from Sausalito, California, many models top three hundred pounds, and personal ads speak of men's yearning to rest their heads on a big, hairy chest. The Black Party in New York, full of mostly white, well-muscled youth, is followed the next weekend by the Blacker Party, where men of color, and all shapes and sizes, celebrate. In Faerie circles from Seattle to Sarasota, slender, skirted men with names like Funbuns and Cypress dance, drum, and make love under the stars (for more on the Faeries, see Chapter 13). On the Internet, where all you need is a scanner and a dream, the "It boys" of the moment often sport a chunky, ordinary masculinity, their thick legs, round faces, and hairy, chewable chests sparking admiration and invitations.

Really listen to gay men sing the body electric and you'll hear more than one tune. Some of us cherish the lanky, the goofy, and the squat. "I for one, love girly boys, though I'm happy not to be one," says thirty-nine-year-old David, a writer from Kalamazoo, Michigan. "My lover scours cyberspace for filthy pictures, a huge portion of whom turn out to be bears. He wouldn't mind if I exploded at the middle, which I frankly am hoping to avoid."

So imagine—and this may not take much work—that you're one of the beautiful men we've all seen staring into the mirror at gyms or on the dance floor. Say you've just finished a workout, a practice with your volleyball team, or a hot round of dancing. What do your eyes scan for as you stare into the glass? Are you looking with satisfaction, appreciating the healthy play of muscles under flesh, the tendons and ligaments that let you make that dazzling turn or superb spike? Does your body look back at you like an ally, a reliable friend? Or do you go right for what is missing, how you've yet to reach the perfect biceps or the chest of death? Perhaps you can't even see yourself, feeling your eyes drawn instead to the hazier reflections of those who stand behind you, the audience without which you may feel nothing at all.

How do you look? The question, no matter how hard we try to make it simple, is always two in one. The first and more familiar one is how you appear to others: how you imagine they see your hair, your skin, your eyes and clothes and body. The second version of the question returns the emphasis to the word *how,* and the responsibility to you. How do you look at yourself or others? Do you use the eyes of the critic, noting defects and softness? Do you go right to comparisons, stacking yourself up against someone else to see who's hotter, better, and why? Or are you more forgiving, more able to see your way, in the mirror or at the local bar, to the inner places that stay soft in all of us? There's a third question that gay men might do well to ask, no matter how hard or soft our bodies are: How do I feel?

Exercise Basics

My father would turn into a different person when he took out the ball and glove. "Hustle!" he'd start yelling, throwing me balls. All his usually encouraging comments were replaced by negative ones. I threw "like a girl." I swung "like a rusty gate." I couldn't "hit the broad side of a barn."

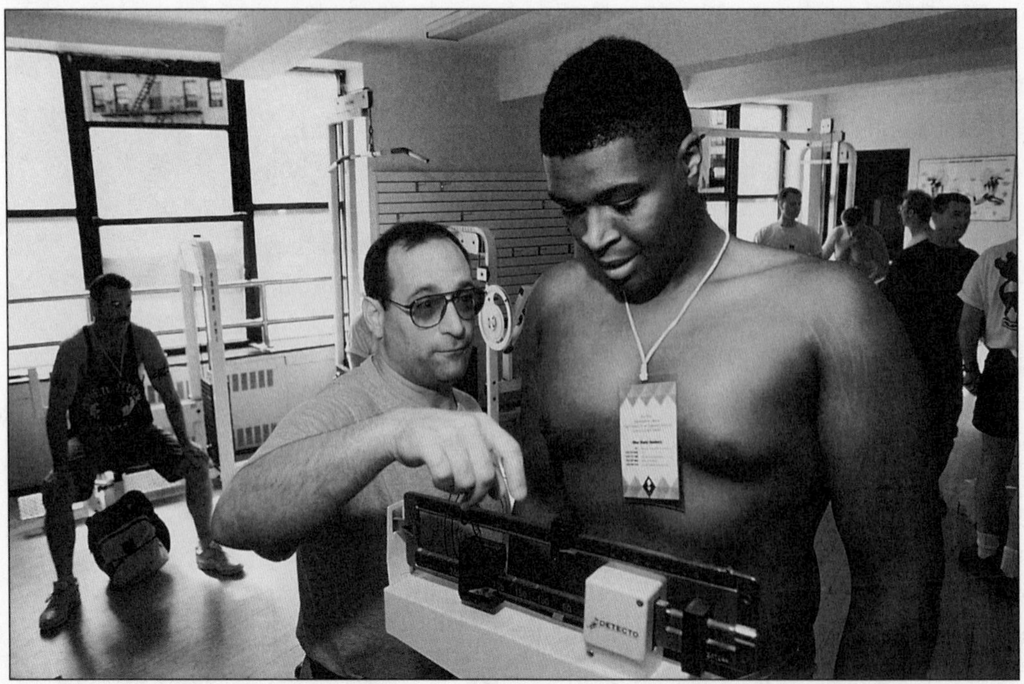

I'm getting to the age where you start to hit things like heart attack, and felt like it was better to start now than not. I chose swimming because I thought it would interest me long-term, and was something I could do in the summer and winter. An added bonus, which I hadn't even taken into account, was the locker room. I had always kept myself out of it at school, for

fear of being taunted for being so skinny and because the possibility of dealing with being sexually attracted to my schoolmates was something I wasn't really ready to deal with. But now I'm a skinny man, not a kid, and even though this pool doesn't have sex, I enjoy the sexual charge. It's nice just to be able to walk around and look, and to feel comfortable being naked in front of other people.

Athletes talk often about the "flow," the place where things click and mind and body operate as one. Gay men who never did sports remember the mind-body connection too, but often in terms of what our bodies managed to reveal, or what we thought they might, about our teenage secrets. But you're a big boy now, the world is changing, and some teenage-era problems seem less pressing, or even pleasant. If you haven't been able to exercise since dangling

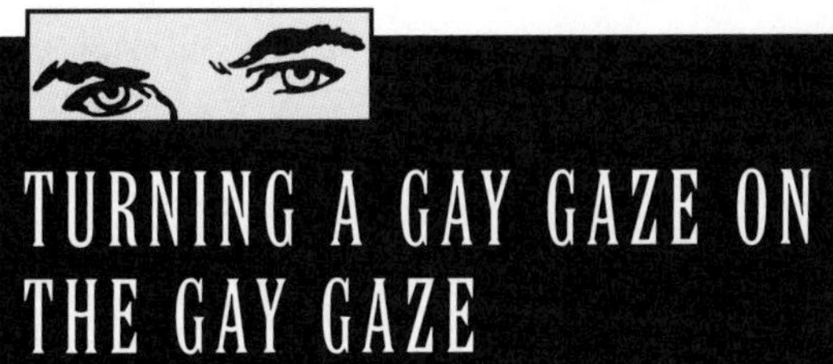

TURNING A GAY GAZE ON THE GAY GAZE

You might say it was just an exchange of glances between strangers, but it was a lot more powerful. We were both on our way somewhere else, which was probably what made it so good. I'd look up, or he would, and we'd catch each other's eye across the train. That was enough. We both got what we wanted, we both left happy, and neither of us felt like he had won or lost. It was like a perfect relationship.

Those trashy fifties novels about the "sad gay lifestyle" are always talking about our eyes, the gaze that stays, searching, for something that seems to make the author vaguely uncomfortable. Today, gay men themselves talk in different terms of the pleasure of the look, the connections you make across a room, or subway platform, or just about anywhere else. "It may not necessarily go anyplace," says Peter, twenty-four, "but you catch somebody's eye and it's just like—click—something falling into place." For Jaime, forty-five, it's not about being seen so much as surveying, exercising your desire: "Sometimes I sit on the bus and go man by man, like a treasure hunt, finding something attractive about every one," he says. Other gazes may be less about wanting than being wanted. "I call it the 'gotcha' game," says Anders, thirty-five, his voice tinged with the knowledge that he is "played" as often as he plays. "He looks at you just long enough for you to be interested, and then his look goes distant, like, 'How could you possibly imagine I'd be interested in you? Gotcha!'"

What are gay men looking for? Is the gay gaze simply another mode of competition, a way of measuring our worth—in the manner of men, and the marketplace—by seeing if we have something someone else wants? Is it a way of tuning up our "gaydar," scanning for safe havens in a potentially hostile environment? Or perhaps we're trying to transform hostility, finding a way to rewrite the old gay story most of us experienced when younger: the fear of being rejected for, or by, the men we most desired. "Let's face it: If you're rejecting, you don't have to worry about being rejected," offers Anders simply. "It's the same thing that happens, say, on a phone sex line, when someone seems interested, you're drawn in, and then, for no apparent reason—beep!—you're over." Isay, forty, from Hawaii, sees another, modern layer in the gotcha game. "AIDS raised the stakes," he suggests. "It's like you're saying, 'If I'm going to take a risk, I have to look really close to be sure you're worth it.' Even when there's no sex, what's left is the concern that you're making an equal exchange, or better still, trading up."

Looks can't kill. But they can hurt, or satisfy, or forge connections.

SPEAKING OUT ON THE GAY GAZE

Joel Beard, who was born with dislocated hips and had polio in infancy, lives with his lover in New York City. The following was excerpted from the spring 1998 issue of Able Together, *a quarterly newsletter for men with and without disabilities.*

The gaze is one of the ways we connect, usually what comes first: I like what you look like, you like what I look like. Sometimes on the street, just walking, there's the look that lingers, you can still feel it on the back of your neck and you turn around and smile. Appreciation, lust sometimes: how I'd like to strip you naked, skin to skin, if only we weren't hurrying in opposite directions.

Bars are definitely about the gaze. You walk in under the light shining over the door and heads turn for a second. It's not the same for disabled guys, of course. How often do you roll into a bar in your wheelchair and feel like one of the crowd? Or does the gaze glance right off you and suddenly it's as if you're not there?

"I never think of you as disabled," he said, meaning well, intending a compliment. There's a pair of crutches directly in your line of vision. Look at how I move. How can you not think of me as disabled?

"But what about fat people," you say, "or anyone else who doesn't fit the young, body-perfect ideal?"

It's very personal, I know that. Everyone fights their own battles. Like the time when I was nineteen. He was a few years older. He had a lover and I slept on the extra bed in the same room. The lover left for work early, and he had the day off. After we had sex, he said, "I was worried I might throw up when I first saw your scars."

Or the one who used to tell me I was sexy from the waist up, that I was sexy in spite of having no ass because of the polio. I'm not sure what I was supposed to think, whether I'd be better off with no legs at all—or even what that said about my cock, which is definitely below my waist.

Just the other day I read some messages left on a gay discussion board on the Web: "Hey, I had this amputee last night. You should try one. That was the most fantastic blow job. I guess they try harder." And a later response: "I'm an amputee, and we do try harder, give me a call."

Yeah, we try harder, and I'm not even thinking about sex here. We work harder just to get through a day. Period. And even though that posting recognizes us as sexual, I'm not so sure about making someone sexy just because he's freakish. I'd rather see something much more inclusive, where the gaze encompasses difference and doesn't set it aside as a specialized minority attraction.

helplessly on the pull-up bar in gym class, maybe you can try again. Getting to a team, or to a gym, or wherever men do sports will be at least a viewing pleasure.

Exercise, though, is pleasing to more than the eyes. Whether you're sixty or sixteen, HIV-positive or positive you've never had a virus in your life, doing an exercise routine tones your muscles, burns fat, lowers cholesterol, boosts your immune system, strengthens your heart, expands your range of motion, elevates your mood, and does about three dozen other good things, none of which necessarily has to do with looking like, or finding someone else who looks like, an Adonis.

Do it in a way that you personally choose, not because you're the dough and the workout is the cookie cutter. Work hard shoveling in the garden or doing push-ups in your bedroom. Join one of the growing number of gay teams doing sports. If you want to go to a gym and get huge, that's fine. Maybe you just want to lose twenty pounds, or increase your physical strength and endurance, or make sure your shoulder gets back to normal after surgery. Perhaps you just want to blow off steam at the end of a rough day at the office, something for which thirty minutes of swimming, running, or Stairmastering can work wonders.

Every good exercise regimen has three components: strength training, aerobic exercise (also known as cardiovascular exercise, or "cardio"), and stretching. How you balance these elements depends on what you want to happen through your exercise. "The quick summary is that if you want to lose weight, stress cardio, if you want to define your body, stress cardio, and if you want to get big, stress strength training," says YMCA trainer Ryan Rivera, summing up the basic approaches and motivators. That doesn't mean, insist Rivera and other trainers, that emphasizing one component means you should ignore the others. A study for the YMCA, for example, found that people who combined weight training with aerobics lost two and a half times more fat than those who did the aerobic exercise alone.

Getting Started: General Pointers for Beginners

Look at gay men girding themselves in muscle as though they're preparing for war, or massing in formation in front of the Stairmasters, and it can be easy to admit defeat. If you're older, or recovering from illness, or not between the ages of twenty and thirty-five, the spandex legions can seem all the more overwhelming. Plus One Fitness, a medically based fitness clinic in New York City, works with various populations, including many men—older, HIV-positive, or just plain scared—to guide them through an exercise routine that works. Below find a few of their tips to make the battle of the beginner a little easier.

1. *Consult a doctor.* Everyone should ask a doctor if, and to what extent, they should start a fitness program, advises Bill Vayo, senior exercise specialist at Plus One Fitness. Among the questions to ask: "How many days a week should I start out at? How long should each session be? How intense?" If you're on the frail side, older, or HIV-positive, you might want to talk to your friends about finding a trainer (or even a certain gym) who has experience with clients with similar concerns.

2. *Start with an activity that you like.* "If you're steered into something you don't enjoy," says Vayo, "your main motivation is going to be fear or a sense that you 'should.'" Enjoyment works better, even if it doesn't exactly match the requirements of a perfect exercise routine. "If going out dancing, or even staying in dancing, is what gets you moving," says Vayo, "then go for it, and have fun doing it."

3. *Find a friend.* "Being alone is one of the main reasons people give up or stop their exercise efforts," says Vayo. "Playing on a team or working out with a friend can keep you going. It doesn't have to be someone you know really well; there's a tradition in sports of helping each other."

4. *Be your own judge of intensity.* That's especially true if you're on any medications that prevent a clear reading of your heart rate while exercising. Base what you can and cannot do on what fitness experts call a perceived exertion rating, a subjective range that puts resting at 0 and extreme exertion at 10. "You know your body better than any doctor or trainer," Vayo says.

5. *Exercise is where you find it.* "Get off your train one stop early, or take the stairs instead of the elevator," suggests Vayo. Even if you want to do strength training, you don't necessarily have to plunk down a lot of money on membership at an expensive gym. Push-ups, chin-ups (aided by a bar you can easily install), and abdominal crunches are just three of many excellent strength-training exercises you can do in your own home, though investing in a few barbells or a gym dramatically increases your options.

6. Even if you're going to be working out at home, try to get at least one or two sessions with a trainer to learn proper training and stretching techniques. Most gyms will give you one session with a trainer for free, and it pays to revisit every once in a while for new ideas and correction. "I can't afford a regular trainer, but I meet with one every six months or so to get advice and new suggestions," says Charlie, who, single at seventy-two, has started going to his gym for the first time in thirty years. "I need help, but also to be sure that someone's watching. It's only recently that friends are starting to notice that I'm looking and feeling better."

7. *Eat, drink, and be conscious.* Focusing on fitness for an hour and then gorging at the dinner table—or getting trashed and staying out until five in the morning—may be okay every

THE ABCD (AND S) OF EXERCISE

Training regimens change from gym to gym, year to year, and trainer to trainer. The good news is, those fitness magazines with beautiful men in nothing but sweatpants will never go out of business. The other good news is that there are so many different ways to exercise that one of them is bound to keep you happy. While an informal poll of personal trainers from gay meccas—South Beach to West Hollywood, Chelsea to the Castro—reveals as many different approaches as a Diana Ross show has costume changes, most agree on the basics.

Aerobics over all. If you only have half an hour, choose aerobic exercise over other forms. "It's the best overall for you," says Leonardo Machado, fitness supervisor at Body Tech gym in South Beach, Miami, "lowering cholesterol, burning off fat, toning muscles, and increasing the sense of general well being." Even if you want to stress lifting, advises Machado, use aerobic exercise to warm up, increase circulation, loosen muscles, and prevent injuries. *Bottom line:* Five to ten minutes of light aerobic exercise before strength training, and thirty minutes or more three times a week.

Breathe. Whether it's yoga, stretching, aerobics, or weight training, don't forget to keep your focus on your breath. "A lot of people tense up, particularly when they stretch," says Sharon Moss, a certified personal trainer and former manager of the nutrition department at Gold's Gym in West Hollywood. "You should try to relax your mind and keep breathing." *Bottom line:* For weight training, breathe out on the difficult part of the movement (think "exhale for effort") and in as you return toward your resting place. Whatever your exercise of choice, consciously return your focus to your breath throughout.

Cool down when done. Don't go from sixty to zero without a transition. If you're doing an aerobic workout, says Moss, simply slow your pace until your breathing is down to its normal rate. If you've been lifting weights or doing push-ups, conclude with some simple stretches of arms, back, and legs. Even yoga stretching or other, less aerobic exercises should conclude with a period of mental cooling down, a conscious return of your body to a more centered, calmer place. *Bottom line:* Take three minutes at the end of whatever you're doing to bring your body to a more normal, resting pace.

once in a while, but it doesn't make much sense in the long term. View what you eat and drink as part of what you do at the gym, not as an entirely different topic (see Chapter 6).

8. *Underdo.* For any one exercise session, there is a threshold of time after which physical exertion starts doing more harm than good. ("It's probably why long-distance runners are more prone to upper respiratory infections," says Vayo.) Sports injuries, too—most common among men between the ages of twenty and forty—tend to happen early in your workout, and when you push too hard. Better to stay in it for the long haul than to play Superman the first week and end up sidelined for months with a sprain or pulled muscle.

Okay, now, towels around the neck, Reeboks laced tight, tank tops formfitting but not trashy, and you're ready to begin.

Drink more water than you think you need to. Drink water before, during, and after your workout, sipping from a water bottle even if you're not thirsty, says Bill Vayo. Contrary to some myths, drinking water just before your workout can prevent cramps, not cause them. If you're properly hydrated, says Vayo, your urine should be clear or pale; if you're peeing yellow, drink some more. "Once you start getting thirsty, it's too late," he says. "Either give yourself a break from your workout that day, or seriously lower the intensity of the exercise." *Bottom line:* Eight large glasses of water or other liquid a day. Milk in your cereal and soup count. Alcohol, tea, diet Coke, or anything else that contains caffeine doesn't.

Stretch. Trainers differ about when you want to do this: before workout to loosen up, in mid-workout to ease muscles while weight lifting, or after the workout to make sure you're not in knots tomorrow. All, however, agree that stretching is essential to prevent injury and retain flexibility, and that it's too often ignored. Never stretch with a bouncing or jerking motion, try to stay conscious of your spine and stomach muscles rather than slumping into the stretch, and breathe. *Bottom line:* Stretch to resistance, not to pain. Hold each one for twenty to thirty seconds—less is too short, and longer makes no difference.

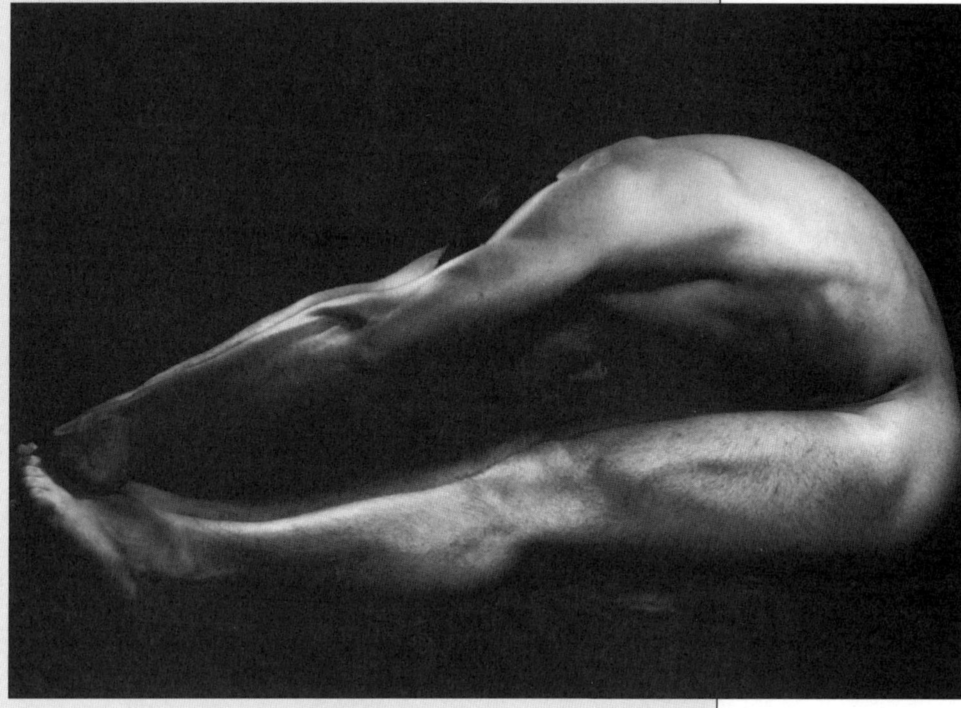

Aerobic Exercise

On Fridays, after that long week of work, I do an extra long session of nothing but cardio. I struggle to get through the first half hour, and then the last thirty minutes is just like this great high, this incredible buzz.

Aerobic exercise does not necessarily mean joining a class of spandex-wrapped beat bunnies bouncing to dance music. The term *aerobic,* used interchangeably with the popular *cardiovascular,* the precise *cardiorespiratory,* or the all-purpose *cardio,* refers to any activity that keeps the heart and lungs working at a steady rate. Though it may be tempting to spend your precious lunch hour pressing toward a bigger chest, many of the biggest benefits of exercise—lower blood pressure, relief from anxiety, better sleep, and a general rush of pleasant feelings that comes from the release of the painkilling chemicals known as endorphins into your bloodstream—come after twenty to thirty minutes of brisk aerobic exercise. Build up to forty-five minutes or an hour, three times a week, says Greg Ryan, a personal trainer at Market Street Gym in San Francisco, and in addition to a rush you'll get a good solid fat-burning, heart-strengthening effect.

So how will you aerobicize? Running on the street or the treadmill? Cross-country skiing? "Slaloming" on a cutting-edge contraption at your gym, or swimming laps in the public pool? It doesn't matter, so long as you are doing it at the appropriate intensity. All fitness training is based on what physiologists call the "overload principle": In order to get benefit from training, you have to force your muscles, or your lungs, or whatever, to work harder than usual. In aerobic exercise, most fitness authorities say, you should work hard enough to raise your heart rate to around 75 percent of your maximum, and then maintain that level for thirty minutes or more. Work your heart too hard, and the benefits diminish. Charles Franchino, D.C., a New York City chiropractor who works with a large gay practice, recommends the talk test: "Do it at a pace that lets you carry on a conversation, but not sing."

If you are using electronic equipment, keep your eye on the heart rate, not the calorie counter. "Pedaling slowly on the stationary bike may burn 250 calories, but it won't give you the full benefit of aerobic exercise," explains Rivera. "Reach the right intensity, and your body continues to burn off fat stores after the exercise is completed." Try combining different machines or different methods. "I keep myself going by finding a 'rabbit,'" says Adam, a thirty-five-year-old aerobics buff from Los Angeles. "I stand behind some really attractive and unattainable man in class and struggle to keep up, like the greyhound at a racetrack." Aerobics classes are also the place where powerful bonds between gay men and straight women are traditionally formed. "I got my current job through a lead from this woman in my step class," says Hans, age thirty-six, a banker in Seattle. "It all started with trading grievances about our thighs!"

Technically, your ideal pace—50 percent to 75 percent of the maximum heart rate—changes by sport and by age. The basic targets recommended by the American Heart Association are summarized on the chart on the next page.

Age	Target Heart Rate Zone (50%–75%)	Average Maximum Heart Rate (100%)
20	100–150 beats per minute	200 beats per minute
25	98–146 beats per minute	195 beats per minute
30	95–142 beats per minute	190 beats per minute
35	93–138 beats per minute	185 beats per minute
40	90–135 beats per minute	180 beats per minute
50	85–127 beats per minute	170 beats per minute
55	83–123 beats per minute	165 beats per minute
60	80–120 beats per minute	160 beats per minute
65	78–116 beats per minute	155 beats per minute
70	75–113 beats per minute	150 beats per minute

These days, many cardiovascular workout machines come equipped with the technology to measure your heart rate as you exercise: Press your palms to the sensors for ten seconds, and the number appears. There's also the good old-fashioned method of taking your own pulse. Lightly place your fingers (not your thumb, since it has its own pulse) to the throbbing artery in your neck and count the beats for fifteen seconds. Multiply by four, and you have your heart rate.

AROMA AND AROUSAL

Strenuous exercise, and the sweat it provokes, may have an additional benefit: sex appeal. Underarm sweat contains a chemical known as androstenol, a pheromone, or chemical signal, which some scientists suspect may be one of the triggers of sexual arousal. "Everyone's familiar with the olfactory system that allows mammals to smell with our noses," says Luis Monti-Block, Ph.D., of the University of Utah. "There is also the vomeronasal system, which allows us to pick up on chemical messengers, pheromones, which have no smell at all." Some perfume manufacturers have gone as far as to isolate androstenol from its most accessible source, male pig slobber, and market it as a man-catching substance. In a totally unscientific but amusing study, ABC News took identical twin women, dabbed one with witch hazel and one with a pheromone-based product, and set both women loose in a singles bar. The witch hazel honey got chatted up by eleven guys; her pheromone-wearing twin was approached by thirty. ABC reporters cautioned against reaching any definitive answers from the "study," and Dr. Monti-Block insists that pheromones are species-specific, with dogs responding to doggie pheromones and humans responding to human pheromones. Both completely failed to mention the most obvious conclusion: Men are pigs.

Pheromones have nothing to do with the conventional sense of smell, so if body odor is an issue for you, consider two things. One, a rose is not a rose; different people like different smells. If you don't like your own smell, or if someone important to you doesn't, careful bathing and a deodorant should do it. If that's not enough, check with a dermatologist; in rare cases, the presence of odor-causing bacteria can be addressed with a topical antibiotic, or you may be able to try heavy-duty treatment with aluminum chloride to reduce the amount your underarms sweat. According to James Green, author of *The Male Herbal* (Crossing Press, 1991), astringent herbs such as white oak, pipsissewa, horse chestnut, partridgeberry, and witch hazel can also help you perspire less, reducing body odor.

Strength Training Basics: Weight a Minute

When I first started, I was really just looking to get acknowledgment from other men, though it took two years before I got any. By then it had also become a major stress reducer, and a way for me to enjoy both my love of food and my love of feeling fit.

My mom was a single mom, and she was always pushing me to sports. I remember she took me to a fortune teller who said what we knew already: "He's no athlete." My mother was so upset, saying, "Oh, why do I keep trying?" It was years later, when I was twenty—actually, it was the year she died of cancer—that I started working out. Seeing her wasting away in the bed, her arms so thin, I think I felt like I had to put some flesh on my own. Or it was like I was honoring her memory, how lucky I felt to have her inside me, as part of me.

People say the gym is a vain place, and I say, yeah? So? If that's what gets me there, what's wrong with that? I'm still being healthy.

Strength training is not just pumping iron and getting huge. Even if you want to be smaller, or more defined, building muscle mass is an essential component of good conditioning, increasing bone strength, muscle definition, and your body's ability to burn fat, even in your sleep. The higher your muscle-to-fat ratio, the more calories you will burn off twenty-four hours a day. It takes between thirty and fifty calories a day to maintain a pound of muscle tissue, while a pound of fat uses up only two calories a day.

As with aerobic exercise, the overload principle applies. Though how you structure your strength training will depend on what you're trying to achieve, change is achieved only by pushing your muscles harder than they're used to working, which means gradually increasing the amount of weight you lift, the number of reps you do (see "Gym Jargon," page 204), or the effort required by the exercise over time. Bookshelves and magazine racks are full of different workout plans, exercises, and approaches. Generally speaking, if you are just starting with weights, says Body Tech's Machado, figure out the amount of weight you can lift for twelve repetitions and then start at just over half that. If you're going to work on more than one muscle group in a day, start with larger ones such as back, legs, and chest first, and then work toward smaller ones such as arms or neck. If you're just beginning, try using machines that make it easier to perfect your balance and form before moving on to free weights, cables, and pulleys. Among other general principles:

- If you're looking to get bigger, do fewer repetitions with more weight. "I usually focus on one body part a day, doing heavy weights for three to eight reps per set, and resting for five minutes between each set," says Paul, twenty-nine, an actor in Los Angeles who says he "set out to move from scrawny kid to serious hunk."
- If you're looking to define what you have, do more reps with less weight. "Pumped up, beefed up, is not my ideal," says Tony, age twenty-four. "I want to stay lean, so I group them up: back, biceps, and legs one day, chest, shoulders, and triceps the next, with ten or twelve reps for each set and only a minute or so in between."
- If you're looking to get leaner, try up to twenty reps, with little rest in between sets. "I use weights almost like another form of aerobic exercise," says Saul, thirty-two years old, a high-school English teacher. "I go at off hours so there's no waiting, and just go right from machine to machine, boom, boom, boom."

"However you do it," says Moss from Castro Street Gym, "remember that for growth, you only need to work out each body part really hard once a week. The real growth takes place when you're resting and the muscles are recuperating, so you've got to give them that time." Except for your abs, adds Machado. Those you can work every day.

PART-Y BOYS?

Some years back a twenty-five-year-old personal trainer in San Francisco died after having a tiny amount of fat liposuctioned from his already well-muscled body. While the postoperative blood infection that killed him was rare, his predicament is familiar to more than one of us who still find that one "bad" body part may threaten to spoil the whole bunch. "We murder to dissect," observed the poet Wordsworth. If you're seizing on your love handles as an excuse to throw all your hard work at the gym out the window, or if you're ignoring your built-up arms to focus on your smaller chest, it may be time for connective measures.

CONNECT TO YOUR PAST

What kind of body did you have before you started working out? How about the other people in your family? No matter what the gay ideal of the moment ("It's all about a big chest and cut stomach," says Tom, twenty-eight), your family history is likely to shape your body as much as any weight training. Swimming against the gene pool is the hardest and most unsatisfying workout there is. "I did it all: protein shakes, power bars, carbo loading, supplements, but I had to accept that I was making myself miserable without really getting as big as my friends," says Abel, thirty-three, who put thousands of miles between himself and his family in Puerto Rico but stands only a few inches above his diminutive mother when she comes to visit. Until the gay clone is a biological reality and not a fashion statement, trying to make your wiry legs into tree trunks or vice versa is an exercise in frustration. In the age of steroids (see "Vial Stuff," page 211), pectoral implants, and Photoshop, that model in the magazine is probably only two-thirds real anyway.

CONNECT TO YOUR BODY

Beneath the clanking free weights or the whir of the Cybex machine, you may no longer be able to hear the old tune reminding you that the thigh bone's connected to the hip bone. Review the connections: the way the hamstrings that run down the back of your legs help support your back, the way your back helps support your chest, and the way that working any one part to excess may throw off the rest of you. "I see a lot of men who have huge chests but have never developed their upper backs, making them vulnerable to shoulder separation," says Dr. Franchino. Walking around like Brutus on Olive Oyl's legs is also asking for injury.

CONNECT FORM AND FUNCTION

Form, rather than pounds lifted or number of reps, is cited most often as the key to successful strength training. Some trainers recommend starting an exercise with virtually no weight at all, and just focusing on the movement. Arching your back as you bench-press or letting your joints lock as you struggle to put another twenty pounds over your shoulder is bad form, and it won't help. "If you're struggling, you're probably just going to stretch your tendons and ligaments without even hitting the muscle," advises Moss.

Franchino suggests cutting back on the poundage and doing the exercise more slowly, focusing on squeezing and tightening the muscle(s) you're working. "My equation is work equals weight over time over distance. So if you lower the weight, you can get equal results by increasing the length of time of each push or pull."

Team Time

I did the sissy sports, the ones you could do alone—swimming, running—and I did them well. But competition on a team was something that had been beaten out of me when I got knocked on my ass in football and was cut from the team. It's only now, at thirty-three, that I've found I like competing physically. I guess gay volleyball's a sissy sport, too, but the team takes it seriously. The coach is very serious. I'm loving it.

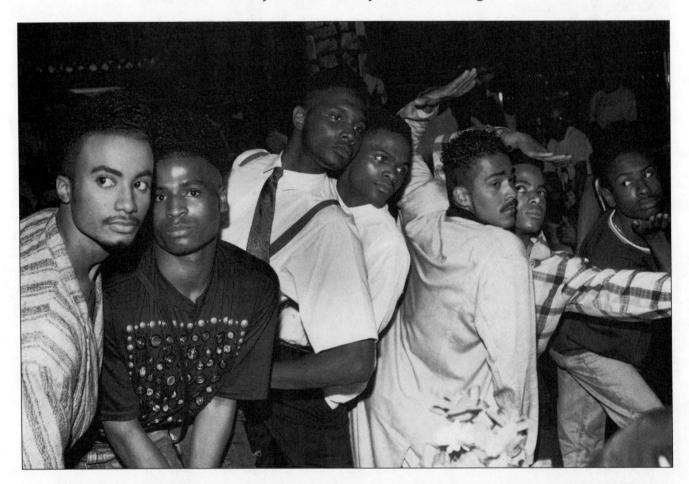

When gay body consciousness seems limiting, remember that working with our bodies has helped heal plenty of gay souls. We're not talking rates of heart attacks, though those too have dropped with fitness consciousness, but ways in which gay men have rediscovered teams, systems of support that let us do things we never thought we could. In the East Coast urban "ballroom" scene, impeccably styled young gay and transgendered Black and Latino men walk and vogue down the runways in their competitions for "realness"—"executive realness," "butch queen," "femme queen," or "European runway model effect" realness—coached and cheered on by friends and "families." In Michigan, members of the gay running club Front Runners lope for miles alongside the Grand River, pushing each other to feel stronger, faster, and more connected. In Utah, the gay aquatics club cuts through the water, and stereotypes, at the Salt Lake Community College pool. In Los Angeles, buff workout partners spot each other while lifting weights and then saunter out of the gym like Jason Priestleys heading for a trauma-free Beverly Hills High they never had. Farther up the coast in San Jose, members of the gay volleyball team practice their spikes in the Wilson Adult Center gym.

Whether ballroom competitions and gay teams are challenging mainstream models of male bonding or just finding gay ways to give in to them depends on you. As with all relationships, it's worth asking if yours to gym culture, or to your team or voguing House, is one that lets you grow or keeps you stuck. The answer may change over time, and with your needs. "The first time I went to the gay games with my water polo team, I felt a sense of togetherness I've never experienced anywhere as a gay man," says thirty-three-year-old Mark. Ryan, also thirty-three, says the support he got from gay men at his local Y helped him lose sixty pounds through diet and exercise, but offers a variation on that theme. "I have a body I never imagined having," he says. "The gym opened up so much for me: new friends, flirtations, a whole new sense of possibility. But I'm also ready to move on a bit, to find something more spiritual."

Plateaus

The first little while, it was amazing. And then I just stopped. I could not skate any faster. I couldn't practice any harder. I was stuck.

I go to the gym, feel good afterward, and then, a week or two later, something comes up, I miss once, and I wait six months before going back.

It can happen in week two, or three years into exercising. Your routine, sailing smoothly for a while, begins to drift, or you miss one practice and suddenly they all seem pointless. Perhaps you go to the gym only to find that you're stuck at the same level, with the only thing you're able to raise being the level of pessimism you feel at your lack of progress.

Plateaus are common, but they can be surpassed. Below, a few suggestions by men who say they still struggle:

- *Are you out of your mind?* "Whatever you do, don't stay in your head, listening to the excuses or the doubts about how it's not making any difference," says Brian, twenty-four years old. "When you hear yourself repeating a negative statement of the you-can't-do-it variety, substitute a positive one. Like 'I'm just going to run one more lap.'"
- *Are you comparing you and him, or you and you?* "There's always going to be somebody who's bigger and more beautiful," says Scott, thirty-five, who's worked out in gyms from Laguna to London since he was eighteen. "The waistline you'd kill for or the cut stomach you'll never have. The only way I keep going is by measuring myself against myself." Keep a notebook so you can remember where you've come from, and the progress you actually have made.
- *Are you varying your routine?* "I don't buy fitness magazines much, but I'll look at them in the bookstore, and since they cycle through the same questions every six months or so, there's always new exercises in there," says Scott. People who work out regularly talk about the "treat" of doing a different kind of triceps exercise, or doing things in a different order, or changing a grip. Try a lot more sets with a lower weight, or fewer reps, more weight, and a longer rest time. Your muscles get as bored as you do; in strength training, "confusion" (see "Gym Jargon," next page) is something you want to encourage.

• *Reach out.* People exercise together not just to compare and despair, but to take advantage of the collective wisdom. If you're exercising alone, consider joining a team or at least going somewhere where there are other people. If you're with others but not talking to anyone, reach out. "I sat on the machines for six months, looking at the free-weight room and thinking those guys were too serious for me," says Ryan. "Once I got in there, people were actually very willing to talk and trade tips."

The Gym: Choosing, Schmoozing, and Cruising

Sometimes I feel like they should put up little tables and serve coffee, it gets so chatty.

I made all my friends at the gym when I first moved here. Whenever I go to a strange city, it's also the first place my boyfriend and I go. It's a way to meet gay men without all the drugs and alcohol, and it makes me feel good.

Gym Jargon: "Spotting? Is That Like Cruising?"

For the newcomer, it all sounds worse than it is. Here are ten terms every aspiring gym goer can use, including a number that aren't what they sound like.

Burn. This is what you feel when you lift a weight past your usual level of exertion; it's a flooding of your muscle with blood and lactic acid. Trainers usually tell you that for something to be effective, you should "start to feel a burn," but the burn is also an indication that you shouldn't go any further. It's sort of like a weight-lifting orgasm, that moment of maximum intensity.

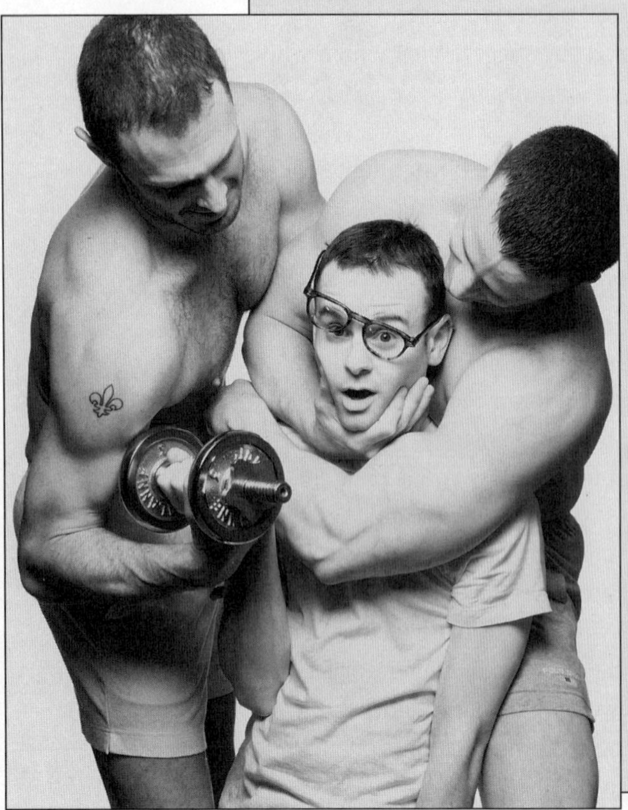

Confusion. What your muscles experience as you constantly change your training routine, switching from barbells to dumbbells and back again, using different exercises on the same muscle groups, varying set length and reps—all of which you should do. Muscles stop growing when they get used to a routine, and you've got to "confuse" them back into growth.

Cut. Meaning very well defined, sculpted, as in his "cut" pecs. Stronger forms of the same idea include "ripped" and the highly complimentary "shattered."

Giant sets. Also known as super sets, an advanced technique to get you past a weight-training plateau. Try four to six consecutive exercises for a single body part—chest, back, front of thighs—with little or no rest between them. You don't want to do it too often, but if you're stuck, giant sets can help you get past the block.

Grunting and groaning. What straight men do at the gym when lifting weights, usually in scary twosomes. Gay men at the gym don't do this, even when lifting three times the amount of weight.

"It's all you." Supportive thing to say when "spotting."

I remember the first time Philip told me that he went to a gym. I just stared at him, thinking, "Why would a gay man want to go to a gym? I mean, what is up with that?" I think the hardest work for me was getting to a point where I could imagine feeling like the gym was a place I'd want to be.

I hate the gym because I never feel my body measures up, and because I think AIDS made all these men want to build their bodies into something I never found that attractive. I miss pre-gym bodies. When we undressed, we really undressed.

The gym has become such a central factor of gay urban life that it's hard to think back to a time when many gay men had no opinion about it all. Today it's a place for catching up with old friends and making new ones, dissing old boyfriends, swapping business cards, torturing yourself with the unattainable and, in what may or may not be a related activity, doing the mating dance. Sometimes, between the social obligations of the gym and their accompanying

someone (see below), even though it may not necessarily be true. Something gay men copped from straight men, along with gym going in general.

Negatives. Each movement has two parts: the positive portion, when you're lifting the weight, and the negative phase, when you're returning it to its starting position. Focus on doing that second portion of the exercise slowly, and you'll get some of the benefits of negative training. For a more intense version, and only if you're working with someone experienced, get a training partner to help you lift a weight that's too heavy for you to raise on your own, and then slowly return the weight to the starting position. This is the source of lots of tendonitis and bursitis, so proceed with caution. "I don't believe in forcing reps of any kind," says New York City trainer Terry Fister. "The reality is that when there's muscle damage, it often occurs in the negative phase."

Progressive resistance. A classic form of weight training in which you start an exercise with a light weight and high reps and then gradually add weight while subtracting reps. For example, on a straight bench press, your first set might be twelve reps at fifty pounds, your second ten reps at seventy pounds, and your last seven or eight reps at ninety pounds. Since the early sets warm up your muscles and the latter sets push them to their utmost, progressive resistance allows you to train hard with less risk of injury.

Rep. Short for repetition, this word describes the contraction and/or extension of a given muscle group against resistance. Translation: moving a weight from a starting position to full extension (don't lock your joints) and then back to the starting point.

Set. A series of repetitions (usually between eight and fifteen). Generally, a brief rest of at least thirty to ninety seconds is taken after each set to allow you to catch your breath and provide time for the targeted muscle group to partly recuperate.

Spotting. When you stand behind someone who is lifting to "spot" them for weakness, providing only as much support as needed for them to complete the set. You may also want to encouragingly count out their reps for them, with the occasional utterance of the aforementioned "It's all you." Getting someone to spot is crucial when you're lifting challenging weights. It's also a great excuse to make conversation.

Working in. When someone asks if he can rotate using a certain machine or set of weights with you—"Mind if I work in?"—and, of course, you graciously concede. And wipe your sweat off the machine with the towel around your neck.

anxieties, such as having the right color and width of racing stripes down the side of one's high-tech-fabric athletic pants, it can be hard to finish even a simple workout in less than five hours. All the more reason why you should know what you want and don't want in your gym experience.

Choosing

If you live in the suburbs or a relatively small city, you may have few choices, or none at all, when it comes to selecting a gym. But if you live in a city such as New York, Los Angeles, Atlanta, or Boston, you know that the choices can be staggering . . . especially when all your friends hop from new gym to even newer gym, and you're left wondering if you should join the "old" gym for a cut rate, or in effect double your rent and join the new one with the DJ booth and the cute staff at the juice bar. "That's why they call it the Y, as in why am I still here," jokes Peter, thirty, a New Yorker who has not yet gone over to greener and more expensive pastures nearby. Most gyms allow you a free workout—or at least a tour—and you should definitely take the time. Visit at rush hour (you can always go off-peak, but you want to know the worst-case scenario) and check the following details.

HOURS

Is it open early enough for you to work out before going to work? Late enough for you to stop in and treadmill away the day's stress when you leave the office at 9:30 P.M.? Is it open Sunday nights, so you can ward off here-comes-the-workweek panic attacks with a good hour of free weights? "I wish they'd encourage more people to come during off-peak hours," says Guillermo, age thirty-eight, a marketing consultant from Atlanta. "That way it wouldn't be so crowded when I go!"

COST

If all you want is a way to get out of your studio apartment, that $99-a-year cinder-block room full of oxidized free weights, a stationary bike, and a few hard-core power lifters may be fine. Maybe you're willing to shell out that $200 sign-up fee alongside $99 a month in return for a five-level gym that looks as though it were designed by Philippe Starck, staffed by the cast of *Baywatch,* and outfitted with an activewear boutique and a consultant who helps you pick out the right hair and clothes to go with your new body. At all but the cheapest gyms, rates are often variable depending on who recommends you and what special is going on, so ask around to find out what other people paid, and don't be afraid to bargain. Many high-end gyms also have peak and off-peak rates. Some cities, such as New York, Chicago, and Seattle, have a few public gyms where membership ranges from $5 to $100 a year.

CLASSES

Does it offer aerobics classes? Spinning? Yoga? Body sculpting? How many times a week? At extra cost? Who are the instructors? In the long run, a wide array of classes can keep you interested, particularly if you're plateauing or not sure you really want to be there.

TRAINERS

Most gyms have them, but do they seem friendly or threatening? Do you get at least one free session with them to set up a workout? Are there gym staff on the floor to answer your questions, help you with your form, or give you a spot? If you're new to the gym and just putting a weight-lifting program together, this can be essential, but if you're already comfortable, then maybe the cinder-block gym *is* for you.

THE PEOPLE

Just like the human beings who go there, gyms have reputations and personalities. No gym employee who shows you around the facility is going to tell you that their gym is "100 percent breeder-free, thank God," or "as straight as we can keep it," so you'll have to exert your own powers of observation and ask friends for the down-low. Is everyone in the weight-lifting room huge, hairy, and scary? Trim, with matching tank tops and baseball caps, and scary? Is the radio on the classic rock station or the dance music station? Do you see anyone who looks like you? Anyone who doesn't? Don't look to a gym to get you over the hurdles you haven't been able to rise above in the rest of your life. "I joined the trendiest, gayest gym in the city, and then couldn't go there for fear of the attitude," says Don, a forty-two-year-old graphic designer. "I was much happier at the mixed gym, where some people had better bodies than mine, some had worse, women and men were together, and nobody was quite sure where everyone else in the room would be later that Saturday night."

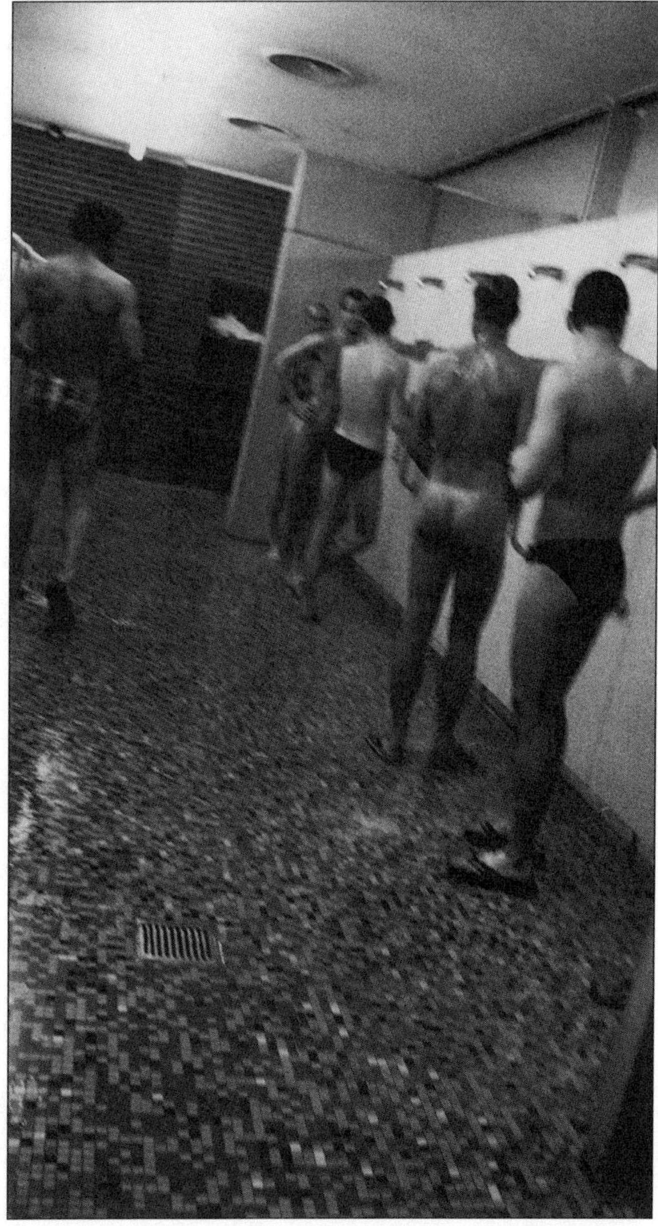

THE FACILITIES

Are the locker rooms, steam room, and sauna (assuming it has them) clean, or better suited for a mushroom farm? Are the showers "gang-style" or private stalls? Which do you prefer? Do you see lots of sign-up sheets, rule boards, or other telltale signs of overcrowding near the cardio machines?

Schmoozing

Networking is a tradition at gyms from Eastern Europe to West Hollywood. Say you need a new job, a roommate, a summer share, or an actor for the play you're directing. Mention your dilemma to someone before climbing aboard the Precor elliptical, and chances are someone will get back to you long before you've started your crunches. But will you welcome their advice? "After listening to all the straight older guys talk politics in the locker room at the top of their lungs, my blood pressure is higher than if I hadn't exercised at all," says Richard, forty-four. "Still, I prefer them to the superattitudinous queens at the gym across town."

Cruising

Athletics and the pleasure of spectatorship are a time-honored gay marriage. It's no accident that the ancient Greeks were the ones who came up with the idea of naked young men running through cheering crowds carrying flaming phallic symbols. In modern times, gym cruising has led to flirtations, friendships, and courtship. And if looking is your thing, then the gym is one of the few places on earth where men are in such proximity to each other while wearing so little clothing. Just don't stare too long, and remember, whoever he is, that you definitely have something to talk about if you want to get to know him. Ask him what muscles he's working with that interesting dumbbell exercise, if that Bulls tank top he's wearing means he's from Chicago, or if he really saw Madonna's Blond Ambition tour, as suggested by his T-shirt with the sleeves cut off.

As for sex in the gym, we've all heard steam-room stories, or maybe even been a character in them. Every city has a gym that's notorious on the gay circuit. But proceed with caution before you extend that hand. One, not everyone present may wish to be part of your steamy scene; they paid too, and it's an embarrassing thing to be hauled out naked or have your membership revoked for "inappropriate behavior." Two, conversations—including warnings about STDs and HIV—are not likely, so be careful about risking your health or his. And three, keep in mind that you're likely to see whomever you play with in the steam room again and again as long as you both go to the same gym. "I try thinking of sex in my steam room as 'gym incest'—when I'm feeling like a steamy experience, I pay the day rate at another family's gym," says Tom, age thirty-two. Finally, beware of making sex the main motivator for your gym visits. If you find yourself spending more time in the sauna than on the Stairmaster, you're probably not doing too much for your health—or your reputation.

Hurts So Good?

I might be kind of sick, but I love the feeling of soreness I get after a good workout. It lets me know my body's there all day.

Postexercise pain can be a sign of health, with muscles "reknitting" after exertion. But there's a difference between a dull ache that hurts so good and the sharp or shooting pain of a pull, sprain, or strain that comes when tissue is tearing or a tendon gives way. "If you get a pain with a certain movement, stop that motion and have a doctor check it out," says Charles Franchino, who sees a large number of gay men—and a large number of athletic-related injuries—in his Manhattan chiropractic practice.

Sprains and Strains

Sprains or strains can be serious injuries. "I sprained one ankle, got up on it too early, fell down the stairs, sprained my other ankle, and spent a month on crutches," says David, a twenty-eight-year-old lawyer in Washington, DC. "And all because I thought an ankle brace would cut down on my mobility." If you do get a sprain or strain, standard immediate treat-

MEAN, LEAN, AND SQUEAKY-CLEAN: SOME TIPS ON GYM HYGIENE

Whether you're protecting a shaky immune system or simply want to know what you "should" be doing and then ignore it, here are a few tips:

• Bacteria and viruses like the warm moisture of the steam room just as much as you do. Keep a towel between your butt and the bench, preferably one you've brought, and bleached, yourself.

• Flip-flops may be a pain. So are toes and nails that are red and peeling with fungus you got off the floor. As for getting someone else's sperm in your athlete's foot, don't panic: No cases of HIV transmission through that route have been recorded.

• Skip the gym-provided bar soap. Use your own, or a liquid soap dispenser.

• Gloves don't just look cool—they protect you from the skin and sweat left on the weights by the last guy. Wear them, or wash your hands before putting them to eyes, nose, ears, or mouth after a workout.

If your T-cell count is less than 200, bring your own filtered or boiled water. As for the portable water bottles with filters built in, as of this writing none were certified to be crypto-reducing, and so probably aren't worth the $25.

ment is the RICE (rest, ice, compression, elevation) approach. Rest the injured part, apply ice for twenty minutes (never on bare skin), use compression (elastic) bandages to hold the ice pack in place and wrap the injury after the ice is removed, and elevate the injured body part whenever possible to be level with, or slightly above, the heart. Some immediate swelling is normal, but any discoloration, numbness, extreme tenderness, or prolonged pain or discomfort is reason to get to a physician.

Back Pain

Back pain is perhaps the most common form of injury of all. Approximately 80 percent of men will experience some form of lower back pain in their lives, and many respond by stopping exercise completely. That, says Dr. Franchino, is one of the worst things to do, since prolonged rest makes back problems worse. Instead, try stretching, low-impact aerobics, and careful exercise of the abdominal muscles to help speed recovery, since those loosen the tissue that tightens up around an injury and send fluid into the discs that cushion the spine.

"Avoiding the injury in the first place is the best," says Franchino, who ticks off familiar but often-ignored advice for better backs. Make sure the chair you sit in all day, if you do, allows you to rest both feet on the ground and keep the spine straight. Safer lifting—whether it's a barbell on the gym floor or the box in your basement—is done by bending with the knees, not from the hips, and standing up slowly with the object close to your body. Stretching

A PAIN IN THE...

If your pain is	And you've recently been	Probable cause	Possible remedy
Above your heel	Stairmastering	Planting your feet fully on the steps.	Standing on the balls of your feet gives a better stretch to your Achilles tendon, says Franchino. So will the calf stretches and the shoes with better heel support.
Above your heel	Running	Overdoing it, resulting in stress to the plantar fascia (the band of tissue that runs from the heel to the toe of your foot).	Getting supportive shoes, lacing them tightly, and using anti-inflammatory drugs if necessary can all help. Ease up on pounding the pavement or walking barefoot, both of which cause the plantar fascia to bow, or in extreme cases, to rupture.
Lower legs	Running or doing lots of aerobics	Hard surfaces are producing shock that your lower leg muscles can't handle.	Stretching and strengthening your calf muscles, and the Achilles tendon above your heel, are both in order, says Franchino. You may also check out a new, more cushioned pair of shoes, and skip the asphalt in favor of a softer surface.
Knee	Cycling	Your seat's adjusted wrong. If the pain's medial (inside), the seat's too low; if it's outside, it may be high.	Dr. Franchino suggests standing next to the bike and putting the seat at the level of your hip.
Lower back	Cycling or stair stepping	Hunching over.	Stay conscious of your stomach muscles and use them—not the handlebars—to hold you up. Abdominal exercises will help, says Franchino. You may also want to avoid straight handlebars and go with the V-shaped ones, suggests Bruce E. Robins, D.C., a chiropractor in Fort Lauderdale, Florida.

the lower back (one simple stretch is to lie on your back, pull one thigh toward the chest until you feel it, hold for thirty seconds, and switch, but there are lots of others) daily will do wonders, as can abdominal crunches. Finally, to protect your back, do stretches and warm-ups *before* you start lifting—most sports injuries, including back-related ones, happen early in a workout—and don't let fear of pain keep you from basic strengthening exercises. Instead, check with a professional about how to proceed.

Chemical Catalysts: Steroids and Supplements

Drinking lots of water, eating something with protein an hour before you work out, and having a complex carbohydrate within an hour after finishing are among the standard recommendations for fueling your exercise regimen (see Chapter 6 for more on diet). But what about that shadowy land beyond turkey burgers and baked potatoes—the shifting terrain of powders and potions, hormones and "health supplements," which supposedly made that skinny guy on the team erupt in muscles within three months while you've worked for a year trying to put a little bump in your biceps?

Vial Stuff: Steroids

History repeats itself: As early as the 1940s men "suffering" from homosexuality were prescribed male hormones by doctors hoping to correct their overly feminine natures. A half century later, gay men are inflicting the same medicine on ourselves, this time hoping to redirect nature's physical, rather than psychological, course. Boldly going where many straight athletes have gone before, gay gym rats are popping pills or putting needles to thighs, using steroids to give themselves the big bodies years of working out and eating protein haven't made possible.

Anabolic steroids include testosterone and synthetic derivatives fabricated to promote the muscle-building effects of that naturally occurring male hormone. They are also illegal unless prescribed by a doctor to combat HIV-related wasting or another medical condition. Steroids have been monitored by the Drug Enforcement Agency since 1990, sale of them is a felony, and possession without a prescription is against the law in many states. Nevertheless, 'roid rage—the name given to the mood swings and superaggressive behavior some steroid users experience as a side effect—could also describe the booming black market for the drugs in high schools, colleges, and other athletic circles across the country, including gay ones. An estimated one million Americans, half of them teenagers, are using steroids. One Massachusetts study found that more than 2 percent of 965 middle-school students surveyed, some as young as ten, were using them. In a gym in Chelsea or the Castro, "Are you on a cycle?" is more likely to refer to a two-month period of intramuscular injections than to the stationary bike.

As with all drugs, the dangers of steroid use depend on whom you talk to, how much you take, and where you get the steroids. Like many who inject illegal drugs, steroid users can rattle off observations about purity and process like amateur chemists or doctors. "I don't do oral since they're more dangerous, always cycle, inject into the upper outer quadrant of the buttock to avoid hitting a sciatic nerve, and keep a close watch for androgenic side effects," says Tom, twenty-eight. Androgenic effects of steroids, in addition to 'roid rage, include changes in characteristics other than muscle mass: balding, testicular shrinkage (think cocktail peanuts), pimples on the back, and an overall complexion that Jordan, a San Francisco gym goer, describes as "like a hot dog someone put in a microwave—slightly swollen, almost blistered and red." Even the most careful users, say doctors and trainers, can find their caution undermined by the realities of supply and demand. "The bottom line is that if you buy on the black market, you don't know what the hell you're buying," says Bill Vayo of Plus One Fitness. "I've heard of some injectable steroids cut with baby oil, and some containing no steroid at all." Packaging is no guarantee, since counterfeit vials can come complete with printed lot numbers, bogus informational inserts, and incorrect dosage information.

If steroids' effects—both bulging muscles and bouts of "bacne"—seem plain when gay men shed their shirts to dance the night away, others are less visible. Deaths from steroids are rare, the result of constant usage over years, but other strains on the internal systems of the body are common. Elevations in liver enzymes, reduction of "good" cholesterol, enlarged liver and prostate, and sterility are among reported symptoms from high dosages. More difficult to measure is "bigarexia," the distortion of body image that comes from feeling you're still too small, or fearing that once you stop your cycle you'll shrink. "The guys I know on steroids aren't satisfied," says Bob, thirty-five, who says many of the men at his gym "stack," combining more than one steroid at a time. "If I tell a friend, 'Oh, you're looking great, you're really big,' and he says, 'Really? I think I'm still really small,' I know he's on a cycle" (see "Exercise Control?" on page 215).

SAFER STEROID USE

If you are determined to use black-market steroids, there are ways to make it safer. Vayo suggests you consider the following:

- ***Be damn sure you know your source.*** "Buying any steroid on the street or in the locker room is playing Russian roulette," says Vayo.
- ***Use clean needles and never share.*** You can get HIV and hepatitis from intramuscular injection.
- ***Cycle.*** Going off steroids regularly, and making sure you start with small doses, can give your body time to recuperate. Also, don't "stack." "Most people think more is better when they start seeing the results, and they're wrong," warns Vayo.
- ***Consider herbs and other supplements.*** Supplements for your liver, such as milk thistle and alpha-lipoic acid, may help your body combat steroids' toxic side effects.
- ***Watch for negative side effects.*** If you're seeing mood swings, changes in skin color, or other undesirable effects, stop and consult a doctor. Remember to hold on to the steroids you were taking for medical analysis. "Even if you don't notice negative effects, you should at least be honest with your doctor if you're doing the things, so they can monitor your blood work and give you a physical on a regular basis," adds Charles Franchino, the New York City chiropractor who treats many gay men for polyarthralgia, a steroid-induced condition in which "every joint in the body aches." Once again, what your doctor doesn't know—and what you're afraid to tell him—can hurt you.

Powders and Supplements

At any health food store and plenty of gyms you can find a vast array of nonprescription products that claim to help you cut fat, increase muscle mass, and boost energy.

Fads for supplements change as often as Madonna's hairstyle, shifting with each report of adverse effects or something better. GHB (gamma-hydroxy butyrate), an over-the-counter powder that was used by many in the '80s to increase release of growth hormone, is now an illegal drug used recreationally (see "Drugs in Partyland," page 269) with sometimes deadly effects. DHEA, the steroid substitute of choice in the mid-nineties, has dwindled some in popularity after reports from users of prostate problems. "Creatine's the product of the moment," says Bob, thirty-five, who is in the initial, four-dose-a-day phase of the supplement.

For various reasons, supplements involve little of the rigorous science associated with prescription drugs (see "Alternative and Complementary Medicine," page 309). Still, say most nutritionists and trainers, in moderate doses (and with a few exceptions such as ephedra, discussed below), supplements may help, and the greatest harm is likely to be to your pocketbook. "Try to get away with a minimum," says Vayo, "since even if cost is no object, danger may increase with higher doses." If you take any of these supplements, tell your doctor, suggests Dr. Scott McCallister of Chicago. "He or she may not know much about them," he says, "but can still monitor your liver and kidney functions."

Below are listed some of the many popular powders and pills on the market. To find more information, see "Further Reading" at the end of the chapter.

AMINO ACIDS

Found in most foods, these chemical "building blocks of life" are being isolated and sold to promote various effects. Common ones for strength training include AKG, the skeleton of the amino acid glutamine, which proponents claim speeds growth and metabolism; carnitine, made in the body by the amino acids methionine and lysine and said to decrease lactic acid buildup and improve cardiovascular endurance; and OKG, from the amino acid ornithine, said to stimulate growth hormone and reduce burning.

Creatine (creatine phosphate), sold in powder and pill form, is thought to enhance strength and muscle by improving the body's ability to break down the energy-producing compound adenosine triphosphate (ATP) and then refuel. Creatine's been studied in small numbers of athletes against a placebo. It's expensive, it tastes bad (even in the Kool-Aid-like, flavored version), and—at least until they ban it or reveal it to be flawed—it seems to work.

EPHEDRINE (EPHEDRA)

Some bodybuilders combine ephedrine, a stimulant (or ephedra, its herbal equivalent), with caffeine and aspirin to burn fat and dull pain during a workout. In 1996, after reports of seventeen deaths and eight hundred illnesses linked to ephedrine-containing supplements, the FDA issued a strong warning and proposed new regulations to alert the public to ephedrine's potential dangers. Ephedrine or ephedrine-containing compounds should not be taken by people with any type of heart disease, hypertension, thyroid disease, diabetes, or enlarged prostate, or by anyone taking MAO-inhibitor drugs for depression or appetite suppression. Using aspirin to dull pain is also depriving yourself of what may be a needed warning sign to stop, adds Vayo. As for caffeine, it's a diuretic that makes you pee out water you need while working out.

CHROMIUM PICOLINATE

This mineral is sold to decrease body fat, increase muscle mass, and lower blood sugar. Studies haven't shown it to do much for the first two, but it does seem to have potential for lowering blood sugar, perhaps helping to avert diabetes.

DEHYDROEPIANDROSTERONE (DHEA)

A hormone thought to build muscle mass, increase energy, and decrease heart disease risk without the nasty side effects of the anabolic steroids (see "Vial Stuff," page 211), DHEA has at least one similar side effect. In some studies, DHEA speeded prostate enlargement. It also helped bulk up sedentary men over fifty who didn't get much exercise. For those younger than that, or whose hormone levels are normal to high, many experts suggests it's useless, or even harmful.

ELECTROLYTE SUPPLEMENTS

Better known as sports drinks, these liquids, such as Gatorade, replenish the electrolytes, including potassium and sodium, that you've sweated out, as well as a fair amount of carbohydrates. Electrolytes are necessary for muscle contraction and to maintain fluid balance in the body, but fruit juice, water, and table salt may well give you what you need.

ESSENTIAL FATTY ACIDS (EFAS)

Linoleic acid and linolenic acid are two essential fatty acids necessary for thousands of biochemical reactions, including the production of testosterone, the decrease of total cholesterol, and possibly the acceleration of fat loss. EFAs are also good for your skin and are available in the form of flaxseed oil (high in linolenic acid), which is often mixed with safflower, canola, sunflower, or soybean oils high in linoleic acid. Primrose oil and borage oil, both used by some bodybuilders, contain decent amounts of both types of essential fatty acids.

PHOSPHATES

Often combined with creatine (see "Amino Acids," above), phosphates are said to increase the amount of oxygen that gets to the muscles and to give an energy boost during exercise.

PROTEIN SUPPLEMENTS, PROTEIN-CARBOHYDRATE SUPPLEMENTS, AND MEAL-REPLACEMENT POWDERS (MRPS)

Almost all of these products come in powders that you mix into milk or water and drink as a supplement to your whole-food diet. Often they have amino acids or other supplements mixed in, as well as vastly different amounts of protein, sugar, and carbohydrates, depending on what you want from them: to be leaner, bulkier, or simply healthier. Protein-carbohydrate supplements are postworkout beverages; MRPs are just-add-liquid meals claiming to provide the perfect balance of nutrients for optimal training. If you have a reasonably balanced diet,

WHO'S ZOOMING WHO? TIPS ON BODYBUILDING SUPPLEMENTS

Mike Kurt and Brett Brungardt, in their *Complete Book of Shoulders and Arms* (HarperCollins, 1997), spend some one hundred pages leading readers through nutrition, stretching, and other fitness basics, proving once again that focusing on one body part involves focusing on the whole. In their review of supplements, they set forward three commonsense principles important to knowing whether you're taking something useful, or being taken.

1. Supplements are supplements—not replacements for food, exercise, or sleep.

2. How much are you taking? If you don't know how much you're taking of something, you probably aren't in a position to evaluate what it will or won't do for you. In particular, advise Kurt and Brungardt, compare what you're buying with what you might get ordinarily in food, since supplements like amino acids are often equally or more available in your diet than in that expensive pill. There's more potassium in a banana than in most specially purchased supplements.

3. How much are you spending? Supplements can add up fast. If you wouldn't go out for a $30 meal but are dropping $10 or $20 worth of vitamins and powders each week, you may be losing perspective rather then gaining weight.

watch out for protein supplements, as protein overdose may cause depletion of glycogen stores (which are converted to glucose, energy-producing blood sugar) in the muscles, and consequently make you more tired.

Exercise Control?

The main reason I get depressed when I'm sick is because I can't go to the gym. I don't want to visit out-of-town friends, either, because I miss it so bad.

Sound familiar? With the possible exceptions of Cher and Chaka Khan, there's always too much of a good thing, even exercise. And although being exercise-obsessed is probably better for you than an addiction to martinis, crystal meth, or Dolce & Gabbana, it's not good for you if it's cutting into other elements of your life, causing physical problems, or leaving you with a perpetual feeling of dissatisfaction because you think your body is too small.

Greg Ryan, from Market Street Gym in San Francisco, sees the preoccupation in many of his clients: "I ask them what their goals are, and they say to get bigger, get bigger, get bigger," he chants. "I tell them that it's not going to happen overnight—it could take years, patience, and major lifestyle changes in their diet and sleep patterns. They want to do it, even if the ideal they're going for is unattainable." Franchino calls this the reverse of anorexia: "I have patients who are getting bigger and bigger, but when they look in the mirror, they still see that skinny little kid who got picked on." Medical researchers have a more precise name for it: muscle dysmorphia.

Is this a gay thing, or would straight men understand it? Harrison Pope Jr., MD, who teaches psychiatry at Harvard Medical School, helped conduct one of the few academic studies of gym-going people that has included both gay and straight gym denizens. He recruited only

EXERCISE YOUR JUDGMENT

Do you consistently exercise more than fifteen hours a week?
Do you feel restless, agitated, and uptight before a workout?
Does missing a day cause you to become even more stressed and agitated?
Do you feel guilty if you miss even a single workout?
Is exercise your only relief from the stresses of daily life?
Does exercise take priority over other activities and social relationships?
Are you reluctant to stop working out because of illness or injury?
Do you feel compelled to work out even when you're tired?
Are you satisfied with what exercising does for you?
Are you having fun?

If you're not always sure about the last two, you're probably human. But if you answered most of the others with a yes, and the last two with a no, try to refocus. One route may be to diversify, doing mind-body work (see next page) or trying counseling (see Chapter 11).

men who said they could bench-press their body weight at least ten times—an indicator that these men had already logged a lot of hours in the gym—and then did research on those with dysmorphia. The result? Equal representation of gay and straight men in both groups, suggesting that pathological preoccupation with body image is not dependent on sexual orientation. Other studies among students in high school and college have found gay men to be more preoccupied with body image than our straight counterparts.

If you beat yourself up for renting *Valley of the Dolls* (or *Rocky*) and staying in when you had been vowing all day to hit that super abs class, you are not alone. That doesn't mean you shouldn't ask yourself a few questions (see box on page 215) if exercise or weight training is your obsession. As with all behavioral gauges, especially the ten-minute-quiz kind in books and magazines, they're not an acid test—just food for the mind sitting atop that ever-thickening neck.

Mind and Body

Paying attention to the body, the breath, I can toss out the scolding, the criticisms, the impatience. I think of it as my real weight loss program.

My partner and I do a few yoga moves, the ones called sun salutations, every morning. Breathing, going through the movements, it's like we're taking an early-morning swim together, floating and taking a moment to let the phone calls and the to-do lists and the work anxieties drift away. Also, my arms are getting bigger, and I like that.

I saw a program on one of those newsmagazines where a hardworking woman had a personal trainer she loved, but she gave him up for another personal trainer who told her how she could do everything in thirty minutes. And I thought, hey, why stop there? Why not find another personal trainer who can blow all your gaskets in ninety seconds so you can spend the rest of your time working working working? The time I spend doing this—as much as an hour and a half a day—is like going on a trip for me, a vacation.

Disciplines that urge a consciousness of mind and body are often labeled "California" or "New Age," but actually it's step classes and Cybex machines that are the new American approach to the body. Yoga, for example, the combination of mindful breathing, balance, and stretches called asanas ("easeful poses" in Sanskrit) has been practiced and developed for more than four thousand years. Chi kung (also spelled qi gong) and tai chi, Chinese forms combining slow, careful movement and meditative breathing, also date to 2,000 B.C. Designed to increase the strength and flexibility of your body and aid the healing flow of energy, these disciplines are seen by some as a complete science of the body's glands, organs, and immune response. Cultivate an awareness of the breath, and the process calms the mind as well.

Yoga

The word *yoga* means "union"—of physical and spiritual self—but neither physical prowess nor spiritual commitment is required. "A lot of us had the bejesus scared out of us by those pictures of a wraith-thin Indian man who could wrap his leg around his throat and through his pancreas, or who had trained himself to lower a half-dozen of his favorite internal organs out of his intestines to wash them by hand," says David Wetter, a volunteer instructor of hatha yoga—which focuses on physical poses—at Manhattan's Integral Yoga center. "But all yoga is not a religion, and doing it does not necessarily mean becoming a wide-eyed, way-too-happy soul in flowing robes or giving yourself over to some bearded, oversexed master." What you *do* need for the practice of hatha yoga, says Wetter, is a willingness to breathe, stretch, and listen to your body. "One of the reasons for yoga's recent popularity at the close of the millennium, beside the increasingly frenzied pace of life full of car alarms and appointments, is that anyone—from children to senior citizens—can do yoga," says Wetter. "There are no prerequisites, no prior work to be done. You can walk into a level-one class and see the widest range of students, from the first-timer who can barely bend forward at all to a regular practitioner with the flexibility of a rubber band."

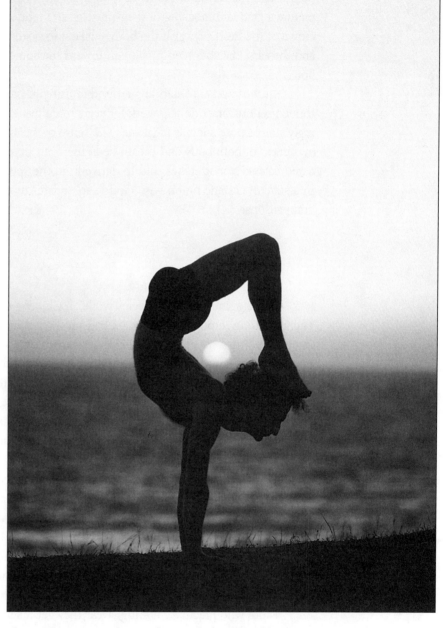

Yoga classes often begin with some simple chanting, often of *om* or other Sanskrit words. If the idea of touchy-feely incantations sends you running for the exit, suggests Wetter, think of the chants as similar to the noises you used to make as a kid, ways of "using your body as a tuning fork." Feeling the vibration, or flow of energy, is something that continues throughout a hatha yoga class, with the movement from one posture to another moving you to a deeper state of relaxation. "The more familiar you become with the asanas, the more able you are to do them with your eyes closed; then you don't have to check out, for whatever reason, that guy at the other end of the room whose muscles have muscles," says Wetter. "Nautilus training may involve pushing yourself to exceed where you were last time, but in yoga the work is *not* comparing, allowing yourself to note where you are while letting go of expectations. You make progress, but gradually." Tadasana, or mountain pose, finds you in a simple standing position, with the feet two to three inches apart, hands open by your sides. Some imagine the spine lengthening in both directions simultaneously: the lower part reaching down through the feet and into the ground like roots of a tree, and the upper part flowing up through the crown of the head toward the sky like branches reaching for the sun. Others picture a gradual unlocking of their muscles and tendons: an elastic band gently drawing the crown of the head skyward, the body relaxing to open a great distance between the shoulders and the ears, the abdomen moving in toward the spine while the tailbone extends toward the floor.

"All those years of standing around cruising in bars? You were doing yoga!" jokes Wetter, though serious practitioners work for years to cultivate a complete awareness of even a seemingly simple pose such as tadasana. The sense of the spine lengthening and a simultaneous awareness of both body and breath lie at the heart of all asanas, including the more complicated balances or stretches said to derive from the spontaneous body movements of people in a state of ecstatic union with God. Can't relate? In yoga, remember, there need be no comparisons.

Chi Kung

Chi kung simply means "energy work" in Chinese, so named because it directs the "chi," or energy flowing through the body. Its cousin, the martial art tai chi chuan, is perhaps better known, and mastery of tai chi's 108 basic moves draws on many of the principles of chi kung. Like yoga, chi kung brings the focus to what it calls "the three treasures of every person: body, energy, and mind." What makes chi kung especially noteworthy, though, is that you can practice it even when you can barely get up a flight of stairs. "We do some classes largely from a seated position, or from few simple, stable standing postures," says Emilio Gonzalez, who teaches a drop-in, $1-a-session class in San Francisco for people with chronic illnesses or anyone else who wants to stay well.

Chi kung movements are slow, stylized, almost hypnotic ones: hands move slowly from before the heart to the forehead and back to the heart, an arm glides out in slow supplication, your waist bends or turns, legs slide in a countermotion as if the laws of physics were slowed down to make an ordinary step a feat of choreography. Unlike the more complicated tai chi forms, a basic chi kung sequence can be learned in two or three classes, says Gonzalez. The name of one of the basic chi kung forms, Eight Pieces of Brocade, gives a sense of the way the slow, deliberate movements embroider the air and soothe the soul.

Those who practice chi kung swear they get relief from stress, improved strength, more energy, and better immune function. "It's like acupuncture without the needles," says Gonzalez, who has practiced the form, as well as tai chi and other martial arts, for twenty-five years. HIV-positive for the last fifteen of them, Gonzalez—and his many students—see chi kung as preventive medicine, a balance to the systems of the body that helps them deal with other, more pharmaceutical approaches. "Health is not just the absence of sickness," says Gonzalez. "I feel like chi kung offers a way to work on it, to keep things flowing and vibrant."

There are dozens of mind-body disciplines, and different teachers often urge the same approach: See how it feels. "Please don't take it from me, because I wouldn't," says Wetter. Then, trading his Bronx, New York, edge for simple candor, he offers what some yogis might call advice for the ages: "Give yourself the gift of trying. You deserve peace. You deserve stillness. You deserve joy."

FOUR MIND-BODY BASICS

1. ***Breath.*** Following the flow of the breath, the energy source for mind and body, is central to most mind-body practice. One basic breath that recurs in many practices is abdominal breathing, what some chi kung teachers call the "return to childhood breath." It starts with the stomach relaxed, and then—inhaling from your abdomen, with air flowing into your nose—you fill your lower belly with air, the way a sleeping child might. "Swimmers and singers who come to the class know how to do it, but most people have forgotten how to breathe," says Gonzalez. Yoga teachers, too, use this method, or build on it for what Wetter calls three-part breath: a slow build (for say, six counts) that begins in your abdomen, fills your lungs, and then rises all the way up to your collar bones. Yogic variations on deep breathing including the ujjayi, or ocean breath, where each breath in and out of the nose has the sigh of an ocean, or the "breath of fire," which is fast, quick panting. Focused breathing alone can still a racing heart, lower blood pressure, and calm the mind.

2. ***Absence of pain.*** While you may feel the difficulty of a stretch, and muscles may strain or shake from holding a pose, the adage "No pain, no gain" has little place in mind-body disciplines. "If you're struggling against pain, your mind is not going to be present," says Gonzalez, "so you ease out of a painful position to a place where you can still be mindful." Many of Gonzalez's students, in fact, arrive complaining of pain or neuropathy (numbness in the arms and legs) related to drug reactions, and with chi kung and acupuncture find their symptoms lessening. The lesson, apparently, is being learned by health insurers: Increasing numbers are offering subscribers free yoga, acupuncture, chi kung, or other forms of energy-based healing.

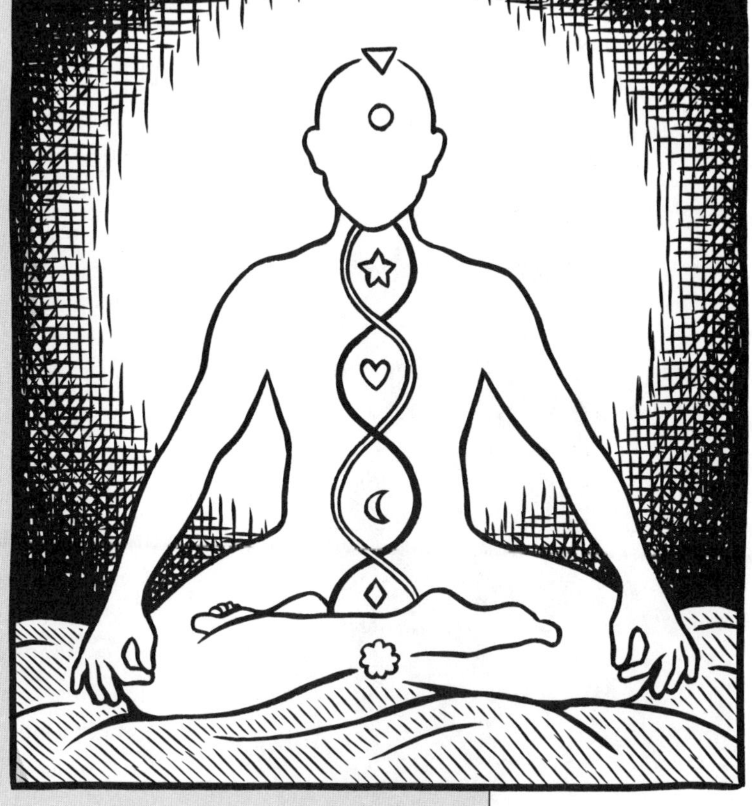

In yoga, too, the object is to relieve pain rather than to work through it. "I had a wonderful teacher," Wetter says, "who used to talk about finding the place between 'take it easy' and 'don't be lazy.' That's what you're looking for."

3. ***Class.*** Concerned as they are with feeling the flow of energy, mind-body practices are greatly enhanced by doing them with others, by a sense of collective energy and motion. "Do postures or meditation in a room with others and you feel the full meaning of why *yoga* means union," says Wetter. Classes also offer the benefit of a teacher, a watcher to straighten out mistakes or inspire you to greater concentration. "I've been working with the same teacher for twenty-five years," says Gonzalez, "and when he comes in the room, I still try harder."

4. ***Visualization.*** In this context, visualization means picturing your own motions and postures in space. Half meditative practice and half mechanism for refining your technique, visualization unites mind and body in a way that leaves you both present and apart from yourself. Imagine your breath as steam that you breathe out and then inhale back in. Feel your tendons stretching down our legs and deep into the ground. Imagine the earth under your back, warm and solid, stretching out in all directions.

Skin Care Basics: Water, Sun, and See

Boasters take note: It's the skin that is man's largest organ. And like that other long one—the gastrointestinal tract—the skin is among the quickest to show strains and stresses. How your outside looks depends greatly on what's going on within: your worries and your diet, what hormones your body happens to be releasing, and how much nicotine or alcohol or adrenaline is in your system. What goes on outside—from the weather to whether you use an oil-based soap or moisturizer—also has its effect. The terrain of skin care is no longer a no-man's-land, with more and more men, including straight ones, consuming a breathtaking array of new cleansers and creams. What to choose and use? The market is vast, but the principles relatively few. Below, find an explanation of the basic three.

Basic #1: Water (Inside and Out)

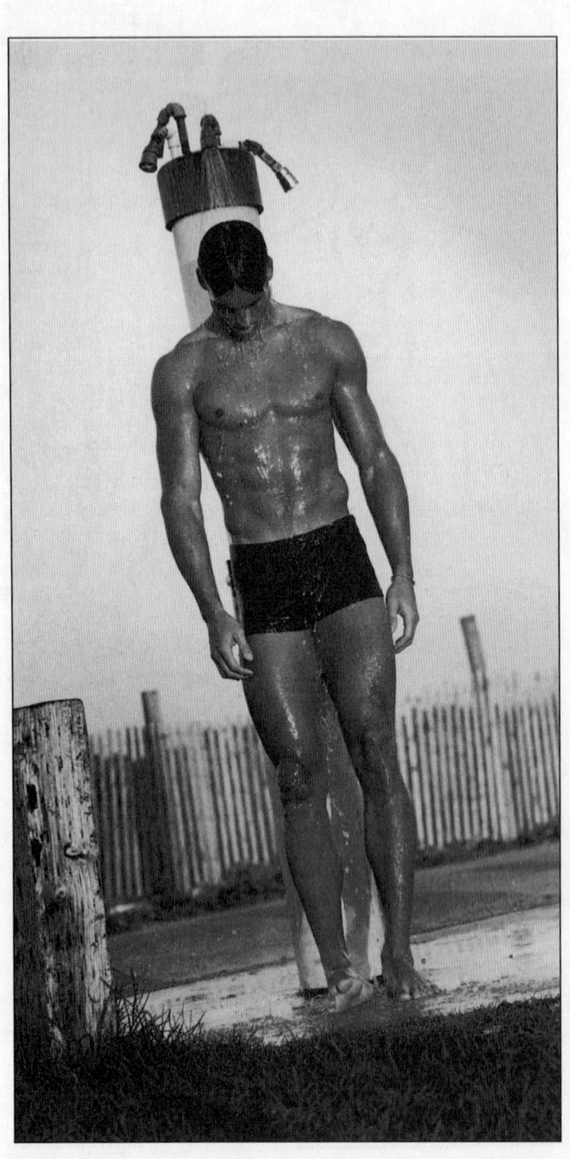

DRINK UP

Once again, drinking at least eight large glasses of water per day (coffee, beer, and soda don't count) is a key to health, moisturizing your skin and helping flush out the impurities that cause blemishes. You can also try taking fish oil or evening primrose internally (check your local health food store). Both are known for helping your body hydrate from within.

SHOWER SHORT

The longer the shower, the less oil your skin has left to keep moisture in. Harsh soaps make the matter worse. "Antibacterial soaps are the most parching, and only work for a matter of minutes before bacteria 'recolonize' you anyway," says Christopher Nanni, MD, assistant clinical professor of dermatology at New York University Medical School and for years the dermatologist at the Whitman Walker Clinic in Washington, DC. Dr. Nanni chalks up a full half of the cases he sees in the winter to the combination of harsh soaps and dry indoor heating.

In fact, adds Jeffrey Roth, MD, a dermatologist in New York City, "the only places most people need to soap are their hair [shampoo], underarms, groin, and buttocks. The body doesn't usually make oily secretions in the other places." If you'd put your face forward as an exception to that rule, see the box on the next page.

MOISTURIZE

Real men, of all skin tones and varieties, *do* moisturize. Products range from the classic cocoa butter to the pricey Crème de la Mer, but Nanni says you don't necessarily need to spend big bucks to get the benefit you need. Lotions tend to be lighter and less oily (avoid petroleum-based products and look for a product that says it's "noncomedogenic" if you're fighting acne), while oilier creams are better for dry skin and nighttime use. Whatever you use, put it on just after you shower, says Dr. Nanni; it'll seal moisture in much more effectively.

FACE FACTS

As with all affairs of the skin, reducing your stress level, getting adequate rest, eating healthfully, and staying away from smoking are key to facial fabulousness. Until you retire to a life of purity, though, there are skin-deep solutions. First, no matter what the issue—acne, oil, flaking, or peeling—lose the I'll-just-pick approach. "If men didn't touch their faces so often," sighs Ernie Benson, founder of the Face Place in West Hollywood, "they wouldn't have to pay me to do it."

If You're Facing:	Action Plan	Why?	See a Doctor If:
Flaking	Wash with a gentle cleanser and use a light moisturizer every time you wash.	The old must make way for the new. Otherwise, you risk shaving cuts, clogged pores, or an ashy, dried-out look.	Scaling and red skin if you're White, or severe darkening of the skin if you're Black, may be eczema, seborrhea, or other more serious conditions requiring antifungal or cortisone creams.
Acne and oily skin	For acne, spot-treat with an over-the-counter 2.5 percent solution of benzoyl peroxide. Wash your face twice a day with a mild cleanser, and don't forget to moisturize. If possible, use disposable razors to avoid spreading bacteria.	The tiny hair follicles all over your face get clogged with oil, and bacteria accumulate. Scrubbing the oil away is fine, but your body just makes more unless you moisturize. Also, fried foods and other oily substances are not in order.	When acne's seriously painful, extensive, or sudden, check with a doctor to determine its cause. Acne medication such as isotretoin (Accutane) can help, but has side effects ranging from nearly universal skin and lip dryness to the less common, but more serious, depression and possible liver trouble.
Acne and dry skin	As above, use spot treatment, a mild cleanser and moisturizer on the dry areas.	Watch where the acne comes: if it's around your hairline, avoid petroleum-based hair gels, and rethink the baseball cap.	See entry above.
Puffy red cheeks, spider veins (rosacea)	Avoid alcohol, sun, stress, and spicy foods, all of which can make it worse. So can physical exertion.	Rosacea is *not,* contrary to popular belief, only a drinker's ailment.	Tetracycline, and some topical ointments, help control it. Delay and you may face a red, bulbous nose—think of Boris Yeltsin, or Tip O'Neill.
Flesh-colored bumps, red, itching bumps, sores around the lips or nose	See the doctor.	Could be anything from a cold sore to herpes, folliculitis, or molluscum. If you just shaved or have curly hair and red bumps, it's probably razor burn or PFB (see "Gay Blade," page 233)	Treatments vary. For more details on herpes or molluscum, see pages 142 and 149.

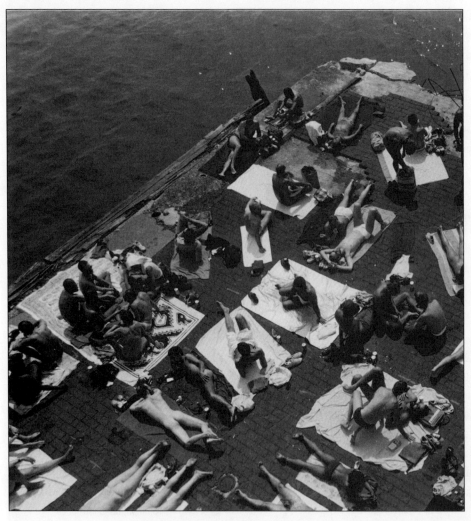

Basic #2: Sun

Gone is a good-sized piece of the ozone layer and the days when emerging from the beach the color of a walnut was considered getting a "healthy tan." Beaches from Mykonos to Miami are still popular destinations for gay travelers, but with the incidence of skin cancer up 25 percent for White men since the mid-1980s, sunshine on your shoulders (or anywhere else) may not make you happy. The danger of skin cancer increases with the fairness of your complexion, with redheads at the greatest risk. While the sun poses less of a danger for those of us who are naturally nut-colored or darker, black and brown men also have to watch out, especially for dangerous melanomas on the soles of the feet, the palms of the hands, or the beds of the fingernails. How something that feels so right can be so wrong for your skin is one of life's unsolvable mysteries, but if you want to avoid problems, including skin as *wrinkled* as a walnut, follow these steps to sun smarts.

AVOID THE SUN AT ITS WORST

This is especially important between 10 A.M. and 3 P.M., says Manhattan dermatologist Jeffrey Roth, or anyplace where reflections from sand, snow, or water increase the amount of ultraviolet radiation you're receiving.

BLOCK AND SCREEN

Never mind the difference: In 1999, the FDA threw out the distinctions, ordering all sun protection products to call themselves sunscreen. The important thing is that you use one, preferably one that contains one of the pantheon of protective chemicals that protects against burn- and cancer-causing UV-B rays as well as wrinkle- and cancer-causing UV-A rays. If you don't think you're up to the white-nosed lifeguard look of zinc oxide, try sun protection products containing "micronized" or pulverized titanium dioxide, or the newer avobenzone (Parsol 1789). As for sun protection factor (SPF), look for the word "high" on the bottle, which can mean anything from SPF 15 to 30, and refers to how many times longer it will take you to

SENSITIVE MEN

Medications from Ambien to Zoloft, with plenty of common antibiotics, antidepressants, and anti-inflammatories in between, can make you more sensitive to the sun. In addition, says Dr. Nanni, sun may make you vulnerable to recurrences of herpes, rosacea, and other problems. AIDS pioneer Marcus Conant, an assistant dermatologist at the University of California at Los Angeles, suggests that long exposure to the sun may boost levels of HIV itself in positive men with low CD4-cell counts. "Use sunscreen even if you're just walking down the street on a spring day," says New York City physician Howard Grossman. "I have people coming in all the time, really red."

Among the medications and herbs causing photosensitivity:

- Sulfa- or tetracycline-based antibiotics, including the anti-PCP medications sulfamethoxazole-trimethroprim (Bactrim or Septra) and dapsone (Dapsone)
- Sleeping pills, antidepressants, and antianxiety medications, including zolpidem (Ambien), sertraline (Zoloft), all tricyclic antidepressants, and St. John's wort
- Anti-inflammatories and antihistamines, including ibuprofen (Motrin, Advil, Nuprin) and diphenhydramine (Benadryl)

burn if you wear it than if you don't. Be generous—underapplying sunscreen can reduce the protection factor by half or more—and relentless. The Skin Cancer Foundation actually recommends sunscreen on all exposed skin every time you go outdoors. You can also get moisturizers that have sunscreens already in them, for a time- and face-saving solution, though these twofers rarely block UV-A damage.

HAT AND GLASSES

A hat with a three-inch brim is best (think Audrey Hepburn in *Funny Face*), as are wraparound sunglasses that protect your eyes from all angles (think Jackie in the White House). The sunglasses don't have to be expensive, but they do have to block 99 to 100 percent of UV-A and UV-B radiation. Before you strike a pose, check the label. UV protection comes from an invisible chemical applied to the lenses.

DID SOMEBODY SAY SARONG?

Lightweight, loose-fitting, long-sleeved shirts and pants, or other garments that cover your skin, are recommended beachwear. Careful, though: A dry T-shirt only offers you an SPF of 6 to 9, rather than the needed 15 or more, and wet ones drop down to around 3. Forget those sexy mesh numbers, too; if you can see through them when you hold them up to a light source, they protect little if at all.

DON'T GET BURNED

If you do, try aspirin, lots of water (not caffeinated or alcoholic beverages), and potassium (orange juice and bananas are good sources) to dull pain and regain pep, says Dr. Roth. Many also swear by vitamin E—break open the capsules and spread the contents on the affected areas. Other home remedies include applying plain yogurt (then rinse it off), aloe vera, apple cider vinegar, and cooled chamomile tea.

Rash, blisters, fever, chills, upset stomach, and confusion are signs of sun poisoning, not sunburn. If you have any of these, see a doctor.

SKIN CANCER DANGER SIGNS

When looking at moles, keep your eye out for the **ABCD**s of malignant melanoma, the most deeply spreading, and dangerous, of the three types of skin cancer:

***A**symmetry:* One half of a mole or lesion doesn't look like the other half.

***B**order:* A mole has an irregular, scalloped, or not clearly defined border.

***C**olor:* The color—whether tan, brown, white, red, or blue—varies or is not uniform from one area of a mole or lesion to another.

***D**iameter:* The lesion is larger than 6 millimeters (about the size of a pencil eraser).

Adapted from the American Academy of Dermatology

If you have rough, slightly raised lesions that look reddish on white skin, or unusually dark on dark skin, they could be anything from a case of psoriasis (see next page) to actinic keratoses, roughened red patches on the skin that may increase your risk of skin cancer.

Any lesions or lumps that start growing, change, bleed, are scabby, or won't heal could be signs of the two "milder" types of skin cancer: the "superficially spreading" basal cell carcinoma and the tumor-causing squamous cell carcinoma. Though less serious than melanoma, even local damage by basal cell carcinoma can include serious destruction of tissue like a nose or an ear, and may require deep incisions to remove it. Get anything suspicious checked out, and if you are diagnosed with even an actinic keratosis, consider a low-fat diet and supplementing your diet with antioxidants such as vitamins C and E (see page 259). A 1998 study published in the *Journal of the American Medical Association* found that getting less than 20 percent of your calories from fat significantly reduces your risk of developing lesions and tumors, and earlier research suggests that diet can also keep your skin cancer from progressing.

A raised violaceous (that's purple to you) lesion may be Kaposi's sarcoma, a cancer commonly associated with HIV and older men of Mediterranean ancestry. KS lesions look reddish purple on light-skinned people and bluish or brownish black on dark-skinned people.

If you do find any of these, advises Dr. Roth, go for total sun avoidance and an immediate doctor's visit.

AVOID TANNING BEDS

They're unregulated, explains Dr. Nanni, and can emit levels of radiation that have been linked to cancer. Even at lower levels, adds Dr. Roth, the UV-A rays they give off are implicated in wrinkling.

Basic #3: See

As you dry yourself after a shower or bath, take a moment to look at your skin front and back, including between your fingers and toes and the soles of your feet. Note rough spots, moles, birthmarks, and blemishes. Do this monthly. Getting to know yourself better is always good, and catching a possible skin cancer early (see box above) greatly improves treatment options.

Remember, though, that not all red, scaly, or itchy patches are life-threatening. Common dermatological problems you may find as you give yourself a going-over include those below.

ATHLETE'S FOOT AND JOCK ITCH

Redness, inflammation, or itching between your toes, around your groin, or around your anus can be signs of athlete's foot (tinea pedis) or jock itch (tinea cruris). Clean the area twice a day with an antibacterial soap, then apply an over-the-counter antifungal cream containing clotrimazole (such as Lotrimin). Even if the itching is really bad, avoid cortisone cream, which will only makes things worse in the long run.

Some of us are genetically predisposed to getting fungus, says Dr. Nanni, so if you're among them, try not to walk barefoot on gym floors, hotel-room carpets, or other public areas. Prevention of future outbreaks, by drying carefully (including between your toes and butt cheeks) and by dusting affected areas with an antifungal powder, is key. A blow dryer, on a comfortable setting, can help dry out nooks and crannies and feels good. "If a rash doesn't respond to over-the-counter treatments in a couple of weeks," adds Roth, "hotfoot it to a doctor."

NAIL FUNGUS

Especially if you have a history of athlete's foot, discolored, thickened, or deformed toenails may be a sign of nail fungus (onychomycosis). This is harder to get rid of than athlete's foot, usually requiring a doctor's visit and at least a three-month course of medication. Herbalists recommend a liberal dose of tea-tree oil, applied to the fungus in question.

SCALING AND ITCHING SKIN

Patches of scaling or itching that fade away into the surrounding skin may be signs of contact dermatitis or eczema. Contact dermatitis comes from contact with irritants from the outside, which could be anything from laundry detergent to a new piece of jewelry to poison ivy. Eczema is skin irritation caused by internal factors, and different types show up on your face, the palms or soles of the feet, or other places on the body. Both conditions can often be soothed by an over-the-counter cortisone cream, says Roth, though it's best to see a doctor if you don't know their cause or if they're on a sensitive place such as your scalp, your anus, or your eyelids. If you've just started a new medication and find yourself with a rash or itching, contact your doctor immediately: You may be having an allergic response with potentially serious consequences.

PSORIASIS

Finding deep pink, raised, itching patches with rough or scaly skin on your knees, elbows, scalp, or elsewhere may mean you have psoriasis. Psoriasis, caused by skin cells replenishing themselves too fast and piling up, can also cause pits in the fingernails, raised pus-filled blisters, and open painful cracks in the skin. Treatments range from topical drugs to ultraviolet light treatments (which ironically may increase your risk of skin cancer) or newer treatments with lasers. As psoriasis is often difficult to treat, some have turned to alternative treatments, including sarsaparilla and an herb called *Coleus forskolii,* said to contain a compound that controls skin cell proliferation.

FOLLICULITIS

If you have red swellings or bumps with pale centers, and if it's not acne, you may have folliculitis, infected hair follicles. A hot washcloth applied to the bumps may help the pus come to the surface, and this common form of infection usually resolves itself within a few weeks.

Staph infection may also be a possibility, so if it seems to be getting worse, see a doctor for some antibiotics.

If you have HIV, infections or inflammation of the hair follicles can spread to include dozens, or hundreds, of locations. As many as ten different bacterial, fungal, or allergic conditions can cause the symptoms, usually lumped together by doctors under the descriptive if not particularly technical name "itchy red bump disease." Its real name is pustular eosinophilic folliculitis (PEF). See your doctor for diagnosis and treatment.

PLASTIC AND BEAUTIFUL?

When human beings have been fascinated by the contemplation of their own hearts, the more intricate biological pattern of the female has become a model for the artist, the mystic, and the saint. When mankind turns instead to what can be done, altered, built, invented, in the outer world, all natural properties of men, animals or metals become handicaps to be altered rather than clues to be followed.

—*Margaret Mead*

Anthropologist Margaret Mead's theory—that using tools to change the face of nature is an essentially male approach—will find surprisingly little argument from the American Society of Plastic and Reconstructive Surgeons (ASPRS). The trade organization says that men, concerned about droopy eyes, sagging cheeks, and lard-laden waistlines, are turning to plastic surgery in droves. From 1992 to 1997 male eyelid repairs rose 57 percent. Face-lifts climbed 81 percent, and male liposuction—now weighing in at a whopping 20,200 procedures annually—more than tripled.

In sixteen years of nipping and tucking, Richard Marfuggi, MD, a board-certified plastic surgeon and author of *Plastic Surgery: What You Need to Know Before, During and After* (Perigree Books, 1998), has watched his clientele swing from majority female to majority male. Though most are lawyers and financial execs—the bills for even the most basic procedures can make your face fall—Dr. Marfuggi's patients range from models to morticians to construction workers. About 80 percent of the men he sees are gay, says Marfuggi, a statistic that isn't scientific but still may be significant. "Like anyone else, gay men want to look their best," says Marfuggi. Like anyone else? Doctor, please: How many of us want to settle for that?

Overeagerness to refinish yourself, however, leaves you vulnerable to unscrupulous doctors or shoddy procedures. If you're determined to proceed, do so with care. The ASPRS (800-635-0635) can tell you if a plastic surgeon is board-certified, which means that he or she has passed the required oral and written exams and has completed five years of general residency, three years of general surgery, and two years of plastic surgery. Personal recommendations, preferably with before-and-after pictures, are also important, as is meeting the surgeon to discuss pros and cons well before the day of your procedure. "If you arrive at a doctor's office and meet the sales rep instead, go elsewhere," advises California plastic surgeon Gary Alter, MD. Also give some thought to the behaviors causing the condition you want to correct. Getting the bags erased from under your eyes isn't going to make that much sense if you stay out all night three times a week, and no liposuction can reverse the effect of daily junkfood binges.

Whether or not gay men have more plastic surgery than other men, it seems safe to assume we talk about it more. Is it guilty deviance from masculine do-it-yourself norms or love of the lady within that leaves us dishing with delight and disdain about chest implants, ear pinning, calf restructuring, or the latest, abdominal etching (strategic liposuction that makes it look like you have six-pack abs)? Get men to talk about their own "work," however, and the conversation starts sounding less like preciousness than like pragmatism. "It's not so much losing the pounds but the shape," says Tony, a forty-something New Jerseyite who recently turned to liposuction to trim his tummy. "Diets just didn't work, and though I exercise, it doesn't get rid of the fat cells for that specific area." Carter, proprietor of Inn Exile in Palm Springs, California, articulates his stitch-in-time philosophy with the prudence one would expect from a desert homesteader of a different era. "The time to consider cosmetic surgery is not when you need it but when you start to see the changes happening—a preventive sort of thing, rather than out of desperation," says the forty-five-year-old, who's undergone a hair transplant and had the skin underneath his eyes tightened. "It's kind of like changing the oil in your car, or repairing a single upholstery tear before the whole chair rips." Carter is now considering facial resurfacing. "The laser results are pretty impressive—smoother and tighter," he says. "There are fewer deep wrinkles, and a lot of the fine ones disappear entirely."

Lasers are remaking the face of many cosmetic procedures, including electrolysis (see "Gay Blade," below), vision correction (laser refractive eye surgery, at roughly $2,000 an eye), teeth whitening, and a host of other operations. Should lasers fall short for you—most do not, says dermatologist Christopher Nanni, MD, remove tattoos as easily as we've been led to believe, for example—despair not. Even newer technology may soon give you what could be *the* makeover option: a total body transplant. A team of surgeons at Case Western Reserve University in Cleveland says the science-fiction-like procedure is nearly fact, though not at all cosmetic. The team has already performed the surgery somewhat successfully on monkeys; it seems the simians could see, hear, and taste perfectly with their heads atop new bodies, though unfortunately they couldn't move. That would certainly give new meaning to just sitting there looking pretty.

SIX-MILLION-DOLLAR MAN?

The most popular cosmetic procedures for men, and their estimated costs:

Liposuction: $1,700–$5,000 per site

Blepharoplasty (eyelids/under eyes): under eyes, $3,500–$5,000; upper and lower together, $5,000–$6,500

Rhinoplasty (nose): $3,800–$4,500

Gynecomastia (breast reduction): $3,500–$4,500 for liposuction only; $5,500–$6,500 with skin resection

Face-lift and neck work: $7,500–$16,000

From Plastic Surgery: What You Need to Know Before, During and After, *by Richard Marfuggi, MD (Perigree, 1998)*

Hair Care, Hair Loss, and Hair Removal

For years I felt my red hair was something I had to struggle to live up to. I mean, my only role models growing up were Lucille Ball and Bozo. I was actually relieved when I started balding young. But no sooner had that happened than I found myself sprouting rich, red hair all over my body.

I love my hairy chest—it makes me feel animal, male, like I'm from some long tradition of strong men used to winters and wars and cradling someone on dark nights in a warm tent.

They say that karma—the history of your past—is in your hair, which is probably one reason why they shave it all off you when you join the army or go to jail. For me, hair has always been about self-definition. When I was younger, I dyed it purple to say, "I'm not like you." Even now, when I'm in a bad mood: haircut.

More than one gay man smiled in amusement in 1997 when Miami police announced that killer Andrew Cunanan was dressing as a woman after they found body hair in his razor. Law enforcement authorities may not know it, but the South Beach fashion police are clear: Body hair is cause for apprehension. If you're hopelessly hairy, take heart; this is only a phase. From the foundation of FAFH! (Fags Against Facial Hair!) in the 1970s to the roar of the emerging bear movement at the close of the millennium, gay men continue to struggle to decide how to grow hair in one place or get rid of it in another. Are Jheri curls retro or retarded? Should we really change our cut from an Edwardian fall-forward look to a George Clooney–esque Caesar? Would we look better as a sun-kissed blonde . . . at least for a few streaks of hair in front of the eyes? And of course, the crucial question: How will we be wearing our chest hair this summer: lush, clipped, or shaved right down to the epidermis?

Hairs are slender threads, but they bind us tight to history. Few other bodily characteristics, advises the Encyclopedia Encarta (Microsoft, 1999), are as reliable as markers of our heritage: Japanese, Chinese, and Native American hair is round in cross-section and almost always black; people of African and Melanesian descent have hair that grows from a curved follicle, and has a spiral twist; European, South Asian, and Semitic hair comes from a straight follicle but is oval in cross section, and spans the spectrum between curly and straight, pale blond and blue-black. If villains in movies are often bald, it may be because hair separates the cold-blooded creatures from the warm: Mammals, us men included, are the only animals who have the stuff.

That's all fine, but what do we do with it? The basics, says Alex Koskos of the trendy Manhattan spa The Service Station, are simple.

- Skimp on shampoo, but never on conditioner.
- Use a couple of different shampoos throughout the week to prevent buildup.
- Get a trim at least once every two months.
- Use a tar- or zinc-based shampoo if you're facing flaking scalp and dandruff.
- Don't wear a hat all the time, since it will dry out your scalp.
- Never let anyone inexperienced color your hair.

The rest is up to you. If fashion seems fickle, it always has been. In ancient Egypt, men and women shaved their heads and put on heavy black wigs on special occasions; by A.D. 100, in Christian circles, wearing another man's hair on your head was a mortal sin. In ancient Athens men wore shorter, curly ringlets, requiring so much attention that the profession of hairdresser was born. Some Native American warriors shaved their heads entirely, leaving only a central tuft. The Renaissance saw the rebirth of the bob, with men wearing their hair rolled under at the neck or ears. By the early seventeenth century, fashionable European men wore flowing locks and short, Vandyke beards; later in the century, so many notables were bald from syphilis that wigs were in again—at least until the French Revolution, which also turned European hairstyles on their head. As for men who love men, history will recall: Our hairstyles have covered it all (see page 230).

Balding Basics

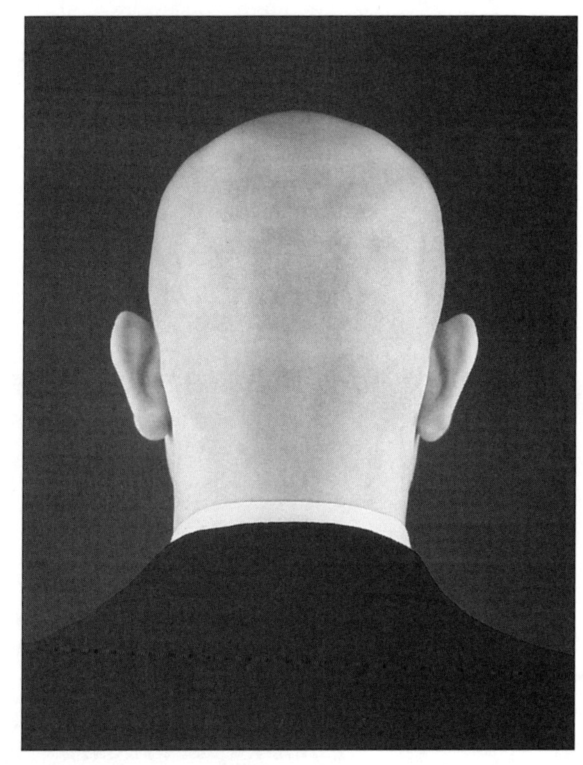

I like my hair, and I regret losing it. Half of me wants to do anything I can to keep it, but it seems to me that all the options leave your hair looking like a field of corn in the Midwest or a cheesy hair weave. So I look in the mirror and say to myself, "Take a deep breath, relax. You're not twenty-three anymore. You're a little bit wiser and emotionally more stable. It's too bad you can't have a twenty-three-year-old body with what you know now, but you can't, and nature has probably structured it that way for a reason."

I think guys with bald spots, providing they keep it short all the way around to blend, are actually really sexy . . . it gives off an air of maturity, so long as you're not neurotic about it. I actually slept with a guy who insisted on wearing his baseball cap the entire time.

Hippocrates, the famous doctor, smeared a sludge of opium, pigeon shit, rose petals, and olives on his head to cure his baldness (history, in this instance, does not record his oath). Others have slathered their scalps with snake oil, swallowed female hormones, hung upside down for hours to stimulate circulation, or endured painful and useless treatments ranging from low-level electric shocks to (no kidding) castration. Today, in modern America, more than thirty-five million men in America are facing alopecia androgenetica, or male pattern baldness, and continue to shell out more than $2 billion annually to reverse it.

Explanations of the cause of baldness have come and gone as quickly as remedies over the ages. Aristotle was convinced that semen was stored in the head; as sexual activity over a lifetime began to use it up, men lost the heat and moisture necessary for hair growth. A more modern shaggy-man story—that baldness comes from a gene passed down through the mother's side of the family—has been replaced by evidence that either side can pass the gene that leads to baldness. The more immediate cause of baldness is high levels of testosterone (or, more accurately, a hormone known as dihydrotestosterone), which cause the hair follicles

GAY MEN'S HAIR CRISIS? GAY HAIR THROUGH HISTORY

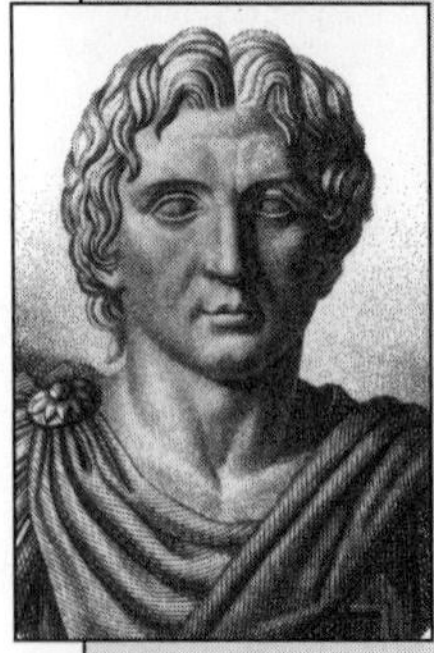

ALEXANDER THE GREAT, CONQUEROR

Was it fair-haired good looks or his military might that made the world fall to its knees?

Tips for blondes: "If you have naturally blond hair, violet shampoos will enhance an ashy or platinum look," says Ennio of Blades Salon in West Hollywood. "If you want to go lighter," Ennio recommends, "the best way is to use three colors for gradation, rather than damaging your hair with bleach. Highlights are even better—they last longer and require fewer trips to the salon."

As for the brunettes who wish we all could be California girls, "don't go all the way blond," says Ennio. "You can get there, but it'll be really damaging because of all the processing. If you really have to do it, make it an extreme cut—I'm talking supershort—to go with the extremeness of the color."

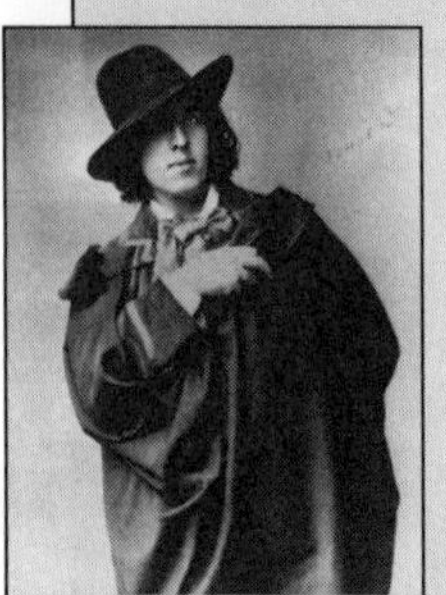

OSCAR WILDE, WRITER

His long, luscious locks defined the dandy; his tongue, the soul of English wit.

Tips for long hair: "No man should wash his hair every day, but men with long hair especially shouldn't," says Manhattan hairstylist Dave Hickey. "The oils and nutrients that your hair produces come from the scalp—they need time to get to the ends. Leave-in conditioners are very important, since they help control frizz and protect hair from damage by the sun, wind, and all the daily wear and tear." As for cuts, Hickey recommends trims every eight weeks to prevent split ends from traveling all the way up to the top, as well as a bit of layering for "flow" and to give body at the top of the head. "That hair has been on your head for at least a year or two," explains Hickey. "It needs care."

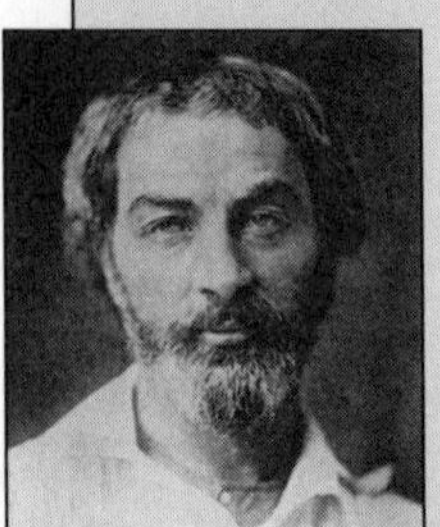

WALT WHITMAN, POET

Champion of brotherly love, he was a forebear of the modern move toward nature-loving, beard-wearing, big-bellied fellas.

Tips for beards: "Goatees are very hot right now, as are 'stingers'—a little tuft of hair, or line of it, just under your lower lip," says Sam Zifferblatt, editor of *GRUF (Great Unshaven Faces)*, an on-line adult magazine in San Francisco (www.gruf.com). "Make sure to moisturize as much as if you didn't have a beard, or even more," adds Koskos from Manhattan's Service Station. "You're not shaving, so the dry skin isn't getting scraped away."

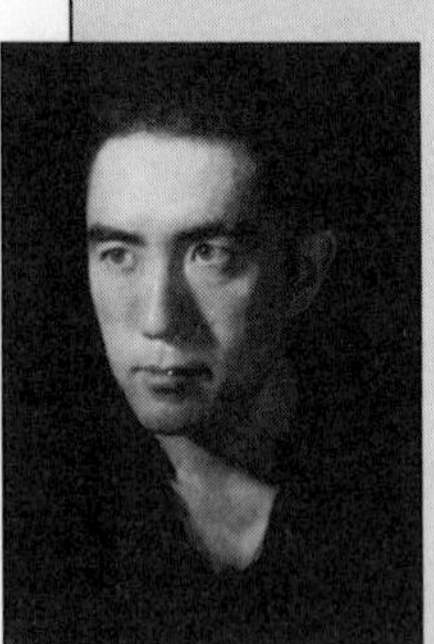

YUKIO MISHIMA, WRITER

Japan's famous lover of all-male brotherhoods, and a die-hard member of the cult of the hard body.

Tips for Asian hair: "The basic misconception about Asian hair is that it's all pokey and straight and hard to work with," says Elizabeth Hartley, West Coast creative director for Vidal Sassoon. "In reality, it runs the gamut from the stereotype of straight and coarse, to very fine, to so curly it grows in ringlets when it's long. One of the beautiful qualities of Asian hair is that it tends to lie flatter, which gives the hair a great sheen and allows for wonderful layering. You can have a shorter shape underneath, with a suedelike texture, and a longer, shiny and silky length on top."

Because it's dark and lies flat, Asian hair "tends to be a bit oilier than Caucasian hair," says Hartley, "absorbing more heat from the sun and oil from the scalp." Regular shampooing will keep oil down and bring the sheen to a manageable, luscious level.

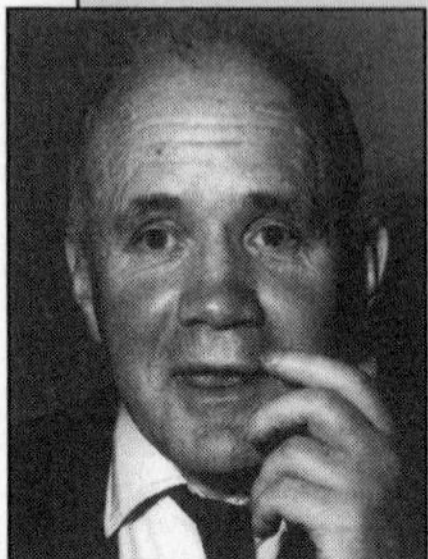

JEAN GENET, WRITER AND FILMMAKER

Our century's most fearless explorer of the intersection between the criminal and the erotic.

Tips for bald heads: "One of the great things about bald heads is that they don't need much care," says John T. Capps III, founder of the bald pride organization Bald Headed Men of America. "Just a little sunscreen and moisturizer and occasionally insect repellent to keep the mosquitoes away." (For more, see "Balding Basics," page 229)

LIBERACE, ENTERTAINER

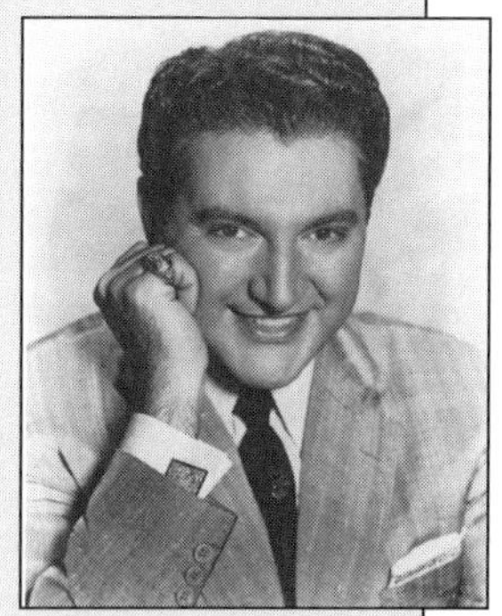

The pianos are smaller in most gay bars these days, but the bold bouffant lives on.

Tips for big hair: "Don't use conditioner or conditioning shampoo—it makes the hair too soft," advises Nancy Wisdom, stylist at Salons in the Park in Dallas. "And your mousses and gels should contain alcohol for maximum bigness." To get height while blow-drying, Wisdom's wisdom includes using a round brush, preferably one with a metal base and short bristles, and waiting until your hair is 70 percent dry to start. If you want to use hair spray, says Wisdom, "pull the hair away from your head with the brush and spray underneath—spraying all over weighs hair down." Among Texan men, she notes, big hair is smaller than it used to be, with more choosing perms and body waves. "Most of the people I do who want it big—the men anyway—are strippers and televangelists," says Wisdom. And you thought politics made strange bedfellows.

SYLVESTER, DISCO SENSATION

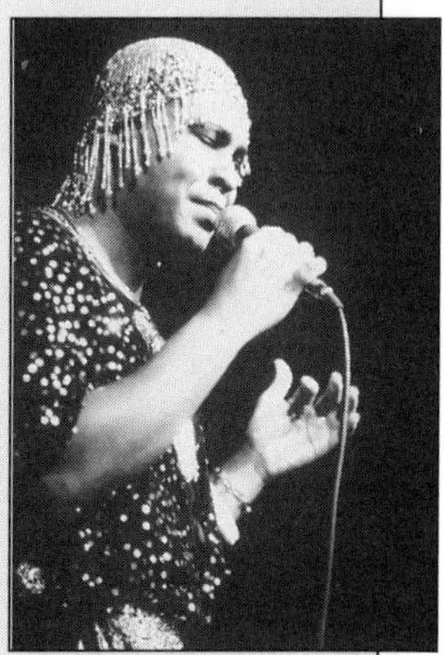

The realest of the disco divas.

Tips for Black hair: If you want to grow "locks," says Shannon Ayers of Turning Heads in Harlem, find a reputable hair specialist who can train your hair to lock through coils, twists, braids, or extensions. "To maintain them," says Ayers, "shampoo them gently through a stocking cap until they lock enough not to fall apart under shampooing," which is usually about two to seven months. If you don't do it yourself, see your stylist every three or four weeks to have them retreated. For more general care, Ayers urges men to stay away from old-fashioned petrolatum or mineral-oil-based pomades that "sit on the hair rather than penetrate," and recommends instead "products made from plant and flower extracts." It'll be worth the extra cost, says Ayers. "For sheen, Aveda's Brillante is brilliant."

QUENTIN CRISP, ACTOR AND SOCIAL CRITIC

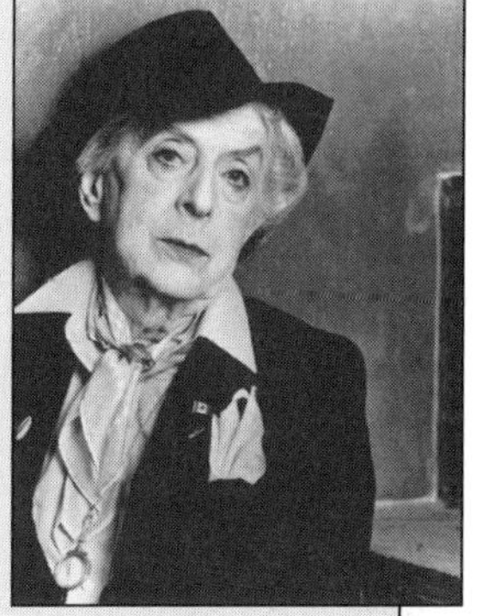

"I loved the blue upsweep," gushes one fan. "His look was as timely as his commentary," offers another. Meow.

Tips for graying hair: "Keeping gray is great, distinguished, and sexy," says Hickey, "so long as it doesn't get dull." Minerals in hard or soft water, or chlorine from the pool, can turn gray to dingy greenish or yellowish, and tar-based shampoos for dandruff may leave an orange-brown tone. "Shampoo, rinse, or toner labeled 'brightening,' with a blue or violet base, can help," observes Hickey, "and pomades and silicone shiners also make gray look dazzling."

If you want to tint or color out gray, we've come a long way since henna or Grecian Formula: "I like something called Slate, but there are a variety of vegetable dyes and rinses that won't give you a hard line at the roots, growing in gradually, and darkening the gray without looking like you're hiding something," says Hickey. "Gray hair is very resistant to color, because the cuticle of the hair, the outer layer, is more closed. If you want to totally cover it up, you're going to have to use a permanent dye."

RU PAUL, SINGER AND FORMER TALK-SHOW HOST

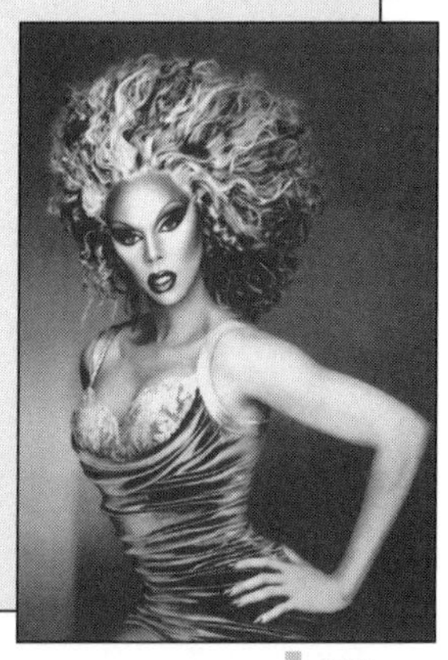

S/he gives new definition to "daring do."

Tips for wig wearers: You better work. Wigs need attention after every wearing. "Make sure to comb from the underside up," says Veronica Vera, dean of students at Miss Vera's Finishing School for Boys Who Want to Be Girls in Manhattan. "Also, learning to tease is important, *especially* when it comes to your hair. With good back-combing skills, you can style like a pro."

HAIR HELPERS? ANTIBALDNESS DRUGS

I think some of the smartest twenty-two-year-olds in the business must have come up with this one. I used it for six months but couldn't tell if it was working, and then was afraid to stop because maybe it was helping me keep what I had. And they say if you stop, whatever you've gained will fall out.

Two drugs with FDA approval—minoxidil (Rogaine) and finasteride (Propecia)—are now on the market to jump-start hair growth. Neither can give bald men full heads of hair, and neither works for everyone. Minoxidil is an over-the-counter product you spray or drip twice daily into your scalp: the new, stronger formulation approved in late 1997 seems to grow 45 percent more hair than the regular-strength formula, according to Upjohn, Rogaine's manufacturer, and works best on people with fine hair and those who start using it before they've lost too much. The results? An average increase of about 39 hairs per square centimeter on your bald spot, the possibility of itching or dryness of the skin or lips, and a wait of two to six months before you know if it's working at all. Even when effective, minoxidil is a lifetime commitment that will cost you $15 to $30 a month, because if you stop using the drug, all your new hair falls out.

As for finasteride (Propecia), it's a once-a-day pill, approved in December 1997, that seems to help about half the people who take it. Preliminary reports showed about 18 percent of men had moderate to heavy hair growth, and another 30 percent had slight increases. What that means in hard, hairsplitting terms? An average of 107 more hairs per circular inch for men with bald spots, and insufficient evidence to say that Propecia works for receding hairlines. As with minoxidil, reports indicate that if you stop using Propecia, you lose your new hair, and you have to use it for a minimum of three months to know if it's working. Cost is estimated at about $50 a month. Since Propecia is also prescribed as a prostate medication, make sure your doctor knows you're taking it before you have a PSA test (see Chapter 8).

Makers of both drugs claim they'll help you hang on to what you have, though that's harder to evaluate. As for all other treatments—hair growth shampoos, "hypnohair" treatments, "magic combs," "intrasound stimulators," and other exotic and ancient "cures"—they're all unproven and probably bogus. Men looking for baldness remedies fork over an estimated $100 million each year for unproven treatments; instead of new hair, most get clip jobs. Still, you may feel better: Even 62 percent of men taking a placebo in the Propecia drug trials thought their appearance had improved. As for those who go for combos, the studies haven't been done, but some swear by a Propecia-minoxidil mix, at least for other people. "It didn't seem to do much for me, but Jeff looked like a totally different person when I saw him on the street," sighs Carl, thirty-three. The hair is always fuller on the other guy's head.

to slowly close, making the hair get thinner and thinner until it disappears from view entirely. In rare instances, high fever, malnutrition, prolonged illness, certain kinds of medical treatments, really tight cornrows, and the disorder alopecia areata—which can cause all the hair on certain parts of your body to fall out—can all cause baldness.

Given that testosterone is its cause, and the difficulty of reversing its effects, some men choose to see baldness as a sign of manliness, or a hallmark of age and experience. "After wondering about creams and chemicals and transplants, you know what I realized? There are other parts of my body that respond better to my efforts," says Douglas, forty-four. "I'd rather cut my hair short and look fit. That seemed better than constantly hearing, 'Don't wear a hat, you'll lose more hair,' or worrying at how much I found in the shower drain."

For those who think it'll be easier to find a hairpiece than inner peace, there is an ever-growing array of hair replacement options, and that doesn't even include ripping out your ex-boyfriend's locks the next time you see him out with some twenty-two-year-old Olympic gymnast. "If you have to go bald, this is the time to do it," enthuses Alex Koskos, listing the array of new technologies that have supplemented the old glue-on toupee, itself greatly improved (and now referred to as a "hair system"). There are microplugs (hair taken from the back and replanted in front, but in a way that re-creates the hairline without the cornfield look), "weaves" (extensions braided into your real hair and periodically retightened), and "flap surgery" (which cuts away the bald skin of your scalp and sews the hairy parts together). Wigs range from a bottom-of-the-barrel $140 model to a handsome, hand-tied product (made to fit your head) that can run about $800, says Dennis of Studio International in San Francisco. Weaves seem to be wending their way toward oblivion, since adhesive hair systems ($325 to over $2,000) have improved so much; Dennis says weaves work only for men willing to wear their hair long or high in order to keep the "track" they attach to from being visible. As for surgery and microplugs, they come with a macro price, from $3,000 to about $15,000. "I figured I'd look better in a new car," observes Mark, thirty-seven, after checking out the options. If you want to check them out too, www.hairsite.com offers a good overview from a balding individual's perspective, and the American Hair Loss Council (www.ahlc.org) is the national trade organization for purveyors of balding remedies.

If you decide to let things fall as they may, Koskos advises cutting your hair short, or if your hair's dark and your skin is light, bleaching to a natural-looking blond to cut down on the contrast between hair and head. As for shaving it all off and going with the Kojak look now making a comeback, Koskos warns that it requires good head proportions and significant maintenance. "We're talking regular shaving, daily sunblock, or wearing a hat winter and summer," he adds, "so you don't get a burn on your head."

As often as not, though, the sting of balding, and what it seems to represent, is felt more deeply within. For more on feelings about growing older, see Chapter 8.

Gay Blade: Some Tips on Shaving Face and Body

Remember the seventies, when letting it all hang out included facial and body hair, and when a push-broom mustache and a chest like a shag rug made you the envy of Polk Street, Christopher Street, or maybe even Main Street, USA? Today, a clean look prevails on many gay faces, and, in more extreme cases, from the neck down too. If you have no time or tolerance for such vanities, or if you wear your face and body hair with the bearish pride of a Walt Whitman or a Burt Reynolds, more power to you. If you think staying on the cutting edge means holding fast to your razor, then at least make sure to change the blade often, shave after you've softened up in the shower, and follow these five often-ignored tips for hair removal.

FOR YOUR FACE

"Nicking your face often has nothing to do with cutting your beard. It's also from cutting your skin because of the accumulation of dead skin cells," says Ernie Benson, founder of The Face Place in West Hollywood. Get rid of those cells with an exfoliating scrub, says Benson, and you'll "stop nicking yourself and improve your shave by 100 percent."

FOR YOUR BALLS

"I shaved them once, which I think many of us can probably say," says Max, thirty-six. "After

RAZOR BUMPS, BLACK SKIN, AND CURLY HAIR

It's the curly-hair part that's responsible for what Shannon Ayers, owner of Turning Heads in Harlem, calls the scourge of Black men who shave: razor bumps. This condition is experienced by men of all races and ethnicities when hair curls back and repenetrates the skin, causing inflammation, soreness, and infection. The official name is pseudofolliculitis barbae, or PFB. It's "pseudo," or false, folliculitis because the irritation takes place where the hair goes back into the skin, not where it comes out. The official cure, says Ayers and skin doctors, is to stop shaving, and use moisturizers and exfoliants. "Whatever you do, don't pull at it!" warns Ayers. "And do see a dermatologist."

If you're dead set against whiskers, or your job won't allow them, Dr. Nanni suggests you use all the tricks for sensitive skin: using shaving gel rather than cream, showering before shaving, and taking care not to shave against the grain of the hair. There are also special PFB razors, which cut less closely than ordinary ones. Some people find electric razors easier to tolerate. Stay away from double-track razors, advises Joseph Bark, MD, author of *Your Skin . . . An Owner's Guide* (Prentice Hall Trade, 1995), because the first blade cuts off the hair and the second often slices off a small bump of skin just below it, increasing infection and scarring. Antibiotic and antiacne creams can help with the small, infected follicles, says Dr. Nanni, and some laser treatments can reduce PFB scars.

living through the aftermath, I'd rather do it to someone else." Whether it's now or forever, using antibacterial soap before you apply shaving cream cuts down on possible cuts and infections, says Howard Grossman, MD. If you're itching terribly as the hair grows back, soothe yourself with over-the-counter cortisone cream. If you're doing it to each other, don't share razors—change the blade or use a disposable.

FOR YOUR CHEST

On this area of the body, cutting with the grain is as important as it is on your face. That's true even with clippers, which Koskos says give a better look than a razor and won't make your hair grow in all itchy and stubbly. If you don't know how, let someone do it who does, or at least use clippers with a guard. If you do use razors, don't share.

FOR YOUR BACK

Waxing to remove hair on the back runs about $50 to $75. (And no, the hair will not grow back softer.) Depilatory creams, like Nair, can also be effective on back and bikini line, says Koskos, but work better if you trim with clippers first.

FOR "PERMANENT" HAIR REMOVAL

The processes that claim to remove hair permanently—electrolysis and laser removal—are expensive and often unreliable.

Electrolysis kills hair by sending an electric current into the follicle. A facial hair, though, may have to be zapped some twenty to forty times to be done away with. Since each jolt can feel like a minor bee sting, writes Joanne Stringer in *The Transsexual's Survival Guide* (Creative Design Services, 1992), and since your face has some fifty thousand hairs, she figures getting rid of your beard is like a million bee stings delivered for between $45 and $60 an hour.

Laser removal, the latest and most expensive strategy, claims to remove hair forever in a single session. Denuding the chest or back takes about forty-five minutes, costs anywhere from $400 to $1,500, and may or may not work as well as the salesmen say. "Only long-wavelength lasers are appropriate," explains Dr. Nanni, "and many types of hair are going to take more than one session. The process can also cause some problems in pigmentation, lightening dark skin and vice versa."

Watch Your Mouth: Oral Health and Hygiene

The same rules you've heard since you were a little homosexual-in-training still apply. "There's no substitute for proper brushing and flossing to maintain good oral hygiene," says Roger Wills, DDS, a dentist in downtown Chicago with many gay clients. Not only can regular dental help keep your breath sweet and teeth white, but it will decrease risk of bleeding gums or other problems that may increase the risk of transmission of HIV and other viruses. If you have HIV already, regular visits to the dentist may detect early symptoms of HIV-related illness, which commonly show up in the mouth before they do anywhere else.

Canker Sores

The white and sometimes painful sores on your gums, the inside of your mouth, or the inside of your lips can appear in response to stress, sweet or spicy foods, or external causes like a hot

HIV-Related Oral Complications

"I don't see these as much as I used to, thanks to the new antiviral drugs," says Wills. "But these complications are often one of the first signs that someone's immune system may be under strain."

ORAL CANDIDIASIS (THRUSH)

Thrush is one of the most common oral problems of HIV-positive people. Caused by variants of the fungus *Candida,* thrush shows up as creamy white patches on the membrane of the mouth and the upper throat, which can be swabbed or swiped away. Thrush is best treated locally, with a cream or lozenge (also called a troche) that melts in your mouth, though it can also be treated systemically with an antifungal drug.

HAIRY LEUKOPLAKIA (HL)

Hairy leukoplakia looks like thrush, with white patches on the tongue, but usually appears only on the sides of the tongue and can't be scraped off. It's called hairy because it has small, hairlike projections, not because it's hard to deal with—in fact, you usually don't feel it at all. HL doesn't necessarily require treatment, but high doses of acyclovir may eradicate it.

RECURRENT APHTHOUS ULCERS (RAU)

This is the name for canker or cold sores that won't go away. These can be painful, though they often respond to topical treatment with a liquid suspension of tetracycline or with steroid solutions.

CYSTS OR INFLAMMATION OF GLANDS IN THE GUMS OR MOUTH

These are a common and commonly missed sign of early HIV infection. See a dentist for assessment and treatment.

piece of pizza or a rough tooth. "Over-the-counter ointments or rinsing with salt water can help dull the pain," says Dr. Wills, "and some men say lysine tablets help clear canker sores faster. They should go away on their own. If they don't heal within ten days, see a physician or dentist."

Dental Floss

Flossing, so often lectured on, is so little practiced. "Once I miss a few days, I give up," says Jerry, thirty-nine, in a common refrain. Some 75 percent of men over thirty-five have some form of gum disease. Dr. Wills urges men having problems with floss not to give up after missing a few days. "It's best to do it as a part of your nighttime routine, so you're not going to bed with a mouthful of debris. But doing it at any time of day is better than not doing it," says Wills. With a little practice you can combine it with your favorite TV show. Recent research shows that healthy gums may help prevent heart disease, stroke, and other ailments. Who knew so much hung by a (waxy) thread?

Bad Breath

Halitosis often comes from decaying food debris, so flossing (see above) is crucial, says Wills, as is brushing both teeth and tongue. Some pharmacies also sell tongue cleaners, U-shaped instruments of plastic or metal with which you drag off that nasty coating. Some over-the-counter pills claim to help "internally." Although they may mask the problem temporarily, says Dr. Wills, "you may also be covering up a serious problem such as periodontal disease, ulcers, or sinusitis. The bottom line: Anytime there's persistent halitosis, see a dentist, and then see a physician if it's not a problem of dental origin."

Mouthwash freshens the mouth only briefly, says Wills. Products labeled "mouth rinse"—among them Listerine—reduce the number of germs in your mouth more significantly.

Straightening

If you're still thinking all these years later about being straight and white—meaning your teeth, of course—cosmetic options are booming, but they'll cost you. Most dentists advise against potentially enamel-damaging, over-the-counter whiteners (big surprise), suggesting instead that they make you custom plates you fill with bleaching paste and stick onto your teeth at night for two to six weeks. Wills says that there are also new, whitening lasers, requiring a mere one to two visits, which may become increasingly popular in the near future. As for other strategies, there are caps (porcelain caps for $300–$1,500 a tooth), veneers (they cover the front only, for $500–$1,200 a tooth), bonding (filling in gaps with white stuff, $250–$700 per tooth), and braces, which are not just for metal-mouth eighth graders anymore. According to Wills, 20 percent of orthodontic patients these days are adults, many choosing lingual (behind-the-teeth) braces or brackets done in porcelain so that people just see the wire. You're still talking two to three years and $2,500–$3,000.

If you're looking into improving your oral health, also examine what you put into your mouth. Coffee and cigarette smoke, for example, are sure to stain your teeth. If you don't brush after lunch, the bread of your sandwich may linger on your teeth all day, turning into sugars that might eat away at the enamel.

In fact, all skin-deep affairs discussed in this chapter—teeth or hair, skin or body—

depend as much on what you eat and drink as on whatever weight training machine you slip into or gloss-enhancing cosmetic you slap on. To really get a sense of your body and what shapes it, look away from the mirror and toward your refrigerator, the restaurant you lunch in, or the corner store in which you buy your daily doughnut. You may not yet know the way to your heart, but the way to your health—at least one important way—is through your stomach.

FURTHER READING

Anderson, Bob. (1997) *Stretching at Your Computer or Desk.* Bolinas, CA: Shelter Publications. Okay, it's a bit of a stretch to call this "reading," but this *is* the skin-deep chapter.

Atkins, Dawn. (1998) *Looking Queer: Body Image and Identity in Lesbian, Gay and Transgender Communities.* New York: Harrington Park Press. Essays by lesbians and gay men on body image and its dangers.

Caine, K. Winston, Perry Garfinkel, and the Editors of *Men's Health* Books. (1996) *The Male Body: An Owner's Manual.* Emmaus, PA: Rodale Press. One of several clearly written, clearly heterosexual guides to male physical health, including simple and useful workout and grooming tips.

Paris, Bob. (1993) *Flawless: The Ten-Week, Total-Image Method for Transforming Your Physique.* New York: Warner Books. A gay bodybuilder offers programs and insights on building up right.

Ulene, Art. (1996) *Really Fit Really Fast.* Encino, CA: HealthPOINTS. A *Today* show–style plan for fitness, complete with charts and checklists.

Weider, Joe. (1996) *Men's Fitness Magazine's Complete Guide to Health and Well-Being.* New York: HarperPerennial. Another of the clear and clearly straight male guide's to health.

Williams, Melvin H. (1998) *The Ergogenics Edge: Pushing the Limits of Sports Performance.* Champaign, IL: Human Kinetics. Information on most of the supplements, shakes, powders, and brews sold to enhance weight training.

CHAPTER 6

You Are What You Eat (and Drink and Smoke and Snort and Shoot)

Thoughts for Food • The Pyramid • Changing Your Orientation • Slimming Down • Bulking Up • Digestive Health • Vitamin Vitae • Smoking, Drinking, and Drugging • Thinking Through Using • Thinking Through Changing • Getting Help • Last Call: Helping a Friend

"When I was growing up, being gay was very connected to being a good cook, knowing something about food—entering a world of sophistication. Café society, all that kind of stuff. And when I moved to a big city in my early twenties, that was absolutely what I experienced.

There was a guy in New Haven we called Mr. Raspberry Chicken. He was a horrible cook, but he learned one recipe. And that was his pickup dish. From what I heard it worked pretty well. Whenever I would meet anyone who went home with him, they would say, "Yes, he cooked me his raspberry chicken."

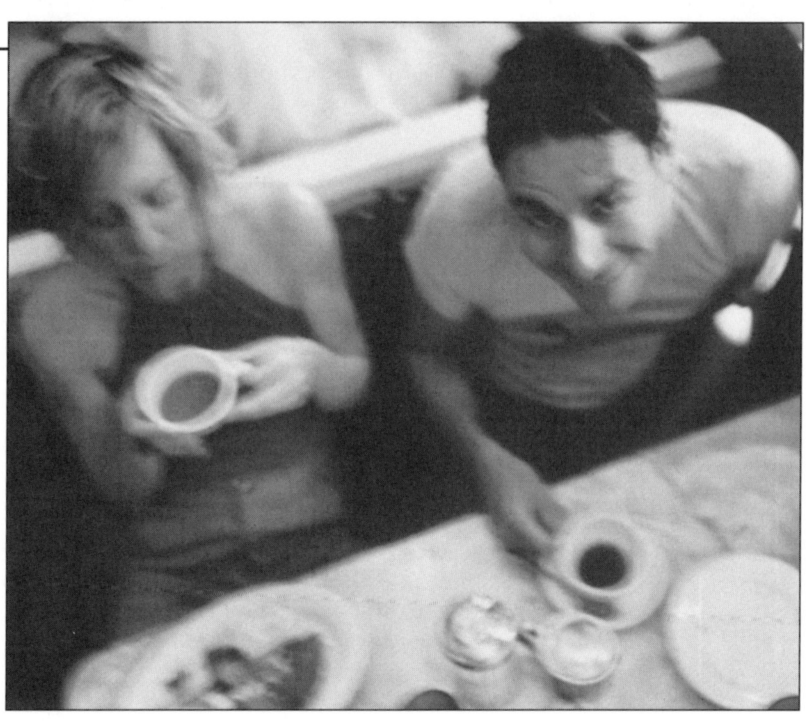

Gay men's rich and complicated relationship with food dates back as far as Plato's Symposium in ancient Greece, where for-men-only evenings of philosophical banter were lubricated by luscious meals and angel-faced boys. In the twentieth century, long before the first explicitly "gay restaurant," we gathered in cafeterias and Automats, or at homosexual homes where we ate, drank, and camped our way toward a world where we retold history instead of being hidden from it. You thought *Boys in the Band* was the last word on dinner parties? In small towns and rural areas across the country, the potluck is still the gay gathering of choice.

Today, gay men have our own dishes (quiche), our own meals (brunch), even our own grudges. Who can eat a Twinkie since San Francisco city supervisor Dan White, claiming one induced a bout of homicidal homophobia, murdered fellow supervisor Harvey Milk in 1978? Have you forgiven the ham sandwich rumored to have lodged in the throat of love goddess and gay icon Mama Cass, taking her from us forever? Behind many a gay gourmet's love of food and drink and our hatred of their long-term effects (why do they call them love handles, anyway, when no one loves them?) lie collective memories of gays gone by: a wasted Liberace claiming his thin face and gaunt body were the result of a "watermelon diet," or formerly wispy Truman Capote turning to fat and feeling compelled to confess: "I was kind of a Hershey Bar whore—there wasn't much I wouldn't do for a nickel's worth of chocolate." He, like many of us, didn't even bother to mention what he'd do for a drink.

Among the trim and proper set, not to mention the many cater-waiters and flight stewards and wine stewards and bartenders and chefs and hotel service staff who play on our team, gay men often claim we've got a deeper love for food, and a higher aesthetic. Science has yet to prove it definitively, but social marketers are sold. "Gay men were probably among the first to serve merlot when it became hot a couple of years ago," says Larry Chiagouris, Ph.D., managing director of the Manhattan-based trend-spotting firm CDB Research & Consulting. "These guys were among the first to eat the mesclun salads, most likely to abandon iceberg lettuce, and earliest to purchase organic. We believe in general that gay men are likely to be a little bit choosier."

No doubt. But beyond pride in our own good taste and some questionable stereotypes about fine dining and DINKS (double incomes, no kids), there is little that's unique about gay men and food. We savor it, revile it, abuse it, live on it and live *for* it, poach it and fry it, binge it and purge it—just like the rest of them. In the early days of AIDS, watching so many friends and lovers shrink to nothing, bulk often seemed like money in the bank, and our bodies still reflect that bias (see Chapter 5). Today, with what St. Luke's–Roosevelt hospital gastroenterologist Donald Kotler, MD, calls "a welcome decline in the grotesque wasting we used to see," lots of us may have to think more of eating well than of eating huge amounts. "Now we know that people who have HIV and no symptoms don't need any more calories than anyone else," says Fred Tripp, MS, RD, CDN, of the Department of Nutrition and Food Studies at New York University. "What they need is a nutritious, muscle-building diet."

THOUGHTS FOR FOOD

John was a glutton. It was one of the things I found studly about him. He would suck the meat off the bones and things like that. It was so manly. Nothing turns me off like an anorexic gay man whining about fat when he doesn't have any.

If I'm by myself, I can eat very simply and sparely, things that are healthy. Get me at an all-you-can-eat restaurant with friends and I'm a three- or four-dessert man. Of course, I know it's bad. I kind of like to be bad. I think my friends like me to be bad. Later, though, looking at my body, I also feel bad, which is less amusing.

Food is one of the great pleasures. Often during my day I think: "Where am I going to get that snack? What will it be? Where should we eat tonight?" Then, when I'm done with that delicious chocolate-covered macaroon that I've walked blocks to find, I'll think, "Oh, God! I can't wait to be hungry again."

Psychologize it into the call of the child, oral fixation, or the pleasure of the mother's breast, if you must. Eating is emotional. Though most of us can rattle off the things we "should" be eating, it's less easy to articulate the way that food and feelings go together, even for men who haven't missed a step on the food pyramid for years. "My mother's obese, and after two decades of really paying attention, I finally feel in the luxury zone of not worrying," says Bill, thirty-six. "My boyfriend, though, still won't eat anything but boneless, skinless chicken breast." The way your eating changes when you go out with friends, go home to visit family, or go from coupled to single or vice versa provides some clues to the ways that self-awareness is linked to a healthy diet. "Eating right, eating good, the whole thing's already so self-righteous," says Andrew, thirty-eight, a teacher in Rochester, New York, who lost a hundred pounds when he first moved away from his family to go to college. "I mean, please, of course it's important to eat right. But what about pleasure? What about feelings? What about the fact that German chocolate cake, Joni Mitchell, and Christian fellowship are the only things that got me through high school? Until I started dealing with what *that* was about, I couldn't deal with food."

Whether the feelings or the diet comes first is a question of—with apologies to the vegans—chicken and egg. The important thing is recognizing the connection. "People tend to talk about diet as an alternative or fringe approach to health, but what's the alternative to eating?" asks New York City nutritionist Maria Baldo, RD. Every day food affects your mood, your energy, and the effectiveness of drugs you take or the efforts you make. Plenty of us use food as consolation, curling up on the couch with a container of ice cream after a fruitless date, or shoring up our sense of control by sticking to Thinny Thin. But while the phrase "my therapist" trips easily off many a gay tongue (see Chapter 11), it's usually not until people get sick—"and usually with HIV or cancer or something else serious," says Baldo—that we consider talking to a nutritionist.

WHO YOU GONNA CALL? As with therapists, people who want to call themselves "nutrition counselors" or "diet counselors" can do so without special license or certification. If you do go for professional advice, think about what kind you're looking for. Although requirements vary by state, in most states the title "nutritionist" requires certification (CN), and usually a master's degree. Registered dietitians, or RDs, have gone through five years of schooling plus an internship. Some RDs, like their unlicensed and less conventionally schooled counterparts, may also specialize in alternative approaches, including vegan and macrobiotic diets, though that is by no means a given. If you're ill, proceed with extra caution and consult with a few people, including a doctor, before making drastic dietary changes.

The Pyramid

Ironically, the triangular shape of the food pyramid doesn't help most of us figure out what point it's coming to. "It's best to use the pyramid to determine goals, not rules, and to recognize that nutritional targets—including the amount of calories and fat you eat—are going to vary with your desired weight, level of physical activity, age, and health," says Professor Tripp.

Basic Building Blocks

To make a long series of questions short, here are a few building blocks:

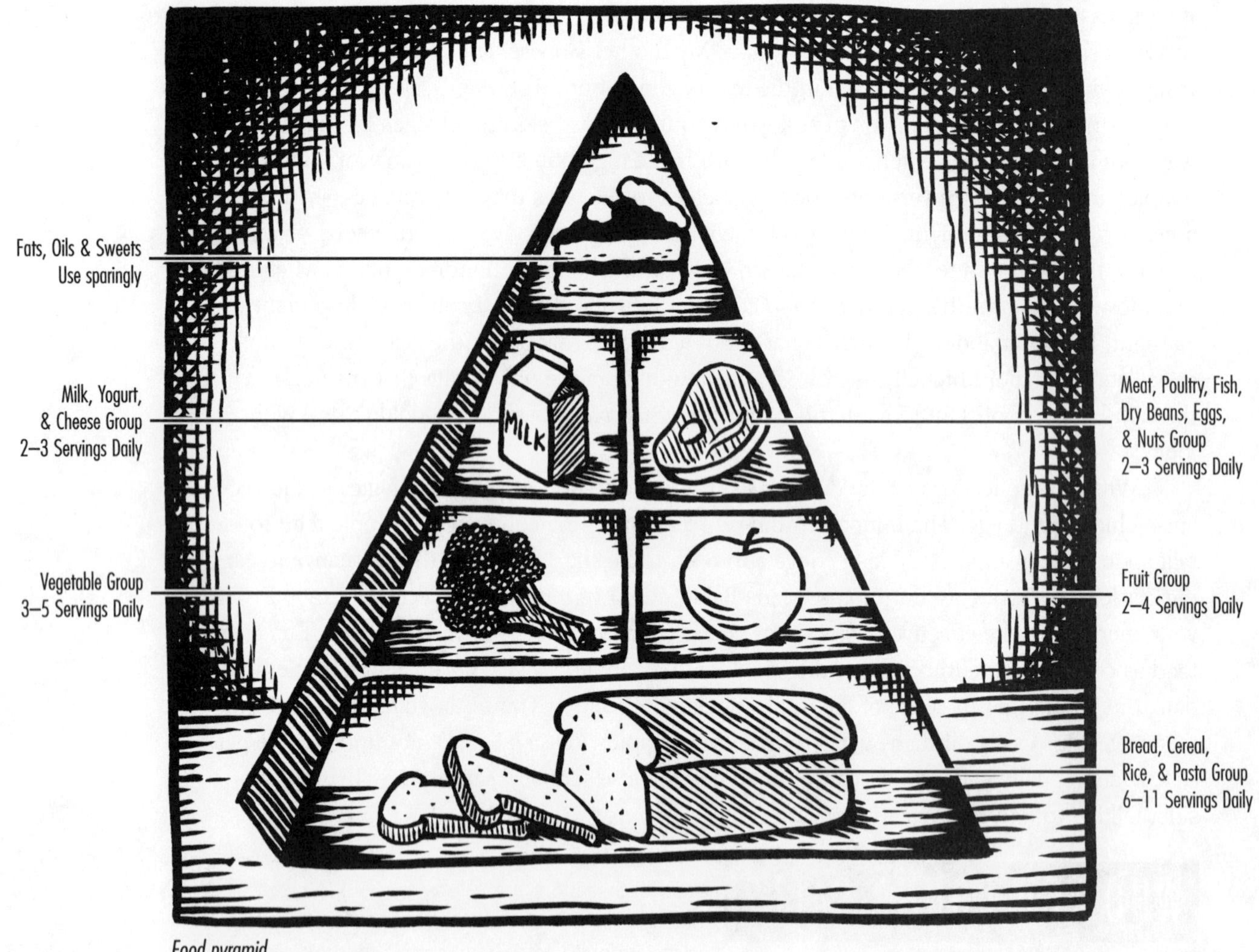
Fats, Oils & Sweets
Use sparingly
MILK
Milk, Yogurt,
& Cheese Group
2–3 Servings Daily
Meat, Poultry, Fish,
Dry Beans, Eggs,
& Nuts Group
2–3 Servings Daily
Vegetable Group
3–5 Servings Daily
Fruit Group
2–4 Servings Daily
Bread, Cereal,
Rice, & Pasta Group
6–11 Servings Daily

Food pyramid

WHOLE GRAINS, YES; WHITE FLOUR, NO

Breads, cereal, rice, and pasta are our major source of complex carbohydrates as well as vitamins, minerals, and fiber. Yet more than 60 percent of micronutrients are removed from flour and rice when it's processed, so go for whole grains: brown rice, brown bread, whole wheat pasta, and the like. These should amount to half your nutritional intake, which is why they take up the entire base of the pyramid.

SIZE DOES MATTER

When it comes to servings, you're looking for small. The reason the USDA recommends eleven servings of complex carbohydrates is that one dinner-size portion of pasta may count for two or three servings. A single serving of meat is about the size of "a deck of cards," says GMHC nutritionist Christine Hannema, MS, RD, while a big ol' steak may actually be three or four. Snack manufacturers understand: Their labels list fat per serving, rather than per package (see "Labels: Read 'Em and Eat," page 246). That package of Twizzlers you gulp down before the movie may really be three servings. The bag of potato chips you polish off during the Miss America pageant is five servings. You get the idea.

SIX TO NINE DAILY SERVINGS OF VEGETABLES AND FRUITS CAN BE DONE

Remember: a serving is small. Have lettuce and tomato on your sandwich and you might make a serving, says Hannema. A hefty helping of spinach with dinner could be three. As with breads and grains, fresh is better than processed, and darker is better when it comes to leafy greens. Spinach, collards, kale, and broccoli rabe are all especially rich in antioxidants and phytochemicals, substances believed to fight cancer, heart disease, and other ailments (see "Vitamin Vitae," page 258).

GO FISH

Most American men consume way too much protein for the body to use. On top of that, all but skinless poultry and lean cuts of meat are pretty fatty, and red meat has been linked to stomach cancer, colon cancer, and particularly nasty-smelling bowel movements. As long as you don't deep-fry it, even the fattiest fish, such as salmon or mackerel, is protein-rich and has less than a third of the total fat you would get in an equal-sized portion of rib-eye steak. Fatty fishes also contain omega-3 fatty acids, which may sound unhealthy but have been linked to a lower incidence of heart disease.

DON'T GOT MILK? DON'T WORRY

One of the recommended two to three servings from the dairy group means nothing more than a thin slice of cheese or a cup of yogurt. Try to have it be the lowest-fat version you can bear. If you're among the many who encounter gas, diarrhea, or other digestive problems from milk products, try lactose-reduced milk or over-the-counter tablets or drops taken with dairy products to help you digest them more easily.

OUT OF THE CLOSET AND INTO HIS PANTRY: PAUL RUDNICK'S BEAUTY TIPS

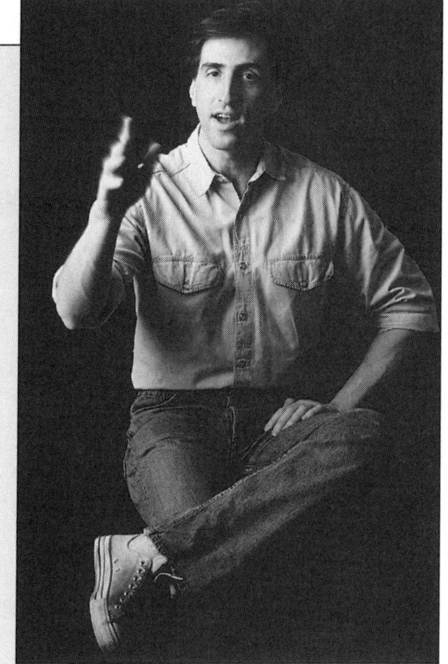

For the award-winning playwright (*Jeffrey*) and the alter ego behind Libby Gelman-Waxner, *Premiere* magazine's bitchiest film columnist, good eating boils down to a few easy-to-follow basics. "Avoid anything that does not contain processed sugar and lard," he instructs. "Make these your four food groups: Scooter Pies, candy corn, Raisinets, and any treat that comes in the classic, mini, and Double Stuf versions." Additional advice:

1. "Carrot cake is a contradiction in terms."
2. "Ignore all serving size directions. A double package of Mallomars feeds one person, especially at breakfast."
3. "Additives are always a bonus. Especially whatever chemical keeps those supermarket chocolate-chip cookies eternally moist 'n' chewy—it's like collagen for snacks."
4. "Pringles are my idea of progress: a food that stacks. Other marks of quality include hot-pink marshmallows, breakfast cereals shaped like the animated characters from *Anastasia,* and anything in the form of a bunny."
5. "An ideal buffet should duplicate the contents of a display case at a movie theater."
6. "White chocolate is not a dessert, it is a soap."

CHANGING YOUR ORIENTATION

Do you eat oysters?

—*Laurence Olivier, sounding out the young Tony Curtis on the subject of sexual orientation while being scrubbed down by him in the bathtub, in the 1960 film* Spartacus

The hardest part of mending your old eating ways is changing your self-image. After all, you eat a certain way because that's what you like. That's who you are! You're a person who eats barbecue ribs. Or four desserts. Or Slenderella plates.

No matter what constitutes your current diet, the biggest mistake you can make is to convince yourself that everything you're doing is wrong and must be changed at once. "That tends to make change seem impossible, and just becomes an excuse to continue what you're doing," says GMHC nutritionist Christine Hannema. If you're just starting to make changes, skip the calorie wheels and the special protein diets. You don't have to memorize long lists of antioxidants or food combinations. You don't have to be 100 percent wheat- or yeast- or fat-free, or eat nothing but brown rice and cabbage soup. Better, says Seattle nutritionist and herbalist Charles Rosenberg, CN, to start with a not-so-simple exercise: Eat when you're hungry, and don't eat when you're not. "Lots of us use food to deal with other needs such as relieving boredom, escaping stress, or suppressing sadness," he points out.

OUT OF THE CLOSET AND INTO HIS PANTRY: SEAN SASSER'S NUTRITIONAL HIGH FIVE

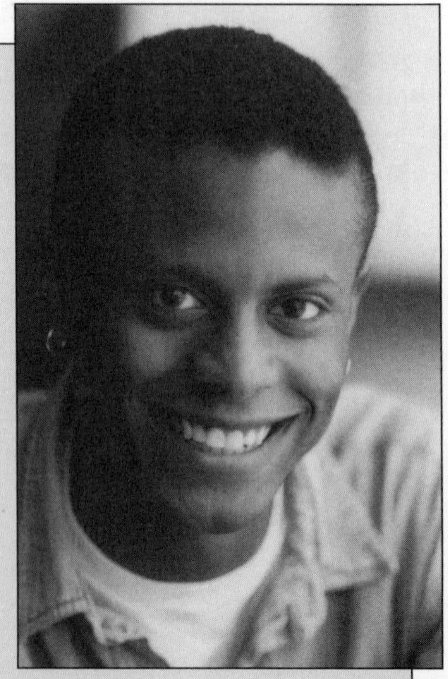

As Sean Sasser and Pedro Zamora dated their way through a variety of San Francisco restaurants, most MTV viewers were too taken by *The Real World*'s first gay romance to notice who was eating what. Pity. Sasser, a former culinary school student (and now adolescent HIV services program director for Health Initiatives for Youth in San Francisco), also knows how to put on a show in the kitchen.

1. ***Come out and play.*** "Outdoor farmer's markets are the best places to explore the food world, especially if there's an organic section with pungent, flavorful fruits and vegetables."
2. ***Veg out.*** "Always have fresh veggies on hand. I'm forever munching raw vegetables—I try to fill up on them—and I like them steamed or barely blanched."
3. ***Diversify your grain portfolio.*** "It's not just about pasta. There are all kinds of grains you can play around with: beans, barley, long-grain rice, couscous."
4. ***Meat and moderation.*** "Fruits, grains, and vegetables should take center stage. Try to view meat as the side dish. I eat out a good deal because you get a balanced meal: correct portions, and a vegetable and starch. On the other hand, for me to say to myself, 'No more red meat'—no way."
5. ***Sweet surrender.*** "Low-fat bonbons? Phooey. This concept of low-fat dessert only encourages people to eat more of it. Dessert is an indulgence, and I indulge—in moderation. I slip up, of course. I've had moments when a carton of Häagen-Dazs was all I needed for dinner. But you should be able to count those times on one hand. Per year."

As for changing what you do eat when you eat, here are six basic principles:

1. *Add, rather than subtract.* "So much of talk about eating is about deprivation," says Hannema. "I think it's much more useful to start by increasing the healthful things you're eating. Each time you have a meal, look down at your plate and ask yourself: Do you have a source of protein, a complex carbohydrate (like a grain or potato), and a fruit and/or vegetable? If not, make your next meal heavier on the missing food category to balance things out."

2. *Water.* "People are used to running around dehydrated," says Hannema. "Half the time, when you think you want something to eat, you're thirsty. Next time you feel hungry, drink a glass of water and wait five minutes. If you're still hungry, you're hungry." Average eight glasses a day, or even more if you're on heavy medication. If your CD4-cell count is under 200, you need to boil it first, or drink filtered water (see "Food Safety," page 255). The liquid in soup and the milk in your cereal both count toward your eight-glasses-a-day goal. Soda, coffee, tea, or anything else with caffeine, which makes you pee a lot, doesn't. Neither does alcohol.

3. *Fat ain't phat.* Small amounts of fat are necessary, but calories from fat should be limited to 25 percent to 30 percent of total intake at most, says Hannema. Some nutrition experts suggest closer to 20 percent; for those with special medical problems, such as heart attacks, best-selling author Dean Ornish, MD, recommends 10 percent. If you don't know how much fat is in your favorite food, check the label, which since 1990 has been required by the FDA to list grams of fat. Lots of products, and not just the healthy ones, even list calories from fat alongside the total calories on the label. What you're looking for is foods where one-third or less of the total calories are from fat. If it's not broken out, you can do the math (see "Labels: Read 'Em and Eat," next page), or just use your head. "Anything too creamy, saucy, or with skin, I won't touch," says Scott, thirty-six. If you do partake, ask yourself if you know what kind of fat you're having (see box on next page).

4. *You're sweet, sugar's not.* If you do succumb to the fat-free frenzy, says Hannema, don't free-fall into a sugary mess. "Lots of fat-free desserts and the like are loaded with sugar in an effort to make up for the taste lost when the fat source is removed. The end result is empty calories with no real nutritional value," she warns. Excessive sugar consumption may exacerbate fungal infections such as thrush or jock itch, worsen diarrhea, and perhaps even weaken your immunity. It will certainly add pounds—fat-free foods are now a major contributing factor to the caloric excess that keep Americans getting chunkier and chunkier.

5. *Haste makes waist.* Waiting until you're so hungry your knees are weak, or allotting fifteen minutes for lunch, are both recipes for bad food choices. You're not going to be bothered walking the extra block to the healthy place or making a salad when you need food *now*. So snack. The ideal is five or six small meals a day rather than three big ones, says Tripp, but at least make sure you always have something healthy with you in your bag or your cupboard to take the edge off. "I buy a piece of fruit every day and don't let myself put my key in the door to go back into the house until I've eaten it," says Tyrone, thirty-five. "Broccoli in the microwave gets jokes at work, but it makes me feel good. And if I know it's someone's birthday in the office and there's going to be cake, I make sure to pick up some grapes or something else before going in." Work your alternative-lifestyle muscles. "Who says you have to eat breakfast food for breakfast?" says Hannema. "A piece of pizza in the morning is more healthful than a doughnut."

6. *No matter where you are.* "Even fast-food places are attempting to offer more healthful

FAT CHANCE: WHICH ARE BETTER AND WHICH WORSE?

All fats are not created equal. *Saturated fats* (any animal fat that turns solid at room temperature, such as bacon grease, chicken fat, steak fat, or butter) are among the least healthful fats, raising levels of LDL ("lethal" cholesterol) in the blood and lowering HDL ("healthy" cholesterol). You already know what "sat fats" do to the pipes in your sink; they clog your arteries in somewhat the same way, except you can't clear *them* with Drano (for more on cholesterol, see page 295). And now, after years of suffering through margarine, studies of heart disease in 80,000 nurses have shown that *trans fats* may be the worst of all. These are often the fats that keep things such as candy bars, commercially produced cookies, or sticks of margarine firm at room temperature, and they're not broken out on any nutritional labels. If the words "partially hydrogenated" or "hydrogenated" appear on a label, you can be sure you've found trans fats, though you don't know in what quantity. Go for the margarines that are softest, or that have the highest levels of liquid oil rather than the hydrogenated stuff.

Unsaturated fats from vegetable and plant oils include mono- and polyunsaturated varieties; these are more neutral or even heart-healthy. Some polyunsaturated fats, such as corn, soybean, safflower, and sunflower oils, reduce total cholesterol, though levels of the helpful HDL may drop as well. Olive oil eaters rejoice: This oil, along with other monounsaturated fats such as peanut and canola oil, may actually boost helpful cholesterol.

Finally, there's the newest entry: the *nonfat fats,* such as olestra (Olean), which taste like fat but aren't absorbed like it. Olestra has "anal spotting" as one of its potential side effects, which does *not* mean a glimpse of killer butt in the steam room; rather, olestra has been known to cause severe cramping, diarrhea, and uncontrolled oozing. Even more seriously, fat-soluble vitamins and phytochemicals, including those helpful in preventing a range of illnesses (see "Antioxidants and You," page 259), may not be absorbed, or absorbed as well, when eaten at the same time or close to nonfat fats.

You want calories from fat to be ⅓ or less of the total. As you can see here, this naughty snack gets half its calories from fat.

Note that it's two servings, meaning all the percentages and counts are doubled if you eat the whole thing. Which you probably will.

Some labels just list this number, not total calories from fat. To figure out total calories, multiply fat grams by 9.

Uh-oh. Partially hydrogenated soybean oil: trans fat alert.

Peanut oil is a heart-healthy, monounsaturated oil

Nutrition Facts
Serving Size 1 oz (28g/about 12 chips)
Servings Per Container 2
Amount Per Serving
Calories 140 Calories from Fat 70
% Daily Value*
Total Fat 8g 12%
Saturated Fat 1.5g 8%
Cholesterol 0mg 0%
Sodium 330mg 14%
Total Carbohydrate 15g 5%
Dietary Fiber 1g 4%
Sugars 0g
Protein 2g
Vitamin A 0% • Vitamin C 6%
Calcium 0% • Iron 2%
* Percent Daily Values are based on a 2,000 calorie diet. Your daily values may be higher or lower depending on your calorie needs:

		Calories: 2,000	2,500
Total Fat	Less than	65g	80g
Sat Fat	Less than	20g	25g
Cholesterol	Less than	300mg	300mg
Sodium	Less than	2,400mg	2,400mg
Total Carbohydrate		300g	375g
Dietary Fiber		25g	30g

Calories per gram:
Fat 9 • Carbohydrate 4 • Protein 4

INGREDIENTS: POTATOES, PEANUT OIL, SEASONING (SEA SALT, CORN STARCH, SODIUM DIACETATE, DEXTROSE, SUGAR, MALIC ACID, SODIUM ACETATE, PARTIALLY HYDROGENATED SOYBEAN OIL, CITRIC ACID).

options," says Hannema. "Go for the roasted rather than fried." If dining usually means a stream of pumpkin ravioli and whipped-cream lattès carried to your table by cute boys with pierced eyebrows, you don't have to stay home and eat melon balls out of a lunch box. You do need to learn a few key phrases, including "Sauce on the side" and "Can you cook that without butter, please?" Order fewer french fries and more vegetables. Be demanding. Cute waiters are very attracted to men with special needs. Really.

Labels: Read 'Em and Eat

Since 1990, the FDA has required food manufacturers to spell out grams of fat per serving, and many a label lists how many calories of the total also come from fat. The label often tells other stories, too: what kind of fat (except trans fats), how much sugar, and the like. Ingredients are listed in order, so if sugar's number one, take heed. At left, a sample from a bag of potato chips bought in an American airport, and some tips on fat-a-matics.

OUT OF THE CLOSET AND INTO HIS PANTRY: TONY KUSHNER LEARNED FOUR THINGS ABOUT BEING SKINNY

In 1995 Pulitzer prize–winning playwright Tony Kushner, author of *Angels in America,* shed 110 pounds in tribute to the late John Candy. "He was three hundred pounds, and I was only forty away from him," he says. Okay, other reasons for the diet included Tony's own high cholesterol, wide silhouette, and empty dance card. Keeping the weight off has been a bigger challenge. His personal strategy:

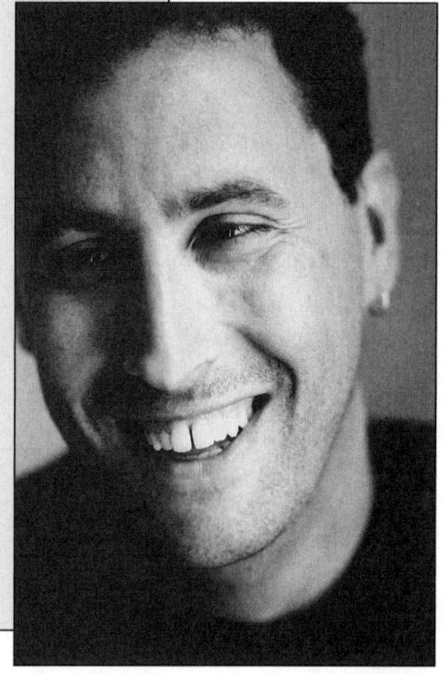

1. ***Eliminate oils.*** "I stopped eating all meat, chicken, and fish, which are high in fats and oils, and essentially became a vegetarian. Now I get my oils from soy products, although I do allow myself some parmesan cheese occasionally."
2. ***Don't give in when dining out.*** "Tell the kitchen to cook without oils and butter. Some are lovely about it; some are terrible. Eventually you'll learn which ones are the most accommodating."
3. ***Cross-country ski.*** "With my NordicTrack, I can listen to opera, follow along with the libretto, *and* get my endorphins going."
4. ***Mourn not the fried chicken.*** "I'll never be able to eat it again. But I'll never forget what it tastes like. Besides, watching someone else enjoy it has become almost as good as eating it myself. It's quite erotic in a way."

Slimming Down

I dote on myself, that there is that lot of me, and all so luscious.
—*Walt Whitman*

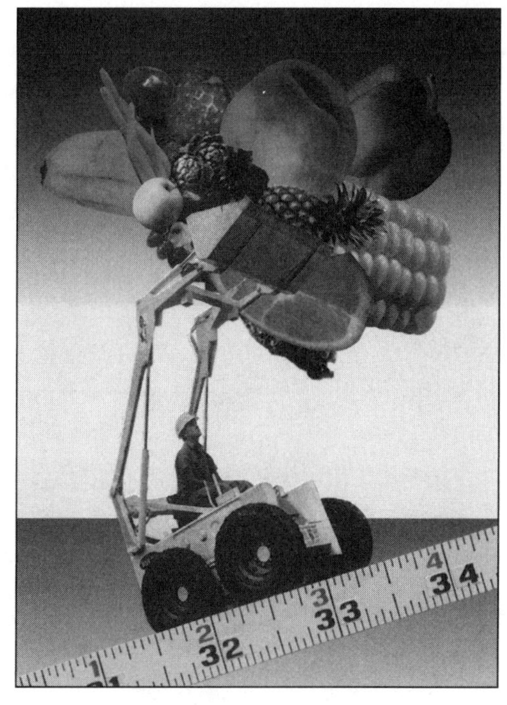

"For most people, the most effective weight loss formula comes down to four words: 'Eat less, move more,'" says Hannema. Instead, though, Americans jump through thousands of different kinds of diets in an effort to take off weight. With national spending upward of $32 billion a year to cope with excess pounds, dieting—Richard Simmons notwithstanding—seems to know no sexual orientation. It also knows little long-term success. "The vast majority of dieters who lose weight on radical diets gain it back," says Hannema, "because long-standing eating behaviors are not addressed." While weight loss is rarely permanent, some suspect the damage done to your body by constantly losing and regaining weight *can* be lasting. The National Association to Advance Fat Acceptance (whose agenda is obvious) cites data from the landmark Framingham heart study showing that the people who had severe weight swings actually lived less long than those who were con-

OUT OF THE CLOSET AND INTO HIS PANTRY: SEAN STRUB BUILDS UP HIS BODILY DEFENSES FIVE WAYS

"In the pre-AIDS world, Spam and Velveeta were my idea of a home-cooked meal," admits *POZ* magazine founder Sean Strub. But since his HIV diagnosis more than a decade ago, Sean has ditched that trashy diet in favor of comfort food and vitamins to boost his energy and immune system. His strategy:

1. ***Keep healthy snacks** (fruit, nuts, and so on)* ***everywhere.*** "I try to have them in a bowl in my office and bedroom. Hopefully, I'll eat that instead of something less nutritious."

2. ***Take antioxidants.*** "With all the medication we're putting in our bodies, anything that does some cleansing is useful."

3. ***Eat garlic.*** "It's amazing what it can do for gastrointestinal stuff."

4. ***Trim the Twinkies.*** "Every time I go to the supermarket, I look at my grocery cart before I get to the checkout and remove some of the processed food."

5. ***Post nutrition notes and tips.*** "Stick them on the refrigerator and medicine cabinet, so you're forced to see them every day."

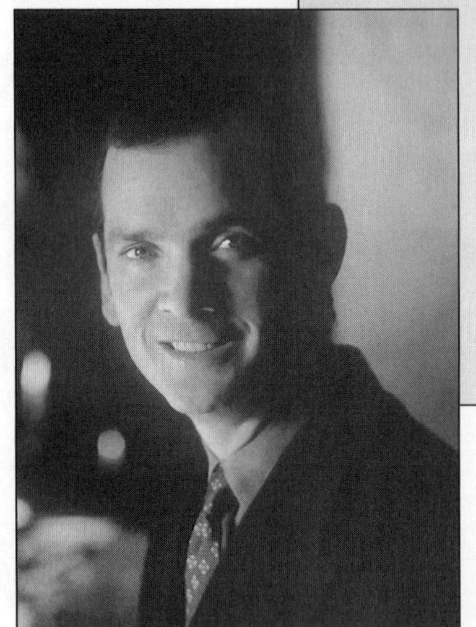

sistently overweight. "Other studies have refuted this," says Hannema, "but even without definitive data, it's pretty clear that the yo-yo syndrome—lose ten, gain fifteen, lose fifteen, gain twenty—is less desirable than long-term, sustainable changes to your diet."

Weighing your genetics is an important step in setting goals for weight loss, say dietitians. If both of your parents are obese (defined as 20 percent above recommended weight), you yourself have an 80 percent chance of being so. According to the National Institutes of Health, where your fat is on your body may also change risk to your health, with those of us who are "apple-shaped" (with bulging bellies) at greater risk for heart disease than the "pears" among us, with heavy hips or thunder thighs.

No matter what your genes, thinking solely in terms of failures and triumphs of the will is not the best approach to dieting. Nor is making your favorite foods off-limits. "No foods should be taboo," says Seattle nutritionist Charles Rosenberg MS, CN. "Restrictions lead to food binges." Instead, if ice cream is your weakness, allow yourself a spoonful now and again. Try one Hershey's Kiss instead of a whole Snickers bar. Work toward lowering the amount of fat in your diet, and get plenty of aerobic exercise (see Chapter 5). And never underestimate the power of reshaping your attitude.

Some Basic Principles for Dieting

ANY SUCCESSFUL WEIGHT-LOSS PROGRAM MUST BE SHAKEN AND STIRRED

A person can lose weight on almost any diet, healthy or unhealthy. But without exercise, nobody can keep it off. Establish a workout regimen that includes thirty minutes of heavy breathing at least three times weekly. Your heart and mind will both thank you for this.

IT'S A FAMILY AFFAIR: WHEN ONLY ONE OF YOU IS TRYING

Sometimes, especially for those of us in couples or families, one person's change for the better isn't always welcome. "All these aunts who had always gossiped about how I needed to lose weight were suddenly in the kitchen pushing food at me and telling me I was too skinny," remembers thirty-five-year-old Tyrone, who went from homeless, heavy, and alcoholic to slim and sober through AA and a low-fat, high-exercise regimen. In couples, or even close friendships, resistance may be more subtle, expressed in snide comments (as in "Would you like some more chicken, or does it fail the standards of the body fascists?"). "Change is threatening," explains Christine Hannema, "especially if you've both gained those extra pounds together. He might not be ready to change himself, so he gets scared and makes you feel guilty for trying." Or worse, he may start killing your effort with kindness, bringing home your old temptations from the grocery store. Sal, twenty-nine, a receptionist, recalls his lover's about-face. "He started saying, 'Honey, would you like some Häagen-Dazs? Have some cheesecake, sweetheart?' when three months before he would have glared at me for ordering it." Equally common, says Hannema, is that your boyfriend or family members are not even aware of what they're up to. "Talk to them," she says. "Explain that this change is important to you, and that you need their help." If it doesn't work, check out other means of support, such as those groups of coworkers you always sneered at who bring in healthy lunches and eat them together.

SAVOR THE FIRST BITE

"If I've really taken the time to enjoy the first bite or two of a dessert, I can push the rest away," says Dave, age forty-one. Stay conscious of ways to savor those first few mouthfuls. Don't eat while standing up or talking on the phone. "Half the time, we're not even paying attention to what we're eating until we snap back into why-did-I-have-this-or-that mode," says Rosenberg.

TAKE A MULTIVITAMIN DAILY

Those who are following a stringent weight-loss program may be missing out on key nutrients that food carries. Fred Tripp, of New York University, recommends adding a simple daily multivitamin covering the standard Recommended Daily Allowances. "Look for a pill with very low levels of iron," he says. "Men don't need extra iron unless we're anemic."

APPRECIATE OVER-THE-COUNTER DIET PILLS AND PRODUCTS FOR WHAT THEY ARE—AND AREN'T

There's herbal fen-phen, Slim-Fast, Trim Maxx, and dozens of others. The number of supposedly weight-reducing products in the supermarket is dizzying, and Americans are snapping them up and swallowing them down to the tune of over $1 billion a year. As for whether they work, Steve Heymsfield, MD, medical director of St. Luke's–Roosevelt Hospital's weight-control unit in New York City, says yes, but not necessarily in the ways you might expect. Most everybody who takes an over-the-counter diet pill will lose weight at least initially, says Dr. Heymsfield, because of the placebo effect—the belief that it's working. As for other kinds of diet approaches, they too will work if you follow them in the short run. "The problem in all cases," says Dr. Heymsfield, "is the long run, when both placebo and severely restrictive approaches

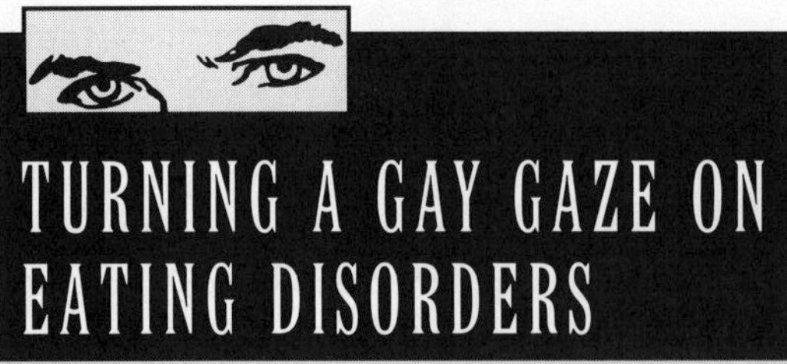

TURNING A GAY GAZE ON EATING DISORDERS

You hear stories in Overeaters Anonymous about the guy who pried the lock off his freezer and ate the frozen steak, or the one who finished seven gallons of ice cream in a sitting. My issues had less of the drama. I'd find myself sleepwalking to the peanut butter jar, or waking up early and eating half of a leftover cake. Nighttime meant a fistful of laxatives. When I finally stopped doing that, especially when I stopped eating sugar, I swear I had symptoms of withdrawal: crying, shaking, the whole thing.

I set out some candy for the neighborhood kids this past Halloween. And a little girl, I swear she must have been eight years old, looked at her treat and said to me, "Do you have anything nonfat?"

Are little girls the only ones who trade in visions of what they want to do for images of what they want to look like? Mention anorexia and the picture you think of is always of a female teenager wrestling with body and control issues, but an estimated 750,000 American men—about 10 percent of total cases—are also suffering from eating disorders. In fact, one of the first cases of the self-starvation and obsession with feeling fat known as anorexia nervosa was diagnosed in a man, says Arnold Andersen, MD, a professor of psychiatry at the University of Iowa College of Medicine and author of *Males with Eating Disorders* (Brunner/Mazel, 1990). In the intervening three centuries, however, Andersen says that theoretical narrow-mindedness (and the relative rarity of cases involving males) has almost squeezed the problem of male eating disorders out of the medical literature. The result is that many treatment centers decline to allow men into their programs, not that the problem has gone away. Men with eating disorders—including anorexia, binge eating, and bulimia, where those binges may be punctuated by vomiting to purge the food—often begin to face them in teenage years, but they can continue for years afterward. Related distortions, such as thinking you're too small and scrawny no matter how much you bulk up (see "Exercise Control?" on page 215) are other, more particularly male forms of body image disorder.

Do gay men, so often compared to women and so often mentioned for our bodily preoccupation, have higher rates of eating disorders than straight men? Many studies have suggested as much, or at least that gay men are more worried about our bodies and eating. ("And for good reason. Has anyone taken a good look at the state of men's bodies in middle—and I do mean *middle*—America lately?" snipes Spellman, thirty-two, from Atlanta.) Most studies, though, suffer from being done only in eating-disorder clinics, says Harvard psychiatrist Harrison Pope, MD, which may tell you as much about gay men's tendency to seek treatment for our ills than how common they are. Pope himself helped conduct a study of men from eight Boston-area colleges, one of the first to use a control group of men without eating disorders. The study did not find any higher rates of eating disorders among gay men, though we were more "worried" about our bodies.

If you find yourself hiding food or your eating habits from others, eating to the point of nausea, or using vomiting or laxatives to control weight, you probably can't bring that under control alone. Often, says Dr. Andersen, eating disorders need to be addressed on both physical and mental levels, since serious anorexia or bulimia can result in electrolyte imbalances, sharp testosterone reductions, dental and gastrointestinal problems due to repeated vomiting, and even death. Mental support—including counseling, examination of family dynamics, and twelve-step programs such as Overeaters Anonymous—are crucial. "I think I'll always have a problem with food," says Richard, who has waged a twenty-year battle with bulimia. "But I refuse to let this thing beat me. And for me, it's the day-to-day, Alcoholics Anonymous model, and a lot of counseling, that is helping keep me healthy."

MASS MOVEMENT? FAT, MUSCLE, AND THE MAGIC RATIO

Starving yourself may make you tip the scales at less, but it can also tip the vital balance between muscle—which you want—and fat, which you don't. Far more important than your weight, say nutrition and fitness experts, is lean body mass, the weight of your body minus the fat content. Average fat levels for men are around 13 percent to 17 percent, and well-conditioned athletes weigh in at more like 7 percent fat. The chart below offers a crude measure.

Measuring Your Body Mass Index

WEIGHT / HEIGHT	105	110	115	120	125	130	135	140	145	150	155	160	165	170	175	180	185	190	195	200	205	210	215	220	225	230	235	240	245	250	260
5'0"	20	21	21	22	23	24	25	26	27	28	29	30	31	32	33	34	35	36	37	38	39	40	41	42	43	44	45	46	47	48	49
5'1"	19	20	21	22	23	24	25	26	26	27	28	29	30	31	32	33	34	35	36	37	38	39	40	41	42	43	43	44	45	46	47
5'2"	18	19	20	21	22	23	24	25	26	27	27	28	29	30	31	32	33	34	35	36	37	37	38	39	40	41	42	43	44	45	46
5'3"	18	19	19	20	21	22	23	24	25	26	27	27	28	29	30	31	32	33	34	35	35	36	37	38	39	40	41	42	43	43	44
5'4"	17	18	19	20	21	21	22	23	24	25	26	27	27	28	29	30	31	32	33	33	34	35	36	37	38	39	39	40	41	42	43
5'5"	17	17	18	19	20	21	22	22	23	24	25	26	27	27	28	29	30	31	32	32	33	34	35	36	37	37	38	39	40	41	42
5'6"	16	17	18	19	19	20	21	22	23	23	24	25	26	27	27	28	29	30	31	31	32	33	34	35	36	36	37	38	39	40	40
5'7"	16	16	17	18	19	20	20	21	22	23	23	24	25	26	27	27	28	29	30	31	31	32	33	34	34	35	36	37	38	38	39
5'8"	15	16	17	17	18	19	20	21	21	22	23	24	24	25	26	27	27	28	29	30	30	31	32	33	33	34	35	36	36	37	38
5'9"	15	16	16	17	18	18	19	20	21	21	22	23	24	24	25	26	27	27	28	29	30	30	31	32	32	33	34	35	35	36	37
5'10"	14	15	16	17	17	18	19	19	20	21	22	22	23	24	24	25	26	27	27	28	29	29	30	31	32	32	33	34	34	35	36
5'11"	14	15	15	16	17	17	18	19	20	20	21	22	22	23	24	24	25	26	26	27	28	29	29	30	31	31	32	33	33	34	35
6'0"	14	14	15	16	16	17	18	18	19	20	20	21	22	22	23	24	24	25	26	26	27	28	28	29	30	31	31	32	33	33	34
6'1"	13	14	15	15	16	16	17	18	18	19	20	20	21	22	22	23	24	24	25	26	26	27	28	28	29	30	30	31	32	32	33
6'2"	13	13	14	15	15	16	17	17	18	19	19	20	21	21	22	22	23	24	24	25	26	26	27	28	28	29	30	30	31	31	32
6'3"	12	13	14	14	15	16	16	17	17	18	19	19	20	21	21	22	22	23	24	24	25	26	26	27	27	28	29	29	30	31	31
6'4"	12	13	13	14	15	15	16	16	17	18	18	19	19	20	21	21	22	23	23	24	24	25	26	26	27	27	28	29	29	30	30

Source: Shape Up America (www.shapeup.org)

If you're too short or tall for the table, figuring your BMI involves three "easy" steps:

1. Multiply weight (in pounds) by 703
2. Multiply height (in inches) by height (in inches)
3. Divide the answer in step 1 by the answer in step 2

While risk changes with other factors, a general rule of thumb for BMI says:

25–26 Low risk
27–29 Moderate risk
30–34 High risk
35–39 Very high risk
40+ Extremely high risk

How to measure the magic number more accurately? Since fat floats, and will displace less water than muscle, the most accurate measure is a special scale that uses submersion in water to see how much you weigh. A more common test is bioelectrical impedance, where they clip a little electrode to two points on your body, such as wrist and ankle, give you an imperceptible zap (fat conducts electricity less effectively than muscle), and get a reading. Your local pharmacy may also stock the home scale that does the same by using two points on your foot, or a much cheaper set of calipers, or plastic clips, that you use to gently grasp the skin at a few crucial points to see how much fat hangs there. It's a more sophisticated version of the wave test some of us use to check out the jiggle of that fleshy part under our biceps ("schoolmarm arm"), but you need to be trained on how to use the calipers to get an accurate reading.

Knowing your lean body mass is also crucial if you're HIV-positive, since it establishes a baseline reading to help detect and take action against potentially dangerous wasting syndrome. That can happen without any serious weight change, and the health consequences can be serious enough to include malnutrition, weakness, and worse (see "Wasting Away Again?" page 411).

OUT OF THE CLOSET AND INTO HIS PANTRY: JERRY HERMAN'S THREE-PART ARRANGEMENT FOR NUTRITIONAL HARMONY

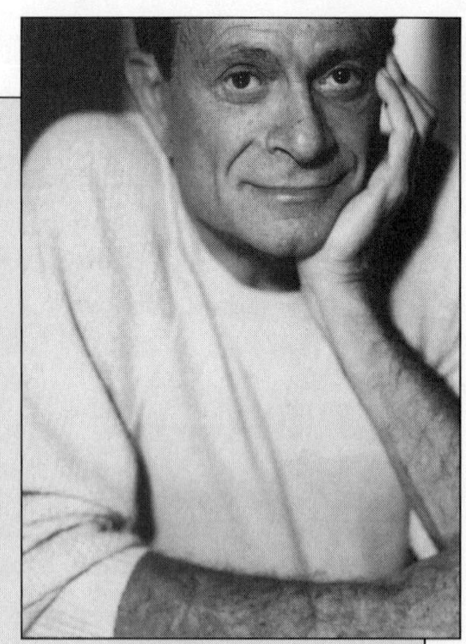

"I have always, since childhood, eaten a sensible and balanced diet," says Broadway composer Jerry Herman. Being HIV-positive and recovering from heart bypass surgery has the legendary author of classics like *Mame, Hello Dolly,* and *La Cage aux Folles* even more conscientious about eating well lately, although an occasional lapse into sin isn't unheard of. "I eat sensibly overall," says Herman, "but I'm a chocoholic."

1. ***Hello deli?*** "My doctor has this theory: Eat a varied diet, including plenty of fruits and vegetables, and my system can afford to go to a restaurant once in a while and just forget about nutrition. I have fish and chicken several times a week because I happen to like it, and enjoy eating a vegetable plate now and again."
2. ***Low-fat could be finer.*** "Since my surgery I've cut down on fats and stopped drinking whole milk. Entenmann's makes a low-fat chocolate cupcake that's absolutely delicious. I eat that cupcake with the same enjoyment as if it were the real thing. In fact, I have a few in my kitchen even as we speak."
3. ***I am what I eat.*** "I take multivitamins and vitamin E twice a day. I'm now past sixty-five and I feel marvelous!"

give way to the same old struggles." If you're using diet products as a bridge to more sustainable changes, that can work. Doug, thirty-three, from Fort Morgan, Colorado, lost twenty-five pounds on Slim-Fast. "I gave it a week, just like the ad said," he says, "and it changed my life." He was able to keep the weight off by paying careful attention to a long-range, nonliquid eating effort. He also cut back his consumption of alcohol—a staggering source of calories.

KEEP THINGS IN SCALE

Water weight in your body can fluctuate by as much as a few pounds every day. "If you don't have a scale," says Christine Hannema, "you don't necessarily have to go out and buy one. Most people are better off judging by the way pants pinch or shirts fit. The scale also won't tell you the type of weight you've lost: muscle, fat, or water. The question should not be how much you've taken off, but rather what." (See box on page 251.)

BE PATIENT

Rome wasn't built in a day. Neither were the Roman gladiators.

DON'T BE A BEAN COUNTER

Those old doctor's tables have been updated in recent years, with the ideal body weight adjusted slightly downward (see box on page 251). "While looking at those charts can be helpful, simple number crunching isn't," says Cade Fields-Gardner, MS, RD, a nutritionist with the Cutting

Edge, a company specializing in nutrition and HIV-related research, education, and patient care. "Large-scale studies have found that it's normal, and healthy, for body weight to fluctuate as much as 10 percent in a yearlong period, no matter what the ideal." If the only movement in your weight is an upward one, year after year, that may be a problem.

Bulking Up

If slimming down means fewer calories and more exercise, bulking up usually requires more of both, at least if you want to add helpful muscle rather than harmful fat to your slender frame. Again, it's about what you put on as well as how much, writes Bob Paris, who warns against the endless-red-meat-and-milkshakes approach to bigger bodies. "In the past, body builders were basically told to worship the god protein," the former Mr. Universe writes in *Beyond Built* (Warner Books, 1992). "We now know this isn't necessarily true. What happens is that the body utilizes the protein it needs for current tissue repair, but the calories that surround it are stored as fat." Endurance athletes need more protein, adds Hannema, "since they usually end up using some of it as a fuel source."

Hannema suggests that athletes and others trying to build up their bodies get between 60 and 65 percent of their calories from complex carbohydrates (that's nearly 20 percent more carbs than the average man takes in) and between 15 and 20 percent of calories from protein. Fats should be kept to no more than 25 percent of total calories. For competitive athletes, dieters with drastically reduced caloric intake, and those of us just beginning an intensive exercise program, protein requirements are slightly higher.

Many of the muscle-building rules also apply to those who are ill, or older, and hoping to bulk up or stave off loss of lean muscle mass, says Fred Tripp of New York University. HIV, though, often complicates the equation, changing the way the body metabolizes fats, inflaming the gut, and increasing lactose intolerance by removing the enzyme that helps break down dairy products. More than a quarter of people with HIV have shortages of certain essential fatty acids, have difficulty absorbing fat, and have diarrhea (see "On the Runs," page 256), and some experience sharp decreases in lean muscle mass (see "Wasting Away Again?" page 411). And while the adult Recommended Daily Allowance is an average 2,000 calories for a man, some nutritionists estimate that those with symptomatic HIV illness may need as many as 6,000 daily calories. Make eating a priority, keep quick and easy foods on hand, get into high-calorie (though not high-fat) ingredients, and drink juice instead of water. "I get really light-headed now if I don't eat," says Gary, forty, who says HIV has taught him the hard way about the need for increased calorie intake. "I didn't before I was infected." Practice the following sentence, useful for friends and coworkers alike: "I'll do that, but right now I need to go eat."

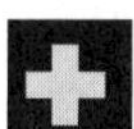

Eat 'Em Up: Appetite Enhancers

If chemotherapy, depression, medication side effects, or HIV are suppressing your appetite and dulling your taste buds, or if you're facing infections that speed up metabolism or slow down your ability to absorb nutrients, try a few appetite enhancers.

OUT OF THE CLOSET AND INTO HIS PANTRY: THE SIX SECRETS TO RUDY GALINDO'S DOUBLE LUTZ

"I try to have muscle tone and stay thin," says Rudy Galindo, the 1998 U.S. men's figure skating champion, in all earnestness. "You really have to be in order to make the jumps." (So *that's* his secret.)

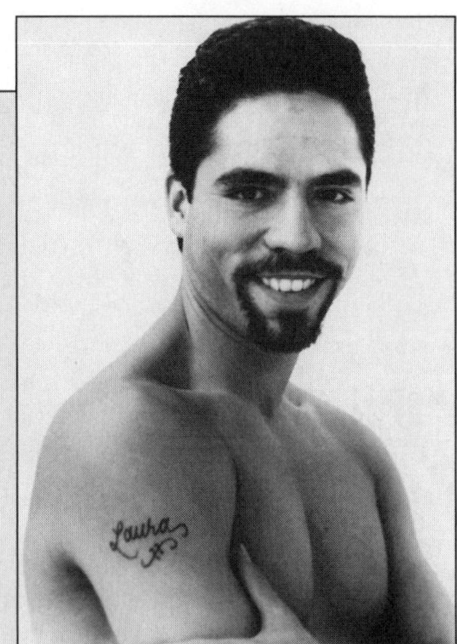

1. ***Be consistent.*** "I pretty much keep my diet the same when I'm on tour as at home: lots of sashimi—raw tuna in particular—fruits, and vegetables." (Raw fish is a no-no for HIV-positive men, though. See "Food Safety," next page.)
2. ***Eat a lot of protein but curb the carbs.*** "I like powder protein shakes, but I go easy on the rice and the pasta."
3. ***Plug-in appliances are our friends.*** "I bring my own blender on tour. That way I can always have a protein shake for breakfast."
4. ***Shun dessert.*** "People are constantly pushing dessert on me, and I'm like, 'No, thanks.' I like my candy, but hard sour candy—not chocolate."
5. ***Alcohol in moderation.*** "I might have a glass of wine with dinner. But *no way* am I going to go out and drink two bottles of wine after a performance."
6. ***Stay away from potato chips.*** "I try. But they're so good."

COMFORT FOODS

You know what yours are: macaroni and cheese, the skin off the top of the pudding, the rice on the bottom of the pan, the cake your mother used to make. Don't try to force them down when you're nauseated (throwing up or feeling sick may ruin the comfort effect forever), but take advantage of those warm memories.

SPICE IT UP

Adding a little more sugar, spice, or other things nice can help you taste things that have otherwise lost their flavor. Remember that sugar is empty calories, so use it as a help, not a way of life.

HEAVEN NOSE

The smell of baking bread, for example, can stimulate appetite.

MARIJUANA?

There's a pharmaceutical derivative, Marinol, that also soothes nausea and stimulates appetite, though men using it say it's hard to control the dosage. Smoking marijuana, for those who are comfortable operating against the law, has helped many. Washington, Oregon, Alaska, California, and Arizona have passed laws permitting marijuana use with a physician's supervision, and thirty-five other states enable some patients to use medical marijuana. They don't protect you from federal prosecution or help you get the marijuana, though buyer's clubs in many cities sell pot for no profit to people carrying letters from their doctors.

Digestive Health

Food Safety

With news reports about *E. coli*–carrying burgers, salmonella-prone poultry, and listeria-filled frankfurters, the rule about not leaving egg salad out in the sun for more than half an hour is starting to sound quaint. But it's still true, says nutritionist Fields-Gardner, and is one of a few essential rules of safe food handling that can avert an inconvenient, or tragic, case of food poisoning. Food, like sex or any other pleasure, always involves some risk, and even food safety experts will admit to sneaking a little sushi at a reputable restaurant or chancing an occasional oyster. If you're ill already, though, you may not want to take the chance. "It's not that the rules are so different for people with compromised immune systems, though there are a few special ones," says Frank Abdale, head of the food service program at GMHC. "It's that the stakes are higher if you do get sick."

"Meat preparation and failure to wash your hands are probably the two biggest sources of food poisoning," says New York City nutritionist Maria Baldo, RD. Minimizing risk of both means making the most of a few simple rules:

Wash your hands with hot, soapy water. Rinse the soap off before you cook, and wash your hands frequently as you're cooking.

Clean your cutting board thoroughly. Use soap and very hot water (or run the board through the dishwasher) after using it for raw meat, chicken, or fish of any sort. Or better yet, have one chopping board for meat, and another for other kinds of raw foods.

Defrost and marinate meat, chicken, and fish in the refrigerator. Leaving it out on the counter, or using the microwave, is not as safe. Cook all meat, chicken, and fish thoroughly; the less raw, the safer.

Keep hot foods hot and cold foods cold. Divide big batches of leftovers into smaller ones, and put them in the fridge right away rather than letting them cool on the counter.

When reheating soups or stews, let them boil for at least a minute. As with defrosting, microwave reheating may be faster, but not as safe.

Use your senses. If it smells bad, comes from a bloated can, or has sat in the backseat of the convertible since yesterday, don't eat it.

Check expiration dates. If it has an expiration date, there's a reason. Don't use food whose time has passed.

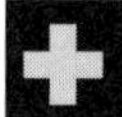 If you have HIV and a CD4-cell count under 200, a few extra rules apply:

Skip the salad and oyster bars. Abdale says it's safer to avoid all clams, mussels, and oysters (they carry hepatitis A) and salad bars with insufficiently hot or cold offerings (they breed the bacteria *Clostridium perfringens,* among others).

Well-done is a must. Don't eat runny or raw eggs (salmonella), raw fish (parasites of various varieties), rare meat (*E. coli* and toxoplasmosis), or underdone chicken (salmonella and campylobacter). Skip raw honey, unpasteurized milk and juices, or unprocessed peanut butter, too.

Drink filtered or boiled water. If your immune system is weak from AIDS or chemotherapy, tap water may not be for you. Some of it contains microscopic oocysts, or egg sacs, of the organism cryptosporidium, which can leave you with intense, profuse diarrhea (six to twenty-six times a day). It's safest to drink water that has been boiled for at least one minute or filtered through a filtration system that's labeled as meeting "NSF standard 53 for cyst reduction" or says it filters to 1 micron. (Brita filters do not do the trick.) Not all bottled waters, whether sparkling or flat, use a small-enough filter; call the toll-free number on the label and ask if their product is crypto-free. Bottled, pasteurized juice is fine, as are bottled teas. Iced tea and soda from a bar, luncheonette counter, or movie theater usually aren't (they're made with tap water). Neither freezers nor coffeemakers kill the crypto, so stay away from the iced cappuccinos and go for your drinks without ice. And don't torture yourself. "If you're sitting in the middle of a hot park and the only thing there is a water fountain, being dehydrated is probably more of a health risk than taking a drink," says New York City doctor Howard Grossman, MD. "And you're never going to shut out every drop of water on a lettuce leaf or in a glass at a restaurant. It's about risk reduction."

For information about the risk of crypto in your local water supply, contact the Environmental Protection Agency hot line at (800) 426-4791 or check their Web site: www.epa.gov/safewater/crypto.html.

Wash fresh fruits and greens well in filtered or boiled water. If you want to be really safe, you can soak them for five minutes or so in a solution of one capful of bleach in a bowl of filtered water (notice you must still use filtered water, since bleach does not kill cryptosporidium). If you can smell the bleach on your food, you've used too much. How does it taste? Not of bleach, if well rinsed. "The flavor evaporates after a few minutes," says Fields-Gardner. "Some people say the bleach actually kicks up the flavor of greens." But it won't do much for that new Moschino shirt.

On the Runs: Diarrhea

Indigestion and *malabsorption* are fancy words for when your food doesn't stay down, won't break down, or rushes out of your body via diarrhea. Too much of that for too long and you can get malnourished, losing weight and crucial nutrients. If you are suffering from chronic diarrhea, fatigue, vomiting, or sweating, you may also be suffering from severe dehydration, whose symptoms include dark hollows under your eyes and throbbing pains in your head.

If you're having more than three bowel movements a day for more than two days, get your ass to a doctor. Anything from stress to a host of different parasites to food poisoning can disrupt the gastrointestinal system. More than 25 percent of people with HIV experience severe diarrhea as the result of the virus or the medications used to treat it. In the meanwhile, here are some things you can do to stand firm.

REHYDRATE

If you're seriously dehydrated, supplement your water intake with electrolyte replacement drinks such as Pedialyte (made for children with the same problem), sports drinks like Gatorade, or diluted fruit juices or nectars. Nonfatty soups and broths, lactose-reduced milk, or, in a pinch, Kool-Aid (though it's sugary) can do. Drink liquid throughout the day, and less at mealtimes.

EAT DIFFERENTLY

If it's a short-term crisis, you can try a modified version of the BRAT diet: bananas, rice, applesauce, and toast. The rice and bread in this instance (unlike in most others) should be white. Caffeine and fibrous whole grains both speed passage of stools, which is not what you need when your bowels have turned to water. In the long run, though, says Cade Fields-Gardner, this pale diet will only make it harder for you to get to the point where you can tolerate regular food, and does little for you nutritionally. Instead, she suggests easily digestible, nutrient-rich foods already broken down by canning or cooking: skinless chicken and tuna in water; canned fruits or vegetables, and instant Cream of Wheat or oatmeal. Stay away from spicy foods (Tabasco, jalapeños), acidic foods (oranges, grapefruits, and the like), excessive amounts of fat (hard to digest), and sugar, which enters the intestine rather quickly, leading to further GI problems. If you have cramping, avoid gassy foods such as beans, cabbage, or broccoli. Eat many small meals, which are easier to digest, rather than a single big one.

LEARN FROM WHAT'S GOING DOWN

Looking at your stool can give you clues about how to help. Floating, greasy, and foul-smelling stools are often the result of failure to digest and absorb fat. Pieces of undigested food can be the result of irritable bowel syndrome, thought to be a stress-related condition, or functional bowel disease, which causes rapid movement of food particles through the intestine. Fat absorption problems can be helped by skipping butter and other fatty foods in favor of lower-fat choices. For severe fat malabsorption, MCT (medium-chain triglyceride) oils, such as coconut oil, may work better when fat can't be avoided, since they're easier for the body to absorb than standard fats. "Your pancreas is crucial to fat absorption," says Fields-Gardner, "and getting your doctor to prescribe pancreatic enzymes may help you digest and absorb things that are giving you trouble." Irritable bowel syndrome and functional bowel problems may be helped by avoiding gastric irritants such as caffeine and by taking soluble fiber (start with a teaspoon of psyllium a night, work up to full doses of two teaspoons one to three times daily, and read "The Fiber Factor," page 35). Acidophilus and thermophilus,"friendly" bacteria found in yogurt (or in a bottle in your health food store), may help with overall digestion. Any yogurt labeled as containing active cultures will do the trick.

INVESTIGATE THE DIAGNOSTIC AND TREATMENT OPTIONS

Stool tests and breath analysis can help detect the cause of ongoing diarrhea, while loperamide (Imodium) is a common prescription medication to slow the flow. Complementary medicine mavens swear by glutamine, an amino acid, usually taken in doses between twelve and forty grams a day. "It worked so much better than Imodium for me," says Michael, age thirty-five, who, like many men battling HIV-related wasting, adds his glutamine to three daily whey powder protein shakes. "Not only did it stop the runs, but I think it's helped to heal what seemed to be a chronic inflammation in my gut." Herbal remedies include teas of ginger root (also good for nausea), meadowsweet, and bayberry root bark. Diethylhomospermine (aka DEHOP, a drug still considered experimental as of this writing), is also getting good reviews.

GET THE (POOP) SCOOP

"My friends and I talk so much about our daily dumps that we joke that we should have a newsletter called the *Stool Pigeon,*" says Eric, who's twenty-five. "It's not too tasteful, but I now know where every public bathroom in the city is, have learned to carry an extra pair of underwear, know when it's something everybody's experiencing as opposed to just me, and know what kind of tests to ask my doctor for if I'm not making progress. I also know I'm not the only one whose liquid interior puts a damper on his sex life."

Vitamin Vitae

Doctors figured out centuries ago that certain foods—such as liver for night blindness, or oranges for scurvy—cured illness. It was not until 1913, however, that the first vitamin was discovered. The importance of focusing on food rather than vitamins is a lesson whose wisdom should be carried forward even into the pharmaceutical age, when researchers have isolated thirteen different vitamins and a range of minerals and trace elements essential to healthy function. "People come in with fifteen or twenty supplement bottles and say, 'Let's talk about this,'" says GMHC nutritionist Christine Hannema, MS, RD. "And I move them aside and say, 'First let's talk about what you're eating.'" While a daily multivitamin remains a basic recommendation, no pill adequately supplies phytochemicals, the hundreds of plant chemicals and compounds contained in a spinach salad or a bowl of fruit. Science has yet to fully understand the interactions and importance of these elements, though they often combine in ways that seem to give vitamins and minerals synergistic or complementary power. "Vitamin supplements," says Hannema, summarizing advice given by many nutritionists, "are just that—supplements—and are almost never substitutes for nutrient-dense foods."

How much to supplement is a thornier question, with some nutritionists and doctors proposing megadoses (from five to five thousand times the Recommended Daily Allowance) to enhance immune function or fight conditions ranging from cancer to the common cold. Use of vitamin supplements, in combination with or instead of certain medications, falls into the realm of complementary medicine (see Chapter 7), with conventional and alternative health care providers often divided about approaches and sharply defending their own. Self-education, and a refusal to swallow orthodoxy of all kinds, is probably the best medicine if you're just beginning to explore vitamin therapy. Whomever you decide to work with or get advice from, try to see if they can provide you with some written material and talk with the other people providing your primary care. Toxic overdoses are a possibility with fat-soluble vitamins (among them A, D, K, and even E), and other problems can arise when one hand doesn't know what the other is doing (again, see "Alternative and Complementary Medicine," in Chapter 7).

If you have HIV, get special advice, since deficiencies in B vitamins are common and certain minerals (such as zinc and selenium) have been associated both with slower progression to disease at relatively low levels and with serious side effects at higher ones. As with any pills or powders, your ability to absorb also determines your ideal dose: If you're constantly shitting or vomiting, or if you can't absorb fat, then that may affect the vitamins you take. It can also be a catch-22, since high doses of certain vitamins, including vitamin C, may themselves cause diarrhea. Proceed with caution before megadosing if you're ill, since the nutrients your body needs may also be nourishing your virus. More is not always better.

Antioxidants and You

Capturing free radicals sounds like something that went out with fondue in the seventies, but it's turning out to be crucial to health and recovery from everything from chemotherapy to sunburn or a hangover. Free radicals are highly damaging molecules that, lacking a particular electron, float around the body getting what they need from other molecules. In the process, they do harm to organs and tissues. During times of infection (such as HIV infection) or after a large infusion of chemicals, legal or illegal, into our bodies, levels of free radicals, and their damaging effects, sharply increase. Attacking cell membranes, they've been suspected in a score of micro- and macro-scale problems, including killing of CD4 cells; cancer in the stomach, esophagus, prostate, and colon; heart disease; inflammations; cataracts; wrinkled skin; and blue Mondays. "I don't recommend people take Ecstasy, since I've seen pretty compelling evidence of potentially irreversible brain damage, but if you're going to do it, I'd definitely recommend taking an antioxidant like vitamin E in hopes of reducing the adverse effects," says Ron Winchel, MD, a New York City psychopharmacologist and a former researcher at Columbia University. "You'd need to do it for several days before, as well as a few days after, to help offset the free-radical activity in the brain."

WHAT THEY ARE

Antioxidants are the vitamins, minerals, or enzymes that neutralize free radicals, giving them electrons and changing them into less harmful compounds. At the heart of many theories about megadosing of vitamins such as A, C, and E is the antioxidant effect these vitamins possess. Vitamin E, linked to a decrease in the risk of progression to AIDS, Alzheimer's disease, prostate cancer, and possibly heart disease, is a fat-soluble antioxidant, meaning it gets into places such as your liver and brain (yes, your brain is partly fat). Vitamin C, the most widely known and widely debated of antioxidants, has been found to reduce HIV activity in the test tube, and has been shown to be helpful (and in some studies, possibly harmful) for things from colds to cancers. Vitamin A and its less toxic relative beta-carotene (which is converted to vitamin A as needed) are both powerful antioxidants. Men with low levels of zinc have been found to progress more quickly to AIDS and die faster from prostate cancer; selenium deficiency has been associated with faster progression to AIDS and heart disease. With both of these elements, doses that are too high can cause serious side effects in people with weakened immune systems.

WHERE TO GET THEM

As with all vitamins and minerals, the more antioxidants that come from food, the better. Carrots and other orange and yellow foods—sweet potatoes, apricots, and cantaloupes, though not Chee-tos—are all good sources of beta-carotene, as are dark green leafy vegetables such as spinach and kale. Vitamin E is found in nuts, wheat germ, whole grains, and green leafy vegetables. Selenium and zinc are in brazil nuts and seafood, respectively, among other foods, but may be among the antioxidants found more readily in the health food store. Another of these is N-acetylcysteine (NAC), which helps raise levels of an antioxidant, glutathione, that helps protect the lymphatic system and stimulate immune response. When glutathione levels drop, as they do with heart disease, arthritis, diabetes, and AIDS, CD4 cells (see "Immune Basics," page 381) cannot function properly.

HOW MUCH TO TAKE

As with many vitamins and supplements, one of the complicating elements is that antioxidants work better together than they do apart. Selenium, for instance, is more effective when combined with vitamin E. Vitamin E is more effective when taken with vitamin C. Such interactions are one reason why nutritionists hope you turn to foods, not pills, for your antioxidants, since the combinations are still poorly understood. At the same time, though, Hannema admits, "something like vitamin E is difficult to get in your diet, especially if you're cutting back on the fats that are its primary source." Check with your doctor, or nutritionist, about possible doses.

SMOKING, DRINKING, AND DRUGGING

Tobacco

The cigarette is the perfect type of a perfect pleasure. It is exquisite and it leaves one unsatisfied. What more can one want?
—*Oscar Wilde*

All they that love not tobacco and boys are fools.
—*Christopher Marlowe*

It's probably a shared taste for dangerous living, rather than an English upbringing, that lent the writers Wilde and Marlowe their appreciation of the dubious charms of tobacco. As early as 1605 England's King James railed against the evils of smoking, calling it "a custom loathsome to the eye, hateful to the nose, harmful to the brain, dangerous to the lungs." James, also a homo, was ahead of his time. It took American leadership until the close of the twentieth century to be distressed enough about the connection between tobacco and ill health to begin to force tobacco companies to foot some of the bills. With the possible exceptions of the Dixie Chicks and fanny packs, smoking continues to be America's most widespread "bad habit," holding one-quarter of the U.S. population in its thrall and accounting for four hundred thousand premature deaths each year from illnesses such as heart disease and emphysema. Among the living, ills attributed to cigarette use include a weaker immune system, reduced lung capacity, faster degeneration of eyesight, hearing impairment, greater risk of memory loss, diabetes, clogged arteries, cancerous cells of various varieties, heart disease, depletion of good vitamins and minerals, introduction of harmful metals into the body, brown teeth, foul breath, $13 billion a year in Medicaid costs, and, of course, a growing social stigma. "The minute I see a guy light up in a bar, he's off the list," says Carey, a thirty-two-year-old New Orleans schoolteacher. "Nothing can kill a romance faster than that foul, smoky taste."

And yet, you probably know all that, even if you're among the quarter of Americans who—handling your cigarettes elegantly like the early Bette Davis or clutching them defiantly like Davis in decline—still smokes.

Understanding why people would spend thousands of dollars and hundreds of hours pursuing a habit that may cause them to lose a lung or their life puts one up against what gay wags such as Wilde and drug counselors everywhere have accepted as one of life's basic truths: What is best for you in the long term is rarely what is most pleasurable right now. And smoking does have indisputable pleasures, reducing anxiety, increasing alertness, and becoming associated in smokers' minds with powerful rewards (or "reinforcers") such as stress reduction, postprandial satisfaction, and, of course, postcoital contentment. "You could say it was a perfect drug," says Barbara Warren, Psy.D., director of mental health services at New York City's Lesbian and Gay Community Services Center and a former smoker herself. "If your body is wired and you smoke a cigarette, it will sedate you. If you're sluggish, it will excite you." Any smoker can tell you the hundred and one ways a cigarette can comfort when nothing else can. "It's so reassuring just to hold it," says Manuel, twenty-six, a bartender in Austin, Texas. "This sounds so pathetic, but cigarettes are my best friend."

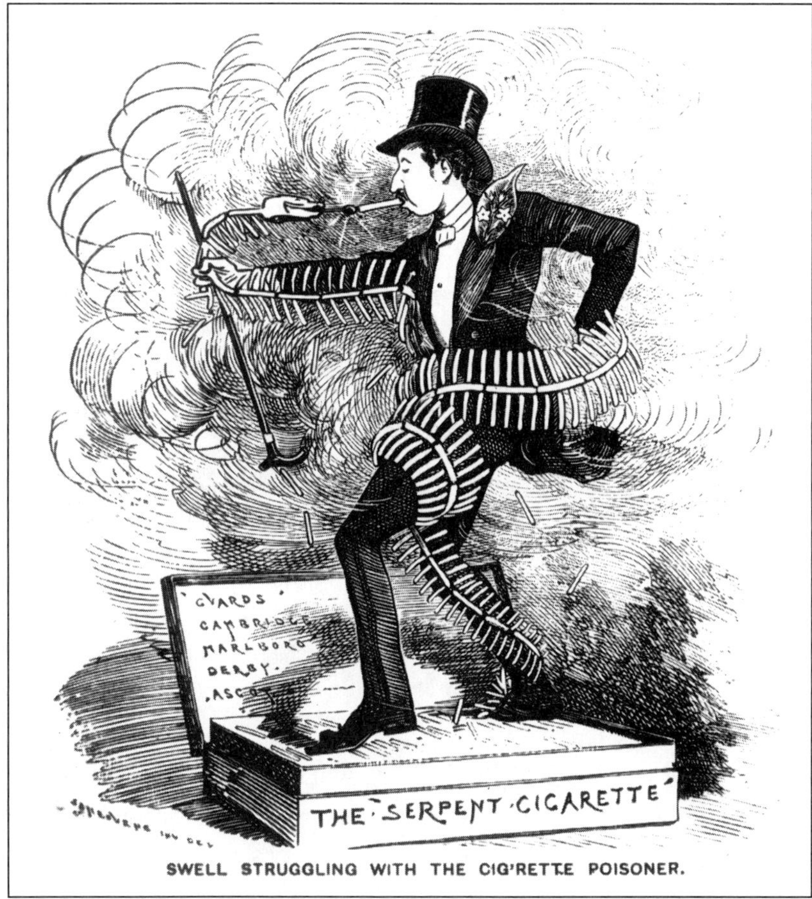

SWELL STRUGGLING WITH THE CIG'RETTE POISONER.

Gay men seem to be in greater need of that kind of company: An estimated 42 percent of us, compared to 28 percent of straight men, light up daily. Among gay men who didn't go to college, an estimated 70 percent smoke, compared to 42 percent of men overall at that educational level. Among gay teenagers, 52 percent are smokers, compared to 28 percent of those who say they're straight.

For all its appeal, the image of cigarettes as a friend in your pocket is probably most appropriate to describe the kind of "friend" who relieves you of your wallet in a crowded city bus. The "bad habit" of smoking has more in common with a heroin habit than it does, say, with interrupting others or an occasional overindulgence in chocolates. It's not simple pleasure that keeps people lighting up, but physiological addiction. While the high may not be as intense, nicotine is in fact more dependency-inducing than drugs such as heroin or cocaine, says Dr. Warren. Like many addictive drugs, the brain's response to nicotine is characterized both by tolerance, the need for more and more of it to satisfy a craving, and by a wicked decline in function of the brain's pleasure centers when you try to stop. "I've worked with a lot of drug rehab people," says Scott Thomas, Ph.D., former administrator of the Last Drag, a Bay Area gay and lesbian smoking cessation program, "and almost every single one says nicotine is one of the hardest drugs to quit." "Plus," says Dr. Warren, summarizing a concern articulated to her by a number of the gay men in her workshops, "you gain weight."

Giving cigarette smoking *its* weight is crucial if you're thinking about stopping. A first step is recognizing that you're more than attached to those little cancer sticks—you're addicted, which means all kinds of associations and dependencies of the physical and psychological kind. Popular contemporary treatments such as nicotine gum or a nicotine patch may reduce your craving, and the antidepressant bupropion (brand name Zyban or Wellbutrin) is now being prescribed to help smokers, including those who feel just fine, get off Tobacco Road. Still, Drs. Warren and Thomas caution against using these methods without other means of support. "If you don't do any work to get your head in the right place, it doesn't work," says Warren. Dr. Thomas thinks stopping smoking "is of the magnitude of ending any significant long-term relationship. You may have to grieve." (For more specifics on how to make it work, see "Can You Make Change?" page 275.)

"DADDY, PLEASE DON'T . . . ": THE STORY ON STOGIES

Whether you're a khaki-wearing daddy or a Gucci-clad guppie, you may well think a cigar clamped between your teeth gives you a special something. Style aside, it does: as much as forty times the nicotine as a cigarette, and the same risk of cancers of the mouth and esophagus. Even if you don't inhale, cigars may be addictive (nicotine, like those B_{12} supplements you should probably be taking if you smoke, gets in under your tongue), and chewing on an unlit stogie can still boost your chances of mouth and throat cancer and heart disease, not to mention brown teeth.

Havana or Ha-*bah*-na—if you think a cigar is the safe alternative to cigarettes, best call the whole thing off.

SMOKING, SEX, AND HIV?

A number of studies have shown that smokers are more likely to become infected with HIV. Though there is some very slender evidence that smoking destroys some of the cells lining the mouth and the throat, which could theoretically open the way for HIV's entry to the body, the research tells you more about the dangers of making easy cause-and-effect declarations based on research. It's probably not smoking that causes easier HIV transmission. It's probably that people who smoke are more likely to take risks in general.

As for whether smoking is especially bad for people with HIV, debate has smoldered for years. A 1993 study in London concluded that smokers with HIV got AIDS (and particularly AIDS-related pneumonia, PCP) faster than nonsmokers, while another study published that same year in Oslo found exactly the opposite. A number of studies have actually found smokers with HIV to be less likely than HIV-positive nonsmokers to develop infections, including the AIDS-related cancer Kaposi's sarcoma, and to be at no greater risk for AIDS-related pneumonia. Smoking in some studies has actually been observed to cause an elevation in the number of white blood cells of all kinds, including CD4 cells. Meanwhile, other studies have found that HIV-positive smokers were more likely to develop oral candidiasis (thrush), oral hairy leukoplakia, and bacterial pneumonia than their nonsmoking HIV-positive counterparts, and that they were at a higher risk for anogenital cancer and dementia.

In the age of "cocktail" therapies and related high cholesterol counts (see Chapter 9), smoking is likely to worsen potential heart problems. And if you are responding well to new HIV drugs, you will have to contend with the possibility of developing the lung cancer and emphysema that are not specifically related to HIV but are still among the deadly privileges of smoking and living into and beyond middle age. "Let's face it," offers Warren, "if you're HIV-positive, smoking is certainly as bad for you as it is if you're not, and that's pretty bad."

Drugs in Partyland

Absolut and tonics in Cincinnati. Long Island iced teas. Poppers in Provincetown, K in Key West, crystal in California, or blunts in Brooklyn. Gay men, like all people, are no strangers to using drugs when we get together to party. What that may mean for you if you choose to join in depends on a number of different factors. Some factors are biological: how much you weigh, how big a dose of the drug you took, how you took it, and how much difference there is with that particular drug between a dose that helps you feel good and a dose that makes you sick. Some are circumstantial: what other drugs (prescription or not) you're on, how much baby laxative may have been mixed into the powder you just paid $25 for, or even whom you're with and where. Some factors might be called psychobiological: in other words, how your mental and physical states combine. If you're in a bout of depression, for example, you're more likely to want to use cocaine. You're also more likely to feel as though the world is ending when you're coming down from a three-day binge.

Alcohol

Not for nothing is alcohol the most commonly used mind-altering substance. It works on the central nervous system in many wonderful ways, easing tension and dissolving inhibitions. Until they start putting Prozac in the water supply, liquor will probably remain the most popular self-medication for mood disorders of all kinds and degrees, whether that's a bad day at work, terminal shyness, or a serious inability to make sense of the world and how to be happy in it.

And now for the bad news: Just because alcohol's popular and legal doesn't mean it's safe. Like tobacco, alcohol (more than a drink a day, that is) can raise your risk of heart attack and worsen high blood pressure. Like tobacco, alcohol is addictive, and can leave you deeply depressed and physically ill when you stop using it. And like tobacco, alcohol's effects can be deadly, with more than a hundred thousand deaths a year attributed to its effects. Among the consequences of alcohol abuse are neurological disorders and mental illness, liver disease and cirrhosis, malnutrition, enlarged breasts, shrunken testicles, and slower response in everything from breathing to putting on the brakes as your car is hurtling toward a telephone pole.

ALCOHOL, SEX, AND HIV

People getting sober often talk about sex as one of the hardest things to do without a drink. "I don't think I ever had sex sober," says Ralph, forty-five. "It took the edge away, the nervousness." You may be among the many who find a drink or two—or five, or eight—a necessary part of foreplay, though whether you can tear the condom open carefully or put it on right after that, even if you want to, is doubtful. If you can't see straight, how are you going to fuck safe?

The effect of alcohol on the immune system of someone who's HIV-positive is unclear. In test-tube and animal studies, alcohol provokes a burst of HIV reproduction, speeds the growth of infectious agents such as *Mycobacterium avium* complex (MAC) and cryptosporidium, and depletes levels of zinc and vitamin E. Consumption of large amounts of alcohol damages the immune system generally, making us more susceptible to, and less resistant to, diseases such as tuberculosis and bacterial pneumonia. Too much alcohol increases the risk of pancreatitis, which can also be a side effect of didanosine, a.k.a. ddI (Videx), and strains the liver, which may already be struggling to process HIV-related (or other) medications.

TURNING A GAY GAZE ON DRINKING AND DRUGGING

Stonewall, you'll remember, was the name of a bar. That gay men spend a lot of our time in bars, drinking heavily, has been a staple of the research "literature" for most of the three decades since patrons of Manhattan's Stonewall Inn turned their bar stools on the cops, showered them with beer bottles, and made it clear, as the New York *Daily News* put it, that the "queen bees" were "stinging mad!" Whether stingers and Manhattans make you think of gay revolutionary spirits or just tall, slender glasses full of alcoholic ones depends on your perspective. The two may not be as separate as they seem: Drugs and alcohol have always been a social lubricant, greasing the way for people to do things—political and personal, wonderful and horrible—we don't dare do sober. A 1998 survey of young men between the ages of fourteen and nineteen, of all sexual orientations, found that 30 percent had had sex while drunk or high on something.

With high new numbers like that, old-fashioned estimates that gay men are three times more likely to be alcoholic than straight men leave a particularly bitter taste. Still, add a grain of salt. "Researchers have found it easiest to sample gay men in bars and clubs, where people are more likely to drink heavily," points out Ron Stall, Ph.D., of the Center for AIDS Prevention Studies in San Francisco. Other studies, such as one of 3,400 readers of a gay and lesbian newspaper in Chicago, found 23 percent of gay men (as compared to 12 percent of the "general population") reported alcohol problems. A household-based study conducted by Dr. Stall among about a thousand men in the San Francisco area found no significant difference between gay and straight men's overall drinking rates. Gay men were no more likely than straight men to be addicted to drugs, either, though we were more likely to combine them and to use a greater variety of substances.

For most straight men, though, the stakes may be a lot lower. Beyond the numbers game is the reality that, whether or not it *causes* unsafe sex or just loosens us up to go after the kind of sex we want in the first place, gay men's drinking and drugging is linked with HIV transmission in study after study after study. Having unprotected anal sex is still the way that most gay men get AIDS, and many gay men are high or drunk when it happens. "If it weren't for AIDS," says Dr. Stall, "substance use would almost certainly be a top-priority health issue for gay men. And there's no doubt that the two epidemics feed each other. We get drunk or high to deal with the pressures of HIV, and in the process bring these two epidemics closer."

Social forces certainly aren't doing much to change the patterns. Much as with other minority communities, for every ad for furniture or cars or community events in the gay media, there seem to be ten for liquor, cigarettes, and blowout parties. "Once I stopped drinking, I wasn't sure where to go to be gay," says Ralph, age forty-five, of Minneapolis, a longtime regular at his neighborhood bar. Chris, twenty-nine, a New York City stock trader, saw his whole social network turn to dust after he stopped using cocaine. "The tension of the trading floor was nothing compared to watching my social life collapse," he says. "My whole 'gay pride' was built around partying."

There are in drinking and drug use, as with all ways of reaching an altered state, incredible pleasures. "My best memories are of the four or five of us together, loose on four or five beers and a line of coke, just standing and swaying together," says Tom, thirty-two. Stephen, twenty-eight, describes his Ecstasy outings with friends as "the closest we get to church." But the fact remains that getting high may also mean getting close to getting HIV, or giving it to someone else. In addition to thinking about what a drug may do to your body, give some serious thought to what you want someone else to do or not do to it—and do that thinking before you smoke, sniff, snort, swallow, or shoot.

Another risk comes not from what you experience on drugs, but from what you don't. "I couldn't use drugs casually," says Bill, thirty-eight, from Pennsylvania. "And doing it seriously took up so much time. Something that was supposed to feel good got to be goddamned boring." If you're using drugs and alcohol often to transform reality, remember to ask yourself what else you may be missing. Time with someone you care about? A balance in your savings account? A needed dose of medication, or a promotion at work?

The Illegals: Coke, Crystal, Poppers, and the Rest of the Gang

In addition to knowing what bodily system a drug works on when determining its risk, there's another important system to consider: the legal system. Even if you're not afraid of arrest, illegal drugs are often coming out of somebody's homemade laboratory—meaning that there is no quality control over the different doses in each pill, potion, or bag of powder, no information about what kinds of mental or physical conditions are incompatible with them, and no way of knowing what else is in them and what that might be doing to your body. "I see all these people who are against Western medicine and pharmaceutical drugs who have no problem doing Special K or Ecstasy," says George Carter of Direct Alternative AIDS Information Resources (DAAIR), a New York City alternative-treatment buyer's club. "And I'm like, 'Hello? Where do you think these things come from? The Ecstasy tree?'" Actually, when researchers have taken Ecstasy off the street and into a lab for analysis, they have found that it came from just about everywhere. Among the things mixed in: caffeine, decongestant, baking soda, dog worming medicine, amphetamines, and MDA (a trippier, and possibly more toxic, relative).

Most drugs used today for recreation began as prescription medications. Once they're made illegal, though, it becomes difficult to get the licenses or the pure drug needed to test them for interactions with prescription medications, and pharmaceutical manufacturers are happy to skip the expense. What that means for you is the added risk, if you're on any medications, of serious side effects. A British gay man died when Ecstasy combined with his protease inhibitor, ritonavir, making two and half hits the equivalent of twenty-two. The impotence drug sildenafil (Viagra), by far the most common treatment for erectile dysfunction, causes potentially fatal drops in blood pressure if used with poppers. GHB mixed with alcohol or even an antihistamine may cause deadly suppression of your central nervous system. You won't find those warnings spelled out on a handy paper insert you get from your friend, liquor store, or drug dealer.

COKE AND CRYSTAL: THE BINGE DRUGS

Most of us have learned to accept that pleasurable things—lying on the beach, or eating chocolate cake, or having sex—have limits. While all party drugs create a sense of pleasure, not all of them are created equal. A few actually are much more powerful at rewiring your brain chemistry, making limits more difficult to accept and creating cravings for more pleasure. These are the binge drugs, the ones you can do for hours or days straight, and they deserve special mention and special caution. Among their features: a distinct tendency to make you feel panicked or paranoid if you use them a lot or go on a long "run," definite depression when you come down, and a special danger to anyone with heart, liver, or blood pressure problems. They also can make it difficult for you to come or get hard, turning would-be tops into inexperienced bottoms too wired to know, or maybe to care, if he's using a condom.

Coke, Blow, Crack (Cocaine)

When it comes to binge drugs, coke is definitely the real thing. Whether you shoot, smoke (crack is the crystallized, smokable version of cocaine), or snort it, coke acts quickly to raise levels of dopamine—a neurotransmitter described as the "pleasure chemical"—in the brain. The initial rush makes you feel alert, confident, and sexy. By the time an hour or two has passed, you're beginning to crash, and your dopamine-flooded cells are calling out for more.

How powerful is the urge to do more cocaine? Put it this way: A laboratory monkey in one of those boxes where it has to hit a lever to get a reward will hit the lever twelve thousand times to get a single dose. "Give it a choice, and a lab animal will keep hitting the lever and taking cocaine to the exclusion of all other things—food, sex, whatever—until it dies of a heart attack," says Justin Richardson, MD, director of Columbia University's Gay and Lesbian Mental Health Program in New York City. Humans, thankfully, rarely have unlimited access to coke, though we show similar persistence when given the chance. And since tolerance builds up, it soon takes more coke for you to get the same rush.

That's not to say that every line of coke leads to a maze of paranoia, bingeing, and craving. Dr. Richardson estimates that about 15 percent of people who use coke end up addicted. Everyone getting high on coke, by contrast, experiences a crash. A crash is like a hangover: Your body, flooded with dopamine, shuts down production of that chemical, and what began as intense pleasure turns into depression and anxiety. That can last for a few days. If you use cocaine a lot, your brain's method of operations changes, with cells requiring high levels of dopamine just for you to feel normal. Then when you stop using coke, you face not only the initial crash but withdrawal: a state of low energy, bad moods, lack of pleasure, and limited interest in what's around you. "Four months later, you may still be feeling depressed," says Dr. Richardson. Faced with that, most of us are no different than the monkey in the box—to counteract those bad feelings, we try to find the lever that will get us more cocaine, and more pleasure. Presto! Dependency.

Continue doing cocaine regularly enough and you'll probably experience some out-of-body side effects, like disturbances in your job or personal life. Medical problems can include feeling as though everyone's out to get you, seizures, heart attack, strokes, and even death. Snorting a lot of coke can cause damage or bleeding inside your nose, and smoking it often leads to burning your lips or mouth. Some reports say sharing a coke straw has led to transmission of hepatitis C (see page 158). Shooting coke comes with risk of abscesses, infections, hepatitis B, hepatitis C, and—if you don't use a new, clean needle—HIV. Both shooting and smoking get coke to the brain fast, within ten seconds, so the high is more intense—but so is the low. The crash begins sooner than if you snort, often within fifteen minutes.

COKE, SEX, AND HIV

Use coke for hours—or days—and you'll get more and more wired, and less able to know your own signals or read somebody else's. In other words, you may be less able to know when to go home alone rather than going for it with someone who won't use condoms. Coke can also make you feel mean or aggressive, or make it easy for you to think of yourself or someone else as just a dick or a hole, rather than a whole person.

If you have HIV already, using coke may lead to AIDS faster. At least one study has shown that cocaine speeds up production of HIV in some blood cells, though the study was in vitro (in the test tube) rather than in human bodies. As with all illegal drugs, what the coke is mixed with can be bad for your immune system. And again, little is known about coke's interaction with HIV medication.

Crystal, Chrissy, Crank, Meth (Methamphetamine)

Crystal is queen of the binge drugs (or is that the "binge drug of the queens"?). Cheaper than coke and longer-lasting, crystal makes people feel energetic, clear, creative, focused, and very horny. It's also highly craving-inducing: People often go on a "run" for three or four days. Like coke, crystal floods the brain with dopamine, causing a definite high followed by an equally definite and often devastating low when you crash. And as with coke, you build up a tolerance, so if you do it a lot, it soon takes more drug to get you high.

As with coke, getting "tweaked"—high on crystal—usually involves snorting, smoking, injection, or a dab on the tongue. No matter how you do it, doing crystal for a long time can lead to not eating enough, spending days without sleeping, and a bunch of possible medical complications, such as the feeling that people are out to get you, depression, hallucinations, stroke, and liver damage. Since the party has to end sometime, crystal can also come with other kinds of consequences, including major complications in your job, finances, or relationships, or the sense that these things aren't even yours. "If I didn't use crystal, I would probably say to myself, 'What am I doing here in this dark room with my ass in a sling and all these men having their arms up my butt? Why aren't I married to a nice man with two cats and living the suburbs?'" one participant told Kathy Reback, Ph.D., a researcher who did extensive interviews with twenty-five gay and bisexual crystal users in LA. "When I'm on crystal I don't think any of those thoughts. . . . I am concentrating on the fantasy of what's happening. This is not me; it's like I'm watching a movie, and I happen to be there."

What you get when you buy crystal often varies. Beware of bunk: a mix of crystal and baby laxative, Epsom salts, or other crap that you definitely don't want up your nose or in your bloodstream. Even with pure crystal, you may experience itching skin, dilated pupils, and diarrhea as well as a faster heart rate and higher blood pressure. Crystal is also processed by the liver, so the added strain may make other medications you are taking, including those for HIV, more difficult to tolerate.

SEX, CRYSTAL, AND HIV

On one hand, crystal users say it's a drug made for extreme sex. In Los Angeles, capital of the crystal kingdom, about half of the men interviewed by Dr. Reback were introduced to the drug through a sexual partner or lover, and all of them eventually used it for sex. It's like "being born . . . like every pore is coming," said one participant of a crystal orgasm, while others used descriptions like "whole-body orgasm" and "every nerve in your body standing at attention." On the other hand, men told nightmare stories: having a ball spreader surgically removed from their rectum three days after a crystal run, or breaking a hand while fisting someone at an orgy ("they moved, I didn't"). Many speed users talk of "crystal dick," a lack of erection or ability to come that makes many a top into a voracious bottom who goes for hours and hours. Which sounds great, but may in fact lead to really rough sex, or condomless sex, or not noticing if a condom is broken. "Some guys try to solve the teenie weenie problem by starting to screw with semisoft dicks, which means they dispense with a condom from the start," says Michael, thirty-nine, a New York City musician. Some guys don't notice that they've had so much oral sex that their mouth is torn or bleeding. A popular crystal story tells of a man who tried to get himself off by masturbating for thirty hours without stopping, not noticing that his dick was hanging in shreds. You get the picture.

While definitive studies have yet to be done, many researchers suspect that crystal suppresses your immune system. Also, whether you're doing crystal for three hours or three days, try to make sure ahead of time that you have condoms with you and are ready to use them. Though the numbers were small, Dr. Reback's Los Angeles interviews found that more than two-thirds of men using crystal sometimes or always had unprotected anal intercourse, and a number of other studies have found strong links between crystal and unprotected sex. Don't be among those who tweak today and freak tomorrow because they couldn't think about a condom.

Poppers (Rush, Butyl Nitrate, Amyl Nitrate)

Poppers get their name from the days when the drug came in small glass tubes, covered with fishnet, that made a popping noise when you broke them open and inhaled. Today—sold in record stores, clubs, and porn shops as "vinyl cleaner," "liquid incense," and "room deodorizer"—the drug comes in small bottles with screw-on caps. The liquid itself can burn your skin, but inhaling the fumes acts as a vasodilator, causing a sharp drop in blood pressure as your blood vessels open wider. Translation? Your heart races and blood rushes to your head, which suddenly feels as light and big as the room you're in. When that room is the bedroom, some people say, doing a hit of poppers makes their orgasms more intense and their assholes easier to open. You are less likely to feel pain while doing poppers, and probably less able to feel self-consciousness for the fifteen seconds to three minutes that the rush lasts.

SEX, POPPERS, AND HIV

In the early days of the epidemic, so many gay men used poppers that some scientists actually thought they caused AIDS. That's been disproved, though many studies have found that poppers are more strongly associated with unsafe anal sex and HIV infection than any other drug. Getting light-headed is one thing, but losing your head and your sense of whether it matters that he's wearing a condom is another. Also, poppers relax smooth muscle tissue (like your anus) and deaden your senses. That may make you unaware of soreness or tearing during sex that puts you at greater risk for HIV. If you're using Viagra (see page 170), poppers weaken your blood pressure so severely you may drop dead. Never combine the two.

Finally, at least one study has found that using poppers even once or twice a week can suppress or weaken your immune system for days afterward.

Thinking Through Using

At first I wasn't even sure I was going out, then when I got there my friends introduced me to this cute twenty-six-year-old DJ who danced with me for an hour. When he asked if I wanted to go home with him to party, I thought he meant sex, but he meant sex and crystal and K and more crystal and more sex. I got home sometime Sunday, tweaked, tired, but with a definite ache in my butthole and no memory of a condom.

I do coke because then I don't have to think. One line and I can talk to guys who'd never give me the time of day. It's like magic.

OTHER DRUGS IN PARTYLAND: A POCKET GUIDE

The pill, powder, or potion	The process	The major downsides	Harm reduction?	Don't use if you have these	✚
Acid, LSD (lysergic acid diethylamide)	Works on the serotonin system, causing powerful hallucinations and distorted, "trippy" sensory perceptions.	One man spent hours trapped by the side of the road by what he thought was a giant spider. You can go from a good to a bad trip in a matter of minutes, or by taking different hits of the same batch. A minority of frequent users get "flashbacks," short returns to the disoriented state, even when they're not tripping.	Don't mix with other drugs, do tell a friend what you're doing, and don't do more than one dose.	Any history or feelings of anxiety, depression, mania, or mood disorders.	Physical dangers of LSD are unknown, as are interactions with protease inhibitors or other AIDS drugs.
Blue Nitro, ReNewTrient, Gamma G (gamma butyrolactone)	Works on the GABA system, master control switch for all kinds of nervous system functions, causing an electric sense of touch, a hangover-free high, and deep sleep.	It was over-the-counter until January 1999. When combined with any alcohol, antihistamines, or many other drugs, it can send you over the top, causing seizures, vomiting, coma, or even death. Similar chemical effects to GHB, below.	Don't mix it with anything, particularly anything that depresses your central nervous system.	Any history of seizures, convulsions, slow heartbeat, low blood pressure, or alcohol in your system.	Unknown as yet.
Ecstasy, X, MDMA (methylenedioxy-methamphetamine)	Increases levels of serotonin, the same "mood chemical" that Prozac and LSD affect, causing intense empathy and openheartedness.	Slight nausea, teeth grinding, higher body temp, dehydration, and later, depleted serotonin, so you-who-were-so-happy-on-Saturday may turn into a bitchy monster on Monday. Also, long-term neurological changes, of unclear effect.	Drink two cups of water or sports drinks per hour, take frequent breaks, get some salt, and don't overheat.	High blood pressure, anxiety.	Potentially deadly when combined with some protease inhibitors.
GHB, Liquid X (gamma-hydroxy butyrate)	Another GABA-system drug. Causes an electric sense of touch, a hangover-free high, and a deep, restful sleep.	Also known as "grievous bodily harm," since when you take too much you fall into a coma or die.	Can be fatal if mixed with alcohol, or even allergy medications, which work on the central nervous system. Start with a tiny amount, don't eat, and wait half an hour.	Any history of seizures, convulsions, slowed heartbeat, low blood pressure, or alcohol in your system.	Unknown.

The pill, powder, or potion	The process	The major downsides	Harm reduction?	Don't use if you have these	✚
Heroin, dope, smack (opiates)	Depresses the central nervous system, dilating blood vessels to make you feel warm, drowsy, and liquid inside.	Short term: itching, nodding out, nausea, constipation, vomiting. Long term: physical addiction, and moderate to severe flulike sickness if you stop. Infections related to injection and impurities in the dope are also common.	Snort rather than smoke or shoot. If you're shooting, always use clean needles and works. If someone you're with gets shallow breathing and cold skin after using, they may have overdosed. Get them on their right side with left knee bent, and call an ambulance.	Liver problems, heart problems.	Heroin itself is less harmful than the impurities it's cut with. Injection brings risks of infection, and liver damage, abscesses, and other problems. Protease inhibitors may also inhibit the high.
K, Special K, ketamine	Also affects the GABA system, causing you to feel as though your body is totally separate from your mind.	Take too much and you're in a "K hole," a state of near paralysis where you can't see, hear, or figure out what's happening too clearly.	Don't combine with alcohol, and wait at least an hour before doing another bump. In case of K hole, tell a friend and wait it out. If you can't breathe, forget what day it is, or start to lose consciousness, get to the hospital.	A history of paranoia, anxiety, mania, or mood disorders.	Protease inhibitors may ramp up dose, increasing intensity and severity of effect.
Pot, marijuana, weed, grass, reefer *(Cannabis sativa)*	Relaxes and intoxicates, causing talkativeness, laughter, hunger, and (in greater amounts) distorted sense of time and sensory perceptions.	Anxiety, paranoia, and (with frequent use) loss of energy, lack of concentration, and psychological dependence. Also, since it's inhaled deeply and contains more than 350 chemical compounds, it increases risk of bronchitis, heart disease, and lung cancer.	Try smoking rather than swallowing, since doses you eat are harder to regulate. And stay away from those fatty snacks when you have the munchies.	Existing or underlying mental illness, lung or heart problems.	Pot relieves nausea and stimulates appetite in people on chemotherapy. Smoking marijuana may put you at increased risk for aspergillosis, a fungal infection dangerous to people with late-stage HIV illness.
	For info on cocaine, crystal, and poppers, see pages 265–268.				

THE CAGE GAUGE

What unwinds one man can completely unravel another. Though there are a lot of different tests to determine if you have a problem with drugs or alcohol, GMHC's Substance Use Counseling and Education program often starts with the CAGE gauge to help gay men at least think about whether they may have some issues around drug or alcohol use.

***C** is for cutting down.* As in, have you tried to at some point? If your drinking or drugging wasn't an issue, you probably wouldn't have made a conscious effort to reduce.

***A** is for annoyed.* When people comment or confront you about your drug or alcohol use, do you feel irritated?

***G** is for guilty.* Do you feel guilty about something you've done, or haven't done, as the result of drug or alcohol use? Do you feel that way a lot?

***E** is for eye opener.* Do you need a little of whatever the drug in question is to "get going," whether that's in the morning before work or in the evening before meeting friends?

Magic has tricks to it. So does getting beyond the illusion that drugs do nothing but make you feel good, and figuring out what drug use really means for you and what it may cost you. You can think through the buzz. Seemingly unimportant decisions may lead to really important ones, particularly if they're about going home with someone when you're high, or mixing drugs without knowing the risks, or ending up with HIV.

Thinking Through the Buzz

I'm very conscious of what my body needs: herbs, vitamins, homeopathy, all these kinds of things. And my mom, she asked me one time, "Why is it that you're a vegetarian, yet you do drugs?" I said, "Mom, that's why I'm a vegetarian." You know, 'cause if I'm going to do things like that I need to take extra care of my body.

Justin, thirty-seven, a Los Angeles man interviewed in Dr. Reback's study of crystal users (see "Crystal," page 267), offered the quote above, but the idea is familiar to anyone who likes drugs and also wants to keep control of his life. Even if you have no intention of quitting or are in that I-will-but-not-right-now place, it may still be healthy for you to make some changes. "Get very clear about your decisions," suggests Bill, who used heroin for five years, took two to quit, but never got HIV or lost his job. "The myth is that you have no choices. The trick is to stop and think about how many you're making."

Twelve Things to Think About if You're Going to Use Drugs or Alcohol

1. *What goes up must come down.* Before doing any drug, give some serious attention to how you're going to feel afterward as well as when you're high. The satisfaction of the cigarette in your hand and the coughing up of phlegm in the morning, the "Xstatic" dance with friends and the depression that follows, the pleasant buzz of the first Bloody Mary and the late-to-work Monday that follows the tenth one: All of these are part of the "drug experience."

2. *Know your own mind.* Really consider that what works for others may not work for you. If you've had anxiety attacks or been depressed, a drug such as K may seriously upset or disorient you. If you're prone to paranoia, crystal may play into your fears. If you feel depressed now, you're really going to be bad coming down from coke. And so on.

3. *Take a body check.* Look yourself over, all over (including inside your mouth), before you start the party. Any cuts or sores that could let in HIV or other sexually transmitted diseases will be harder to feel once you're wasted.

4. *Avoid mixing your medicines.* Mixing drugs is self-prescription, with lots of complicated cross reactions and unknowns. It's much safer not to mix. If you're on prescription medications, don't take any party drug, including alcohol, without a doctor's advice (yes, your doctor can tell you about what the effects might be of taking a little less-than-legal medicine).

5. *Think twice before the second round.* Have you really waited long enough to know how high you're going to feel from the first one?

6. *Avoid shooting and smoking.* Except in the case of poppers and marijuana, swallowing drugs is usually the safest, since it lets them work their way into your system gradually. Snorting is riskier, and shooting or smoking drugs rushes them to the brain, which can make them more addictive and put you at greater risk of overdose (not to mention HIV, hepatitis, and other complications of needle use).

7. *Treat yourself right.* Think about how you act toward others, or how you let others treat you, when you're high. Do you even know? Do you have a friend or lover who can tell you honestly?

8. *Consider another way.* How do you hope to feel on the drug? Are there any other times or ways you can get that feeling without getting high? Pursue those with the same focus it takes to find drugs.

9. *Stay flexible.* Leave yourself the option of staying home or of doing the party without doing the drugs if it doesn't feel right. Real friends will understand.

10. *Missing something?* If you're on HIV medications, especially protease inhibitors, you're not likely to stay on schedule if you're tripping for eight hours or sleeping off eight Bud Lights. Missing doses makes the virus stronger.

11. *Remember HIV.* Doing drugs can bring down barriers. Plan ahead, and don't let a latex barrier—a condom that can save your life or someone else's—get lost in the process.

12. *Don't be afraid to ask for help.* If you're in trouble while you're drunk or high, find a friend or a friendly face. If you have questions about the ways you are combining drugs, alcohol, and sex, you can make changes. You don't need to be an alcoholic or a drug or sex addict to get the information you need. By talking about the things you're doing, what they mean to you, and what they may cost you, it is possible to make partying—and sex—safer.

Thinking Through Changing

"Do you smoke?" and "Do you drink?" are not necessarily yes-or-no questions. In recent years, addicts of all kinds, and the professionals who work with them, have been recognizing that behavior change is more complicated than an on-off switch that rests in one position or another. Whereas most of us, and many treatment models, look at the endpoints—"Do you or don't you?"—another approach, pioneered by the psychologists Carlo DiClemente, Ph.D., and James Prochaska, Ph.D., recognizes that there are a lot of steps between abstinence and indulgence. Times when we "spiral" backward, known as slips and relapses in conventional addiction treatment, are not actually failures but opportunities to reconsider our strategies before we move forward again. Similarly, stopping isn't the end of the process, as DiClemente and Prochaska see it, since maintenance of that decision is one of the crucial steps that often gets ignored.

SAFER INJECTION

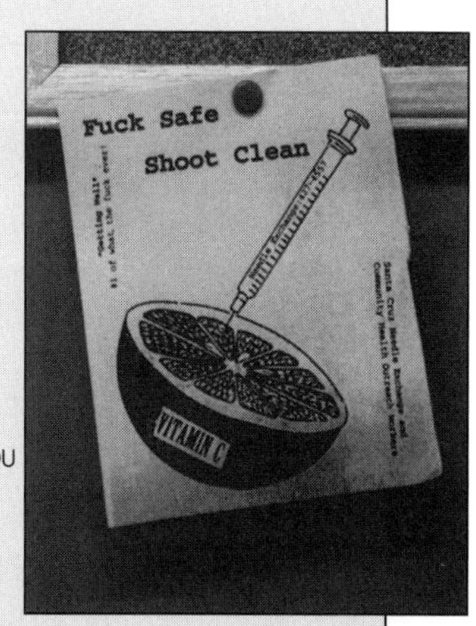

Two guys are sitting together, and the first shoots up and passes the needle to the second one. "Isn't it dangerous to share?" the second guy asks. "It's all right," says the first one. "I'm wearing a condom."
—Old gay joke, circa 1988

If you shoot drugs, getting clean, sterile needles from a local needle exchange program is the only way to be sure you won't get HIV from injecting. Sharing cookers, cotton, or works can place you at risk. If you can't get clean needles, then clean your hands and injection point with soap and water, don't lay your needle down on a dirty table or newspaper, and bleach your works. While this won't totally protect you from HIV or hepatitis B or C, it can cut down on the risk.

A word on bleach—it only works to kill HIV if you leave it in for a full two minutes, which is a long time when you're dope sick. One study showed that people cleaning their works tended to leave bleach in for only eighteen seconds on average between shooting. Go slow. It may set your teeth on edge, but it could save your life.

To remember the details of how to clean works, think 3-2-3, and see the illustrations below.

SAFER INJECTION: HOW TO CLEAN A NEEDLE

STEP 1: WATER (DO THIS THREE TIMES)

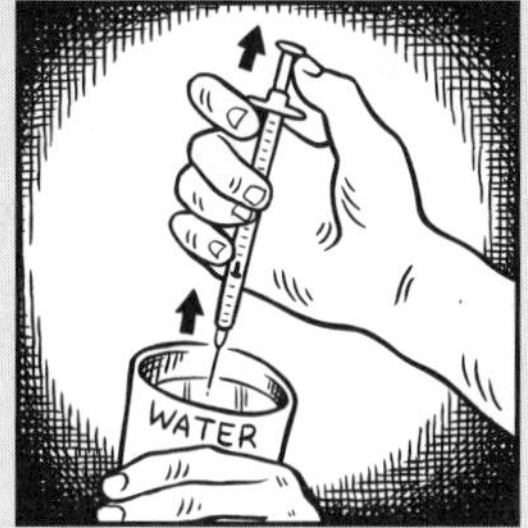

Draw clean water up into the needle, all the way up to the plunger.

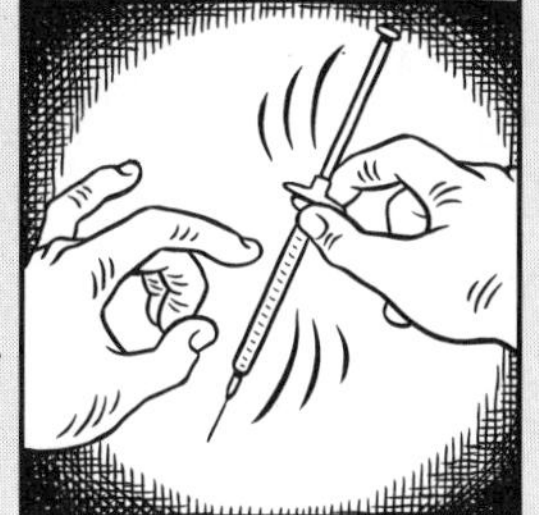

Shake or tap the syringe to loosen any dried blood, and let the water sit for a minute or so.

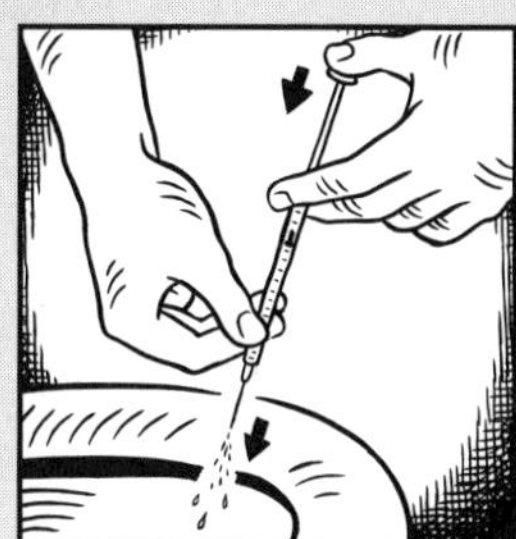

Squirt water out.

STEP 2: BLEACH (DO THIS TWO TIMES)

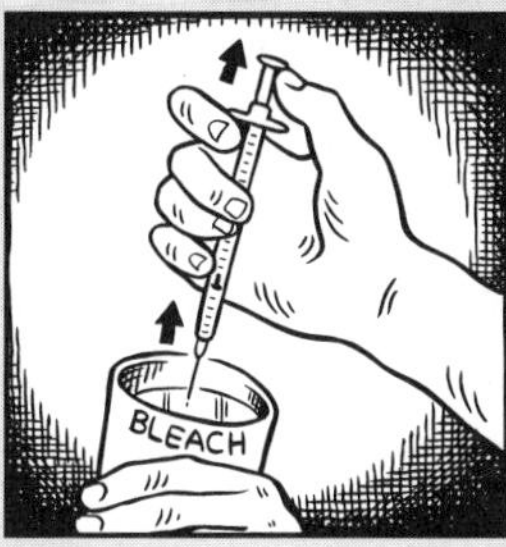

Pour 100% bleach (like Clorox) into a cap or glass, and draw it all the way up into the needle.

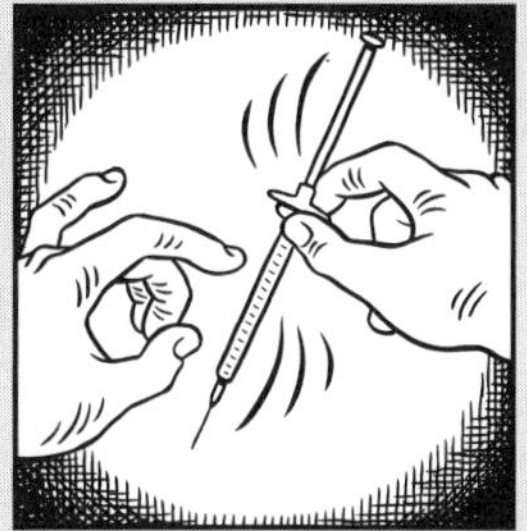

Leave the bleach in for a full two minutes: ten or twenty seconds won't do it.

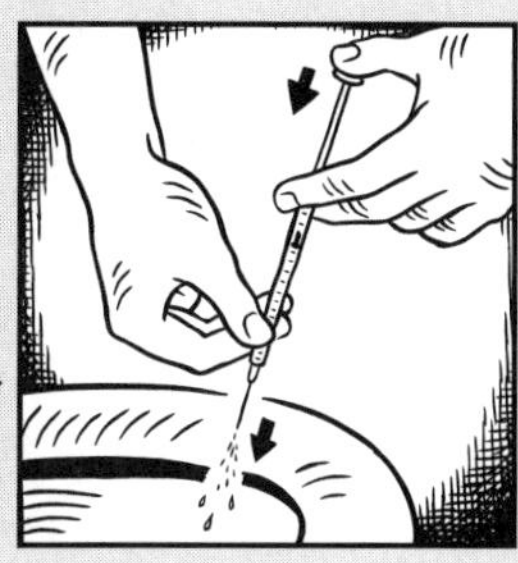

Squirt out the bleach, but not back into the cap or glass.

STEP 3: WATER AGAIN (DO THIS THREE TIMES)

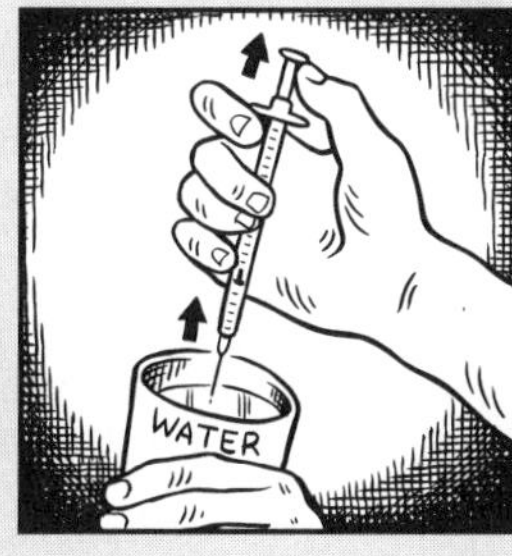

Draw clean water up into the needle, all the way up to the plunger.

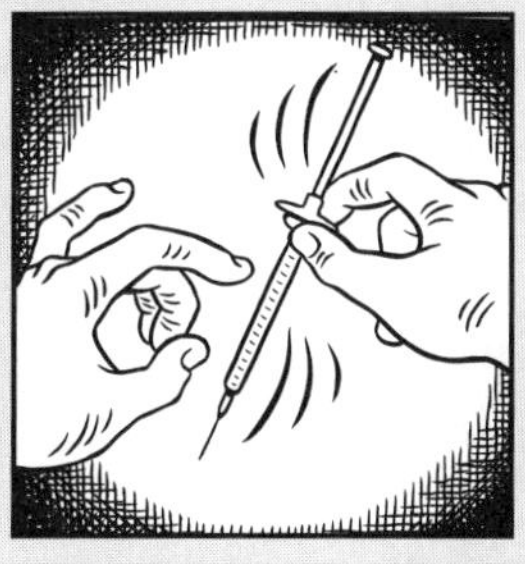

Shake or tap the syringe to loosen any dried blood, and let the water sit for a minute or so.

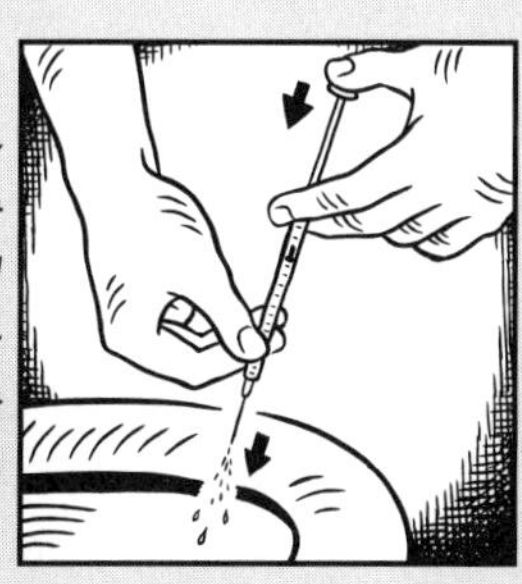

Squirt water out. Clean your cooker by rinsing it out with bleach, and never share or reuse cotton—it can't really be cleaned.

Stages of Behavior Change

In their excellent book, *Changing for Good* (Avon Books, 1994), DiClemente and Prochaska identified six phases common to the process of overcoming self-defeating behavior. Where are you with the various behaviors you, or those around you, wish you could change?

PHASE 1: PRECONTEMPLATION

It's not that you can't see the solution. It's that you don't see any problem. In this phase, what bothers you is not what you're doing, but the reactions of the people around you. You'd just as soon change the subject.

PHASE 2: CONTEMPLATION

This is the feeling-stuck stage: You're thinking about solutions, you're just not doing any of them. "I know I should" (eat less sugar, go to the gym, stop smoking, or whatever) is the refrain of this stage, which often lasts years. Among smokers Prochaska and DiClemente worked with, this was typically a two-year process. It's a step, though. It "counts."

PHASE 3: PREPARATION

This is when you're about to take action, and you announce, for example, that you'll stop using drugs on Monday, or that after the Christmas holidays you're definitely going to start eating healthier. Prochaska and DiClemente note that this phase usually is accompanied by a certain amount of behavior modification: drinking only on weekends, for example, or cutting back to one pack instead of two. Rush this phase by going cold turkey, says Prochaska, and you greatly reduce your chances of success. Recognize that making a plan is a part of change, and that you need to talk to people and enlist support for this phase, not just for the moment you decide to stop (see box on next page).

PHASE 4: ACTION

This is what most of us think of as "deciding to stop." You do it: throw away your cigarettes, give away your booze and go to AA, trash the dealer's beeper number, or decline to order a dessert. This is when support is often highest, but it's not the only time it's needed. It too is only a phase. Most quick-change "crash" programs, say Prochaska and DiClemente (as well as the people who try them), are ineffective precisely because they mistake this stage for the whole battle.

PHASE 5: MAINTENANCE

In order not to gain back the weight, pick up a pack, or whatever, you need what Prochaska calls "an active and intelligent" maintenance plan. This includes replacing old habits with new pleasures, identifying and avoiding triggers for the undesirable behavior, and other tips for quitting. Your support in this stage often helps determine whether you return, as many do, back to the precontemplation or contemplation stage.

PHASE 6: TERMINATION

Whether or not you can "terminate"—move to a point where you no longer desire the behavior or substance in question—depends on you and the behavior. Some people never want

CAN YOU MAKE CHANGE?

Your relationship to drugs and alcohol, like those to people you love, may need to be reworked. If you are trying to make some changes in those patterns, here are some tips:

- *Think about it.* Take some time to think hard about why you're doing what you're doing—not everyone else's reasons, but your own. What are the downsides of the behavior for you? What are the pleasures? What are you going to do to replace the pleasures if you decide to stop? "I couldn't stop using until I had something else—in my case, ACT UP—to transform my life in some way," says George, thirty-four.
- *Don't overhaul your whole life at the same time.* "People make this vow that they're going to quit smoking or stop drinking, lose sixty pounds, go to the gym every day, get a better job, and make more money all at once," says Dr. Warren of the Lesbian and Gay Community Services Center in New York. "Have realistic expectations."
- *Prepare yourself for what's to come.* "Know that you're going to have a lot of mood swings, that you're not going to be yourself," says Warren. "You might have crying jags and feel tense. You might need to do certain things, like sleep later or take a walk. The first six months I quit smoking, I needed twelve alarms to wake me up, cried a lot, and felt sluggish." To reduce cravings for drugs and alcohol, consider alternative methods of stress relief, such as acupuncture, or mind-body practices such as yoga.
- *Who you gonna call?* Whether it's a special group, your friends, your family, or your lover, someone should be there to turn to for support. "If you're in a relationship, your partner may in fact not want you to change," says Warren. "What's in it for him? Talk about ways he can help you with it. Help him understand that you're going to go through some stuff, and that it gets worse before it gets better." It's common to ask a friend to exercise with you. See if you can ask someone to stay sober with you on a hard evening.
- *Look for triggers, and then replace them.* Think of the things that make you want to use drugs or alcohol—chocolate; feeling hungry, angry, lonely, or tired; certain people (going home to visit your family is a classic trigger)—and try to plan accordingly. Maybe you could have coffee instead of a cigarette after your meal, or make sure, for the first few months you're not doing cocaine, to have a friend with you while you get cash out of the ATM. Maybe you could meet your friends at a no-smoking café instead of in a smoky bar. Or try bringing a friend home for the holidays. If they won't cooperate with any of this, maybe it's time to make some new friends.
- *Use counteractive behavior.* When you feel the urge to go to a bar and you don't want to, do something else. Exercise. Call a friend. Eat a succulent piece of fruit. Where you'd usually take a smoking break, says Thomas, "don't just sit there. Get up and move. Go get a treat at the corner store. Don't try to be a goody-goody by switching to carrot sticks and sitting in your chair meditating." Dr. Warren advises prioritizing pleasure. "Remember," she says, "it's much easier to take something away if you replace it with something else you enjoy."

another cigarette again, while others still crave them after thirty years. The same holds true for lots of other things we simultaneously want and do not want to do.

Even if you've stopped a "bad behavior," say Prochaska and others, remember that relapse is the rule rather than the exception. Rather than denying the whole thing or just feeling ashamed, try to consider what you can learn from the lapse. Why did it happen? What were the circumstances? How might they have been avoided or prevented? Even "precontemplators," those of us who really aren't interested even in talking about change, are not beyond its reach. Prochaska and DiClemente, for example, found that programs to end smoking drew only a tiny percentage of those who smoked, or even of those who were thinking about quitting. Holding an informational group for "smokers who didn't want to stop smoking," however, drew crowds. When tested on people who had been smoking more than two packs a day for an average of twenty-five years, Prochaska and DiClemente's approach proved twice as effective as programs used at the time by the American Cancer Society and the American Lung Association.

Getting Help

You know how you go to the gym and you don't see any change? When there's nothing to hold you there, to hold the change? That's how it was for me quitting drinking. I could never see any change. But when I was in a room with other people, people who admitted they had a problem and still had their shit together, I could see them getting better even if I couldn't see it in myself.

The hardest thing I've ever done, the most force I've ever had to expend in my life, is to pry my fingers off a glass or away from a syringe. Everything else has seemed easier than that for me. I couldn't do that for fifteen years. I did some embarrassing, terrible things in that time. I called up people I hardly knew for money. I borrowed my rent three times over and was still broke. I mugged someone, a gay guy, and set other people up to be mugged. I punched my best friend in the face.

Although people will urge you to stop, or not to, only you can choose how much or little drugs or alcohol to use. If you've lost the sense that you *have* any choice, look for support—whether that's a doctor, a counselor, or the observations of someone else in the same predicament. One of the best and most accessible sources of help is Alcoholics Anonymous (AA). With between two million and three million members worldwide, free meetings almost everywhere in the world, and no commercial sponsorships or affiliations, AA is a miracle in community organizing: an international fellowship of individuals who share a common struggle to stay alcohol- and drug-free. The basic tenets of the group, known as the twelve steps (see next page), have become the organizing principles for many other spin-off groups, including Cocaine Anonymous, Narcotics Anonymous, and Overeaters Anonymous, as well as for groups for people involved with alcohol and drug users, such as Al-Anon (for partners of alcoholics) and ACOA (Adult Children of Alcoholics).

If all these groups, or the twelve steps' talk of spirituality, set off warning signals, you're not alone there, either. "I and most of the other gay men I know would sit in those meetings and cringe when we heard the word *God*," says Raoul, thirty-five. "I'd never prayed for anything except maybe to die. It was probably the angry God of my childhood that helped me feel that way. It was only by showing up and seeing people who cared about me that I could imagine a spiritual force that was loving."

As higher powers go, AA's is a flexible one: Every member defines it however he or she wants to, and there are even AA groups for agnostics. As gay men go, AA is also a more welcoming group than most, and was that way long before it was fashionable to be so. The first gay AA group formed, briefly, in 1949; another was formed in 1968. Today, with more than five hundred groups, gay AA is the fellowship's largest subgroup, and many cities have gay AA meetings, or even more specific ones: meetings for gay survivors of incest, or gay men sober for less than ninety days. The chant of the clean-and-sober contingent in various Gay Pride parades across the country—"Two, four, six, eight, we remember who we date!"—draws smiles and, apparently, new members. The New York AA contingent is one of the largest in the parade.

Dating, though, is not what early AA meetings are about. Sex with other AA members is discouraged for your first ninety days of sobriety, as are relationships with other AA members in your or their first year. Staying sober, however you can—calling another member, going for coffee, finding an alternative to Saturday night bar visits and happy hours, and getting through the first few months—is the point. Meetings are free, and are either open (the interested and curious may attend, whether or not they're alcoholic) or closed (alcoholics only). If drugs rather than alcohol are your problem, you're still welcome, or you can join a Cocaine or Narcotics Anonymous group. New members often get a sponsor if they want one (another person who's been through the challenges of early recovery from drugs or alcohol), and every meeting has somebody getting up and sharing a personal "drunkalogue" before the group. You don't need to say anything at all if you don't want to; no one will comment on or criticize what you do say, and though they encourage you to try a bunch of meetings at first, you're free to leave at any time. "Take what you want and leave the rest is what they say, and I did, over and over and over," recalls Duane, now twenty-eight. "It took me quite a few months to get sober, actually. I wasn't ready. Now, three years later, I just got my first sponsor. I listen to him talk and I still get those feelings, those cravings, that tell me I have work to do. But it feels good to imagine that I could sponsor someone someday and give something back."

AA'S TWELVE STEPS

1. We admitted we were powerless over alcohol and all other mind-altering substances—that our lives had become unmanageable.
2. Came to believe that a Power greater than ourselves could restore us to sanity.
3. Made a decision to turn our will and our lives over to the care of God *as we understood Him*.
4. Made a searching and fearless moral inventory of ourselves.
5. Admitted to God, to ourselves, and to another human being the exact nature of our wrongs.
6. Were entirely ready to have God remove all these defects of character.
7. Humbly asked Him to remove our shortcomings.
8. Made a list of all persons we had harmed, and became willing to make amends to them all.
9. Made direct amends to such people whenever possible, except when to do so would injure them or others.
10. Continued to take personal inventory and when we were wrong promptly admitted it.
11. Sought through prayer and meditation to improve our conscious contact with God *as we understood Him*, praying only for knowledge of His will for us and the power to carry that out.
12. Having had a spiritual awakening as the result of these steps, we tried to carry this message to addicts, and to practice these principles in all our affairs.

Reprinted and adapted with permission of AA World Services, Inc.

For those who find AA too cultish, there are other options, among them the Rational Recovery movement. Frankly hostile to AA, Rational Recovery urges individuals to look more closely at their thought patterns rather than surrender to the idea of something more powerful than themselves. Its primary technique, called the Addictive Voice Recognition Technique, involves identifying your addiction as something outside yourself, and realizing when "IT" is speaking. You say to yourself, "IT wants a cigarette, but I don't," or "IT really wants to go to the bar tonight." For more information, check out the group's Web site at www.rational.org/.

Other Roads to Change

Besides AA, a variety of alcohol and drug treatment programs have sprung up all over the country, both gay-specific and for the general population, for-profit and peer-led. Some of these programs integrate AA's twelve-step model; others, such as harm reduction programs, focus on helping you set your own goals for change even if you're not ready or able to stop (see "Thinking Through Changing," page 272). The gold standard of treatment, the twenty-eight-day inpatient treatment program that combines therapy, peer support, and medical monitoring, is increasingly unaffordable, often gone the way of private health insurance (see Chapter 7) and mental health care generally (see Chapter 11). If your life feels as though it's bottoming out so badly that you need to get out of it to get clean, managed care plans prefer to pay for seven to twenty-one days of inpatient treatment to allow you to detoxify, and follow it up with counseling. "Therapeutic communities" still operate across the country, allowing addicts to go away to live, work, and undergo intensive peer and professional counseling and training for a year or longer.

The move to medication that marks the rise of the HMO and the end of the millennium has brought increasing numbers of pharmaceutical options for help, too: the older methadone, to block cravings for heroin; disulfiram (Antabuse) which makes you sick if you take alcohol; and newer antidepressants such as fluoxetine (Prozac), sertraline (Zoloft), or paroxetine (Paxil), which can sometimes make withdrawal from alcohol less painful (see "Clean, Sober, and Medicated?" on page 486). Drugs to block the effects of cocaine are now being tested. For the many people who are combining drugs, legal and illegal, some of these may mess with your experience of others. Methadone, for example, may cause you to experience a greater rush from cocaine, says Dr. Richardson from Columbia University. The tuberculosis medication rifampin (Rifadin) reduces the amount of methadone you metabolize by as much as 85 percent, leading to painful withdrawal symptoms, and certain protease inhibitors or other AIDS drugs may also change your methadone experience. And no matter how many pills you take, recovering from addiction to drugs and alcohol always involves some psychological work if you're going to stay clean.

If you're doing that work in a hospital or therapeutic community setting, try if at all possible to find a gay-friendly one, or go to one of the few, such as the Pride Institute in Minnesota, specifically geared to gay men and lesbians. "Some treatment centers will say, 'Oh, you're not here to deal with your gay issues, you're here to deal with your drug issues,' as if they were so easily separated," says Joe Amico, the Pride Institute's executive director. "If you appeal to your insurer, though [or to your employee assistance program if you're working someplace that has one], you may be able to get placed in a setting that allows you to bring your whole life in." While the Pride Institute runs five such programs across the country, they also maintain a list of others, and can be reached at (800) 54-PRIDE.

Last Call: Helping a Friend

Once I got sober, I remembered which people had the courage to tell me I was letting them down. Those people—not the ones who said nothing but started avoiding me—were the people I most wanted to see later. What seemed intolerably painful then seemed afterward like love.

I came close to killing someone who ripped me off because I thought he'd stolen my dope. Instead I tried to kill myself with an overdose. My sister found me. She paid for one of these places where you go and your family and friends are there and talk to you. I remember it was called Freedom House. I think my family was getting ready to "detach with love," or whatever those people from Al-Anon call cutting you loose, except I'd burned so many options I was looking for something. So I said, "Fine, I'll go into treatment." The woman from the institute was really nice; she said I could go that day or in a few days. I said, "No, let me get high today and I'll go today."

"Confronting the drug or alcohol use of someone close to you takes place on two different levels," says Richard Elovich, founder of GMHC's Substance Use Counseling and Education program. "One has to do with giving the person with the problem a reality check, but the other has to do with you. What issues does the way this person is behaving bring up for you? How similar is it to other relationships in your life or your past?" It's easy to focus on "fixing" the drug or alcohol user without looking at yourself. Refuse to do so and you may find yourself doing what the new language of codependence calls "enabling": consciously or unconsciously making it possible for the alcoholic or addict to go on with their harmful behavior. If you find yourself providing money, shelter, or excuses for someone whose activities enrage or disappoint you, or expressing anger to the person without ever following it up with discussion of the consequences, then you may be acting as an "enabler" instead of being a real help.

Five Tips on Intervening

Hesitating to get too deeply involved in the personal business of someone you think is in trouble is a common reaction, but rarely the constructive one. If you are going to confront somebody, here is some advice for that not-so-happy hour:

- *Give data, not diagnoses or prescriptions.* "Point out that this is the third time the person hasn't shown up in a month, or that they keep borrowing money without paying it back, and spell out how this affects your relationship," says Elovich. Don't get lost in making demands about what they should do. You often help create resistance when you go too fast or make conclusions for them.
- *Consider yourself.* Is this a pattern for you? Is there always someone in your life you're taking care of who's not functioning or who's drunk or who's not being honest? How is tend-

ing to them protecting you from looking at your own life? "This doesn't have anything to do with your conversation with the substance abuser, and is better done without the person present," says Elovich. Groups such as Al-Anon and Adult Children of Alcoholics (ACOA), which have free and frequent meetings in most places in America, may be helpful.

• *If you threaten consequences, stick to them.* "Don't say you don't want to see the person again while they're drinking if you don't mean it," says Elovich. "Going back on threats just makes it seem as if you too are doing the same kind of double-talk you're probably objecting to in them."

• *Don't get too invested in what they do next.* "Think of the conversation as a reality test, not another opportunity for them to disappoint you," says Elovich. Part of calling attention to substance abuse involves recognizing that there is a powerful, or too powerful, relation between the person and the drug. It may be more powerful than you, and there's nothing you can do about that. If you're having trouble accepting that, go back to the second point above.

• *Power in numbers?* Joining with other people who care about the person and are familiar with his or her behavior can reduce the "gaslight" effect, where the drug or alcohol abuser convinces you that you're the problem. It can also cut down on the dynamic that casts you as the critic and another family member or friend as the understanding one. Everyone, though, needs to stick to the suggestions above: one weak link, and the person will find it. They don't call it tough love just because it's tough on the addict—it's hard on all of you. Elovich strongly recommends finding a neutral third party, with training, to facilitate the discussion. "You don't want it to turn into a hammering session," he says. A number of organizations actually make this kind of intervention their business. Again, Al-Anon meetings, or local drug and alcohol abuse counseling programs, may be able to help you find one.

Confronting someone is a brave and difficult act. So is remembering that often, when it comes to drugs and alcohol, change comes after the person has exhausted other options. "The hard part is hoping that they won't hurt themselves, or others, on the way," says Elovich. "That, and remembering that all change is self-help. Much as you want to, you can't do it for somebody else."

FURTHER READING

Anderson, Arnold E., ed. (1990) *Males with Eating Disorders.* New York: Brunner/Mazel. The leading text on a rarely explored subject.

Bredenberg, Jeff, et al. (1996) *Food Smart: A Man's Plan to Fuel Up for Peak Performance.* Emmaus, PA: Rodale Books. A no-nonsense, easy-access guide to basic principles of nutrition aimed at straight men. Heavy on the bachelor-who-can't-cook rhetoric, but fine for gay men too.

Prochaska, James O., et al. (1994) *Changing for Good: A Revolutionary Six-Stage Program for Overcoming Bad Habits and Moving Your Life Positively Forward.* New York: Avon Books. Goes way beyond "just stop already" to suggest how deeply personal change works and how you can effect it.

Romeyn, Mary. (1995) *Nutrition and HIV: A New Model for Treatment.* San Francisco: Jossey-Bass Publishers. Accessible information from one of the doyennes of AIDS nutrition.

Rustim, Terry A. (1996) *Get Ready: Clean and Free Workbook 1; Get Set: Clean and Free Workbook 2; Go: Clean and Free Workbook 3.* Center City, MN: Hazelden. Aimed at smokers, but useful for thinking through changes in smoking, drinking, and drugging. The publisher has lots more good titles where these came from.

CHAPTER 7

What's Up, Doc?

Dr. Right • Making the Most of Your Visits • Symptoms You Shouldn't Ignore • Five Tests and Vaccines No Gay Man Should Go Without • Alternative and Complementary Medicines • Health Insurance • Managing Managed Care

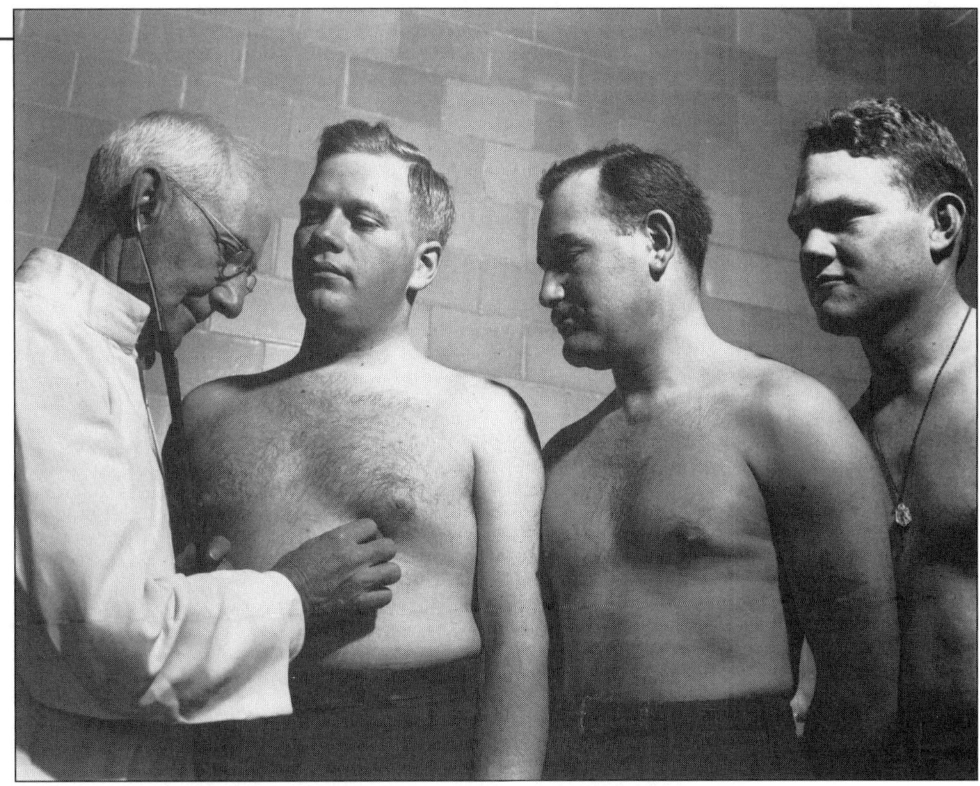

Whether you're struggling to hold on to two T cells or feeling too healthy, wealthy, and gay even to think of doctor's visits, you're in the midst of a health care crisis. America's big hospitals and managed care organizations are fighting for their lives and profit margins, merging, dividing, and dying off much like the cells in the human bodies they now compete to treat. Ads by doctors and dentists, banned until the late 1980s, now confront the consumer like white blood cells clustering around a foreign object, appearing in buses, subways, phone books, and even in newspaper supplements laid out to look like genuine articles. Pharmaceutical companies, which got legal clearance to circulate their advertisements directly to patients in 1997, now spend millions buying television ads, pages in magazines, and even names and addresses off drugstore computers. The "good" news is that the gay press is more stable than it used to be, supported by all those full-color ads of fit-looking men with HIV throwing javelins or climbing mountains. The bad news is that these heights of marketing can be dizzying, with health care costs climbing steadily, choices in doctors plummeting, and serious questions—such as whether or not you really want a drug company getting your name from your Prozac or protease inhibitor prescription—hanging in the balance.

Despite this medical information explosion, one of the most basic and important rules of health care remains unadvertised and ignored by many gay men in spite of (or perhaps as a result of) our long history of caring for others in the hospital: If you can possibly afford it, you should find a primary-care doctor—a first line of assistance with medical problems—before you get sick.

Why find a doctor before you seem to need one? The tired but true advice that an ounce of prevention is worth a pound of cure still applies: Diabetes, HIV, heart disease, and other ailments can all be treated better if you find them earlier. In an era of high patient loads and other managed care madness, first appointments can often take a month or more to get; follow-up visits for existing patients, on the other hand, are easier to schedule. Having a doctor look at you when you're healthy can help him or her gauge what to do if you get sick, putting your health in a context no single visit can provide. And necessity—as in "I can't swallow, I have a fever of 103, and I'm not sure who to call"—is the mother of desperation, leading to loss of control, expensive emergency-room visits, and unfamiliar doctors who may treat you poorly, particularly if they know you're gay.

TURNING A GAY GAZE ON THE PHYSICIAN-PATIENT RELATIONSHIP

I went to a doctor recently for treatment, but got a lecture. "You have anal warts," he said after he'd burned what felt like half my ass away. "And if you want to stay healthy, I'd advise you to never, ever put anything else up there again. Is that really so difficult for you guys to understand?" On the bus ride home, the pain was so intense I thought I'd have to get off. I'd been given neither warning about the pain nor medication for it.

"Doctor means 'teacher' in Latin," says Birgit Pols, MD, former medical director of the Michael Callen/Audre Lorde Community Health Center in New York City. "If they're not teaching you, they're not practicing medicine." Unfortunately, until gay activism and the formation of community-based clinics such as Callen/Lorde forced change, the lessons gay men learned from doctors were mostly of the thanks-but-no-thanks kind. The history of modern medicine is littered with "remedies" for homosexuality: aversion therapy, where doctors gave gay men electric shocks or nausea-provoking drugs while showing us sexy images of men; hormone therapy, where we were prescribed testosterone meant to reverse our supposed excess femininity; or even "psychosurgery," a lobotomy that, claiming to destroy the parts of our brains that gave rise to homosexual desire, destroyed much of the rest of our brains in the process.

The American Medical Association, the trade organization for physicians, has slowly changed its practices, and the last references to sexual orientation disorders have been removed from its diagnostic manual. Abstinence and moralism, though, continue to be prescribed by many doctors, particularly for ailments that stem from sexual activity they don't practice themselves. "No one would ever dream of calling pelvic inflammatory disease 'heterosexual copulative disorder,'" remarks Michael Scarce, author of *Smearing the Queer: Medical Bias in the Health Care of Gay Men* (Haworth Press, 1999), "or advise a heterosexual man with penile herpes to stop using his penis. Yet we still see references to 'gay bowel syndrome' in the medical literature, or hear STDs used as pretexts for lectures on the unhealthiness of anal intercourse."

Medicine is actually quite sensitive to sexual needs when it wants to be. "Male health clinics" treating erectile dysfunction often include a psychologist on staff. Gay men with anal

Dr. Right

I look to him for advice on how to stay healthy, but there's an emotional component, too. I don't want to disappoint him by being sick. Sometimes I have to fight to make him realize that I'm reading and researching, and I'm not just going to sit back and take orders without explanations.

My face was a mess. She took one look at it and snapped, "You've got herpes!" "Oh, my God," I thought. I put my hand to my forehead in disbelief, and she snapped: "Don't touch your eye. You could get herpes there and go blind!" Then it was like a movie: My head started spinning and I fainted. The good part was that she must have realized I was a human being, not just a symptom, because when I came to, she was transformed into a much warmer, more motherly force and has been that way with me ever since.

TURNING A GAY GAZE ON THE PHYSICIAN-PATIENT RELATIONSHIP

problems, however, are more likely to need therapy as the *result* of seeing a doctor. Surveying the two thousand gay and lesbian physicians across the country who make up its membership, the Gay and Lesbian Medical Association (GLMA) found that respondents used terms such as "rough," "brutal," and "violent" to describe the treatment and examination of gay patients. With what the report called "remarkable similarity," more than one respondent echoed the words of a Florida physician who said he had seen staff and surgeons "being particularly scornful and physically brutal to gay male patients," especially those requiring anal exams.

Gay male health, though, involves more than our anuses, and prejudice is not limited to the assholes who perform intentionally rough anal exams. Many of the gay and lesbian physicians surveyed by GLMA, whether closeted or out at work, diagnosed some of their fellow health care providers with good old-fashioned cases of homophobia. "One nurse expressed concern to her superior about whether I should be allowed to examine male patients without an escort," a gay West Coast physician recounted. Other doctors told of being shoved, passed up for promotions, ridiculed for their dating habits or general demeanor, and being labeled as people who would "attract undesirable patients" or "infect patients."

If that's how doctors are treated, how about the rest of us? Nearly 70 percent of the 700 respondents to the GLMA survey reported knowing of lesbian, gay, or bisexual patients who had received substandard care or had been denied it entirely because of their sexual orientation. Eighty-eight percent reported hearing nasty cracks about gay patients. "One of the residents supervising me in my fourth year in medicine spoke of a gay man with HIV in the ICU," wrote one medical student. "He told me that he believed HIV was God's punishment and that, in fact, all gay and lesbian people should be dead." Insights of the gays-are-going-to-die-anyway-so-what's-the-point variety were repeated with frightening regularity in the GLMA survey, and not exclusively about gay men with AIDS.

Given the amount of prejudice in the field, it may be no small wonder that more than half of doctors surveyed remained in the closet to most of their work colleagues, and that many gay men are reluctant to reveal their sexual orientation to their doctors. Still, says Pat Dunn, policy director of the Gay and Lesbian Medical Association, the best strategy is "not to shut up or give up, but rather to make sure to find a doctor you can trust."

I was HIV-negative, and he started giving me some kind of lecture about safe sex and yelling at me like I was some kind of criminal. "Do you use a condom when you have oral sex? You've got to!" And I said, "Excuse me, you're not talking to me. You have no idea what my sexual habits are. You're just giving a public service announcement." He stopped, smiled, and said, "Yes, okay, you're right." Later, when I discovered that he died of AIDS, it became more sad.

Even when they're nice, I don't like seeing doctors. It's like going to a judge or priest: They're authorities, they always know and you don't. I went to a naturopathic doctor, and it was a whole different experience, because he talked to me for forty-five minutes before recommending anything. For the first time, I felt listened to.

"When you've got your health, you've got just about everything" is a stand-in for a more complicated truth: that health, and finding a doctor to help you keep it, can often be about almost everything *but* bodily function. "From the minute you walk through the door, ask yourself whether this is someone who clicks for you," Dr. Pols suggests to gay men in search of a new doctor, her advice ringing the truer for sounding as though it could apply equally well to assessing romantic potential. Though there are some important differences between going to see a doctor for the first time and a blind date (some dates are definitely less intimate), both feature the same awkward blend of deeply revealing and highly formal exchanges. Sickness and the fear of sickness are some of the most personal matters in our lives. At some point in your dealings with your doctor, he or she will touch something in you that reminds you of a parent, a teacher, a boyfriend you want to please, or one that you hated. You're not always going to be comfortable, because plenty of medicine isn't. But if you're not open—if you can't share important questions or speak honestly with your physician—then you probably need to be going to someone else for help.

Finding Dr. Right?

In Norman, Oklahoma, fresh from a vacation in San Francisco, a twenty-five-year-old named Mike was cruising the University of Oklahoma student union, saw a local florist, and decided to take a chance—on a physician referral. "I thought since the florist was always making deliveries to the hospital, he'd know who the good doctors were," he remembers. "And I figured neither he nor the doctor he recommended would be shocked that I was gay."

As it turned out, the doctor the florist recommended wasn't the least bit shocked—but he didn't exactly inspire confidence, either. "After I told him I'd had sex with a number of men in San Francisco, his first question was, 'Are you heterosexual?'" Mike recalls, "which I guess was his way of not having to say 'Are you homosexual?' But he was very pleasant and clear in his instructions, and he never acted like he wanted to turn me away."

Mike had a better experience five years later, when he moved permanently to San Francisco. There he went to the same doctor a high-school friend—also a transplanted gay Oklahoman—was seeing for HIV treatment. "Everyone knew Dr. Bob was gay, and so were all his patients," Mike recalls, "so we talked freely about everything." When Dr. Bob left private practice, the doctor who took over for him made no unwarranted assumptions about his new patients. "On my first visit, he asked me, 'Are you gay, straight, or bisexual?' and 'Are you monogamous or not?'" Mike says. "Later, when I saw him, I told him about my new relationship and he said, 'Oh, let me make a note of that!'"

SPECIAL TREATMENT

There are doctors whose specialties come from what they do: a pathologist examines tissue, blood, and other body products to identify disease; a radiologist performs and interprets X rays, magnetic resonance imaging (MRI) scans, and other "pictures" of the body's organs. There are those whose expertise is in a certain phase of life or kind of training: the geriatrician specializes in care of older people, the oncologist is a cancer expert. Most specialists, though, focus on parts or systems of the body. If you need confirmation that every part of you is special, here it is. But chances are it'll cost you.

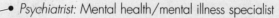

The reality is that Norman, Oklahoma—like most of America—is always likely to be light-years behind San Francisco in terms of gay awareness and acceptance. Still, thanks to the Internet, the HIV epidemic, ACT UP, the rise of patient advocacy groups, and general cultural exchange (you know, like *Ellen*), there is likely to be a doctor somewhere near you—whether you live on the buckle of the Bible belt or in a gay metropolis—who not only is unfazed by your "lifestyle," but may even be supportive and relatively informed about it.

Five Steps to Finding Dr. Right

I went to the dermatologist with a bright red bump over my eyebrow, and he took only a quick glance. "Either it's a blood blister or you have AIDS," he pronounced. Then he proceeded to tell me how good he was at recognizing AIDS-related skin problems and how he was the envy of his colleagues because of his diagnostic skill. I hadn't told him I was gay, and he was completely oblivious to my reaction—I was reeling, terrified. I went to my regular doctor and had an HIV test, which came back negative. I never confronted the dermatologist, but I never went back to him, either.

1. Know Your Priorities

Beyond a basic level of technical skill and personal rapport, what do you want in your doctor? Someone who is businesslike and efficient, or with a warmer, more personal touch? Someone like you, or someone like the kindly straight parent you never had? Do you feel more comfortable with a man or a woman? Some of us like to be told what to do; others want to be given information and explanations and weigh decisions ourselves.

Doctors, like their patients, are more than just their sexual orientation. While somebody gay-friendly is a must, a gay doctor probably is not. "There are nongay doctors who are terrific and open-minded, and there are gay doctors who suck," notes Scott McCallister, MD, longtime director of the Howard Brown Clinic in Chicago. "I don't want a gay doctor, I want a good doctor," agrees Miles, thirty-seven, a journalist in New York City. "I get plenty of gay affirmation and information in my life. Frankly, if I saw safer-sex posters on the wall of my doctor's office, I'd probably run out screaming." Others, outside of New York, find their doctors are the ones doing the screaming about safer sex, and say they'd welcome more open-mindedness.

2. Ask Around

A list of gay clinics around the country appears on page 571 of this book, and the Gay and Lesbian Medical Association will also refer you to gay doctors in your area. Call or contact them through their Web site (www.glma.org), and they'll give some local options. Gay-friendly doctors can also be found through local AIDS service organizations, local gay and lesbian hot lines if there are any, or even local hospital or HMO lists. "You won't see things like sexual orientation or race in print, but if you ask doctors flat out, they may tell you," says Dr. McCallister. Referrals from friends, florists, travel agents, or even strangers in a bar—it's not the sexiest conversational opener, but it can work—are all potentially helpful. Use the (pink) triangle method, asking until the same physician is recommended by three different people. Other standard rules, such as never going to doctors who advertise, can also be bent in this case, since doctors who advertise in gay publications are likely to be sensitive to your concerns. Maybe too sensitive: "I had to stop going to my dentist because I couldn't stand listening to him sing along to Barbra for an hour," says Michael, forty-four, a Los Angeles actor. Again, though, many gay men—and many doctors—wish they had that option.

3. Be Assertive

Once you have a short list of doctors, do your own checkups. Most people interview a few people before hiring a contractor or a mechanic, so be at least as careful with your body as you would be with your house or car. If your budget and doctor allow this, meet for an initial appointment, though you can also ask the office staff for names of a few patients willing to talk.

4. Trust Your Instincts

You don't need a stethoscope to listen to your heart. Is this someone you feel comfortable with? Does he or she inspire trust or fear? Remember, though, that no doctor is perfect. Doctor shopping is fine; doctor hopping is not. And beware of deciding on a doctor because of one factor—that he's gay, that he's near, or that his office manager is cute.

5. Tell It Like It Is

Pay particular attention to your feelings and the doctor's responses when gay-related health concerns come up. If you're thinking they don't need to come up at all, think again—and if

DOCTOR DISH: WORKING THE NETWORK

If you are practiced in the art form of gay gossip, now is not the time to stop. Find people who've seen your potential doctor, and pursue finding out about the experience with the same attention given to weighty questions such as how many times your ex-boyfriend tried to sleep with your best friend's brother, or whether Leo DiCaprio really is Titanic down under. Things to find out:

- Is the doctor friendly or reserved? Pressured or relaxed? Available by phone?
- Does he or she explain a procedure before performing it, including the reason for it and what you can expect to experience while it's happening?
- How long do you usually have to sit in the waiting room? How about the examining room?
- How friendly and helpful is the office staff? Gay? Gay-friendly?
- Is there a nurse or physician's assistant who helps with routine care when the doctor is out? Is he or she available by phone?
- What kind of payment is required at the time of the visit, and how does that compare to what insurance reimburses for?
- Are most of the patients there for a particular reason?
- Do you see the same doctor every visit, or just whatever doctor in the group is there?
- Does the doctor stop, look, and listen, or is it wham, bam, thank you, Sam?
- How well does the doctor answer questions? How well does he ask them?
- How does the doctor react when patients express strong emotions: fear, grief, anger, or anxiety?
- What do people like most and least about this doctor?

necessary, find another doctor where that fantasy is out of the question. "Doctors can only be as good as the information the patient provides them with," notes Ben Lipton, MSW, former director of clinical services at GMHC. "If it's someone you're seeing for a single visit, that's one thing, but in the long run staying in the closet with your doctor can definitely be hazardous to your health." Recognizing that being out can also be dangerous, some men in small or gossipy communities choose to segment their care, going to one doctor for routine things and supplementing with an occasional visit to a city or more anonymous clinic for gay-specific —or HIV-specific—concerns. Though that's not ideal, the important thing, says Lipton, "is that you have a doctor, somewhere, with whom you can talk frankly about what you do with your body and whom you do it with."

If it's your responsibility to come out to a health care provider, it's his or hers to make that easy. Scan the doctor's office, and the demeanor of the staff, for clues of gay-friendliness. Do intake forms allow for the possibility that your partner might be a man, or is there only "married" and "single"? Does the doctor ask you about your "lady friends" or simply ask if you sleep with men, women, or both? However it's phrased, a doctor's questions and attitude should make it comfortable for you to explain that you have sex with men, or at least want to.

George, a Philadelphia financial analyst worried about discovery by homophobic colleagues, figured bringing up his nervousness might gauge the doctor's own. "I said, 'I'm apprehensive about talking about this. Could you leave the fact that I'm gay out of the chart?' My doctor was completely relaxed, saying he'd write it so that only he would know what it meant, and then went on to ask if my anxiety had anything to do with worries about AIDS." Some doctors are also willing to leave substance abuse information out of the chart in case an

SICK QUESTIONS: SPECIAL THINGS TO LOOK FOR IN A DOCTOR WHEN YOU'RE ALREADY ILL

• ***Hospital admitting privileges.*** Hospitals decide which doctors can admit patients into their facilities. Find out which hospitals a potential doctor works with; some are a lot better at treating particular kinds of illness than others. One study, done before the approval of combination anti-HIV therapy but still telling, found that people with AIDS were more than twice as likely to die if they were treated in a hospital inexperienced in treating their conditions.

• ***Board certification.*** While not every problem you have falls into an officially designated "specialty"—there's no AIDS certification, for example—board certification shows that your doctor has been trained and tested in a specialty. To find out if a doctor is certified, and how long ago it's been since he recertified, check with the American Board of Medical Specialties at (800) 776-CERT or www.certifieddoctor.org.

• ***Location.*** Along with a recommendation from a friend or family member, this is the single most important factor for most Americans. If you're going to be visiting the doctor often, traveling across town can be exhausting. On the other hand, a little inconvenience may seem like a fair price to pay for seeing a doctor who knows a lot about your condition.

• ***Money matters.*** Many of us feel embarrassed asking about the cost of a procedure recommended by a doctor. Your insurance company or lab has no such hesitation in asking you to pay for it if it's not covered. If you're short of money, and most sick people are, make sure to discuss potential costs. "Every time I asked my doctor, he looked at his beeper, until I became sure he was faking getting calls," says Solomon, forty-four. "After I kept insisting, he finally told me to ask the office manager."

insurance company reviews the records. If you're feeling too tongue-tied to ask such things, Dr. McCallister recommends these ice-breaking questions:

1. Do you have gay patients in your practice? (You want them to say yes.)
2. Do you think there's a cure for homosexuality? (You want them to say no.)
3. Are you knowledgeable about gay men's specific health concerns? (They'll all say yes, but you want them to answer calmly and openly. If they rush to the sink and start washing their hands, wash yours of them.)

Dr. McCallister also adds a plea for patience. "Talking about specific sexual practices can sometimes be uncomfortable for anyone," he says. "If the interaction you have with your doctor isn't perfect at first, give it a little while to see if a rapport develops. Remember, before we're doctors, we're human beings with all the failings everyone else has."

Making the Most of Your Visits

I treat my doctor's office just like an airport. A few hours before, I call ahead, make sure I'm going to see him, and ask how late he's running.

The days of the leisurely exchange of information and the house call are largely over, at least for mainstream medical practitioners. Time and money pressures are bearing down on doctors as well as patients in the health care system, and you can help relieve both, and get better treatment, with a few simple steps.

1. Arrive Prepared

If it's a first visit, have medical records sent from your old doctor, or bring a copy and a list of all medications you're taking (including dosage) with you. Take a few minutes before you go to refresh your memory of your medical history—significant illnesses, injuries, or operations you've had, medications you've taken or are taking, allergies, and anything else that may be pertinent—as well as your familiarity with your family's health history.

2. Bring a List

It's common, even for smart people in a friendly doctor's office, to feel confused or to forget to ask something important. Start with the most important things first, and outline things in as organized a way as you can. If you're sick, think about how you can describe your symptoms precisely. Is your headache dull and constant or sharp and stabbing? Is the pain in your back concentrated in a single spot or generalized through a large area? Doctors love symptom logs—simple notes of when a symptom started, went away, how painful it was on a scale of 1 to 5, and what might have brought it on. Doctors hate "by the way, Doctor," syndrome, where you save important information until you're on your way out the door.

If you've seen other doctors for the condition, don't hide that fact. Tell them briefly what the previous doctor did and when. If you're still seeing someone else, ask if this doctor might give your other doctor a call. If you've had tests, bring in the results.

3. Bring a Pen or, if You're Sick, a Friend with a Pen

Going in with someone else can help keep you calm, show a doctor you're serious about getting help, and—if your friend is willing to take some basic notes—leave you free to focus on understanding what the doctor says. That extra shoulder to lean on might be your lover's, though you may want to save him for home care and get a friend to go. Even if you're alone, write down information, since it's hard to remember everything. Always ask for more information if you don't understand something, and remember that follow-up questions can help remind the doctor, and you, to explore the options. Good follow-up questions, suggests New York City doctor Howard Grossman, MD, include:

- What's the name and cause of the illness?
- What happens if I don't do the treatment?
- Is there anything else I could do to feel better?
- What kind of side effects are there from the medication, and what should I do about them if they happen?
- How long should I expect this condition to last?
- What changes or symptoms should I report to you?
- When's the best time to call with questions?
- What should I do in an emergency?

4. Get to Know the Office Staff

Whether it's the nurse who can write a refill of a prescription or the receptionist who will (or won't) put you through on the phone, a doctor's staff is his or her support. (Why else do they call them the staff?) Ask them for help, and be nice.

5. Do What You Agree to Do, or Let the Doctor Know When You Can't

Doctors assume you're taking your medication and, often, that the medication they have prescribed is working. If one or both aren't the case, let them know and explore other options. Don't be surprised if they act irritated, but don't be intimidated, either. They'll get over it. There's often more than one way to treat something, and you're supposed to be working together.

Dance with a Stranger? The Doctor-Patient Dynamic

In the end, I've discovered that being liked is not the same as being helped. I ask, even pressure, to make sure that I'm getting the attention I need. I tell my doctors that treatment isn't something I let people do to me anymore; they need to do it with me.

My friend Paul was a doctor, and when he was sick and in the hospital, he had a big sign put over his bed for the people who drew his blood all day: "First try is free. Second time, we work together. Third time, I demonstrate on you!"

In 1978, at the end of the let-it-all-hang-out era, the *New England Journal of Medicine* let down a little hair of its own. An article titled "Taking Care of the Hateful Patient" spelled out four types of patients that drove doctors up the wall. As revealing as the stereotypes were the descriptions that followed them. Doctors, their training and our expectations aside, turn out to be human, decidedly full of likes and needs and insecurities.

In 1994, at the end of the AIDS activist heyday, New York City health care providers Judith Rabkin, Robert Remien, and Christopher Wilson published *Good Doctors, Good Patients* (NCM Publishers, 1994). Drawn from their own experiences and extensive interviews, the authors explored health care issues from both patient's and doctor's perspectives. Consistent throughout was the sense that when the doctor-patient dynamic was working, it was about working together.

A lot has happened since 1978 and 1994. The idea that doctor knows best has been challenged seriously by patient advocacy groups, on one hand, and accountants concerned with rising health care costs, on the other. Anti-HIV drugs that appear to be suppressing HIV have also eroded some of gay men's skepticism toward the medical-pharmacological system. Still, things that make doctors uncomfortable haven't changed so much. The new AIDS drugs are failing more than originally reported. And the things that work for patients with terminal illness and few options still set a standard worth consideration.

Symptoms You Shouldn't Ignore

Men go to doctors less often than women even when we're sick. Whether you're toughing it out or trying to be the best little boy in the world, ignoring symptoms comes with serious consequences. "Showing up three months into a diarrhea spell that's left you thirty pounds lighter makes things harder for patient and doctor," says Dr. Grossman in New York City. "In general, if a symptom lasts longer than two days, have it checked out."

Symptoms That Should Send You for Emergency Medical Care

- Crushing chest pain, particularly if it radiates down your left arm
- Sudden disturbance in vision, such as seeing sparks or large black spots, or developing partial blindness
- Sudden disturbance in speech
- Persistent numbness in any part of the body, especially concentrated on one side
- Vomiting blood
- Difficulty breathing
- Any intense, unremitting pain that makes activity impossible

Symptoms That Should Be Checked by a Doctor as Soon as Possible

- Weight loss of more than 10 percent of your body weight without reason
- Diarrhea (three or more bowel movements a day) that lasts for more than two days
- Unexplained lump or growth on any part of the body
- Difficulty swallowing
- Skin rashes that last for more than a few days, a change in a mole, or unusual-looking new moles or skin growths
- Constant thirst
- Frequent urination
- Blood in your bowel movement

What doctors say they hate	What doctors say they like	Things to think about
From "Taking Care of the Hateful Patient" (*New England Journal of Medicine,* 1978) **The "Dependent Clinger"** This seems to be the doctor's version of what in certain sexual circles is known as the "bottom-less bottom," someone whose needs seem never to be satisfied. These patients, claimed the *NEJM,* "escalate from mild requests for reassurance to repeated, perfervid, incarcerating cries for explanation, affection, analgesics, seda-tives and all forms of attention imaginable."	From *Good Doctors, Good Patients* (New York: NCM Publishers, 1994) **The "Good Patient"** Observes and reports symptoms to the physician promptly. Keeps track of prescriptions and understands their purpose. Considers physicians trustworthy working partners with whom he can be open and honest.	Look twice at what you're gaining by being polite. If you're resisting calling or going in, why? Is your desire to be "good" masking a reluctance to find out what's really happening? Does being the "perfect patient" really mean being endlessly patient? If you demand an emergency appointment, it had better not be for a hangnail. At the same time, you deserve to be respected. If you leave a message saying it's urgent, the doctor should return your call promptly.
The "Entitled Demander" This type tries to get needs met by intimidation. "Moreover, such patients often exude a repulsive sense of innate deservedness as if they were far superior to the physician."	Is informed about and keeps current on changing treatment recommendations. Expresses appreciation on occasion to a physician who is caring and concerned.	In health care settings, bullying or threatening is unlikely to do much except get you labeled as a problem. Calm, determined advocacy—by you or someone close to you—can do wonders. One study trained patients to ask questions and express feelings, and then compared their progress to those with no such training. The assertive patients did bet-ter, lost fewer days from work, and improved faster.
The "Manipulative Help Rejecters" These patients "feel that no regimen will help . . . When one of their symptoms is relieved, another mysteriously appears to take its place. Apparently, what is sought is not relief of symptoms. What is sought is an undivorceable marriage to an inexhaustible caregiver."	Accepts, and seeks, help when necessary. Takes responsibility for and charge of his or her health. Is "vigilant" (keeping on top of symptoms and reporting them promptly) but not "hypochondriacal" (imagining they're sick at the slightest chance). Complies with agreed-on treatment regimens. Practices a healthy lifestyle.	Sometimes it really is the approach, rather than your attitude, that's not working. If your treat-ment's going nowhere, consider talking to other people—doctors and patients—who have pur-sued alternative or complementary strategies.
"Self-Destructive Deniers" These patients' "main pleasure is defeating the physician's attempts to preserve their lives. They may represent a chronic form of suicidal behavior; often, they let themselves die."	Has realistic expectations, but continues to set and work toward goals. Devotes sufficient time to medical care.	Increasingly, even sensitive doctors don't have time to be so. If you're having trouble "complying" with a treatment, having safer sex, stopping smoking, staying sober, or doing other things your doctor rec-ommends, seek support from other people going through the same thing. To go only to doctors for help may be wasting your time and theirs.

Five Tests and Vaccines No Gay Man Should Go Without

My doctor keeps telling me to take a cholesterol test, and I say, "Yeah, right—I'm forty-two years old, I'm single, and I live in a gay urban center. I should be so lucky as to die of a cholesterol problem."

Take heart. Or bloodstream. Or colon. Add forty or fifty years of function, and you'll be in line for a number of important tests—most of them painless—to make sure that things are working as they should be. Though the AIDS epidemic has tended to obscure this fact, gay men are subject to the same causes of death or illness as straight men. Many of these—heart disease, prostate cancer, colon cancer, and diabetes—can be detected through common tests and in some cases prevented by lifestyle changes.

The next chapter in this book, "Coming of Age," details some of the tests most important for men forty and over. If you're not above the usual translation of pronouns (from *she* to *he* each time a sexual partner is mentioned), the bookstore shelves are also groaning with books, many of them excellent, that detail some of the basic methods to warn of—and perhaps ward off—men's leading causes of death.

Five tests and vaccines, in particular, are vital for all of us, young and old. They aren't all especially for gay men, though mainstream male health publications tend to pay less attention to those that are. All of them can make the difference between serious illness, a needed warning, or no illness at all.

1. Cholesterol

WHY?

You've heard the word a thousand times, but do you know your levels? An estimated 75 percent of Americans aren't sure what their cholesterol levels should be. Most don't know that men have higher cholesterol than women, or that the National Cholesterol Education Program recommends we be tested at least once every five years starting from age twenty-one. That goes extra for smokers, which we gay men are sharply more likely to be than our heterosexual counterparts (see page 260). As for the HIV-infected among us, new drugs may well keep us living long enough to have to worry about things like heart attacks, and maybe sooner than anybody thought. Among the common side effects of protease inhibitors is lipodystrophy syndrome, whose symptoms include an accumulation of fat around the stomach, mild diabetes, and high levels of triglycerides, all of which are markers for increased risk of heart disease (see Chapter 9).

If you've long suspected that your picky diet and relentless gym-going make you bad boyfriend material, don't be too harsh: Your heart is probably getting *something* that it needs. Fatty meat, eggs, and dairy products are bad for more than girlish figures, since if you get too much of the soft, fatty animal product known as cholesterol in your blood, the stuff starts to build up on the walls of arteries, blocking the blood flow to and from our body's most important organs. Most harmful is the "bad" cholesterol, otherwise known as low-density lipoproteins, or LDL (think *L* for *lethal*). In ways not totally understood, aerobic exercise seems to reduce LDL levels, apparently by increasing production of "good cholesterol" (high-density lipoproteins, or HDL; think *H* for *healthy*), which seems to take the bad LDL back to the liver for processing.

CHOLESTEROL LEVELS

Most of us, with the exception of men with advanced AIDS or other serious illnesses, produce virtually all the cholesterol we need to function properly without eating any fat at all. The question is, how much extra do you have? "If your total cholesterol is over 200, I recommend you have your test broken down by good and bad cholesterol levels," says Dr. Ulstad. "LDL levels, along with any additional risk factors you have, are what determine your treatment decisions." To figure out what levels of cholesterol are harmful for you, Dr. Ulstad recommends you start by assessing additional risk factors and consult the table at left.

If you have	You want your LDL cholesterol to be
No risk factors or one risk factor	Less than 160
Two or more risk factors	Less than 130
If you have vascular disease	Less than 100

RISK FACTORS

- High blood pressure
- Diabetes
- Heart disease in family
- Smoking
- Age forty-five or older

Other measurements, such as the ratio between your total cholesterol and HDL (you want it to be less than 4.5:1), are also thought to correspond to increased risk of heart disease and may be particularly important for men on HIV medications (see "Protease Paunch?" on page 413). The correlation between cholesterol levels and disease is admittedly rough rather than precise, with doctors disagreeing and some people living vastly longer or shorter lives than expected with supposedly unhealthy levels. "Just as we have no clue how to describe the varieties of sexual orientation, we have yet to determine the varieties of the ways cholesterol is metabolized in individuals," acknowledges Dr. Ulstad. "Still, the evidence is pretty overwhelming that when LDL levels are high, you need to take preemptive action."

Too much of the bad without enough of the good and you risk a partially clogged artery to the heart (causing chest pain known as angina), a totally clogged artery (causing a heart attack), or a narrowing of blood vessels to the brain (causing a stroke), among other arterial diseases.

Once you pass the age of seventy, the risks of cholesterol recede. Until then, if you're facing high levels, go for a low-fat, high-fiber, smoke-free lifestyle to heighten HDL and lower LDL. Weight loss and exercise over the course of a year can boost good cholesterol, and a small amount of alcohol —one glass of wine or one drink a night—seems to reduce the risk of heart attack. Finally, various studies conducted throughout the 1990s, as well as a meta-analysis by Harvard investigators of twenty-nine thousand people on the anticholesterol drugs known as statins, found the drugs to lower the risk of heart attack, stroke, and associated deaths by 20 to 35 percent. The drugs aren't cheap, $1,500 or more a year, and may need to be taken daily until you hit seventy. They also may interfere or interact badly with protease inhibitors processed by the same liver enzymes, so if you're on anti-HIV drugs, investigate alternatives such as gemfibrozil (Lopid) or atorvastatin (Lipitor), which are processed differently by the body. Exercise and diet are generally healthier than medication, though if those aren't working, talk to your doctor about the possibility of medical intervention.

HOW?

The coin-operated machines in the drugstore or the supermarket give you only total levels of cholesterol, which won't tell you how much of your total is bad and how much good. Some doctors prefer blood tests ordered in a doctor's office, says Val Ulstad, MD, cardiologist at the Minneapolis Heart Institute and former president of the Gay and Lesbian Medical Association. These tests measure total and HDL cholesterol, or, if necessary, may even break down HDL, LDL, and triglyceride levels. To get an accurate reading, you should fast, eating or drinking nothing but water, coffee, or tea (with no cream or sugar) for nine to twelve hours before the test.

One point worth noting: experts do not agree on how often tests are necessary, or when they should start. While the most conservative guidelines call for testing every five years starting at age twenty-one, others suggest waiting until age thirty-five to start, unless you have two or more risk factors (see box on previous page). Similarly, some suggest retesting every five years only if you have risk factors or are on the threshold of a cholesterol problem. Once again, reasonable doctors disagree.

HOW MUCH?

A cholesterol workup showing LDL usually costs about $30.

2. Blood Pressure

WHY?

High blood pressure, also known as hypertension, sounds familiar to any gay man walking through a crowd of high-school boys or hostile construction workers. Actually, tension is *not* the cause of hypertension, with stress causing only a temporary rather than a consistent elevation of blood pressure. And though blood pressure does go up with age, high-school students are not exempt. One out of three adult American men between eighteen and seventy-four has hypertension. Among Black men, the figure climbs to 38 percent. While some 5 percent of high blood pressure is caused by hormonal abnormalities or other conditions, the cause of 95 percent of it is unknown, attributed to everything from genes to diet, water supply, salt consumption, smoking, weight, or even processed food. Since hypertension often causes no symptoms until it leads to some kind of organ damage, yearly testing is especially important.

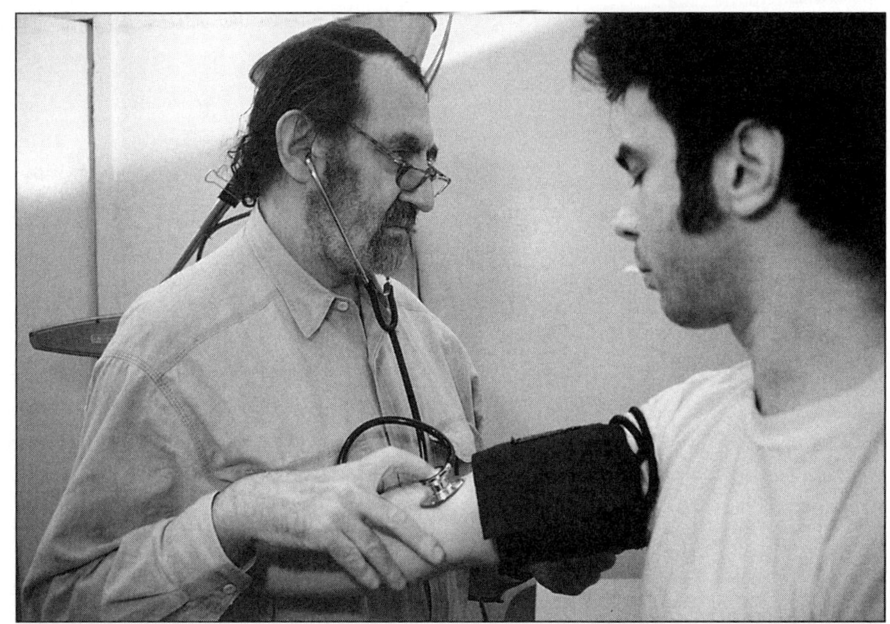

Blood pressure is usually described by two numbers, one on top of the other (it's what the staff on hospital shows are talking about when they shout "BP 120 over 80"). The top number is systolic pressure, the pressure when the heart is pumping blood out through your arteries; the bottom number is diastolic pressure, the force of the blood in the arteries when the heart is at rest. Systolic pressure above 140 or diastolic pressure above 90 qualifies as high blood pressure. As with cholesterol, there are grades of seriousness and of risk. Men with severe hypertension are more than ten times as likely to have a stroke, and five to six times as likely to have a heart attack, than those with normal blood pressure.

With the ill effects of hypertension so similar to those caused by cholesterol, the first lines of defense are also similar. Exercise in consultation with a doctor, throwing out the cigarettes, and changing to a low-fat, high-fiber diet can all help. Weight loss can lower blood pressure an estimated ten points for every twenty pounds lost. In addition to a low-fat diet, says Dr. Ulstad, it helps some people, though not all, to cut the salt. "This is especially true for African-American men," says Dr. Ulstad, "who may be more sensitive to the effects of sodium than White men are." More important still, for all men with high blood pressure, is to scale back on alcohol consumption. Goodbye, margaritas. Hello, virgin Mary.

HOW?

Virtually every physical exam in a doctor's office includes a blood pressure test, done with a cuff tightened around the arm and a stethoscope. You can also get free tests at some local chapters of the American Red Cross, at neighborhood health fairs, or on occasion at your local fire department, mall, or drugstore. Next time you see those nice volunteers with stethoscopes and blood pressure cuffs, shake hands, sit down, and roll up your sleeve. Since blood pressure often goes up when we're nervous—for example, when we're at the doctor's office—those places may be better anyway. Blood pressure fluctuates, says Dr. Ulstad, and so it's best to get three readings before deciding if it's an ongoing problem or just a bad day.

HOW MUCH?

Anywhere from free to the price of a doctor's visit.

#3. Hepatitis A and B Vaccines

I spent four days over Thanksgiving wandering around my grandmother's house like a vampire, feverish, with constant projectile vomiting, piss the color of iced tea, and a strange itching all over my skin.

WHY?

If you're gay and haven't had the liver infections known as hepatitis A or B, you may be a liver illness waiting to happen. While you can do your best to avoid the oral-fecal contact that transmits hepatitis A, many a gay man—including those who do not put their mouths "down there"—has found himself with yellow eyeballs, flu symptoms, vomiting, and other signs of this liver illness (see "Fecal Foes," page 152, for details). Some men choose to lay the blame on the fact that we eat out a lot (we're talking restaurants) or on our delicate preference for salads (contaminated water, produce, or hands handling the produce are major sources of hepatitis A). Whatever the cause, hepatitis A epidemics have been detected among gay men in Boston, Denver, Houston, New York, Seattle, and San Francisco, as well as in several cities abroad, over the last few decades. A vaccine that will protect you for a period of at least seven to ten years has been available in the United States since 1995, and in Europe for years longer. Have you had yours?

Hepatitis B (HBV) is more serious than hepatitis A, involving the risk of permanent liver damage and chronic infection as well as symptoms of the type associated with hepatitis A (see "The Condom Containables," page 156). It too is sexually transmitted—passed in the same ways as HIV, but a hundred times more easily. Hepatitis B is in many ways the original gay epidemic: Studies among gay men in the early 1980s showed rates of HBV exposure to be as high as 50 percent of men sampled. Safer-sex practices have since brought the numbers down to an estimated 20 percent, but the best way to stop infections—the vaccine—remains unused by many of us. Among young gay men in San Francisco, the CDC reported in 1996, fewer than 3 percent had been vaccinated. Those same young men—and any of the rest of us who have more than one sexual partner in a six-month period—run an estimated ten to fifteen times greater risk of HBV infection. Have you been vaccinated?

There's no vaccine for hepatitis C, most serious of the three. For more information on that illness, see page 158.

HOW?

Protection from hepatitis A and B requires two steps. The first is to get a blood test to see if you've had a "silent infection," a case of hepatitis A or B that had no symptoms. If you have had hepatitis A, you won't get it again, so you don't need a vaccine. In most cases hepatitis B, too, will leave you protected against future infection but without further complications. Between 5 and 10 percent of people get a chronic hepatitis B infection and need regular monitoring and

TAKE A SHOT: IMMUNIZATIONS FOR ADULTS

Some vaccines can spare you potentially deadly illnesses such as tetanus, nasty flus, and bacterial pneumonia. Make a note somewhere when you have them, so you don't unnecessarily repeat them. If you're moderately or seriously ill, or if your immune system is very weak, check with your doctor before getting vaccinated.

What?	When?	What you need to know if you're HIV +
Tetanus, diphtheria	Even if you had the recommended shots as a child, you need a booster every 10 years.	Same as everyone else.
Pneumococcal vaccine (bacterial pneumonia)	Once in a lifetime at age 65, or sooner if you have certain chronic illnesses.	All people with HIV should have one; a booster at five years may be needed.
Influenza (flu) vaccine	Once yearly in the fall for adults 65 and older, or for those with weak immune systems.	Recommended for all people with HIV, though some doctors say it may not be effective, and may stimulate HIV production, if you have under 200 CD4 cells.
Chicken pox (*Varicella zoster*) vaccine	Series of two shots, spaced 4–8 weeks apart. If you've never had chicken pox (or the vaccine), have this.	Not recommended for people with HIV. A *Varicella zoster* immune globulin shot may help prevent infection if administered within 96 hours after exposure, but it's expensive—often around $600.
Measles, mumps, rubella (MMR) vaccine	Recommended for all those born in 1957 or later if not previously vaccinated	Recommended for people with HIV who are not severely immune-compromised.

Adapted from Immunization Action Coalition (www.immunize.org)

possibly treatment (again, see page 156). If you've had only one or neither of these two kinds of hepatitis, there should be a vaccine in your future. If you find out about hepatitis because your partner has it, and you think you may have been exposed, talk to your doctor: The vaccine, or shots of immune globulin followed by the vaccine, may be your best course of protection.

The hepatitis A vaccine is a two-shot deal, administered in the arm, with the second given six to twelve months after the first. The hepatitis B vaccine can be administered at the same time, though it involves an extra shot, for a total of three shots spaced out over a six-month period. Both vaccines are safe for men who are HIV negative and positive, though they may be less effective if your immune system is weak. One study found that 25 percent of men with HIV received no protection from the hepatitis B vaccine.

HOW MUCH?

The vaccines can be pricey, as much as $75 a shot. Many insurance plans, from private ones to Medicaid, will pay for the blood tests to see if you have been exposed to hepatitis, and the treatment if you are chronically infected, but not for the vaccine to prevent the illness. "If they refuse, have your doctor remind them that the CDC recommends that sexually active gay men be vaccinated," says Howard Grossman, MD. "Sometimes I have to send a strongly worded letter, but in the end they give in." A number of gay and STD clinics in major cities around the country also offer vaccines at reduced or no cost. Contact your insurer to see if they cover the vaccines, or ask your local health department, gay clinic, or STD clinic about free or low-cost options. A local AIDS service organization might also know. Borrow the money if you need to. Your friends will prefer that to bringing you soup for weeks as you lie, yellow, nauseated and feverish, in bed, or watching you struggle with potentially serious liver damage.

#4. Testicular Self-Exam

WHY?

By the time most of us get around to reading those books on how men can live longer, we're old enough to have missed the most important years for this painless process. Testicular cancer, which self-exams help detect, is the most serious of testicular ailments. It most commonly afflicts men between the ages of fifteen and forty, or those in whom one testicle descended late or had to be surgically brought down. If your father or brother has had it, you also run an increased risk. If you *are* a brother—meaning of African or Caribbean descent—you're safer, since the cancer is least common in Black men and most common in Whites. Even so, testicular cancer

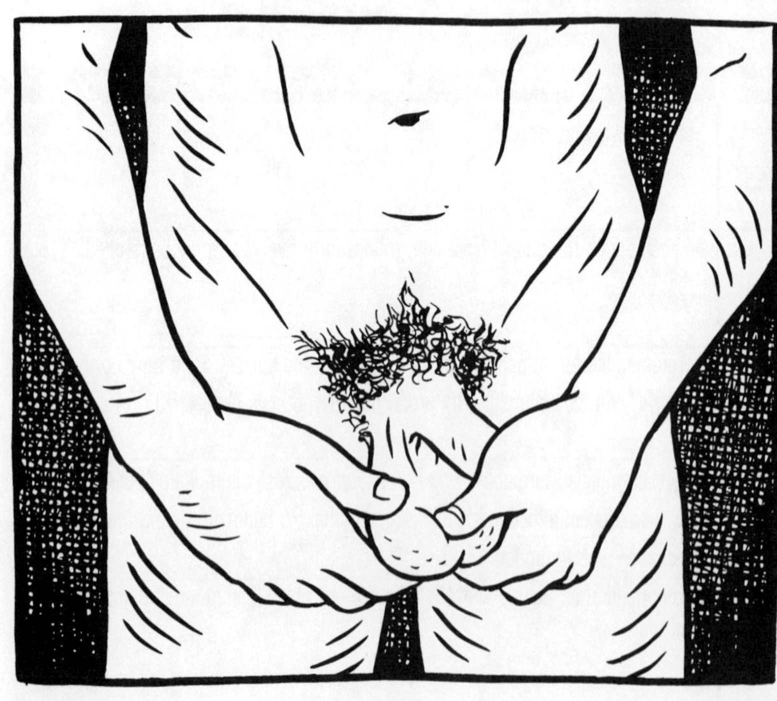

Testicular self-exam

is unusual—according to the National Cancer Institute, only 7,600 new cases are expected in 2000.

There's nothing particularly gay about this kind of self-examination, but it is crucial. "For young men, testicular cancer is *the* cancer," says Todd Yancey, MD, of the Bentley-Salick Center in New York City. "If detected early, treatment is removal of the testicle with an outpatient surgery that takes forty-five minutes. You can go home that day [with an implant if you want one], and there's a 100 percent cure rate." On the other hand, says Yancey, "treatment after testicular cancer has developed means all the radiation and chemotherapy they can throw at you, and removal of lymph nodes from the groin to the bottom of the diaphragm." While cure rates for testicular cancers are still high—an estimated 75 to 90 percent, depending on the type of cancer—you can take things in hand and spare yourself lots of difficulty. A doctor may examine your testicles during your annual physical, but he rarely knows as well as you do what they're like over time.

HOW?

Here's how to give yourself a testicular self-exam:

1. Choose a time when your sack is slack. Sperm die when they get too hot, so your scrotum rises and falls to keep your testicles and the sperm they contain slightly cooler than the rest of the body. It's best to feel your way around after a warm bath or shower, when your balls are loose and hanging low.
2. Weigh each testicle in the palm of your hand, and look at each. Don't panic if one hangs lower—in 85 percent of us, the left one does. The two should weigh about the same, and you want to be able to tell if one is larger than usual.
3. Take each ball between your thumb and first two fingers, with the thumb on top. Roll gently, looking for lumps, tenderness, and changes in consistency. Spend a minute or so. The slightly squiggly tube you feel is the epididymis, and the ridge in it is probably the tube that carries the sperm toward the urethra, the vas deferens. What you're looking for is not these, but a lump, usually pea-sized or so.

Even if you do find a lump or growth, it's unlikely to be cancer. One quick method doctors use for distinguishing between tumors and other kinds of growths is to shine a flashlight behind the testicle in question. Solid masses, like your testicle itself or a tumor, block the light, while fluid-filled or other less dense growths let it shine through. Even solid growths are often benign, though the doctor will send you for a sonogram. "They put moisturizer on my balls and rubbed a magic wand over them" is how Greg, a San Francisco advertising executive, described the painless process, which uses sound waves to give a picture of the testicle on a video monitor and costs around $300. His lump was a varicocele—one of a number of minor and, to his enormous relief, benign testicular ailments (see "Balls and Beyond," page 21). Any kind of lump should be reported to your doctor immediately. Waiting won't help.

HOW MUCH?

Two minutes of your time each month.

#5. HIV Test

Actually, I didn't decide. I went to enlist in the navy and during the physical they took my blood. Three days before they were going to put me on the boat, they came with the papers that said I'd been medically disqualified. They didn't give me any information, they just discharged me. I'd much rather have found out willingly.

As much as you can say, "Oh, I'm not positive," if you're going to do something with someone you love, you want to make sure it's the truth. Testing thrusts you into the present, into reality. For us, it forced us to decide what to do next.

Not knowing seemed like another kind of closet.

I was mentally prepared for being positive—I had it all planned out. When I got my result and I was negative, I was relieved, but in a strange way I was also kind of sad, because now I had to start planning over.

In the beginning you say, "Okay, I'm psyched, I'm ready." Then so many things go through your mind. It took a month to even call to make an appointment, and three tries before I felt like I could go back for the result.

WHY?

In 1989 the New York City Department of Health began to produce an HIV-testing campaign under a headline advising "Take this simple test." Gay and AIDS activists promptly slapped stickers over the posters, advising readers to think again. Facing discrimination isn't simple, they countered. Facing expensive, toxic medications of uncertain effectiveness isn't simple. Learning that you have a potentially fatal disease when you may have no access to health care or no clear idea of what to do next isn't simple. Stress isn't simple. Nothing about HIV is simple.

That was then. Now, the HIV test remains a complicated and stressful step to take, with lots of issues to think through before you rush to a testing site or send your blood into a lab from home. But things have changed—for the better. Now an overwhelming body of scientific data suggests that treating HIV before you show the symptoms of AIDS can alter the course of the disease and improve and lengthen your life. Now new technologies are making it easier to monitor the course of HIV and giving people more information about treatment decisions. Leading AIDS researchers like David Ho, MD, of New York City's Aaron Diamond Research Center, have claimed amazing success in beating down HIV by getting people onto treatment in the first months after they were infected, in some cases while people still had "symptoms of seroconversion" (see next page). "People need to make their own decisions about the hit-early-hit-hard strategy," says Dr. Todd Yancey. "But I can tell you that if I thought I was infected, I would use the fastest test available, and get treated before my HIV levels had time to shoot up." (For more on when or whether to start treatment, see Chapter 9.)

Most of us, apparently, are missing that message—and the opportunity for early treatment—entirely. While activists and public health officials argue about how early to take medications or about whether people's names should be tracked when they have HIV or only when they have AIDS, for the vast majority these questions are academic. Researcher Andy Bindman, MD, associate professor of medicine and acting chief of infectious diseases at San

TURN FOR THE WORSE: SYMPTOMS OF SEROCONVERSION

You don't always know when you've been infected with HIV. But as your body struggles to fight the virus, you often feel like you have a bad flu. As many as 50 to 90 percent of people newly infected with HIV experience symptoms that doctors term "seroconversion illness" or "acute retroviral syndrome," symptoms of which can include:

- Fever
- Feeling tired and weak
- Swollen glands or lymph nodes
- Skin rash
- Headache
- Sensitivity to light

If you have these symptoms shortly after having risky sex or sharing needles, get to a doctor immediately. Tests now available may be able to detect the virus even before you turn positive for antibodies, and treatments may help you be able to keep HIV at low levels for a long, long time (for more on this strategy, see "Game, Set, Match? Treatment for the Newly Infected," page 384).

Francisco General Hospital, surveyed testing data from confidential and anonymous HIV testing sites across the country. He found in 1998 that on average people had only one or two years between when they tested positive and when they developed AIDS. "What makes this all the more appalling," says Jeff Levi of George Washington University's Center for Health Policy Research, "is that people should have ten years, since that's how long it takes on average for HIV to progress to AIDS." Other statistics from the CDC offer sad punctuation to the fact that most of us are testing eight years too late: Each year, thousands of adults and adolescents are diagnosed with *Pneumocystis carinii* pneumonia (PCP), an AIDS-related pneumonia that is often deadly—and often preventable if you know you're at risk.

Taking the HIV test isn't simple. It *is* terribly important. When it comes to HIV, what you don't know can hurt you and your sexual partners.

Things to Think About Before You Test

Panic, fear of discrimination, worries about telling your employer or your family or your lover that you're positive: Is it any wonder that a third of the people tested at clinics and doctor's offices don't come back for their results? Thinking through the issues before you give your blood, or lose your cool, can help you decide whether to test and how to stay calm while you wait for your result. Things to think about include:

1. *Your risk.* Check out reality before you press the panic button. How likely is it that you're infected with HIV? If you've never had receptive anal sex without a condom or shared injection drug equipment, chances are very good you're not infected. If you've sucked someone without a condom, you're still at low risk (though not no risk). While testing is important, so is trying to get a sense of what you expect and what you might do if you were positive—before you get your result.

2. *Your support system.* Whom can you talk to before you test who might have good

advice or information? If you have to wait a week or two for your result, whom will you talk to in that period? How about if you test positive? Negative? Who cares enough about you to be of help?

3. *Your basic knowledge.* Do you know what the test is looking for? How about the difference between HIV and AIDS? Calling hot lines or a local AIDS organization to answer questions can help if you're not sure.

4. *Your boyfriend* (or spouse, partner, lover, copilot, significant other, or whatever you call him). If he exists, presumably he's part of #2, above. But if you haven't talked with him about the fact that you're testing, you're setting your relationship up for a shock. Similarly, taking the test just because he wants you to isn't always a smart idea. "I tested mostly because Tom was so freaked out about the idea of HIV," says Stanton, thirty-two. "And even though I was negative, I hated him for it and swore I would never, ever be put in that position again."

5. *Your basic health care.* If you don't have health insurance, it's a good idea to try to get it before you test. Insurance companies can make new enrollees wait six months or more for coverage of HIV-related medical care. If you can't afford insurance at the moment, see if your state offers you the option of testing anonymously (so no insurance company knows you know) to leave your options open.

6. *Your method.* There are a number of different kinds of HIV tests and a number of different places to get them. Anonymous testing, offered at health clinics, by some gay and lesbian health organizations, or through a home collection kit, allows you to be tested without ever giving your name; you're assigned a number and either go or call in for your result. Confidential testing, most common in doctor's offices and some state clinics, means you give your name when you get the test, but that the doctor or clinic does not tell anyone else (with a few possible exceptions—see next item) the result.

7. *Your rights.* The results of your HIV test are confidential by law. The doctor or clinician can reveal them only to people who "need to know." What this means can be tricky, since various studies have shown that for an average hospitalized patient, between 75 and 120 different people in the hospital claimed a "legitimate" need to see a patient's medical records. Your insurance company doesn't need to know, but if you ask for reimbursement for HIV-related care or lab tests later, they'll find out. Many states also require that the names of people who test positive be sent to the state health department, which in turn sends it to the CDC in Atlanta. Neither the CDC nor your doctor, however, is allowed to reveal your HIV status to your employer, your friends, or your family. Doctors are permitted to tell your sexual partner(s) if they know them, think you're having risky sex with them, and don't believe you will tell them yourself.

Some states offer voluntary partner notification programs, where they will contact people you've had sex with to warn them, without using your name, that they might be infected (see "Talking HIV," in Chapter 3). Some states make this mandatory by law, though if you don't "remember" the names of your sex partners or if you make up names, they're not going to throw you in jail. If you're relying on the state or city for help, make sure to ask how far behind they are, since it may take them months to reach someone you were hoping would find out right away.

In fourteen states doctors can test you without your informed consent. Other states require you to sign a separate form and get counseling; still others include HIV testing in

HIV TESTING AND REPORTING LAWS

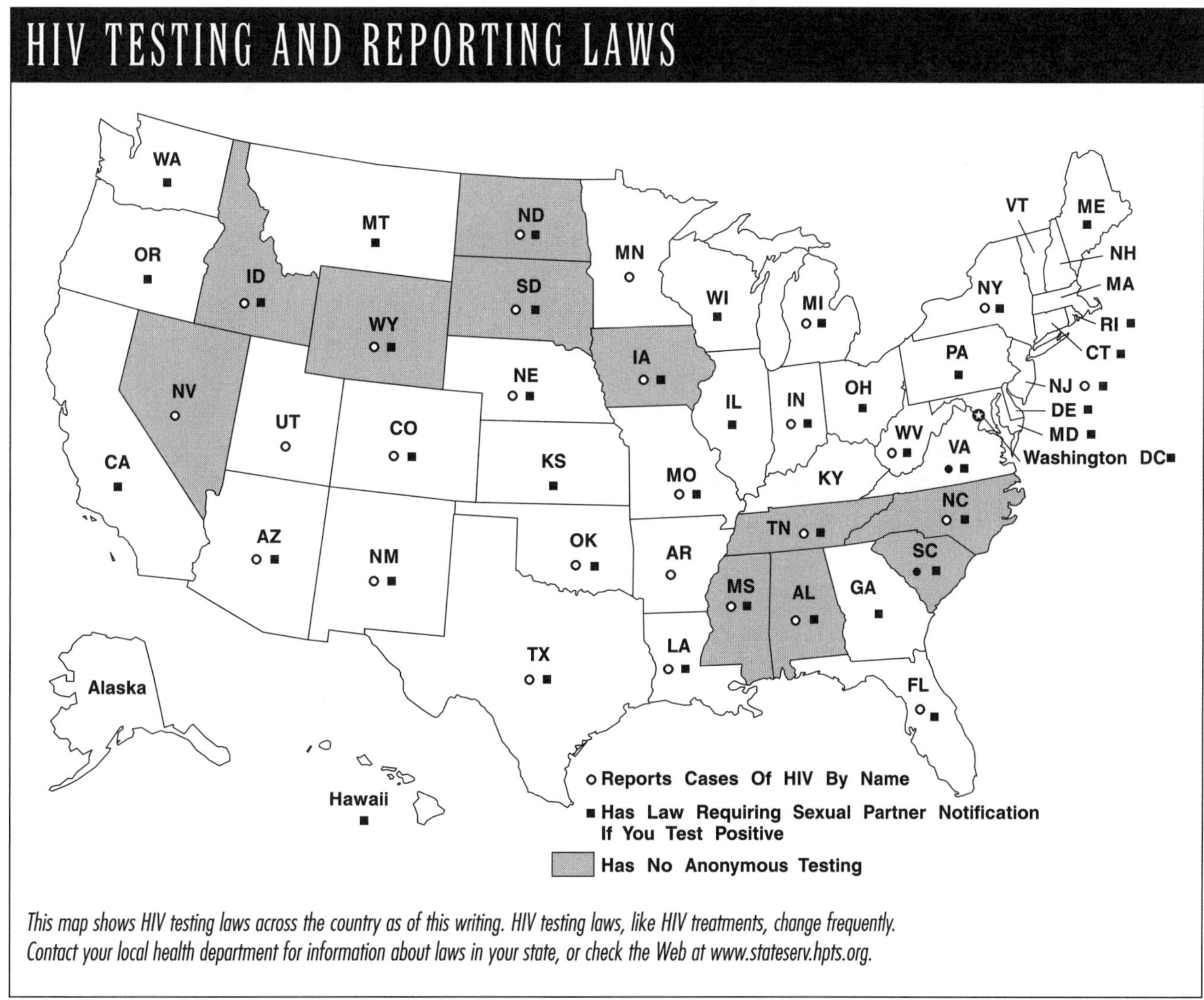

This map shows HIV testing laws across the country as of this writing. HIV testing laws, like HIV treatments, change frequently. Contact your local health department for information about laws in your state, or check the Web at www.stateserv.hpts.org.

larger consent forms at the hospital. People applying for life insurance, to give blood, or to join the military, Job Corps, or Peace Corps are almost always tested without being asked. So are prisoners and applicants for "green cards."

HOW AND HOW MUCH

The HIV-1 Antibody Test

When most people say they took an HIV test or "tested positive," this is the test they're talking about. It's not a test for the virus itself, but one that looks in your blood for the antibodies that your immune system produces to try to control HIV after infection. The lab usually does three tests of your blood before they can tell you're positive: two ELISA tests, which register antibodies to HIV and some other diseases, and another test called the Western blot, to confirm that HIV infection and not something else caused the positive ELISAs. When two ELISAs and a Western blot confirm your HIV infection, the result is accurate 99.7 percent of the time. False negatives are virtually unknown, though a tiny fraction of tests are "inconclusive," and about three of every thousand people gets a false positive result. HIV testing is now "among the most accurate diagnostic tools in medicine," writes Seth Kalichman, author of *Preventing AIDS* (Lawrence Erlbaum Associates, 1998).

It's also slow. Men who come to GMHC and other testing sites say the one- to two-week waiting period can be intensely stressful. A few centers offer testing buddies—people who check in with you during the wait to make sure you have the information and the access to support you need. If your local testing center doesn't offer such a plan, consider creating your own, asking a friend to see you through the two-week period. Quite a few people choose another way to manage stress—going on the prowl for sex—and find that by the time they get their test results, they're wondering if they need to have another.

In New York City, public testing sites have also begun to test for HIV-2, a strain of the virus most common in Asia and Africa but increasingly detected here in the United States. If you have any possibility of having been infected while in those regions, or by someone who's spent time there, talk to your doctor or local health department about HIV-2 testing.

As for how long after risky sex or needle sharing you should wait to test, the ELISA test is more sensitive than it used to be. For 99 percent of people, says Sara Beatrice, Ph.D., director of the Bureau of Laboratories for the New York City Department of Health, the "window" between the time you get infected and when you test positive is now only three months. Even that's generous, since somewhere around 95 percent of people will show antibodies within a month. Still, if you test negative a month after a risky encounter, it's best to test again a few months later, just to make sure.

Costs for the standard HIV-1 antibody test can range from free (at public test sites) to around $100 in your doctor's office.

The bDNA Test

This is a test licensed to measure levels of HIV in your blood (see page 387), not to see if the virus is present in the first place. Still, many doctors interviewed for this book said that this is the test they would use if they suspected they had just been infected, since it can register HIV in your blood even before antibodies have even had time to develop (meaning within two to three weeks of exposure). Whether you gain anything by knowing a week earlier is a complicated question (again, see "Game, Set, Match? Treatment for the Newly Infected," page 384). This test is more expensive than the HIV antibody test (often around $160), not deemed completely reliable as a diagnostic measure, and may not be recommended by your doctor. It is also not usually covered by insurance for diagnostic purposes, though if it turns out you're HIV-positive, they might pay.

The "Rapid" HIV Test

Gay magazines in urban centers now sport ads for a "fifteen-minute" HIV test, made to spare you the agony of a two-week wait. The CDC, too, concerned about how many Americans tested with a standard antibody test doesn't come back for the results, is encouraging use of this test. What they don't tell you is that you get your result in fifteen minutes only if you're HIV-negative; if they think you might be positive, they usually have to send out for a confirmatory Western blot (which will take at least a few days) to separate out the false positives from the real ones. Even if you get a negative result, it may be less reliable than the standard HIV antibody test, warns Dr. Beatrice. The test used at these testing centers, known as the Murex test, has to be done within fifteen minutes. With well-trained and adequately supervised lab technicians, excellent facilities, and no distraction, this isn't a problem. In the real world, even a phone call or a bathroom break can throw the process off. If the test isn't done again (and it's expensive, so some offices don't repeat it), then the human error isn't picked up, and neither is your infection.

Waiting for three or four days with the gnawing fear that you might be positive can also be as bad as (or worse than) waiting a week without having any idea. Finally, the test can be costly: 1999 prices in New York, Los Angeles, and San Francisco ranged from $95 to as high as $150.

The Oral Test

This test collects a sample of "oral mucosal transudate," collected by placing a small pad on a handle between your lower cheek and gum for two minutes. One downside is that you have to think about the fact that there is something in your body called oral mucosal transudate. Another is that the test is available only in doctors' offices and a few clinics. An upside is no needles or drawing of blood. The pad is sent to a local lab or the manufacturer for analysis, and testing is as accurate as the HIV antibody test above. You can get a negative result back in as little as twenty-four hours, but, as with the fifteen-minute test, if it's positive, you need to wait for a confirmatory Western blot test. The oral test costs doctors about $100 for three tests, including lab work. How much they charge you is up to them.

The Home Test

Actually, it's a home collection kit: You prick your finger, dab a little blood on the special area of the paper, and send it overnight to the lab for analysis. You retrieve the results by dialing a toll-free number and punching in a personal identification number (PIN) you've been assigned with the kit. If you pay extra, you can get the result in three days; otherwise it takes a week. The advantage, so long as you don't leave the wrapper sitting out in your trash, is that you can get tested without anyone else's knowledge. The disadvantages include the fact that you get no face-to-face counseling before the test, have to shell out $39.95, and get your result on the phone. They do offer counseling and supposedly up-to-date referrals to local services, though talking to someone in Kansas when you're in Montana may not be enough to stop you from hanging up and jumping out the window. "For people who've thought through the issues, it may seem like an easy option," says Beth Gery, MD, a psychiatrist and HIV testing expert in New York City. "But I'd be hard-pressed to recommend it in the best of circumstances."

A further consideration with home tests, as with many for-profit ventures, is that their ads aim to sell a test rather than to make you think seriously about what taking it might mean. Home Access Health Corporation, the manufacturer of the Home Access HIV test, launched a campaign in men's magazines with the dubious slogan "Why Women Find a Little Prick Attractive." The text then went on to explain how much more aroused your girlfriend would be when she learned that you were responsible enough to take the test. Needless to say, "her" relief, or yours, will really be greater only if you're negative, since "You're positive? I love it, let's screw!" is rarely anyone's response, regardless of gender. If you've been at risk for HIV, don't be swayed by appeals to how relieved you'll be at your result. Perhaps that's one reason why the company didn't run the same ad series in gay magazines. Or maybe "Why Men Find a Little Prick Attractive" sounded like too much of a stretch.

HOME IS WHERE THE TEST IS

Recognizing our need for privacy, our dislike of long waits in the doctors' offices, and the fact that we are a nation of do-it-yourselfers, hundreds of companies have followed where the humble home pregnancy kit began. Today, more than three hundred home test kits are licensed by the FDA, from strep throat tests to do-it-yourself IQ assessments. Besides the home-collection HIV test (see previous page), some of the more common include:

The Test	The Method	The Warnings
Cholesterol	You prick your finger, dab it on a pad, and watch what happens. Fifteen minutes later, if the colored columns on the chemically treated paper rise past a certain point, your cholesterol's high.	Doesn't distinguish between good and bad cholesterol (HDL and LDL), meaning that you could have acceptable overall cholesterol levels and still be in danger of a heart attack.
Blood sugar	Used especially by insulin-dependent diabetics, this test allows you to prick your finger and test your blood sugar level.	Not for first-time diabetes detection and no substitute for a doctor's exam if you're experiencing the extreme thirst, hunger, frequent urination, or sudden weight loss that may be indicative of adult-onset diabetes.
FOB (fecal occult blood test) test for colorectal cancer	Test manufacturers know the (fecal) matter at hand, at least when it's *in* hand, is nobody's favorite. For this test, you drop a pad into the toilet, and if it turns a certain color, it's positive.	Misses an estimated one out of three cancers, which don't bleed, and gives you a false positive if you have a hemorrhoid, have just eaten rare meat, or had high doses of vitamin C. For more on colorectal cancer, see the "Tests You Need" section in Chapter 8.
Hepatitis C (HCV)	As with the "home" HIV test, only the blood collection happens at home. You send the sample in to a lab and call in for results and, if necessary, for a medical referral.	Tells you if you've had HCV, not if it's chronic or still doing damage. For that, you need a doctor and probably a viral load test.

Home tests are a little like vitamins—they're designed as a supplement to, not a substitute for, the main course (in this case, course of treatment). If a test does detect a problem, make sure to see a doctor.

Finally, doing these tests at home is better than buying them there. Though reputable companies do use the Internet and the mail, a lot of fraudulent companies use the Web to market unlicensed tests, particularly to people who may be anxious about going someplace for a test relating to sexual behavior or other potentially embarrassing subjects. Among the offenders reported by callers to GMHC's hot line, or flagged by the FDA, in the last few years alone: unlicensed chlamydia tests and hepatitis A tests, eight different HIV tests that falsely promised to give you the results at home, and a test claiming to see if you have the genetic mutations that may protect you against getting infected with HIV.

When you call companies on their misrepresentations, the Web site often vanishes, with no way to trace it. If you're wondering about the legal status of an at-home test kit, get the name of the test and its manufacturer and call the FDA's Consumer Information Inquiries Line at (888) 463-6332. HIV tests are classed as "biologics," and all the others are "medical devices."

If you test positive, however you decide to test, you'll have many questions about what happens next (see Chapter 9). If you test negative, you may also feel confused instead of relieved, or have mixed feelings you didn't expect. Increasing numbers of AIDS organizations now offer support to HIV-negative men struggling to stay that way. Call to see.

Alternative and Complementary Medicines

If there's anything gay men share, it may be a certain amount of skepticism toward the idea that accepted wisdoms are always wise. That grain of skepticism has no doubt helped nurture an affinity between gay men and practitioners of "alternative" medicine (chiropractors, acupuncturists, naturopaths, herbalists, and a host of lesser-knowns), who also tend to question accepted truths and find themselves marginalized by the powers that be. Years of being told AIDS was hopeless and having to search out new ways of thinking about and treating the disease also strengthened support for alternative medicine in certain gay communities. Some of us supported it in the first place, having an affinity with the women who carried the folk remedies—whether that was Coke syrup to quiet an upset stomach, meat tenderizer for a bee sting, or chamomile tea bags to soothe a sunburn—to the rest of the family.

Alternative medicine can refer to other systems of medicine, such as homeopathy, or to specific treatments used as alternatives to Western drugs (such as taking Saint-John's-wort rather than Prozac for depression). In either instance, the name "alternative" is outdated. Mainstream medical practitioners were shocked when the *New England Journal of Medicine* reported in 1993 that annual out-of-pocket expenditures on alternative care had reached over $10 billion, nearly as much as Americans paid for their own hospital care. While Americans made 388 million visits to primary-care doctors, they made 425 million visits—37 million more—to alternative-care providers such as massage therapists and acupuncturists. With an estimated 42 percent of Americans now using some form of alternative care, "complementary" medicine—meaning therapies pursued in conjunction with Western (also called allopathic) approaches—is probably a more appropriate name. That's not quite right, either, since many Americans seem to suspect that their doctors don't want them to take a complement. More than 70 percent of those who used complementary therapies in the *NEJM* survey admitted they didn't tell their allopathic doctors about them. "There's a long tradition of antagonism between what's called alternative medicine and so-called allopathic or Western medicine," says George M. Carter of New York City's dietary supplement buyer's club, Direct AIDS Alternative Information Resource (DAAIR). "Sadly, this artificial divide keeps people from understanding the benefits and risks of more integrated approaches, to everyone's detriment."

False Profits? Alternative Medicine, the Pharmaceutical Industry, and Science

"People who talk loudest about complementary medicine historically fall into two camps," says Bob Lederer, senior editor at *POZ* magazine in New York: practitioners, who accept its claims without question, and conservative researchers, doctors, and self-proclaimed "quackbusters," who dismiss it all as nonsense. Supporters often point to individual success stories: healing far beyond what Western medicine can explain or deliver, accomplished by herbs, therapeutic touch, visualization, or any combination of holistic healing methods that address mind and body. Detractors take refuge in a basic principle of Western science: that the individual story proves little beyond the fact that people think they know what causes changes in their lives, and that only controlled scientific trials can separate intuition from facts. The only thing on which everyone seems to agree is that herbal medicine and other forms of alternative treatments have yet to be studied adequately.

Why certain things get studied and others don't is a question less often asked but equally important when it comes to alternative treatments. Herbal medicines and relatively low-tech, low-cost medical procedures such as acupuncture are often held back by the force behind the science: the patent-and-profit motive. "It's going to be difficult to get a company to assemble the two tractor-trailers full of paperwork and $100 million minimum needed for drug approval in this country to test something unpatentable like garlic," says Michael Onstott, executive director of the National AIDS Nutrient Bank in Guerneville, California. "At the end of the process, any other company can come in and say, 'Thanks for making this possible. Now we'll market it, too.'" Similar forces structure our approach to medicine as a whole, says David Gilden, longtime editor of GMHC's journal of new and experimental AIDS therapies, *Treatment Issues*. "American medicine's emphasis on intervention, rather than prevention, has an economic structure," he says. "Packaging highly technical knowledge into medications and equipment that doctors and drug companies can charge patients to dumbly apply is a lot more profitable than instructing people on how to live healthy lives."

With potential profits even greater than the high development costs—the anti-HIV drug nelfinavir (Viracept), for example, grossed more than $56 million in the first four months after its approval in 1997, while the erectile dysfunction remedy sildenafil (Viagra) topped $300 million in the same period—pharmaceutical manufacturers and the medical system have a definite interest in protecting their turf. "Traditionally, the organizations most vocally opposing alternative medicines have strong ties to health insurers, conservative doctors, and other professional groups who make money by keeping things the way they are," says Lederer. While the National Institutes of Health have formed a National Center for Complementary and Alternative Medicine and an Office of Dietary Supplements, the two act more to coordinate research efforts and synthesize results than they do to conduct groundbreaking investigation. Their combined budget was only $52 million in 1999—easily less than the minimum necessary for the kind of research required for FDA approval of a single drug.

Even if funded to move more herbal products into the realm of accepted drugs, though, researchers of many alternative methods might not be able to meet FDA standards. "Western approaches put a premium on breaking things down to their smallest organizational level, the cause of a problem at the level of a cell or particular body part," says Gilden. "We pay specialists who look at a single organ or system far more than we give to primary-care doctors charged with caring for our body as a whole." On a pharmacological level, the FDA requires that manufacturers seeking approval of a new drug be able to identify a single active agent and its mechanism of action, a stipulation nearly impossible to meet in traditional herbal medicine. "Within a particular herb or plant, there are multiple compounds," says Lederer, "and Chinese formulations not uncommonly include as many as ten different herbs. With that many complex interactions, it's difficult to conduct a study that will even get you in the FDA's front door."

Instead, dietary supplement manufacturers have taken their business elsewhere, lobbying successfully to be allowed to market their products as food supplements outside FDA jurisdiction. The approach, supported by health food shoppers across the nation, successfully beat back attempts to remove the products from the shelves in 1993, and achieved the passage of the 1994 Dietary Supplement Health and Education Act. The law allows products to be sold, but bars them from making explicit claims about their ability to treat specific health conditions. So long as the claims can be substantiated, companies can say "immune-boosting," for example, but not "AIDS-fighting." In the eyes of many, it's an imperfect advance. "Traditional holistic medicine, with its concern with different bodily systems, environmental factors, and diet, is less about magic than about care and rigor," says Gilden. "Now, instead of articulated systems like Chinese or Ayurvedic medicine, we're seeing more 'alternative' medicine that really isn't holistic at all, but uses plant products for a quick, pharmaceutical-style fix. Just because something's natural doesn't mean we know it's safe—let alone effective." Onstott echoes the concern, pointing to the lines of "herbaceuticals" and "nutriceuticals" now jostling for position on health food store shelves. "Chinese practitioners never prescribe astralagus without combining it with several other herbs," he says, citing one of many such products, "and the concentrations contained in each of these [health food store] capsules would be impossible to attain through ordinary, nonpharmaceutical means." His solution? Reexamination of the magic-pill approach to health, a more European-style research effort that allows for greater flexibility (they've used homeopathic remedies for years), and extensive consumer education.

Lesson number one, says Lederer, may be that industry is industry. "I was one of the naive ones who thought that persecution of the dietary supplement companies meant that they were blameless, but there are good and bad supplement manufacturers," he acknowledges. Some, he says, have voluntarily done what their lobbying made them exempt from: monitoring quality of their products to ensure that they are not contaminated and that each capsule or jar contains the same amount of product. Others haven't bothered, stressing marketing over quality control. "The FDA has finally moved to set up good-manufacturing-practice guidelines for herbal products," says George Carter of DAAIR. "But it remains to be seen if they'll make any reasonable or systematic effort to enforce them."

With an estimated 106,000 annual deaths and 2.2 million illnesses from adverse reactions to Western medicines (and that's just in hospitals, for medications that were properly prescribed), the hype around the handful of recorded deaths and bad reactions from potentially toxic plants such as ephedra, comfrey, or pennyroyal may seem overblown. Indeed, alternative treatment experts point to incidents such as the 1988 removal of the amino acid tryptophan from the market to fault the FDA for an intense preoccupation with dietary supplements and an ignorance of the problems brewing in its own labs. "The fifteen hundred or so people who got sick or died from tryptophan did so as the result of a contaminated batch, not because the product as a whole was harmful," says Carter. "It would be like looking at the thousands of deaths reported each year from aspirin and saying, 'That's it, no more for anyone.'"

Until there is better data on interactions between drugs and supplements and better physician education, says Onstott (who combines protease inhibitors and a complicated regimen of Chinese herbs, amino acids, and other nutritional supplements to keep his own HIV wasting at bay), self-monitoring and consultation with a good alternative practitioner will have to do. That herbs, supplements, and other complementary approaches have healing power seems beyond question to him and many thousands of others who have studied Chinese, Ayurvedic, or homeopathic medicine to learn alternative ways of healing. For those interested in such disciplines, the rise of the alternative medicine that's not a real alternative—the take-two-Saint-John's-wort-and-call-me-in-the-morning approach—is a more bittersweet pill to swallow.

What's Your Alternative?

My roommate came out and said, "What happened to you?" My skin was bright red, I had a 104-degree fever. It turns out I had an allergic reaction to the flu medication. Of course it could always happen, but I decided then that I didn't want to feel like a test animal anymore. I didn't want to give up that power, to let other people put things into my body without understanding, at least somewhat, the risks and benefits.

At my regular doctor, if my appointment is with him at 9:00, I sit until 9:30, go into another room and change, and sit there until 10:00, and then the doctor shows up for ten minutes. My Ayurvedic physician costs me more, but if my appointment is at 9:00, then I am in with him at 9:00 and have his undivided attention. He'll start out by asking, "What's new in your life? What's been going on?" Sometimes he'll start with any physical problems, or ask if I'm still at that job, or what kind of exercise I'm doing. I feel like he's actually checking up on me in the best sense, peering into my life. I use him as a guide to see how well I've been taking care of myself.

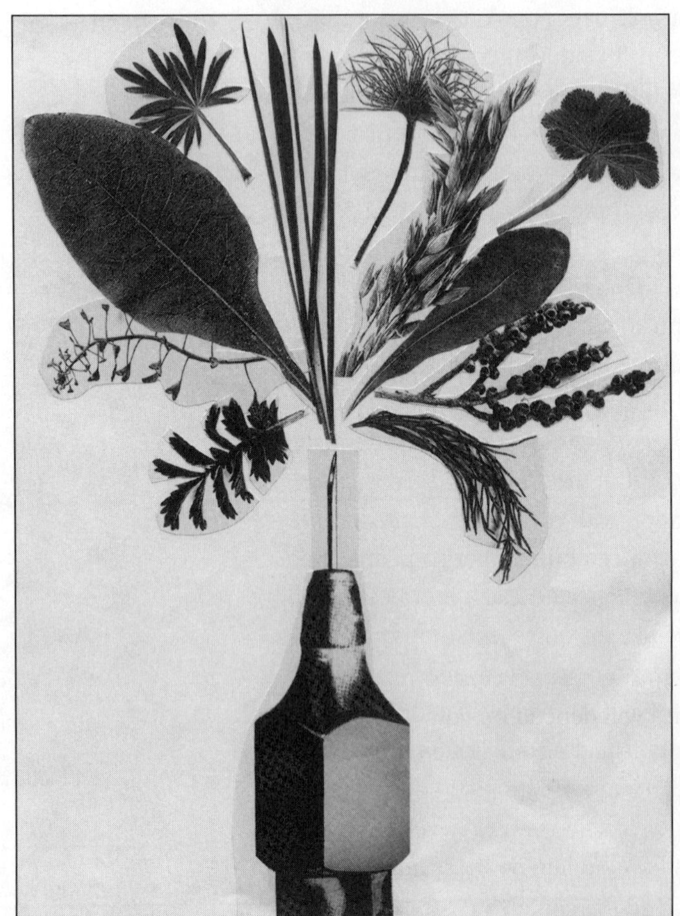

It's not just plants and meditation and diet. When my doctor needs to, he'll say, "You know, I think we're going to need to treat this with antibiotics." But when he does that, he also tells me about how I might change my diet, and about taking acidophilus to replace the flora and fauna the medicine kills off in my gut. Armed with that information, the antibiotic was painless: I had none of the gas or bloating or pain that I'd gotten before.

My attitude is I'll try anything if it'll help, but the medicine my doctor gave me for my liver didn't help. It gave me chills. It made me sick. It made my hepatitis viral load not show up on tests, but it turned out that the virus was still attacking. I decided I was going to attack in a different way, too, and investigate my options.

With increasing numbers of insurance companies paying for acupuncture, yoga, and meditation, and with medical schools increasing the number of hours their curricula devote to topics such as nutrition and herbal therapies, the divide between approaches is closing. "There's an evolution, or revolution, closing the gap between the Western get-the-bug-with-the-drug approach and the holistic approach that addresses both the bug *and* its host," says Carter. The number of osteopathic physicians (DOs rather than MDs), whose academic standards include training nearly identical to that of MDs and up to an additional three hundred hours of training in body manipulation and hands-on healing, will have grown from twenty-five thousand in 1989 to an estimated forty-five thousand by the year 2000. Enrollment is rising steadily in certified naturopathic medical schools, whose four years of training in nutrition, homeopathy, physical medicine, and counseling, followed by a series of board exams, now qualify graduates to be licensed health care providers (and in some cases, to write prescriptions) in eleven states. Just outside of Seattle, home of Bastyr University's school of naturopathic medicine, the first public health clinic in the country to use natural medicines and receive funding from tax dollars opened in 1996. "Things have come farther in the last five years than I ever thought we would in my lifetime," says Rick Elion, MD, a Washington, DC, physician, herbalist, and acupuncturist who works to educate conventionally trained physicians about complementary medicine.

Others among the seven hundred thousand or so traditionally trained doctors are recognizing that having books in their offices about complementary methods of healing makes for good patient relations, if sobering bedtime reading. There are more and more to choose from: *Ageless Body, Timeless Mind,* by Ayurvedic physician Deepak Chopra, MD; *Spontaneous Healing,* by physician and herbalist Andrew Weil, MD; and *Anatomy of the Spirit,* by medical intuitive Caroline Myss, Ph.D., were all huge best-sellers in the late 1990s. Each took on Western medicine in terms that might make more than one old-school doctor rush to the medicine cabinet to pop a few tranquilizers. "Maybe if other doctors seemed more interested in healing, there'd be fewer of us who feel like we need to go outside of traditional medicine," says Robert, who at forty-five has nursed nearly a dozen friends through AIDS and his father through open-heart surgery. "I can't buy all the white-light stuff or the people who say they've cured themselves of AIDS with licorice root. But I know that our achievements with technology and medications aren't enough to give people all the help they need to feel cared for. When my father was in the hospital, there were doctors all over him, measuring and testing but not healing or caring. It was almost like they were going to measure and measure until they finally looked up and said, 'The machines say there's nothing here. He's dead.'"

Somewhere between the accusations that Western medicine is all poison or claims that alternative medicine is hogwash lies what DAAIR's George Carter calls "the commonsense truth." "Patients, as well as practitioners, feel reassured by creating a polarity between this way or that way, but it's a false divide," agrees Dr. Elion, who often makes two appointments with patients: one to discuss Western approaches and one for complementary medicine. General guidelines about the appropriateness of various approaches can be helpful: Bacterial infections and acute medical crises such as heart attacks, diabetic comas, and bowel obstructions are particularly helped by Western medicines, while holistic approaches that look at diet, herbs, and vitamins are often better suited to management of "incurable" viral infections or chronic diseases like arthritis. Still, how you integrate the approaches will depend on you. "Thinking 'and/and' rather than 'either/or' is probably healthy," says Dr. Elion, whose prescriptions for patients with AIDS are likely to include both antivirals (for HIV) and milk thistle (for the liver problems the medications can cause). For sinus infections, Dr. Elion favors not only antibiotics but garlic and a dairy-free diet. "If your doctor doesn't know how to blend, then it may fall on you to learn," he says. In the absence of an herb-friendly doctor, buyer's clubs—non-profit distributors of information and alternative medications—often offer fact sheets and low-cost supplies. In New York, DAAIR (www.daair.org) offers and excellent info-pack, and links to other groups.

One part of consumer education is to stay skeptical of all sources of information, and watch your wallet. "People frame it as a struggle between the overzealous, pharmaceutical-friendly FDA 'protecting' the public from products that can help them, and the multibillion-dollar supplements industry interested primarily in making a buck," says Carter. "Both characterizations are pretty dead-on." Even the most committed complementary-treatment providers, those who sit down and work with you for amounts of time that seem unprecedented, are often reimbursed little or nothing by insurance companies, leaving you with hefty charges for their time. This does not make them disreputable (for information on how to separate out the frauds from the princes, see "Hope from Hype II," page 436), just expensive. As with other doctors, you have every right to ask what costs a course of complementary treatment may involve. "I went to a wonderful man, trained in China, who gave me a great acupuncture treatment and some vials of superconcentrated garlic extract he'd imported, and told me I should come back every two weeks," says Donald, thirty-six, who was grappling with chronic fatigue syndrome. "Then I went to the receptionist, who asked for $185 on the spot, none of which insurance reimbursed. I couldn't show up for the next appointment."

Alt.med

Systems of alternative medicine vary depending on the traditions from which they are drawn, though all tend to treat the whole person rather than just the disease. In Ayurvedic medicine, for example, a medical system that has been practiced continually for more than five thousand years, physicians use a combination of examination techniques to determine which of three constitutional "types" you fall into, and then prescribe diet, movement, herbal remedies, aromatherapy, meditation, cleansing techniques, and other approaches to maintain balance. Homeopathic medicine, based on the ancient principle that "like cures like" and refined several hundred years ago in Europe, uses highly diluted solutions of the natural substances that make you sick (such as pollen for allergies, for example) to heal you. Traditional Chinese medicine uses herbs (often in the form of decoctions, or strong brewed teas), acupuncture, and energy work (see "Mind and Body," page 216) to restore balance and health to the body. Naturopathic medicine synthesizes a number of the approaches above, using herbs, homeopathy, nutritional advice, stress management, and Western screening techniques to help individuals stay healthy.

Western evaluation of these systems has tended to focus on the individual components, rather than the system as a whole, at times confirming the effects of the methods even as it discards traditional explanations. Following are descriptions of a few of those methods. Resources for further information are found in Appendix A.

ACUPUNCTURE

Especially effective for: Pain, nausea, stress, drug-related cravings, asthma, stroke rehabilitation, and carpal tunnel syndrome.

Chinese medicine involves the study of the flow of energy along twelve pathways, or meridians, each associated with a particular organ system or function. Symptoms result from disruptions in the energy flow; acupuncture, through the insertion of ultrafine needles into specific meridians, seeks to restore the balance. Practitioners also spin the needles or apply mild electrical current or heat to enhance the effect. Educational requirements for becoming a licensed or certified acupuncturist vary from state to state, though a single agency, the National Commission for the Certification of Acupuncturists, ensures competency of practitioners.

BIOFEEDBACK

Especially effective for: Anxiety, nausea, pain, high blood pressure, asthma, migraine headaches, grinding of teeth, irritable bowel syndrome, and urinary incontinence.

You don't have to be a yoga master to ease muscle tension, slow your heartbeat, deepen your breathing, improve blood flow, or control other physical responses that we often think of as involuntary. Biofeedback turns technology to the study of mind-body relations, hooking you up to a machine that measures heart rate, electrical activity in the brain, and the like, letting you see how mental focus can achieve bodily results. Lights blink or beeps sound as you successfully raise your body temperature, for example, open blood vessels to ease the pain of a migraine, or relax smooth muscles in the bronchial tubes to allow more air to enter. After eight or ten feedback sessions, you can often remove the machinery but keep the effect. Two hundred hours of formal training and a degree in a related field is required for certification by the Biofeedback Certification Institute of America.

BODYWORK

Especially effective for: Joint and muscle pain, circulation, tension headaches, digestive disorders, stress, and musculoskeletal disorders.

This is really many practices in one category, ranging from the adjustment of joints and misaligned bones of the body, done by chiropractors, to your basic massage to remove toxins and increase the circulation of oxygen (and pleasure) in the body. Theories vary with the practice, though most are based on the idea that removing blockages (whether physical or "energetic") allows for freer movement of muscles, joints, nerve impulses, and sensation. Ironically, the chiropractors regularly denounced as quacks in the 1950s are now among the most accepted bodyworkers in the American medicinal system, often covered by insurance and trained in an accredited four-year training program. Since the nervous system is linked to all different organ systems in the body, chiropractors often treat holistically, assessing and suggesting ways of diet, exercise, and stress reduction.

Eighty different forms of massage are currently taught and practiced in the United States, and sixty of them were developed in the last twenty years. Massage therapists are licensed in different ways from state to state through the accreditation program of the American Massage Therapy Association, though many forms of bodywork—from the Alexander Technique to acupressure—have independent professional associations and standards of certification. Anyone, as is evident from the back of your local gay rag or porn magazine, can call himself a masseur, so ask around to figure out what you want and how likely it is a particular practitioner will give it to you.

HERBAL MEDICINE

Especially effective for: Chronic conditions such as fatigue, depression, anxiety, viral infections, nausea, arthritis, digestive problems, elevated cholesterol levels, and thousands of other conditions for which over-the-counter or prescription medications are commonly employed.

Somewhere between a quarter and a half of commonly used Western medicines are derived from plants. Aspirin came from white willow bark, and the heart medication digitalis is still derived from the foxglove plant. Many more drugs are synthetic copies of naturally occurring plant compounds; ephedrine and pseudoephedrine, for example, are laboratory versions of compounds from the herb ma huang (*Ephedra sinensis*). The basis for most traditional medicine in the world, herbal medicine generally uses plants with medicinal properties in a less distilled or processed form than those prepared by pharmaceutical companies. Capsules, teas, decoctions (very strong teas), and tinctures—concentrated herbal extracts suspended in alcohol or glycerin—are among the common routes of administration in the United States, though the eating of plants or drinking of their juice, herbal enemas, and intravenous herbal extracts are all used in Europe for medicinal effects. So, increasingly, are "herbaceuticals" or "nutriceuticals," pills or capsules whose highly concentrated contents are isolated through chemical means. Though these are more concentrated, whole plants in some cases are more effective, says Charles Rosenberg, MS, CN, a Seattle herbalist and certified nutritionist. "Medicinal plants contain hundreds of active compounds that act together, many of which have yet to be identified," he explains.

Using plants themselves rather than chemical extracts found in pharmaceuticals has its downside. The earth is not as controlled an environment as a science lab, and soil and climate conditions, time of harvesting, and storage all affect the power of the plant. "Buying organic herbs from a reputable manufacturer can help with quality control," says Rosenberg. Fortunately, most herbal treatments are safe enough that you can adjust your dosage within the guidelines on the package until you achieve the desired effect.

Is it safe to self-treat with herbs? Rosenberg says it is, within reason. "Any ailment you would treat with an over-the-counter medicine—a cold, upset stomach, allergy, or general aches and pains—is appropriate to treat with herbs you buy in health-food stores or pharmacies," he says. For more serious disorders, a variety of herbs may help, but they should be used in consultation with your healers, including MDs.

Mind-Body Therapies

Though die-hards still dispute it, increasing numbers of studies show that mental techniques, from creative visualization to hypnotherapy to prayer from afar, are effective in helping with physical healing. Some of the earliest evidence of these therapies' effectiveness came from Herbert Benson, MD, founder of the Mind-Body Institute at Beth Israel–Deaconess Hospital in Boston, who showed in the 1970s that people who practiced a relaxation technique similar to meditation twice a day were able to lower their blood pressure, reduce chronic pain, and overcome insomnia. Most mind-body therapies, including guided imagery, hypnotherapy, and healing prayer, seek to allow the mind to regulate not only the autonomic responses such as heart rate and blood pressure, as well as cellular activity and immune response. Shorter recovery time from surgery, less need for pain medication after surgery, and less nausea and vomiting from cancer chemotherapy have all been documented. Studies now under way are exploring the effectiveness of guided imagery, which involves visualizing physical processes in symbolic terms (diseased cells as weeds being replaced by healthy ones in the form of lush, green grass, for example), to improve immune function.

Many large hospitals and medical schools now have departments of behavioral medicine that may be able to help you locate practitioners of mind-body medicine. Pain clinics, cancer

HOW DOES YOUR GARDEN GROW? TEN HERBS FOR YOUR MEDICINE CHEST

Aloe vera gel for burns, chamomile tea for indigestion, and ginseng to stimulate: These remedies are well-established parts of even urban American folk medicine. The powerful immune booster echinacea (not recommended, by the way, for people with HIV, since it may also boost viral activity) and its domestic partner goldenseal are now right up there with orange juice and chicken soup as classic cold remedies and flu fighters. Consultation with an herbalist or licensed naturopathic physician can help you get back to the garden for almost all your cares and woes, says nutritionist Charles Rosenberg, as well as give you advice on what form of herb may function best. If you're going it alone, you're probably safer choosing a good book on herbal medicine and store-bought formulations, reading carefully for expiration dates and following instructions. If you're being treated by an MD, remember to talk to him or her before you start.

Garden delight	If you're fighting	Taken as	Tips for use
Garlic *(Allium sativum)*	High blood pressure, high cholesterol, or chronic infections of various varieties, including colds and flu	Fresh, capsules, coated tablets, or liquid to be drunk or used as an enema	In lower doses, fights cholesterol and cuts down on heart disease. The compound known as allicin has been used to fight infections from Lyme disease to cryptosporidium.
Saint-John's-wort *(Hypericum perforatum)*	Depression (mild to moderate)	Tablets, tinctures	Like other antidepressants, it takes a few weeks to work, and may make you sun-sensitive. Don't mix with pharmaceutical antidepressants since side effects are possible. May decrease levels of protease inhibitors.
Turmeric *(Curcuma longa)*	Digestion problems (especially with fats), muscle or joint aches	Capsules, spice in cooking	Anti-inflammatory and antioxidant, stimulating liver and gall bladder.
Ginkgo biloba	Memory loss, or problems with sexual desire or erections	Capsules	Boosts blood flow to the brain (and, some say, to the penis). Now in the headlines for its help with Alzheimer's.
Feverfew (*Tanacetum parthenium; Chrysanthemum parthenium*)	Migraines (and related nausea)	Tea, capsules	Can also relieve ordinary headaches.
Bitter melon *(Momordica charantia)*	HIV	Enema, tea, juice, capsule, or fresh	Blocks HIV in the test tube. Used by many to fight wasting and HIV-related skin conditions.
Milk thistle *(Silybum marianum)*	Liver problems	Capsule or tincture	Improves liver function and brings down elevated enzymes, whether from steroids, party drugs, HIV medications, or hepatitis.
Licorice root extract *(Glycyrrhiza glabra)*	Liver problems, HIV, herpes simplex	Tablets	Blocks HIV in the test tube. Not for people with weak hearts, high blood pressure, or low levels of potassium. Used topically for herpes.
Ginger	Nausea and motion sickness	Fresh tea or capsules	Tea works best, but capsules can also do wonders before that boat or bus trip.
Valerian *(Valeriana officinalis)*	Nerves	Tea, capsules, or tinctures	A mild sedative useful for insomnia and anxiety.
Saw palmetto *(Serenoa repens)*	Prostate enlargement	Tea, capsules	Works as well or better than the medication finasteride (Proscar) to ease the prostate condition that is one of the hallmarks of advancing age (see Chapter 8).
Siberian ginseng *(Eleutherococcus senticosus)*	Stress, fatigue, immune deficiency	Tincture, capsule	Helps support the adrenal glands, and enhances immune activity.

referral centers, and cardiac rehabilitation centers can be valuable resources as well. You can also consult books and tapes and learn on your own.

No matter what approach you follow, see what works. Many doctors and patients are doing so already, working toward a time when the idea of alternative medicine fades away and leaves just medicine itself. That's the real traditional approach. After all, the words *heal* and *whole,* though they may often seem worlds apart, come from the same root.

Health Insurance: You're Gonna Pay for This

If your eyes glaze over when conversation turns to copayments or deductibles, that's the way insurance companies want it. Health insurance is actually concerned with three of life's most fascinating topics, money, control, and choices, but the less you pay attention, the more of all three go to the insurance companies. View it like a board game. Your opponent, unfortunately, is usually the insurer, whose goal is not that different from a bank's: Capture as much money as possible, earn interest on it, and pay out as little as possible. Your goal is to learn enough of the rules and methods of the game to become a skilled player, get care, and not lose everything else trying to keep your health.

To understand the game, start by taking a few steps back from all the fine print and thinking about the larger strategies. What drives insurers is the principle of *avoiding* as much risk as possible. An entire discipline, actuarial science, is devoted to helping insurers predict the risks and avoid the payouts. The world we live in, though, is shaped by other, less-than-mathematical elements. "All the negotiations and rules and exclusions and new models of health insurance in recent years boil down to a game of 'who's got the risk,'" says Ruth Finkelstein, head of the Office of Special Populations at the New York Academy of Medicine. "On the one hand, you have ordinary men and women trying to get insurers to protect them;

LIMITED ENGAGEMENT: HOW INSURERS AVOID YOU

Charging more. Most states allow insurers to charge you more if the people in your group (whether that's group of employees, your union, or however else you get insurance) are old, ill, or likely to become ill or injured.

Medical underwriting. This is a nice name for requiring a physical exam, blood test, or questionnaire to make sure you're in good health, and jacking up the price of your coverage or denying it outright if you're not.

Information sharing. Every insurance application to a private company (Blue Cross and HMOs don't count), and all your medical claims to those companies, go into a massive database at the national Medical Information Bureau (see "Information Nation," page 320). This is one way insurers keep you honest and track who's a good or bad risk. If ever you're tempted to lie on an insurance application, don't. If they find out later, they can cancel your coverage, ask for their money back, or even threaten to sue you for fraud.

Preexisting-condition clauses. To guard against having sick people sign up for insurance soon after they discover they need it, insurers use preexisting-condition clauses. These make you wait a certain period of time before they'll cover costs for medical problems you had before you joined them. For people who buy their own insurance, the waiting period can be anywhere from several months to several years.

✚ TO BE REAL? HIV AND THE PREEXISTING-CONDITION CLAUSE

In the case of HIV, the question of what you know and when you know it can make the difference between whether an insurer denies you coverage for a year or simply bites the bullet and pays up. It's a question worthy of a philosophy exam: If you were infected when you were twenty-five but had no symptoms until you were thirty, is your HIV-related illness something new or "preexisting?" If you never had an HIV test, did you have a condition, or is it *knowing* about it that makes it exist? For people who get group coverage through work, preexisting-condition rules now apply only to those conditions you had diagnosed or treated within the last six months. For people buying coverage as individuals, though, rules vary from state to state or even from insurer to insurer. "Some plans consider being positive and symptomatic a preexisting condition," says Karen Timour of the advocacy group New Yorkers for Accessible Health Coverage. "Others say a condition starts from your first symptom."

The bottom line: If you can, get health insurance before you get an HIV test. That way, at least, the question is a little less confusing.

on the other, you have insurers who don't want to cover anyone they think will cost them money; and in the middle you have the government, trying to balance the demands of the two." The equation is further complicated by the intermediate players: the employers who provide most health insurance to Americans, and the doctors who provide the care. Managed care models, for example, particularly those that pay doctors a flat fee per patient regardless of whether the patient comes to see them, are an effort by insurance companies to shift risk to doctors long used to an I'll-do-the-work-and-you-pay-for-it approach.

Figuring out how to "cherry-pick," or take the sweetest customers and leave the sick or sour fruit (don't take that personally) behind, is at the heart of the private health insurance market. Linking health care to work is one roundabout method, since if you're working full time, you're not that likely to be seriously ill. Go to buy a policy on your own (see "Do You Get It?" page 321), and you may be tested for illnesses, asked to pay more, or forced to wait longer for

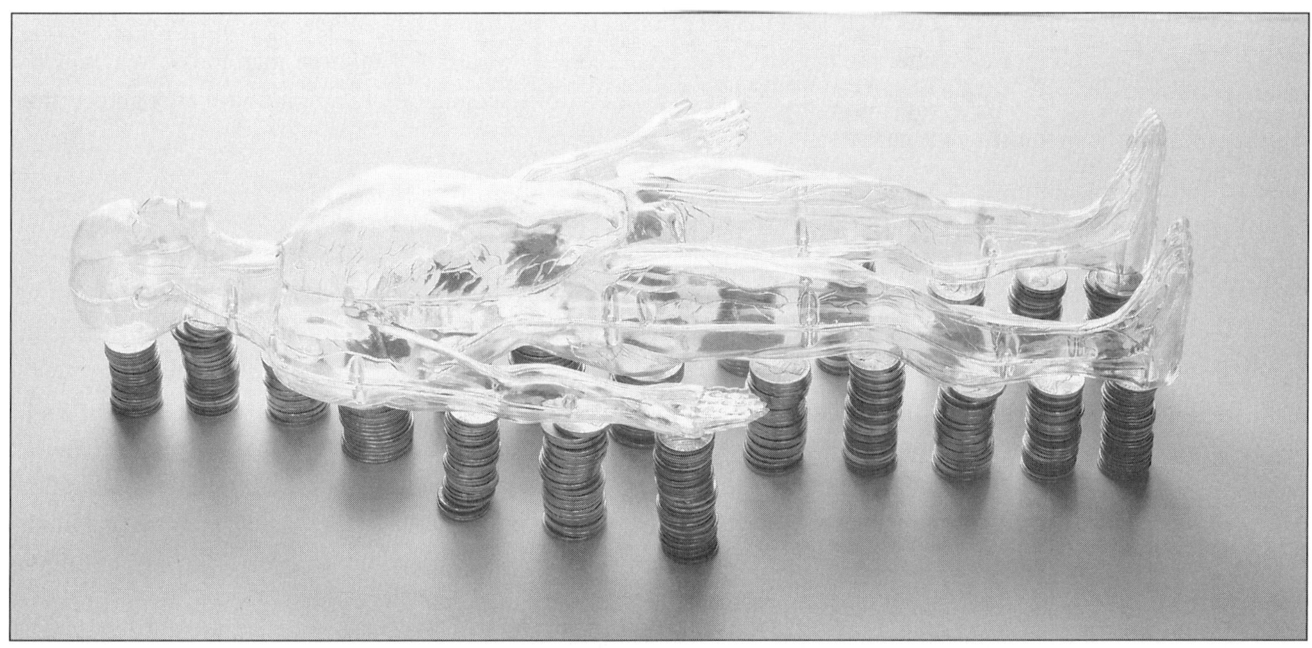

coverage. Add family members to your coverage and insurers get edgy: Kids have accidents, and accidents cost money. As for families of gay men, even domestic partners or those who've taken marriage vows, forget about it; though a handful of big companies and insurers cover gay couples, most save family benefits for heterosexuals. Some insurers, where it's not against state law, go further, barring coverage for single men who live in certain suspiciously gay zip codes or work in "gay" businesses such as hair salons or travel agencies. In "insurance-think," gay men often have AIDS, and AIDS costs money. Don't feel singled out: window washers, older Americans, and inner-city residents of all sexual orientations can't get health insurance, either.

Since insurance regulations vary from state to state, every question has fifty answers. In general, though, there are a few important methods of how insurers limit risk that you should understand (see box on page 318). If you have questions about your options or the legality of an insurance practice, call the insurance commissioner in your state capital.

Health care advocates, public outrage, and premium-sick employers have forced some recent changes. With the passage of the federal Kennedy-Kassebaum bill in 1997, many insurers' favorite risk-avoidance strategies no longer apply to those of us who get our insurance through our jobs. Thanks to the law, insurers of employee groups cannot charge a sick individual in a group more than the rest of the group members. They can also only call conditions for which you received diagnosis or treatment in the last six months "preexisting." So long as you signed up for insurance as soon as you started work, the longest they can make you wait before they cover any condition is a year. Nor do you have to wait another year for coverage, the way many of us used to, each time you switch jobs and insurers. If you've been continuously covered (with less than a two-month gap), you're entitled to what they call "portability": coverage without an interruption. Even if you don't qualify, you still get credit for the months you've already waited for coverage on a prior plan.

If you don't have a job that gives you health insurance, or feel like you're losing the game to keep coverage, you're not alone. "There's a three-word summary for gay men's biggest health care problem," says Dr. Pols, "and that's 'access to care.'" There are no studies to prove or disprove it, says Dr. Finkelstein, "but the exclusion of gay men and lesbians from family policies likely leaves higher numbers of us uninsured." Where we lead, many follow, since even after the managed care revolution of the late 1990s, more than forty-three million Americans have no insurance at all. Another fifty-six million of us don't have enough coverage to get us the care we need.

Information Nation

In theory, the managed care model means better coordination of care, with any doctor or nurse who sees you able to track your treatment, and all of its important details, at the touch of a computer key. Practically, that convenience may be more scary than helpful, with your medical information traveling places you yourself never dreamed of going. Beyond reports of individual abuses—the guy who brought a disk with the names of people with HIV to the local gay bar in Florida, or the enterprising medical student who decided to sell hospital records to a malpractice lawyer—lies a growing industry that trades publicly in medical information most would rather keep secret. U.S. companies now buy and sell an estimated $40 billion worth of medical information each year.

Private insurers have long had a central record-keeping database, the Medical Information Bureau. Make a claim with one company, and all the others will know why. Though managed care companies don't take part in the MIB, they are increasingly being bought, sold, and merged into large health care networks that include hospitals, pharmacies, mental health providers, and other formerly separate parts of the health care system. While most states have laws requiring that insurers or health care providers not release mental health, HIV, and substance abuse information to outsiders without special authorization, this gradual conglomeration may soon replace the idea of an "outside" with one big, information-rich health care family. If all that raises boundary issues, it should. Some major pharmacy chains decided in 1997 to bolster their special relationships with certain drug manufacturers by handing over the names and prescription histories of their clients. Once patients started getting ads in their home mailboxes for antidepressants, the pharmacies confessed and promised they'd stop.

Unless you can pay for everything out of pocket, there are no secrets, but as of this writing advocates are pushing Congress to pass more comprehensive legal protections for medical information. At a minimum, new proposals will allow patients to receive a copy of their medical records and correct any mistakes, require health care organizations (including doctor's offices, pharmacies, and insurers) to give patients a clear, written explanation of how they will use information, give individuals the sole right to authorize the release of medical information that could be linked back to them, and establish civil and criminal penalties for improper use of medical data.

Do You Get It? Insurance Sources and What You Should Know About Them

IF YOUR EMPLOYER OR UNION IS PROVIDING YOUR INSURANCE

In this case, you have something in common with more than 90 percent of the other Americans who don't get health insurance from the government. Some employers offer a choice of different health insurance options to employees, and some don't. The choices may vary, from an indemnity plan (where you pick the doctors, pay them, and wait for reimbursement from the insurer) to a managed care plan (which requires you to use a doctor on a specific list) and variations in between. The basic question you need to ask yourself remains the same: Can you get your insurance to cover the work of a doctor you like and who is sensitive to your needs? In general, about 85 percent of Americans who get insurance through work are now on some form of managed care. Also in general, if you have the option and can possibly afford it, it makes sense to try to leave yourself the option of seeing a doctor outside of the managed care network. "There's no reason that a good, gay-sensitive doctor won't be on your managed care list," says Susan Dooha, GMHC director of health care access, "but there's no reason to assume that there will be one there, either. And if you get sick, you're going to want as much choice as possible."

If you do get insurance through work, you should ask if your employer is self-insured. Over 90 percent of companies with more than a thousand employees, and an increasing number of smaller companies, now insure themselves by establishing a fund to pay their employees' health claims, says Karin Timour of New Yorkers for Accessible Health Coverage. This is yet another strategy to limit risks: Self-insured companies pool only their own employees, and so don't mix with thousands of other employees from other companies who they think might be sicker. Self-insurance is also a way of controlling costs and administrative complications, since self-insured plans are regulated under a single federal law, rather than many different state laws, and can limit or exclude types of care (such as prescription drugs for HIV, or treatment for alcoholism) in ways that other plans can't. They're not allowed, though, to single out gay or any other employees for special exclusions. Federal law requires that they be equal-opportunity discriminators.

You can't necessarily tell if your company self-insures by looking. Many companies have their paperwork handled by other insurers such as Guardian or Prudential, so it can look like regular, old-fashioned indemnity insurance even when it isn't. Your employer, however, can tell plenty about *you* from your insurance claims, since self-insured companies can review an employee's health care claims. Some people, especially those who don't want their mental health or HIV status to be known at work, go as far as paying out of pocket for things like therapy or anti-HIV medications to protect their confidentiality.

IF YOU'RE LEAVING A JOB WHERE YOU HAD INSURANCE

In this case, make sure you take COBRA, the eighteen-month extension of group coverage offered to all employees whose company has more than twenty employees. In some states, COBRA is available to you even if your company has as few as three employees. You pay the premiums your old employer paid, plus another 2 percent in administrative costs. If you're disabled when you leave, or within sixty days of your departure—and you obtain a letter from Social Security saying so—COBRA stretches to twenty-nine months (see box on page 424). COBRA is likely to be cheaper and better than the coverage you'd get on your own, and you'll have more options—including the guaranteed right to buy individual coverage, without a waiting period, at the end of your eighteen months.

IF YOU'RE BUYING YOUR OWN INSURANCE

If you need to obtain your own health insurance, you're in the minority and need to be a savvy shopper. Hospital shows on television, for all their grit, put forward a common fantasy: that a previously unknown individual wheeled into the hospital will be embraced and cared for by the health care system. The reality, at least at the level of the insurance company, is that the unknown individual is the least welcome of entries. Many individuals remain uninsured because they decide it's not worth paying the high premiums; if you want to pay for insurance, insurers are afraid there's some reason you need it. If you have been chronically ill, insurers in many states deny you coverage outright, or leave you to wait for it through the high-risk pool (see below).

Even if you can get it, individual insurance is so expensive that almost no one can afford something more than managed care coverage. There are, however, a few resources, or administrative tricks, that may help you in your search.

Insurance Agents

These are licensed professionals who can work hard to get you the best coverage possible. They are also salespeople, operating on a commission from the insurance company, so be truthful but careful about what you tell them. If the policy does not ask explicitly about HIV, heart disease, or chemical dependency, don't blurt it out. And don't be pressured into an on-the-spot decision; think on it overnight, or ask a friend or lawyer for advice.

High-Risk Pools

If you have a chronic illness or disability, this is your only chance for private coverage in many states. Some states require that you be rejected for another policy or be offered coverage only at prohibitive rates (or with a long or permanent preexisting condition waiting period), before you're eligible. Others ask only for a doctor's confirmation that you have one of a list of diseases. You still may have to wait up to six months for a policy that's more expensive than coverage for people who aren't sick.

"Groups of One"

If you're self-employed or a small business owner, you may have the option of buying a policy as a "group of one." Some insurers consider "groups of one" more attractive than individuals, because they are businesses that may "grow" more business, and because working people are more likely to be healthy. To find out more, call a few insurance agents and ask for quotes.

Managing Managed Care

Managed care plans are the latest effort to control risks and costs. There are plans with different names and initials and structures (HMOs, PPOs, IPAs, and so on), but all of them make doctors partially accountable to the for-profit health insurance giants who pay the bills. Cost cutting takes different forms. There's capitation, where the doctor gets a fixed amount per patient no matter how many visits that patient might make. There's withholding, where plans maintain a profile of how often certain tests and referrals should be performed, and withhold part of doctors' salaries in case they exceed what the company thinks is appropriate. And there is fee-for-service, where the doctor is paid for each service performed, but at a low rate determined by the insurance company. In all of them, the company retains a way to reduce its costs or the amount of care provided.

All managed care plans give you a list of doctors and ask you to choose a primary-care provider, or "gatekeeper." This doctor coordinates your care, whether in the office, through specialists, or hospitals. You pay a small fee (copayment) for office visits and prescriptions (usually between $2 and $20), which is supposed to encourage regular visits. The theory is that the doctor should notice small problems before they become big, expensive problems, ever mindful of the price tags for specialists, sophisticated tests, and emergency room visits. Part of managed care's popularity grows from the theory that the plans will provide you with preventive medicine earlier and more often. But call them, since they won't call you. And since they're busy, the rule about going to see a doctor to establish a relationship before you get sick strongly applies.

Do They Care? Questions to Ask a Managed Care Plan

I've always been a dizzy queen, but when I realized that managed care meant I'd have to manage the care, I got out my attitude, my boa, and my five-inch pumps and told my administrator HMO meant "Honey, move over!"

If you're getting a managed care plan through work, you must be offered a choice of two different plans. Even if you're buying as an individual, ask the company a few hard questions before you choose. If they won't answer—in a 1998 survey, for example, 80 percent of the largest plans in New York State refused to provide even the basic information required by law—ask the state insurance commissioner.

Good questions to ask a managed care plan include:

• *Can you go outside the network of doctors they recommend?* How much will this cost? If they say they reimburse for 80 percent of "reasonable and customary charges," can they (or anyone else you know) give you any sense of what that complicated formula means in dollars and cents for certain typical visits or procedures?

• *Will you be told about all treatments, even if your plan doesn't cover them?* Some plans "gag" doctors from discussing anything but the care the managed care plans cover.

• *How do they handle prescriptions?* Some plans cut deals with certain drug companies or pharmacies and have lists of medicines (formularies) and pharmacies that they require you to use. Find out if they substitute their own drugs for ones your doctor prescribes, whether they force you to go to certain faraway pharmacies, and what the procedures are for approving medications not on their list. How much are copayments for prescriptions? Can you use cheaper, mail-order companies for your drugs?

• *How do they handle case management?* Some HMOs have case managers for people with chronic conditions such as HIV, diabetes, asthma, and other chronic conditions. Good case managers can help you through red tape on matters such as getting a drug that's not on the formulary or getting a larger number of pills so you don't have to lay out copayments for repeated prescription refills. Bad ones just throw up obstacles between you and what you need.

• *How do you get to a specialist?* For people with chronic illness or more than one health problem, going to see two doctors each time you need to see a specialist costs you time and money. Some plans will let you have a specialist as your primary-care provider, or will give you a "standing referral" that allows you to go directly to the specialist you need to see. Some won't.

• *Are there annual or lifetime limits for benefits, prescription drugs, or conditions?* This is especially important if you're facing chronic illness.

• *How do they handle emergency care?* Some plans deny you coverage if you rush to an emergency room for something that turns out to be a false alarm. Some will cover it if it seemed reasonable at the time.

• *What should you do if you get sick when you're out of town?* If you travel, you want a plan with branches across the country, or reciprocal arrangements with others outside your area.

• *Do they pay for mental health services?* Some plans pay for limited numbers of visits to a therapist, make your therapist write long reports every few sessions to justify continued care (see Chapter 11), or only let you see a nurse or social worker rather than a doctor.

• *How do you complain?* Do you have to put it in writing? How long does it take before they respond? Can someone represent you in the process?

• *Is it quality care?* Most plans track quality of care, but they probably won't tell you much about what they find. A basic gauge, controlled by the insurance industry but more objective than a plan's own promotional materials, is the National Commitee for Quality Assurance (www.ncqa.org) in Washington, DC. The Center for the Study of Services (www.consumercheckbook.org), a non-profit group in Washington, publishes an annual ranking, including disenrollment rates (the number of people who dropped out), of more than three hundred managed care plans. And CareData Reports, a private New York group, publishes the results of their consumer surveys on their Web site (www.caredata.com)—including ratings by people in poor health, who are the ones who know the flaws in a system best. Unfortunately, CareData charges a hefty $12.95 per plan, which means that seeing the results for plans in your region could run you as high as $155.

And finally, the two most important questions to ask yourself:

• *Who else do you know who uses them?* Friends or colleagues are the absolute best source of information on how long you have to wait for customer service, how long reimbursement takes, and so on.

• *Is there a doctor you like on their list?* Make sure he or she is still participating—these lists change constantly—and that the doctor you choose is accepting new patients.

Appealing Behavior

I think calm and clear and with a little sense of humor works best. It's hard. I was talking to a nurse in the administrative office who said, "Thank you for very much for telling me that, but I don't really need information about your physical condition." I thought, "You don't? Silly me, I thought that was important." And they're always saying things like, "That's too bad, but that's not our problem." I mean, you'll say, "My eyes are falling out," and they'll say, "That's a shame, but we don't cover eyes."

My lover had a stroke at age forty-three. The doctor said he was a great candidate for occupational therapy to learn to walk and talk again. The HMO approved twenty days of therapy, but the next day they changed that to a custodial nursing home. I got suspicious, questioned them, and finally ended up hiring an attorney. After a month of wrangling, we forced them to approve therapy, but he suffered permanent damage during that time. We were too trusting. Next time I'll start fighting immediately.

I needed a wheelchair that had footrests that folded down so I could get up against a desk or sink. They sent a physical therapist to come see me, but he just kept telling me what I couldn't have. He kept saying they "wouldn't pay for a scooter," which wasn't what I wanted anyway. It turned out they also wouldn't pay for the chair I needed. At first I accepted it, but then it really started to bother me. I mean, they pay to put people on life support when they don't even want it, or to give someone radiation for potentially fatal cancer. I had salespeople come to my house until I found the chair that worked for me. I wrote letters explaining how I wanted this to make me more mobile, to keep me working rather than collecting disability and bedsores. I threatened to file a complaint against the physical therapist. I think I probably have a scarlet letter for troublemaker in my file. But eventually I saw another physical therapist who was nice and who recognized that I did need to be able to do my work and my dishes like other people, and that this chair would do it. They paid for the whole thing.

If there's one rule of dealing with managed care plans, says Susan Dooha, director of health care access at GMHC, it's that you don't have to accept their decision. Just to be safe, keep a record of all your phone conversations, including the names of anyone you spoke with, as well as copies of any correspondence you send to or get from them. If you want to file a grievance, do it in writing, and if possible get a letter of support from your doctor. "Medicaid and Medicare managed care organizations [see "Medicaid," below, and "Medicare," in Chapter 8] have special routes of appeal," says Dooha, "but privately insured individuals should also complain whenever they feel like they've been denied needed care." Go to your state insurance or health department if you don't get what you want, and if you feel comfortable discussing it, get your employer's human resource department involved. Thomas, forty-two, a seasoned health care consumer, offers some guerrilla advice: "Know what you're entitled to, know how to file a grievance with the insurance department, and have the names of three health care reporters in your little black book," he advises.

MEDICAID

If you have been disabled for two years or have reached the age of sixty-five, you are automatically entitled to the fairly comprehensive government health insurance program known as Medicare (see Chapter 8). For the rest of the uninsured, losing almost all your assets is virtually the only way to qualify for the safety net the government provides to the needy, known as Medicaid. Since Medicaid is supposed to be for people who don't have other options, the government can't really screen out deserving applicants; instead, they strive to control costs. They usually put a maze of bureaucracy between you and the care you need: The longer you take to get through it, the more they save. Increasingly, Medicaid patients are required to enroll in managed care plans and undergo "utilization reviews" that try to rein in care. And though government insurance is meant as a safety net, it's very easy to fall through the cracks.

Many people find themselves in transition once they get sick, moving from employed to not, and from comfortable to financially strapped. If you do lose the job that gave you your coverage, especially if you have few or no assets, you may not have to lose your private health insurance—in some states, Medicaid will pay those private premiums. Others just offer straight Medicaid coverage, which includes hospital and clinic visits, some home health care, and prescription drugs, lab tests, and doctors' visits (at pharmacies, labs, and doctors' offices that accept Medicaid). Six states impose monthly prescription limits.

Regulations are complicated and vary state by state, though you're not going to get Medicaid anywhere unless you have limited income and virtually no assets besides your home, car (not too swanky), and a burial account of up to $1,500. Since welfare "reform" in 1997, Medicaid is generally available only to citizens, some legal permanent residents, and a handful of others for whom they make special exceptions.

Details, Details: Medicaid Facts You Should Know

No matter who you are or how long you've been here, it's good to go to a public entitlements advocate, hospital social worker, local AIDS organization, or local aging office for help untangling the complicated web of regulations surrounding Medicaid. If you do apply, you'll need to assemble proof of who you are and how much money you make, including your birth certificate, a copy of your Social Security card, your last four bank statements, and pay stubs (see "Paper Tiger," page 425, for hints on applying for government benefits). Here, however, are a few additional things that most people don't know about Medicaid and which they may not leap to tell you at the government office.

• *If your income is too high, you may still qualify if you have high medical bills.* "Most people don't realize that Medicaid will often count your medical bills against your income," says Tom McCormack, author of the *AIDS Benefit Handbook* (Yale University Press, 1990). This is known as Medicaid "spend-down" or "share of cost." It allows you to deduct bills that you've paid (or in some states, bills you've incurred and not yet paid) from your income. If you get a letter from Medicaid saying you have $600 too much income to qualify, for example, you can reapply and get coverage when you have $600 worth of medical bills in a given eligibility period (they run from one to six months). Think of it like a deductible on private health insurance, except that it may have to be met as often as every month instead of every year. "Of course, in the next eligibility period you have to start all over again," warns McCormack. Twelve states do not allow Medicaid spend-down.

• *Even if you're making money now, you may be able to apply for Medicaid coverage retroactively.* It's possible to ask for Medicaid coverage for up to three months prior to the date of your application. "Say you're now back at your job that doesn't give you health insurance, but last month you spent two weeks in the hospital and didn't work at all," says McCormack. "You could apply for Medicaid just for that month you didn't work, and get them to cover at least part of the bills."

• *You can buy your way in.* States may allow working people who make too much money to qualify for Medicaid, but less than 250 percent of the poverty level ($19,740 in 1998), to buy their way in. Additional measures were approved in late 1999 to enhance the ability of states to offer Medicaid buy-ins to disabled people who have returned to work. The premiums vary, and only some states offer the option, but it's much cheaper than private insurance.

• *Appeal.* If you're denied treatment under Medicaid, or denied Medicaid itself, ask for a "fair hearing," to review the decision. "If you can, do it within ten days," says Tom McCormack. If you're in the hospital and feel as though you're being discharged too early, appeal then and there and you may delay or block the discharge. Every state has an appeal mechanism for people on Medicaid.

FURTHER READING

Boston Women's Health Book Collective. (1998) *Our Bodies, Ourselves for the New Century: A Book by and for Women*. New York: Touchstone. Probably the single most important book in the history of self-care. There's lots here for men to learn from, too.

Chum, Nathan. (1996) *Take Control: Living with HIV and AIDS*. Los Angeles: AIDS Project Los Angeles. People with AIDS need all kinds of medical care, so this clear, fact-filled resource can help anyone engaging with the health care system. The benefits information, though, is California-specific.

Dossey, Larry. (1993) *Healing Words*. New York: HarperPaperbacks. A (slightly) critical survey by a physician of the many studies linking healing to the power of prayer, with lots of references and suggestions for further reading.

Goldberg, Ken. (1993) *How Men Can Live as Long as Women: Seven Steps to a Longer and Better Life*. Fort Worth, TX: The Summit Group. Pitched at straight men, of course, but filled with clear, helpful information on everything from cholesterol to erectile dysfunction.

Green, James. (1991) *The Male Herbalist: Health Care for Men and Boys*. Freedom, CA: The Crossing Press. For those who'd rather skip the pharmacy in favor of the herbalist.

Hoffman, David. (1996) *The Complete Illustrated Holistic Herbal: A Safe and Practical Guide to Making and Using Herbal Remedies*. Rockport, MA: Element Books. One of the few peer-reviewed herbal guides, with clear explanations.

Hoffman, Ronald L. (1997) *Intelligent Medicine: A Guide to Optimizing Health and Preventing Illness for the Baby-Boomer Generation*. New York: Fireside. Words from a doctor who takes on many of medicine's myths and sacred cows.

McCall, Timothy B. (1996) *Examining Your Doctor: A Patient's Guide to Avoiding Harmful Medical Care*. Secaucus: Carol Publishing Group. Like it says. Written by a doctor.

Scarce, Michael. (1999) *Smearing the Queer: Medical Bias in the Health Care of Gay Men*. Binghamton, NY: Haworth Press. A keen academic analysis of how the medical and research establishment has handled, and too frequently mishandled, the gay male body.

Weil, Andrew. (1996) *Spontaneous Healing: How to Discover and Enhance Your Body's Natural Ability to Maintain and Heal Itself*. New York: Fawcett Columbine. From one of the best-known practitioners of the "new" integrated medicine.

CHAPTER 8

Coming of Age

Ageism • Midlife and More • Off the Gaydar? • Body Talk • Tests You Need • AIDS and Older Men • Prostate Primer • Prostate Cancer • Medicare • Gimme Shelter • Parenting Your Parents • A Political Agenda for the Ages • SAGE Advice from Your Elders

"You exaggerate."
"This is not exaggeration."
"It is. The only trouble is that you exaggerate the bad points only."
—Carlos Castaneda, *The Teachings of Don Juan*

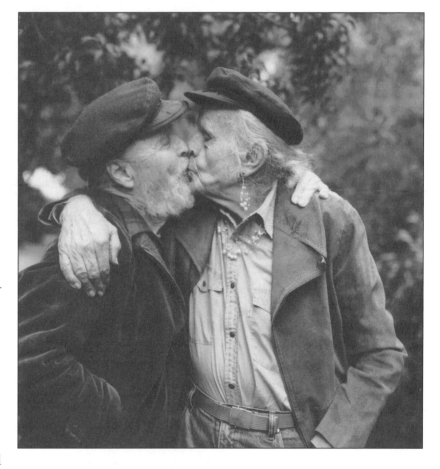

Richard Huskey, MD, forty-nine, has no problem with gay stereotypes. It's just that he's not going to waste one moment of the time he has left buying into the myth of the lonely old queen. "Think about it," he says, his stream of statistics and hyperbole making it hard to tell where seriousness ends and creative license begins. "Why is the rate of suicide highest among older, straight White men? They're facing the realization, all those years later, that the kids' weddings didn't help. The grandkids' weddings didn't help! Getting old means confronting the myth that the all-embracing family is enough. Their wives may be getting old or sick at the same time they are. Their siblings may be gone. But you know what? Lots of gay men have already discovered the limitations of the family myth! We've already been alone but then sought out new friends! And while straight men had some kids, took to the couch, ballooned up, and didn't move again except to be put into their coffins, a lot of us have been up and out, doing things and taking care of ourselves. Even the brain studies, like that one in California where they cross-sectioned gay men's and straight men's brains, show that there are more neural pathways joining the lobes of our brains, allowing us to be creative and intuitive *and* regimented and calculating. Which means that we're going to be leading the parade in aging fabulously. I just hope that we go slowly enough so everyone else can catch up!"

As chair of the Washington, DC, Board of Nursing Home Administration, Huskey knows well that his visions of gay elder care—including "theme wings" in nursing homes, where leather queens do it their way while butch dykes with dogs and lumberjack shirts shoot pool across the hall—is at this point just another fantasy. But as one of a relatively small number of gay geriatricians (doctors who specialize in health care for old people) and one of the only doctors in DC who makes house calls, Huskey knows better than to sit around waiting for conventions to catch up. "Congress would have us all think like Osler [the Johns Hopkins physician], who wrote that everyone should take a sabbatical at age fifty-nine and a potion to kill themselves at sixty," he says. "Of course, Osler changed his mind when he got older himself. But down there in the Federal Reserve Bank or in the Capitol, with all those discussions about cutting Social Security and reducing Medicare, they are not getting that we are going to have to make some fundamental changes to be able to accommodate our aging population. Life doesn't shut down at sixty-five anymore! We have a lot of time left. And we need to have the support systems in place to provide an enjoyable life for the massive numbers of people who are going to be old, old-old, older than most of us ever thought possible. Women have been working on these aging issues for decades. But where are all those powerful male CEOs? When all the movers and shakers get old, they get shaken loose from their moorings and just drop away."

And who, in Huskey's view, should be leading the charge to join our sisters and remake society? Take a guess. "We do have to deal with our obsession with the loss of youth," Huskey concedes. "But gay men have so much to offer not just other gay people, but society at large. We are incredibly adaptable. We know how to come to our fellow man, pause, and find a way to take the tired old conflict issues and replace them with something sensible, namely, living lovingly. Straight men haven't mastered that."

For final, microcosmic proof of his big-picture generalizations, Huskey turns to what disability insurance companies and professionals who work with aging populations call the essential activities of daily living, including grooming, eating, and "ambulating" (getting around). "We're immaculate, and you know we cook better than straight men," says Huskey. "Just look at what we've done with brunch." As for getting around? "If we've been getting across town in high heels for years," asks Huskey, "don't you think we're going to be more gifted when we're older?"

But seriously, folks. None of us likes to be described by that most blistering of designations, an aging queen. But you are, Blanche. Each of us is growing older every day. Maybe you're not getting around in high heels, or otherwise, as much as you might like. Maybe you're coping with a sense of growing invisibility in the gay community, or a nervousness about not having a boyfriend as you edge toward middle age. But if you've survived till forty, or fifty, or eighty—with all you've seen and all the AIDS and discrimination and anxiety that's been arrayed against gay men—you have some incredible staying power, and likely some amazing stories. You also have a future that appears to be growing longer by the minute. Overall, male life expectancy went up six months in 1998 alone. AIDS deaths among gay men are sharply down. And most important of all—though like so much talk about age, it quickly sounds clichéd—the quality of whatever life you have left is more important than the quantity. "I'm having more fun at sixty-seven than I've ever had in my life," says Charles, in San Francisco.

"If the good Lord said to me, 'You can change one thing. What will it be?' I'd say, 'Let me go back and do what I did, but let me enjoy doing it as much as I am now.'"

This is not a rehearsal. This—are you ready?—is the first day of the rest of your life. And you, dear reader, have the tools for becoming gay and gray fabulously.

Ageism

I do trainings, so I'm constantly being evaluated by people in writing. And I still remember the day when this twenty-seven-year-old, very bright guy who had clearly enjoyed himself wrote a comment saying I reminded him of Yoda. Now I know he was a Star Wars *fan. And I know there aren't many gay role models as elders. But was I bitter? You bet.*

We were at this picnic and my friend Mark, who had been up all night doing lots of coke and drinking, was feeling disappointed about not picking someone up. I wish I could remember why, but we were joking and I called him an old hag. And he got this look on his face and he came over and bit me on the cheek and said, "Don't you ever call me that again." Now, he was coming down from a two-day coke binge. But he's only thirty.

I call it "gaygeism." I mean, have you looked at the personal ads? "Fifty, looks forty"; "Thirty, looks twenty"; "Sixty, feels twenty." Younger is always better.

The Greeks told the story of Tithonus, a man in love with and loved by Aurora, goddess of the dawn. Unable to bear the idea of parting, Aurora begged the gods to grant her mortal man eternal life. They obliged, with mixed results. Tithonus got eternal life, but not eternal youth. Aurora found herself riding off to make the sun rise every morning, leaving behind a lover whose body grew more and more decayed.

The word *ageism* may have a nineties ring to it, but the debate over whether old age is a curse or a blessing has been in the collective consciousness for more than two millennia. There's an ancient Egyptian papyrus that begins: "How to change from an old man to a young one." While gay men are quick to blame bar culture and our own superficiality for our horror of the aging body, broader explanations (and a huge volume of literature) point to forces greater than ourselves. Some look to the rise of Christianity—with its emphasis of the Son's transformative power over that of the Father, and Christ's death at the ripe young age of thirty-three—as the beginning of the end of honored old age. Others blame the move from cyclical, agricultural society to more industrial modes. "Modern technocratic society thinks that knowledge does not accumulate with the years, but grows out of date," wrote philosopher Simone de Beauvoir in *The Coming of Age* (W. W. Norton, 1968). More than thirty years and eight versions of Microsoft Word later, the newer-is-better logic of the marketplace is more in place than ever, and with it a popular distaste for those who appear to drain the market rather than enrich it. Fat people, welfare mothers, gay people, those with too many children, and those with none: All are singled out for hostility.

Age, though, is inescapable for everyone, and so—like a memory people would rather forget—is put down with special force. "Think of 'old _____,' and what gets filled in," says Phillip Piro, supervisor of group services at Manhattan's Senior Action in a Gay Environment

(SAGE). "There's 'old coot,' 'old fart,' 'dirty old man,' 'old and gray,' 'old troll.'" "Wise old man" is the exception, though it generally requires the addition of a younger person to make the picture real: a child being dandled on Granddad's knee, or a young adult listening attentively to explanations of the lessons of the past.

As for those of us having a gay old time, we're there, but less visible. While we have worked successfully to beat back certain forms of social prejudice, this oldest of prejudices against the old remains a part of the gay community, particularly since older people often have less money, and "gay culture" begins to get pretty thin once you remove bars, stores, restaurants, and other pay-to-play establishments. A few gay men and lesbians are working to reclaim the label "old," refusing to be called "elderly," "seniors," or "aged." But many feel their blood pressure rising, not from age, but the way the younger gay men treat them. "Ageism is epidemic in the gay male community!" shouted one man, his voice full of rage, at a conference on gay aging—the first national conference of its kind—held by SAGE in 1998. "Our obsession with youth and beauty is making us invisible! It's epidemic!"

An irony is that the lessons of the other epidemic we have lived through can be a partial map through the maze of ageism. For most gay men over the age of fifty, the journey toward a healthy gay identity that the Rev. Malcolm Boyd referred to as the trip "to hell and back" has included many stops at stations traditionally visited by much older men. "I'm living with full-blown AIDS, and why I'm surviving, I don't know," said one of the younger attendees at the SAGE conference. "I do know this: I relate to the aging process a lot, because that's what my body has already done. I have low energy levels, and I experience fatigue, and I find it hard to remember things. And for the last fifteen years, my mentors and the people I've looked up to in the gay community have been dying." The infrastructure of AIDS organizations—the experts in will writing and Medicare negotiations, the bereavement counselors, and the volunteers helping the homebound—may have great usefulness as more gay men grow old. "I often fantasize, if we ever find a cure for AIDS, that we'll take these incredible resources we've developed and turn them toward helping gay men age healthily," said Lew Katoff, an early GMHC volunteer and program director who died of AIDS himself before the age of forty-five. Had Lew lived longer, he might have seen the divide between the concerns of AIDS and aging organizations begin to close even in the absence of a cure. New AIDS medications are prolonging people's lives, but their side effects—high cholesterol, risk of heart attack, thickening around the middle, osteoporosis, and potentially fatal interactions with other drugs—are eerily similar to those associated with old age generally.

Also common to both AIDS and aging, and more welcome, is the sense of personal transformation that can come from knowing that your time is limited. At sixty-seven, Mark, a retired textile designer, sounds distinctly as though he's on the better side of hell, and like many whose mortality has forced a sense of confidence as well as crisis. "I don't put up with the bullshit anymore," he says. "I don't have to. If I'm tired, I go to bed. If I don't like someone, I don't see them. I have fewer friends, but the ones I have I trust. In your twenties, there are so many decisions to make. I'm so happy to be done with all that goofiness, to have most of the decisions made." On the broader social level, too, the transformations of AIDS and aging are cross-pollinating. The Gray Panthers—the intergenerational activist group who wheeled a gurney into the American Medical Association's annual meeting in 1974 to demand that the "dying" health care system be resuscitated—has joined forces with AIDS activists to press for health care reform, lower drug prices, and rights of the disabled. Civil disobedience trainings, rallies for medical marijuana use and against HMO abuses, and plans for a "Gay Panthers" group are now in progress.

So if the first sight of gray hairs makes you see yourself as an old troll in progress, ask yourself if the vision is really yours. The idea of the dirty old man, like that of the morally diseased gay man with AIDS, is more about young people's anxiety over loss of power than it is about being sick or old. With AIDS, gay men took back that power psychologically even as we lost it physically, showing a heroic willingness to call attention to what was happening, an unrelenting humor in facing it down, and a persistence that turned pity into admiration. "AIDS was like an X ray into the steeliness of his character," says Brad of his friend Howard, who, like too many men, went through repeated bouts of getting sick and getting well before he died from AIDS at thirty-four. You have only to open one issue of the magazine *Diseased Pariah News,* published for more than ten years during the worst of the AIDS epidemic, to see how often that kind of steeliness was tempered by humor, and the playfulness that came in part from being gay and dying young.

In the same way that we have led the way past victimhood to youthful dying, gay men may now lead the way to aging youthfully. "I don't think I dared think about aging before this, or certainly didn't dare to talk about it," says Bill, now thirty-nine. "I mean, what was I going to complain about while everyone was dying? How little I had in my 401(K)?" With AIDS deaths down, spirits are up. Conversations about aging are open. And *Dirty Old Fag News* may be right around the corner.

Midlife and More

Why do people only talk about age in terms of the body? You'd never describe childhood only in terms of mumps, measles, and chicken pox.

I've had a boyfriend for eight years. That just wouldn't have been possible for me when I was younger.

I was forty-three, married with three children, and dean of the Episcopal cathedral in Springfield, Illinois. Eleven years later I'm an innkeeper with my partner, Ted, in Hyde Park, Vermont. Even with all that change, I don't miss my thirties and forties at all. There was so much pain and confusion then. Now, it's everyday stuff, trying to make a living, stay ahead, and run a business.

One of the reasons I like AA over forty is because we're over forty. I don't want to spend hours listening to a thirty-year-old talk about "I want a boyfriend, I don't want the boyfriend I have, I don't like my job, why isn't my apartment bigger than it is, how come I don't have any fun when I have to stay sober . . ." I can't relate.

Just as when it's paired with AIDS, the word *crisis* no longer neatly captures the complexities of midlife or beyond. There are now so many definitions of midlife that it may make more sense to refer to it as the "middle ages." Chronologically, you can take the life span of the average American male (seventy-two years) and divide it in half to find the midpoint: thirty-six. If your work's your life, you might take the midpoint of an average work span (from

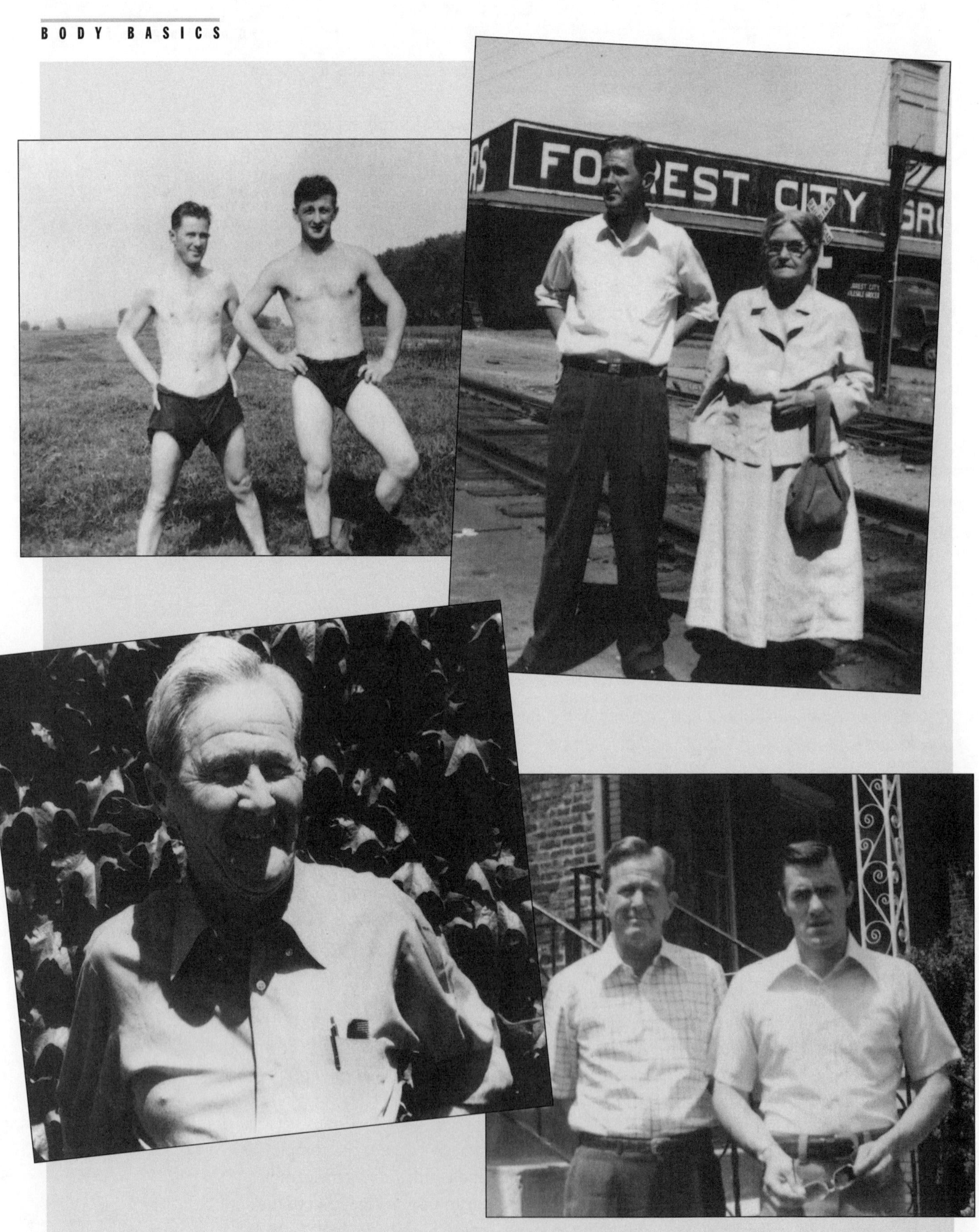

Cliff, 1925–1985

twenty to sixty-seven, say), and arrive at forty-three or forty-four. For those of us for whom the party scene is life, middle age might begin as soon as you begin to be invisible—a point, some argue with conviction, that begins at thirty-two. "I sometimes stare at myself and see that wrinkle in my forehead as a valley," says Drew, age thirty-four, "or say, 'Don't smile anymore—you don't want more lines.'" He's not the only gay man for whom the arrival of middle age is defined as the moment they no longer turn heads (see "Off the Gaydar?" page 341).

Turning your own head around to see the positive as well as the negative is part of coping with middle age. The idea of "midlife crisis," coined by psychologist Elliott Jaques in the late 1950s, originally referred to one of many opportunities to do that kind of self-assessment, a critical moment when you faced a developmental "challenge" to get to a new phase of personal development. Swiss psychologist Erik Erikson conceived of eight such crises occurring across the adult life span. Most of the other academic and popular theorists of aging—sociologist Bernice Neugarten, psychiatrist George Vaillant, researcher and author Daniel Levinson, and others—refined the terms but stuck to the general principle, enumerating various "tasks" or "phases" that we go through to get to a healthy old age. How and when you go through them varies—as Tina Turner says in her version of "Proud Mary," there's doing it "nice and easy," and there's "rough"—but just pulling your baseball cap down tighter, squeezing yourself into a Tommy Hilfiger tee, and pretending none of this is happening is only a temporary option. Thou shalt not ignore the need to think through midlife transitions, warns Levinson in *The Seasons of a Man's Life* (Ballantine, 1978), considered one of the bibles of male aging. Doing so, he says, means paying the price with "a later developmental crisis, or a progressive withering of the self." Carl Jung, granddaddy of the stages-of-life theory, was even more dour. "Whoever carries over into the afternoon of life the law of the morning," he wrote in a 1933 essay, ". . . must pay for it with damage of his soul."

How all us angels of the morning make it smoothly into the afternoon of life is a question that is burning more brightly as we increase in number. In 1900 only one in twenty-five Americans were sixty-five and over. By 2030, one in five of us will be. The huge number of baby boomers (people born between 1949 and 1964) now hitting middle age and beyond is one of the reasons why writer Gail Sheehy, who calls these life transitions "passages," has been able to turn study of them into a series of best-sellers. In her latest book on the subject, *Understanding Men's Passages* (Random House, 1998), Sheehy interviewed hundreds of men, including some gay ones (though their sexuality is not really explored in depth), to glean a list of what she calls "exit events": occurrences when a door slams on your life progress and makes you realize that you need to take a different route. Among the common passage-provokers she lists are loss of a job, death of a parent, divorce, loss of a mentor, children leaving home, and death of a peer.

The neat lines of these passages are more blurred for gay men. Some of us lost mentors when we came out. AIDS made most of us lose peers, while most straight men were feeling nothing but invincible. As Robert Kertzner, MD, an associate clinical professor of psychiatry at Columbia University, points out, our passages, like the bars most of us came out into, are often less brightly lit than those of straight men. "Heterosexuals have traditions and rituals, however insufficient, for their life passages," says Dr. Kertzner, whose research has included extensive interviews with gay men at midlife and beyond. "Wedding anniversaries, your child's sweet sixteen, becoming a grandparent or an elder in the church: While none of these are barred to us, they're not so often celebrated, either." Without those "magic markers," most gay men are left to sketch our own plans for the future, often following the thin, barely visible line of those who've gone before. "It's so important to have role models for aging, and most of us don't," says Don, sixty-four, in Santa Monica, who attributes his lack of midlife crisis partly to the fact that he spent time with a lover thirty years his senior. "He showed me how it was possible to grow old without scaring the shit out of me," says Don. "I saw him writing another book in his seventies and said, 'Well, if he can do it at his age . . .'"

Some of us find plenty to learn from men who aren't gay. "For lots of us, the years after coming out are all about highlighting our sexual identity, shoring it up, declaring our difference," says Dr. Kertzner. "Entering midlife, other concerns also come bubbling up: the hunger for deep connection, ambition in work, questions about your partner if you have one. Those are things that are more similar for all men than they are different."

Many people in their forties or fifties feel as though they're waiting for a signal to set them moving down a different track even as they shoot forward on the one they're on. "You know how the *Inferno* starts, where it says, 'I found myself, midway through our life's journey, lost in the middle of a dark wood'? That's where I am," says Paul, forty, who recently left his native California to take a high-pressure, high-profile job as a public relations director in New York City. "This job's the biggest opportunity I've had, and I've never been a planner, but now I find myself wondering, 'What's the plan?' I've been in the same line of work since my twenties, have enjoyed it, but now I'm asking myself, 'Is this what I'm going to do forever?' And today I got a phone message saying my cholesterol is high. If this isn't midlife, what is?"

San Francisco therapist Rik Isensee, LCSW, author of *Are You Ready? The Gay Man's Guide to Thriving at Midlife* (Alyson, 1999), says that many of his gay male clients start their midlife reassessments with something straight men also do, what he calls the try-harder mode. "If you're not happy at work, you work more," he says. "If you're worried about changes in your body, you work out more. If you're scared not to have a boyfriend, you go out more to clubs." Of course, there's nothing wrong with taking better care of yourself or getting out more, but sometimes "trying harder" is just more of the same and ultimately unsatisfying. For Isensee, the question is both what you'll do differently—change jobs or go back to school or rework your relationship—and how you'll do it.

Adjusting for Age

Deciding to leave your lover of twenty years and move in with your nineteen-year-old intern, or saying you're going to Staples to pick something up and never returning to work, falls into what Isensee calls "evasive action," a make-up-for-lost-time approach that usually just loses you more. What's often needed is a way to recognize that something new inside you is pressing for acknowledgment. Following are some of his and others' suggestions for slower, sustainable change.

BREAK FREE

Daniel Levinson calls this "becoming one's own man" and identifies it as the early edge of midlife, the first stirrings of what lies beyond. It may mean disagreeing with a boss to whom you've been subservient, or breaking—sometimes messily—with a mentor or authority figure. It may mean leaving your job for self-employment, or giving up an image that served some function that's no longer viable. "I think I had a gay self I adopted to come out," says Drew, fifty-three,

TURNING A GAY GAZE ON THE MYTH OF THE LONELY OLD QUEEN

Harry would be private about these things. We always had two single beds, but he still disliked it when people came to visit. It made him uncomfortable. My sister stayed with us and she said once, "What's all that noise coming out of the bedroom?" It never occurred to her that we were having sex. I guess it was because he was a doctor.

I am so delighted to see the young people do what I couldn't do. I couldn't walk down the street with my partner arm in arm. I mean, they just walk right into gay bars. But we had more mystique. In my day, you looked this way and that way, and it was almost like a speakeasy—you had to knock on the door. You were sneaking in. It was like you were one of a chosen few.

Social science researchers have suggested that older gay men are no more depressed than their straight counterparts, which is itself remarkable when you consider how much extra stress they've dealt with. Some researchers, such as Raymond Berger, author of *Gay and Gray* (Haworth Press, 1995), have actually found that older gay men are happier, our aging made easier by a "crisis competence" we acquired when we were young. But though older gay men may be just as satisfied as straight men with their life's work, don't expect them to pour into community centers, don pink triangles, and lecture the young about the bad old days and how they got beyond them. "The young people want to *out* everybody, make everyone identify as gay or lesbian. But we are the don't-ask-don't-tell generation, and that isn't going to change," says George Roosen, men's coordinator for Gay and Lesbian Outreach to Elders (GLOE), a San Francisco social services organization. Roosen, who himself is seventy-four and definitely out, works with gay men from their sixties into their late nineties ("a generation that doesn't want help from anybody") to connect them to existing programs and, more important, to each other.

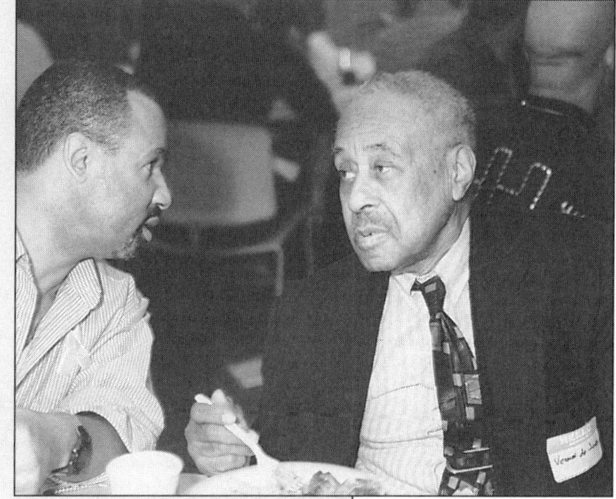

Roosen says he's part of a generation of gay men who came to San Francisco and other cities after World War II, drawn by the relative freedom and safety of urban life. These men still had to take jobs in homophobic industries, though, and step gingerly through the antigay hysteria of the 1940s and 1950s. "I remember a closed life of dinners and parties, all very home-based," says Roosen. Others tell of shock therapy, police raids on bars, and chemical castration attempts. "I was given drugs for ten years that completely erased my sexual drive, which I guess in their minds made me 'straight,'" says Craig, sixty-five. "They were productive years, but I lost ten years of sexuality." When gay liberationists leaped out of the closets and into the streets, many older gay men stayed in their dining rooms. AIDS widened the gap, destroying the generation that bridged the divide between older gay men and younger, more public ones. "It was natural for men ten or fifteen years younger to be our connections to the gay world, and they were the hardest hit," says Roosen. "So even some of us who had been out got paranoid, went home, and locked the door."

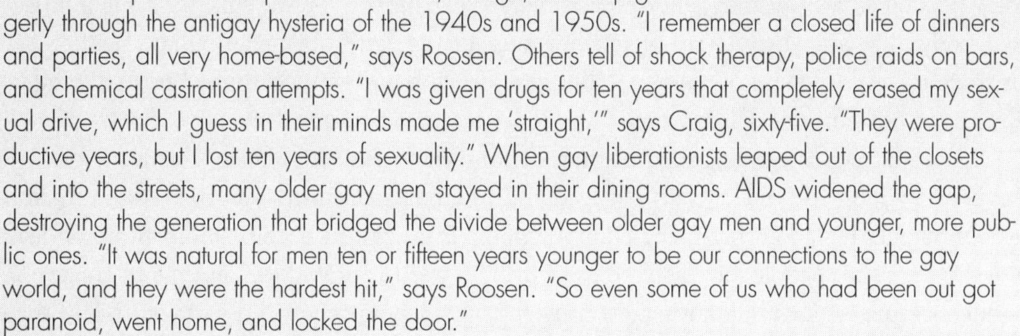

Is it possible to heal the generational rift and bring our elders into the embrace of a loving and nonageist gay and lesbian community? Maybe if younger gay men and lesbians engage in work with the aging more broadly, and listen more carefully. "You can't just throw away fifty years of history and hiding," says Roosen. "What we need instead is to be supported in the choices we've made. Give us that, and we have a lot to give back."

an interior designer. "I liked being on the party lists, with the right clothes and the right apartment. 'A-gay,' you know? But around about forty, things changed. It's not just that people stopped looking at me the same way. I wasn't looking at them the same way, either. I didn't want to be a leatherman or a daddy. The question was, what *was* I?"

2. EMBRACE YOUR OPPOSITE

Jungians might call it your shadow side, though you may think of it just as the type of person or the part of yourself you can't stand or who makes you nervous. "When I was younger, I defined myself by who I wasn't," says Darwin, thirty-eight years old, a Middle East expert. "I wasn't a femme-y queen. I wasn't superficial. I was political, not a mindless clone in a gay ghetto or one of those we're-just-like-everybody-else churchgoing conformists. And then you get older and you realize all those declarations cut down on your options. Maybe church does offer something. Maybe it's not so important to be able to pass as straight." Herman, forty-six, an educator, says his self-image took a beating as his waistline, and responsibilities, expanded. "I always liked having a little boy's body," he says, "being kind of androgynous. It was part of being an outlaw, neither gay nor straight, neither man nor woman. Now, in a job with authority, with my body growing heavier, I'm not outside it all anymore."

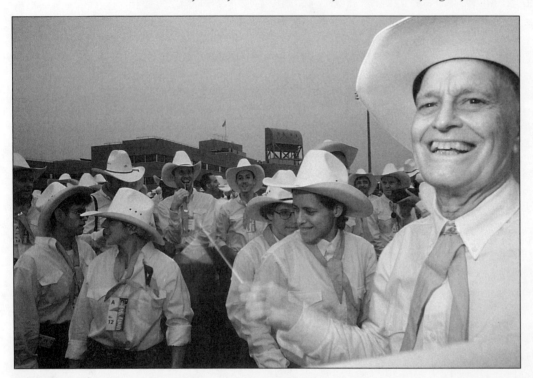

Levinson sees integrating the polarities of yourself—male and female, creative and destructive, young and old, socially engaged and internally sustained—as one of the principal tasks of midlife. It's about balancing contradictions: Even as you become more aware of death or of the ways that people have acted destructively toward you, you feel an urge to create products or take actions that advance your well-being or help others. Loss of youth, and the qualities that come with youth, creates relief *and* despair. Being old makes you feel stable *and* empty, accomplished *and* impotent. Finding a way to hold on to the vital in both, rather than denying one in favor of the other, is what Levinson sees as groundwork for future aging. Rik Isensee suggests that embracing your opposite includes developing an ability to see the positive in the negative, a kind of healing tolerance for yourself. "See if you can find the interesting or good qualities in precisely those things you've avoided," he suggests. "Instead of caving in to bitterness and then hating yourself for it, look at what you can learn from it. What can you be taught, for example, by the bitter queen within?"

STEP OUT OF THE BOX

What kind of person are you? Once you've answered the question, try doing a few things that don't fit. "Let experience teach you what your mind can't," suggests Paolo, who at fifty-five has found himself spending more time outdoors for the first time. Go to an opera. Take a dance lesson. Join a book group. Whatever it is, make sure it's "against type." If your friends would be surprised to hear you did it, that's a good start.

Prioritizing what really moves you over what you always imagined would move you can be liberating. Levinson talks of "de-illusionment"—not disillusionment, but the happier process of letting go of long-held and little-investigated assumptions about yourself or your life structure. That's best paired, he says, with "modification," the process of making changes to allow for new ways of living and experiencing things. "When my brother died I left my job and went back to school," says Jack, an investment banker turned health care policy analyst. "Instead of having middle age happen to me, I decided to happen to middle age. I make half the money. I have twice the satisfaction."

THINK FUTURE GENERATIONS

Erikson saw this stage of successful adult development as the battle between "stagnation" and what he called "generativity," which many have interpreted primarily as parenting. You may be a father already (see "Parenting," page 522), but for gay men—and in fact, for men in general—generativity might be best defined in wider terms: mentoring relationships, collective action, or creative efforts. "The question is, what are you doing that will last longer than you will?" asks Kertzner. Conventional wisdom, attributed to everybody from Plato to the ancient Chinese, captures the idea with the oft-repeated formula "Have a child, plant a tree, or write a book." Providing a place for younger gay men to watch the ball game, or helping to organize a community garden, may also work. "In my neighborhood, there was always a mother hen, an older guy who let the young gay kids hang out at his house," says Charles, forty-two, from Washington, DC. Tony, forty-seven and in a longterm relationship, says he looked into getting a straight friend pregnant, though "the idea of three people raising a family ended up being too complicated for all of us. So I've been spending more time with my nephews, and getting satisfaction from supervising my younger colleagues at work."

COME TOGETHER

For some gay men, aging edges them toward the dream deferred: coming out. "I did indeed have a midlife crisis," says Tom, a fifty-seven-year-old gardener. "At forty-two, after twenty years of marriage and three kids, I told my wife that I was gay. Next to telling my father that my mother was dead, this was the hardest thing I've ever had to do." For those of us who've been out already, a way toward a happy old age may be found by what Dr. Kertzner calls "coming together"—finding a way for different parts of your life to coexist within a single narrative. Erikson's phrase for this final stage of development in old age (which was around age sixty-six when he was writing) was the struggle between "integrity and despair." Integrity does not mean pretending that working as a bartender at the Swamp for thirty years was the best possible choice, or that your five-city, ten-year tour of American gay neighborhoods was without a downside. It does mean, in Dr. Kertzner's phrase, "recognizing that in much of the past you did the best you could, and that you even learned from the times that may have seemed like wasted opportunities."

Mending fences is often a big part of this stage of development. "I've found myself calling old college and high-school friends," says Matthew, who's sixty-eight. "There's a lot of lost history there I'm hoping to recover." Forgiving the flaws and accepting the benefits of one's parents, too, is common in this period. "My father still asks me about a girlfriend I had thirty years ago," says Peter, fifty-five years old, "and I've stopped caring. There's only so many times you can go to a dry well and expect to drink. But I have let my parents know I love them, and they've responded with love." If you're lucky, the reconciliation may even take place before one or another of them wants to move in, which is a whole midlife journey of its own (see "Parenting Your Parents," page 365).

Erikson, Levinson, Sheehy, and other best-selling authors on aging, however, are silent on what many gay men say is their deepest problem in trying to build a continuity with the past: a recognition of how much of it has been destroyed or forcibly removed from us. What intolerant families may have started, AIDS has made much worse. "There was a whole group of men I came out with, made a family with, and was expecting to grow old with," says Howard, forty-six, who's lived in Italy, England, Colorado, Minnesota, and New York. "Wherever I went, they were a base I returned to. Now it's like *The Wizard of Oz,* as if a tornado picked up my house and set it down somewhere else, squashing them in the process." Pete, forty-eight, is one of the many gay men whose Rolodexes contain more dead than living. "I've been to more than a hundred memorials," he says. "It's easier to count who's alive." Even when the sense of loss is less personal, it's pervasive. "In the 1970s it was so easy to come out, because there seemed to be so many other people doing it," says forty-seven-year-old George. "I was joining something. I never imagined then that I'd feel so much on my own when I was growing older."

SEEK SUPPORT

Most theorists of the psyche imagine man as an individual and pay less attention to the social settings that contain us. But if embracing your opposite, stepping out of the box, thinking big and all the rest sound like awfully tall orders just as life is feeling short, you don't have to go it alone. "If ever there was a time when being gay was not just about the gay community, this was it," says Tony, forty-seven, who says he's turned to "conversations with straight peers with whom I reveal much more than I used to, and family." Spirituality (see Chapter 13) provides a great sense of something larger, and interest in it often increases as we age. Gay community, too, is broader than the bars, where you don't get noticed so quickly anymore. Explore some of its other sides (again, see Chapter 13).

NONE OF THE ABOVE

Other famous analysts of the human condition, and their less famous followers, find hope of happy resolution and integration to be colossal self-delusion. "All this self-help stuff," says Peter, fifty-seven, in Rochester, New York, "is trying to deny the feelings of mortality and loss that are the most important, realest part of life." Philosopher Jean-Paul Sartre saw the existential crisis, the moment when "the stage set falls apart" to reveal both your mortality and your complete isolation, as the beginning of true awareness. French psychoanalyst Jacques Lacan identified alienation and insufficiency, fueled by the idea of a perfect "other" who has what you are somehow lacking, as the most basic building block of the human psyche. "It's realizing that the sense of loss can never really go away, I think, that makes you truly human," says Peter, who admits that even talking about his own aging causes him considerable pain. "Once you recognize that frustration and loss are part of life, it can help prevent the destructive fantasy that you should be feeling otherwise, or that everyone else has what you don't."

That approach may work for you. It is, as Tina Turner says, definitely doing it rough.

Off the Gaydar? Sex, Invisibility, and You

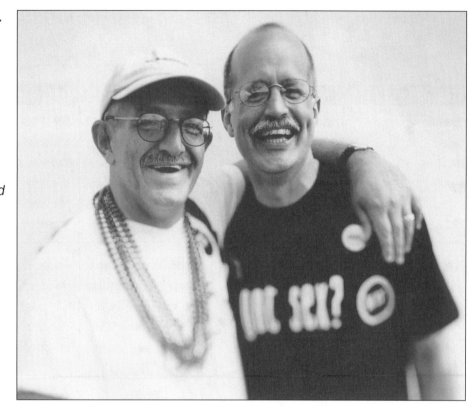

I've become invisible. Dismissed. It's totally unconscious, they don't seem to realize they're doing it. I notice it because I used to be a head-turner. It gives me a sense of anonymity now, which I find rather exciting.

What have I learned? I've learned that I don't need to put up with second-rate crap. I've learned the difference between having sex and making love. I don't want to go through all the dating and the "keeping my options open." I just want the deep stuff.

My lover and I broke up a year ago, but we achieved a truly profound physical relationship that feels like enough to coast on for the rest of my life. I'm not looking now, though that's the surest way to find someone!

People always talk about how your desire drops away when you get older. But they don't talk about what an incredible blessing that is. I have so much time!

That the hunger for deeper connection and making a mark comes at precisely the moment when many gay men feel themselves on the threshold of invisibility is an added pain of growing gay and gray. Talk to gay men about aging, and you often hear discussions of growing distant, vanishing in a sea of back-turned baseball caps and sculpted bodies. "When I was in my twenties, I remember I'd look past the older guys at the bars and think, 'What's that old fart doing there? Why isn't he home gardening or something?'" says Charlie, a participant in a San Diego workshop on aging. "Now I'm the one who's being looked past." For George, from Washington, DC, it's not the newness of invisibility that stings, but its seeming irreversibility. "The truth

SEX THROUGH THE AGES

When it comes to sex, "You're as old as you feel" doesn't quite do. For one thing, it's not just *you* that's feeling, which may spice things up or complicate them terribly depending on how you and your partner treat your aging body (see Chapter 3). "My body's far from firm or perfect, and I think about that fifteen times a day with Peter," says Sam, fifty-seven, whose lover is twenty years his junior. "On the other hand, I'm way past that frantic fumbling of youth. I'm working with the wisdom of the ages."

Part of that wisdom is what Jeffrey, age fifty-five, calls "knowing when I'm just as happy going home to a book than spending hours looking for sex." Part is appreciating what Henry, eighty, calls "the pleasure of seven hours of foreplay, rather than two minutes of orgasm." Part may be knowing the difference between not pursuing desire and not having any. For some older men, falling testosterone levels may be at the root of a dwindling interest in sex, and if you're over forty, you should have your levels tested annually (see "Tests You Need," page 345).

	Age 18	Age 35	Age 55	Age 75
Erection	Springs up constantly, whether you want it to or not.	Works like you want it to, with occasional lapses in judgment or function.	Half of men have some erectile dysfunction (hard-on problems). Also, the angle of your dangle changes; over time, your erection sinks groundward.	More hands-on stimulation is needed, and your erection gets softer.
Ejaculation and orgasm	Like an automatic weapon with a hair trigger. 20% of men Kinsey studied could have orgasms in rapid succession.	Multiple orgasms are within your reach, but unless you're among the lucky 8% who can come repeatedly, it will take some training (see "Tao and Tantra," page 111).	The size of your ejaculation shrinks, and the amount of time you require between orgasms increases. Your control, though, and knowledge of pleasure are probably peaking.	Same as 55 if you're lucky. If you've had surgery for prostate enlargement, which many at this age have (see "Prostate Primer," page 350), you may experience "retrograde ejaculation," where your cum goes into your bladder instead of out your penis. If you've had a prostatectomy, orgasm is strictly internal.
Anal pleasure and the prostate	Who knew what they were back then?	*P* is for *pleasure,* though prostatitis (see page 39) is most common between 30 and 50.	Prostate enlargement (see "Prostate Primer," page 350) occurs. For anal intercourse, though, back pain is probably a bigger problem. Choose a comfortable position (see "Anal Sex," in Chapter 2)	Same as 55, though you're more likely to have had prostate problems or surgery that diminish pleasure.

is that I was never very successful at catching people's eye in the street or in the bar scene," admits the forty-three-year-old AIDS worker. "But now I know consciously that I never will be. Of course I know other things are more important. But it's still painful."

Acknowledging the pain is part of getting past it, though some gay men are carving themselves a new niche in the sexual marketplace. Prime Timers, a social club for older gay men, now has some forty-seven chapters across the country. *Chiron,* a monthly magazine, features centerfolds who often top fifty or sixty. "When I was younger, older men were not admired or considered as attractive as they were today," insists Peter, sixty-three, a magazine editor in Washington, DC, who says his older years are definitely sexually golden ones. "But just go online and visit chat rooms like Men 4 Older Men and they're always full." Then again, Peter has recently been appointed editor-in-chief of a major consumer magazine—and power has always enhanced attractiveness.

A different, more lasting aphrodisiac may come from the realization that you know things a younger man can't hope to. "Mark has a potbelly, is balding, but he has other things I definitely don't," says Ralph, twenty-one, of his "mad affair" with a man thirty years his senior. "He knows what he's doing, in bed and out of it." Leonard, seventy-five, in New York, says three-quarters of a century and two hip operations have left him confined at home but quite free in spirit. "I still get my legs up in the air, with the right help," he recounts with a grin. "I belong to a club called Swan in California, where men correspond and get together. And I have telephone sex. I'm a hot sister when you pull my bloomers off."

As you grow older, the age of your sexual partners may seem as important as whether you're having sex at all. Old men obsessed with youth is the stuff of literature, of movies, and not infrequently of fantasy. What happens on-screen or in books is different than when you're really grappling with love and death in Long Island, Venice, or anywhere else. "To be honest, I love going downtown to the local strip joint, running my hands over some beautiful young boys' bodies, and putting dollars in their jockstraps," says Cameron, sixty-seven. "I know a lot of them now. I'm not looking for a life partner, I'm looking for fun." Take the boys home, and the distinction can get blurrier. "I love young hustlers," says forty-nine-year-old Vincent, who says he's had three or four "roommates" who broke the loneliness, but also broke the bank. "Some older men feel a thrill at having a young man on their arm," says SAGE's Phillip Piro, "the excitement of having a date who's dashing. Even if there's no sex, it's great fun, since being touched is so essential to human survival." At the same time, Piro acknowledges, men at SAGE often tell stories of "roommate" relationships gone wrong, with older men feeling hustled by younger ones for money, drugs, or even their apartments.

Weighing the difference between fantasy and reality has always been a juggling act in sex, but the weight grows heavier as you grow old. "I think for me part of aging has been accepting the fact that I have always fantasized about much younger men. At the same time, my lover, who's my peer, offers me things they don't," says Larry, fifty-five, who ended a relationship with a dancer fifteen years his junior before meeting a lover only slightly younger than himself. "The idea of being with someone young is great. The reality is more banal." If you feel like you're looking for love in all the wrong places (see "Cruising for What You Want," page 125), try to go to places that make you feel you have something to offer, and don't return to places where others don't treat you right. Even more important, say some men, is not going to negative places in your head. "I had to change some of the company I kept, and put up a sign that says 'Complaint Department Closed,'" admits Lawrence, age sixty-six, a retired home health care worker who's weathering not only the death of a lover but the landlord's attempt to evict him from the apartment they shared. He apparently has not retired from the arena of self-definition and adventure: He got cruised by a man his age in

MY CHART BELONGS TO DADDY? GENETICS AND YOUR HEALTH

Every time I go home, people tell me how much I remind them of my grandfather. We walk alike, we talk alike, we're both "ready for a fight" or "solid in a storm."

After twenty years of no contact with him, I've been seeing my father in my body. My hands are his hands.

Even if you haven't spoken to them since they refused to invite John to your sister's wedding or told you they would pray for you, look back to your parents and grandparents—not just in anger, but to see what health lessons can be plucked from the family tree. Heart and prostate problems, colon cancer, diabetes, blood pressure, and depression—the majority of health challenges as you age may have a genetic component. Know your past and you can help protect your future (see "Tests You Need," below).

church last Sunday, and both his forearms sport the pink-hued brightness of brand-new tattoos. Lawrence says they're part of his "old-age madness," but the twinkle in his eye makes it seem as though there might be some gladness in there, too. "I wasn't going to put them on the cheek of my ass," he says. "After all, I'm not sure who wants to see that."

BODY TALK

Sometimes I think aging is the new AIDS. There's Viagra for your penis, statins for cholesterol, Prozac for your mind, Proscar for your prostate, Propecia and Rogaine for your hair loss, testosterone for your sex drive. You'd almost think that if you took enough pills, getting old was a syndrome you didn't have to catch.

Is there anything to set aging gay men apart, physically, from other men? "I think the difference in concerns is more psychosocial than physical," says Jonathan Appelbaum, MD, medical director at the Fenway Community Health Center in Boston, after some deliberation. "But the research just hasn't been done." We know about men in general, for example, that the chief causes of death for men sixty-five and over are heart disease, cancer, stroke, and accidents, in roughly that order. But do gay men run a higher risk of stroke or heart attack because of the stress of living in a gay-hostile world? We know that married men live longer—significantly longer—than single men, but does that include men in a long-term committed relationship with another man? How about gay men with close friends they see regularly? Will all that accumulated grief and loss from AIDS mean faster aging and shorter lives? For those of us with HIV, even if we're "responding" to treatment, doctors are now suggesting that it may take twenty years to eradicate the virus from the body. What is the health prognosis of someone aging for three or four or five *decades* with HIV?

Until there's hard data about gay men's similarities or differences to other men, all we have is careful observation of our bodies. Chances are you're paying attention already, since our awareness of age often begins with the sense of something physical. You may feel the cellular spare tire that seems to be slowly inflating around your midsection, or notice that the typeface on this page is looking smaller than it used to. Most of us can recall a lifetime of bodily reminders of age: the first time a child's mother refers to you as "the nice man over there," the first time a student calls you "sir," and the moment when you realize what dental floss was supposed to be preventing. And somehow, even with all that, many older men have moments where they look in the mirror and can't quite put together the image they see with the picture they carry in their minds. Ram Dass (also known as Richard Alpert), the former Harvard professor turned spiritual seeker, author, and—lately—openly bisexual man, described his trepidation at buying his first senior-citizen ticket on a train. "What I'd felt when I was eighteen years old and went into a bar and said, 'I'd like a beer,' the great trepidation that he wouldn't serve me, that's just the same feeling I had with the conductor," he said in a lecture taped and distributed under the title *Conscious Aging* (Sounds True, 1992). "When I said to him, 'Don't you want to see my ID?' he said no. And I was shocked. Until I was fifty, I think I saw myself as twelve or fourteen."

If you feel like an adolescent again as you pass fifty, it may not all be your imagination. Society—just as it does with teens—is ready to warehouse you with others your own age rather than confront what your struggles raise for the rest of them. Your body is also going through more hormonal changes than it has since you were fifteen. You need less food. You see less well. Your prostate swells. Your body mass decreases. Your ears are hairier. Coffee keeps you up.

Generally speaking, the rules of living well—a low-fat, high-fiber diet, regular aerobic exercise, and enough sleep—can help you stay healthy in a body long into old age. Paradoxically, so can baby aspirin. A low dose of aspirin a day, in consultation with your doctor, can lower your risk for heart attack, stroke, cancer of the colon, cataracts, dementia, and other scourges of old age. Many antioxidants—increasingly hailed as the cure-alls of the vitamin world (see page 259)—are being associated with a reduction in a number of the same conditions. Less definitely studied, and more aggressively hyped, are "age-retarding" dietary supplements such as the hormone DHEA and the jet-lag fighter melatonin.

No pill, though, can substitute for seeing a doctor. "The main thing gay men have to worry about as they age is the same thing other men have to worry about," says Richard Huskey, MD, the Washington, DC, geriatrician. "We don't get checkups." It's one of many reasons why overall life span is longer for women. Older gay men need all the same vaccinations and tests as younger men—among them vaccination for hepatitis, flu shots, testicular self-exam, and an HIV test (see page 295). Regular blood tests, including blood pressure checks and the series of workups known as a complete blood count, or CBC, are also in order. And since the body, like any essential appliance, gets a little cranky with extended use, some extra attention must be paid.

Tests You Need

What tests you should have as you age, and how often, is something upon which virtually no two doctors or medical associations seem to fully agree. Add the gay factor, and the disagreements become even more common. Often gay doctors recommend earlier testing for things like prostate and colon cancer than some professional associations. "We just want to keep you in shape so you can be out there enjoying yourself longer," comments Dr. Huskey with a smile. Suggestions offered by him and other geriatricians who treat gay men include those listed on pages 346–349.

YOUR BODY THROUGH THE AGES AND THE TESTS YOU NEED TO MONITOR IT

Condition	Family ties	Things you can do	Special info for men who are HIV-positive ✚	Tests you need
Heart disease *Cardiovascular disease* is the leading killer of American men, so make sure you check:	Risk of sudden cardiac arrest goes up 50% for people who have a parent or sibling who has had a heart attack.	Low-fat and high-fiber diet, aerobic exercise, and not smoking all help.	If you're on protease inhibitors for HIV, diabetes and high cholesterol (triglycerides) can be side effects. Protease inhibitors may interact badly with some common anticholesterol medications.	Get an electrocardiogram (EKG or ECG), a test that measures the electric activity of the heart, at 40 and at least once every ten years thereafter.
Blood pressure (see page 297) More than 60% of Americans over 60 have high blood pressure.	A history of high blood pressure among close relatives can double your risk of developing the condition.			Get a complete blood count, including cholesterol breakdown and blood pressure test, every year after age 40.
Cholesterol (see page 295)	One in three men inherit a disposition for high cholesterol, increasing heart attack risk threefold.			
Diabetes Over 18% of Americans over 65 have diabetes. Diabetics are 2–4 times more likely to have heart disease than nondiabetics.	Approximately 11% of African Americans, 25% of Mexican-Americans and Puerto Ricans, and up to 50% of Native Americans have diabetes.			Get tested for diabetes annually after age 40 if your weight, blood pressure, or cholesterol is high, or if a family member has the condition. Otherwise, get tested once every three years after age 45.
Colorectal health 90% of cases of cancer of the colon and rectum are detected in people over 50. Colorectal cancer is almost always curable if detected early, yet fewer than one-third of Americans are properly tested.	If an immediate family member had colorectal cancer, you're three times more likely than average to have it yourself.	Experts are divided about the protective effect of a high-fiber diet, but it probably helps. So may exercise and avoidance of fatty foods, particularly red meat broiled or grilled at high temperatures. A multivitamin containing folic acid, and, in some studies, an aspirin a day, may also help.		Have a fecal occult blood (FOB) exam yearly after age 40 (the American Cancer Society recommends it after age 50). The FOB looks for blood hidden in your stool, but misses one in three cancers. Get a sigmoidoscopy—examination of the rectum and lower colon with a fiber-optic tube—every three to five years after age 50. Most effective of all is colonoscopy, where a tube is snaked up the rectum to view the whole colon, and if necessary, to biopsy growths. Get one of these every ten years after age 50.

YOUR BODY THROUGH THE AGES AND THE TESTS YOU NEED TO MONITOR IT (CONT'D)				
Condition	**Family ties**	**Things you can do**	**Special info for men who are HIV-positive ✚**	**Tests you need**
Prostate From age 50 to 85, studies show a fortyfold increase in the prevalence of prostate cancer.	If you have three close relatives (father or brothers) who had prostate cancer, or two who developed it before the age of 55, then you're five times more likely than average to get it. If only one brother or your father had it, your risk doubles. Even if a grandfather or uncle had it, you're one and a half times more likely to be at risk. Black men are at greatly increased risk.	Try a half an hour of sunshine a day (with sunscreen), and a low-fat diet that includes green and yellow vegetables as well as green tea. The tea's protective effect is probably related to the antioxidants it contains (see page 259). Other antioxidants, particularly selenium but also vitamin E, zinc, and lycopene (an antioxidant in tomato sauce), have all been associated either with lower rates of prostate cancer or lower mortality once diagnosed. Soy may also have a protective effect. Tofu lasagna, anyone?	Testosterone treatment for wasting may speed prostate growth.	Many gay doctors suggest a digital rectal examination yearly after 40 for gay men. (The American Cancer Society suggests one yearly after 50.) While medical societies remain divided about the prostate specific antigen (PSA) test, some doctors recommend a PSA test yearly after 40 for men at high risk, and after 50 for the rest of us (see "Prostate Primer," see page 350, for details).
Vision One in six adults age 45 and older reports some form of vision impairment. By age 75, one in four of us does. Common problems include age-related macular degeneration (AMD), a breakdown of the central part of the retina; and glaucoma, a buildup of fluid and pressure behind the eye.	15% of AMD patients have a parent, sibling, or child with the disease. White men get it more often than Black men do, and people with lighter eyes may be at greater risk. Glaucoma runs in families. If you're over 40 and have two or more immediate family members with the disease, you're at higher risk and should be tested yearly. With Black Americans three times as likely as Whites to develop glaucoma, the disease is now the leading cause of blindness among African-American men.	Antioxidants, particularly those found in carrots, spinach, kale, and other green leafy vegetables (see page 259), can protect against macular degeneration. Smoking can make it worse. If you are suffering from visual impairment, use the many devices—magnifying glasses, large print books or books on tape, big-button calculators, etc.—that can help.	Certain HIV-related infections, particularly cytomegalovirus, manifest themselves in the eye. Have an annual eye exam. If your CD4-cell count is under 200, have one every three months.	Visits to the ophthalmologist at 40 and every two years thereafter until the age of sixty should include tests for AMD and glaucoma, as well as examination of the optic nerve. After sixty, get an exam yearly.

YOUR BODY THROUGH THE AGES AND THE TESTS YOU NEED TO MONITOR IT (CONT'D)				
Condition	**Family ties**	**Things you can do**	**Special info for men who are HIV-positive**	**Tests you need**
Hormones Decreased testosterone may cause "manopause": reduced energy, decreased sexual desire, and increased depression.		Many swear by DHEA, an over-the-counter pill that boosts levels of a precursor to estrogen and testosterone. Scientific evidence is inconclusive, though there is a theoretical danger that DHEA could boost the risk of prostate cancer.	Some 30% of men with AIDS have lower-than-normal testosterone levels. Many AIDS medications, such as ganciclovir (Cytovene, Vitrasert, DHPG), ketoconazole (Nizoral), and megestrol (Megace), may further depress levels.	Get a test yearly after age 40 to determine changes. Ask your doctor to test your "free testosterone" levels, meaning how much is freely circulating in your blood, rather than just the total. Labs and doctors vary widely on what they consider normal. If your testosterone is high, don't go out and punch someone in celebration. You may have twice the risk of prostate cancer, and should monitor that carefully.
Muscle-mass/fat ratio Men lose as much as 30% of their muscle cells between the ages of 20 and 70, while average fat goes from 18% to 38% of total body weight. Obesity triples the risk of high blood pressure and adult-onset diabetes, and increases risk of coronary artery disease.	A family history of obesity makes your chances of being obese two to three times higher.	Aerobic exercise and strength training can both help, no matter how old you are. One recent study found that frail men and women in their 80s and 90s were able to increase their weight-lifting ability by 118% over a ten-week period.	HIV can also cause wasting of lean muscle mass. For more on wasting, see Chapter 9.	Get a yearly body mass index test after the age of 40. For more on the test, see page 251.
Hearing A third of men over 65 experience some level of hearing loss. High-frequency hearing is the first to go.	One study found that 62% of people with adult-onset hearing problems had hearing loss in their immediate family.	Avoid loud events, stop smoking, and consider B_{12}. Nearly half of men with hearing problems have a deficiency. Ginkgo biloba, known for increasing memory function, has also shown promise in circulation-based hearing disorders. 85% of adult-onset hearing problems can be helped by amplification technology.		Have a hearing test with your annual physical if possible. 80% of primary-care physicians do not screen patients for hearing loss.

YOUR BODY THROUGH THE AGES AND THE TESTS YOU NEED TO MONITOR IT (CONT'D)				
Condition	**Family ties**	**Things you can do**	**Special info for men who are HIV-positive**	**Tests you need**
Cognitive function and depression An estimated one in six Americans over 65 has some level of clinical depression. As many as 50% of Americans over the age of 85 experience dementia: consistent and at times pervasive mental confusion. Depression and dementia can sometimes be a result of drug interactions. Make sure your doctors and pharmacists are aware of all the medications you are taking to monitor for harmful interactions.	Depression is three times more common in children whose biological parents suffer from depression.	Crossword puzzles, game playing, and continuing education can all increase IQ and enhance cognitive function for those over 65. The more you do with your mind, the more you'll have of it: Remaining mentally active has been shown in many studies to improve mental agility and cognitive function. The herbal supplement ginkgo biloba has been shown to increase circulation in the brain, and by extension cognitive function.	AIDS-related dementia, as well as Alzheimer's, can only be truly diagnosed at autopsy, so ruling out other causes of distraction and absentmindedness is crucial. Simple tests are proving increasingly accurate. One study found that HIV-infected gay and bisexual men were two-thirds more likely to die if they suffered from chronic depression.	A yearly evaluation for depression and cognitive function once you're over 65 is crucial. Somewhere around 75% of cases of depression in older people aren't detected because the doctors don't ask.

AIDS and Older Men

I'm feeling great, never better. I just got promoted. I'm seeing a new, wonderful, younger lover. And yet last weekend I let him make love to me without a condom three times. What was I thinking? That was the first time that had happened since the start of AIDS.

When was the last time you saw a man over fifty on an AIDS prevention poster?

Charles, sixty-seven, is philosophical as he serves tea in his New York City living room. Once richly appointed, the apartment has little left save a few pictures of a time when he was an events planner, their ornate frames contrasting sharply with the wires dangling from the walls where lamps ought to be. "Medicare doesn't pay for medications, so I sold the fixtures to get money for medical bills," he says, gentle in his expression and physical presence. Yet it is perhaps his gentlemanliness that misleads health professionals, and the public, into believing men his age with AIDS do not exist. Just because Charles is unlikely to say "fuck" does not mean he is unlikely to do it. And doctors uncomfortable with talking about sex to young people are more than happy to skip the topic altogether once you're older.

Mention new AIDS cases in 2000 and most think of youthful folly, men in their twenties and thirties. Men over fifty are in some ways a forgotten generation, assumed to be dead, educated, or out of danger's way in a sexless or monogamous relationship. "There's a sense that since most of us who were going to die from AIDS already have, we've been reached," says Doug Goldschmidt, MSW, who leads older gay men's groups on sex and sexuality at SAGE. However common that sense may be, it's not correct. From 1991 to 1996 AIDS cases among adults over fifty rose 22 percent, twice the rise in rate for young adults through that same time period. "While doctors and most prevention campaigns focus on younger folks, one study showed that men over fifty are six times less likely to use a condom and five times less likely to be tested for HIV than younger people," says Nathan Linsk, cochair of the National Association on HIV over Fifty, a Kansas City, Missouri–based group of people with HIV and people who care about them. If you have AIDS already, the risk of stigma may also increase by multiple factors. "All the stereotypes kick in," says Marie Nazon, the former director of the New York AIDS and Aging Task Force. "Now you're the dirty old man with AIDS."

Another reason for the rise in AIDS cases among older men may not be new infections, but rather faster progression to AIDS. Getting care is more complicated when AIDS and aging are combined, both because old people tend to be poorer, and because symptoms may mask and confuse each other. "Men say, 'I'm tired, my memory's going, and I don't know what's age and what's AIDS,'" says Goldschmidt. According to several large studies presented at recent international AIDS conferences, age is one of the most important factors determining how fast you get sick. "One Australian study even found an increase in progression linked to CD4 count and being over thirty!" says David Moore, DO, director of the AIDS program at the Illinois Masonic Medical Center in Chicago. Studies of the new AIDS drugs in the elderly, and the ways their effects on cholesterol and blood sugar levels mask those caused by age or vice versa, have yet to be done.

Older men with AIDS say it's what is *unmasked* by illness—society's deep impatience with people who are old and sick—that is most disturbing. "If you're in a wheelchair, people talk to the person wheeling you as though you can't hear or speak, and address you like a child," says Peter, age sixty-seven. Charles says doctors were reluctant to test him for HIV even after he suggested it, and they often seem unconcerned with pursuing care aggressively. "I've had them say, 'Well, at least you've lived a full life already,'" he says, "and certainly, looking around at all the younger men who are suffering, I agree. But shouldn't everyone be able to live longer, and with dignity?"

Until doctors feel comfortable asking you about sexual risks with the same ease that they recite behaviors affecting heart disease or blood pressure, getting prompt testing and treatment may depend on your ability to ask for it. If you're in need of care, or help caring for someone older with AIDS, your local AIDS organization may be a place to start. "There tend to be more younger people at AIDS organizations," acknowledges Nazon, "but the issues of shame, discrimination, and access to care are similar." Goldschmidt suggests looking to local gay community centers, gay advocates for the aging, and the Internet. SAGE New York offers information and support (www.sageusa.com), and can be reached by phone at (212) 741-2247. There's also Chapters 9 and 10, which may help.

Prostate Primer

While straight men often say that they didn't even know about their prostates until something went wrong with them, we're far more likely to have made the acquaintance of the little gland that nestles around the urethra and under the bladder. If you've lived till middle age without experiencing the pleasure of pressure on your prostate, it's not too late (see "Making Friends with Your Prostate," page 32). Aging, though, brings with it special strains on the prostate that have nothing to do with a well-placed finger or penis. Prostatitis, or inflammation of the prostate (see page 39), occurs most commonly in men age 30 to 50. About half of men have experienced a gradual enlargement of the prostate, known as benign prostatic hyperplasia (BPH), by age sixty. More seriously, an estimated one out of five older men in America is diagnosed with prostate cancer, which can vary in severity from easily treatable to potentially fatal. Around 185,000 men were newly diagnosed with prostate cancer in 1998. Nearly 40,000 died from the disease.

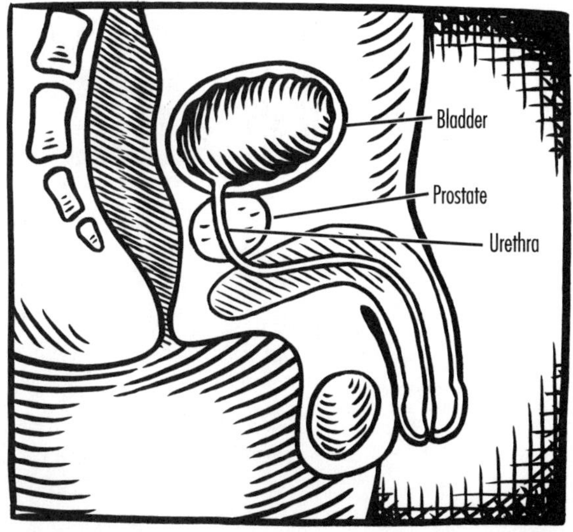

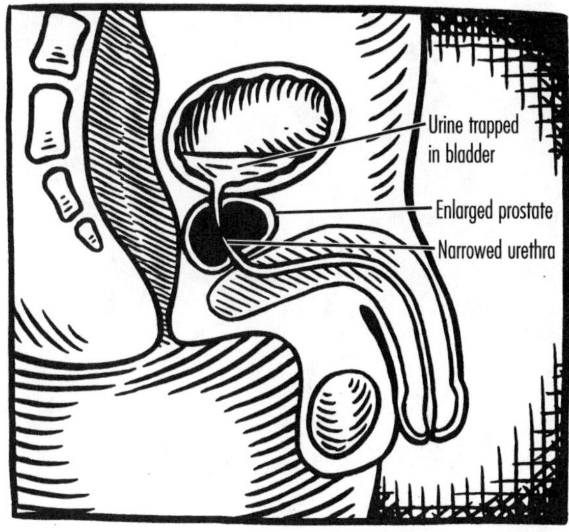

Enlarged, the prostate presses the urethra closed, causing urine buildup

As with so many things male, testosterone seems to lie at the root of BPH and prostate cancer. The hormone is what activates the inert, marble-sized gland you had as a boy, and causes it to grow into the walnut-sized ejaculate factory that becomes so handy after puberty. The problem is that, as long as the testosterone keeps flowing, the prostate keeps growing. By the time you're in your fifties, your testosterone-producing testicles have started to lose some of their vitality, but the prostate, the Energizer bunny of the body, just keeps going. Depending on where the growth is, the new cells may begin to press in on the urethra, which runs through the middle of the gland, gradually narrowing the tube and restricting urine flow. This is the cause of BPH, whose effects, felt by half of men by age sixty, are experienced by 90 percent of us by age eighty. "Less than half of men," says W. Bedford Waters, MD, professor of urology at Loyola University Medical Center in Maywood, Illinois, "will require some kind of medical or surgical treatment for the condition."

A feeling of fullness in your bladder, dribbling and urine stains in your underwear, a weak urine flow, and pain upon ejaculation are all common symptoms of BPH. Other frequently noticed symptoms—for example, having to get up to pee more often at night—may or may not be related to BPH. Even if you do have BPH, *benign* is the key word here; the condition does not mean you're going to get prostate cancer. It's good to go to a doctor to rule out other potential problems, and this is no time to be pee-shy. Describe all the symptoms in detail. "It's amazing how reluctant we are to talk about anything to do with our penises, including urination," says Dr. Waters. If you can't pee at all, he warns, skip the conversation entirely and get to an emergency room: "Obstructed urine, easily remedied, can cause bladder stones, kidney damage, or other serious complications if ignored." For more on treatment of BPH, see page 353.

The PSA Test

Whether you have symptoms of BPH or not, a digital rectal exam (see page 352) is a must every year after forty. But since the DRE misses an estimated 70 to 75 percent of prostate cancers, many doctors are also suggesting a more sensitive approach to cancer detection: the

TURNING A GAY GAZE ON THE DIGITAL RECTAL EXAM (DRE)

A rectal exam is standard for all men over the age of fifty, when the risk of prostate and colon cancer begins to pick up. For gay men, though, or any men whose rectums and prostates are, as Dr. Huskey puts it, "organs of love," having this exam from age forty on is recommended. Given the increased risk of anal cancers in men with HIV, increasing numbers of doctors suggest this regularly for all men with HIV. "I recommend DREs for all sexually active gay men with HIV I see," says Howard Grossman, MD, a New York City doctor with a large gay practice.

The process, where a doctor slides a greased, gloved finger into your anus and gently massages the prostate, sends some men straight into a "homosexual panic," writes Steven Morganstern, MD, author of the heterosexually-oriented *Prostate Sourcebook* (Lowell House, 1993). Worried that he will appear to be enjoying it, "the man resists the probing finger and feels consequent pain." Years of experience with homosexual panic may make many of us calmer but not necessarily less resistant during the exam, since bending over for the doctor is not everyone's idea of what gets them going. For gay men, though, it's homosexual panic on the part of the doctor that can be a source of additional pain and problems. A national survey of members of the Gay and Lesbian Medical Association found that gay male patients coming in for rectal exams were the objects of rude jokes, rough treatment, and crude remarks about how gay men "like" rectal exams to be painful.

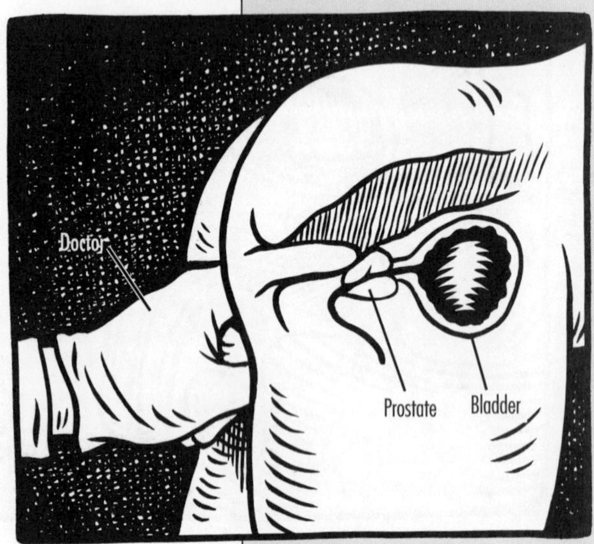

Even if you suspect infection or inflammation of the prostate known as prostatitis (see page 39), BPH, or another prostate problem, the exam should not hurt much, or last too long. In addition to feeling the prostate for tenderness, bumps, or enlargement, the doctor may massage your prostate until a small bit of fluid comes out of your penis. You've probably done something similar yourself, but this takes only a second, produces only a drop of fluid to be put under a microscope, and isn't nearly as much fun. "It's all very clinical," says Ed, fifty-two, "unless you're dating the urologist." The doctor will also get a tiny bit of fecal matter on the end of his glove to test for occult (hidden) blood that may be a sign of cancer, or send you away with a test to do that at home.

If the doc proposes a follow-up sigmoidoscopy, an examination of the lower colon that is among the most effective tests for detecting colon and rectal cancer, he or she should use a flexible instrument. If anyone comes at you with a rigid, old-style proctoscope, ask for another doctor (and if you're feeling feisty, suggest that your old one get some anal sensitivity training).

prostate-specific antigen test, or PSA. The PSA test measures levels of the protein specific to the prostate in the blood. As with other diagnostic tests, like anal Pap smears for men or mammograms for women, doctors hotly debate the whens and whys of its use. PSAs miss cancers as much as 20 percent of the time. Benign conditions like prostate enlargement, prostate infections, and noninvasive cancers can cause higher PSA levels, which means the test may lead to unnecessary biopsy, discomfort, and expenses for conditions that wouldn't hurt you in the long run. Most important, doctors remain highly divided about whether early detection of prostate cancer has any effect on treatment.

The weight of urological opinion, meanwhile, falls clearly on the side of using the screening test and being clear about its defects. "Wait for a digital exam to find prostate cancer and it's no longer curable, but the majority of cancers detected by PSAs can be treated successfully," insists Dr. Waters. "That makes the PSA the single best tool we have for predicting cancer. The fact that you need skilled use of a tool doesn't mean you throw the tool away." Many PSA supporters point to a 1999 study in *The Journal of Urology* that found that prostate cancer deaths declined by 22 percent after screening was introduced in one county in Minnesota. Skeptics point to the Mayo Clinic, also in the area, and say the lower death rate probably had as much to do with the high-quality care available to cancer patients there.

If you do decide to have a PSA, your score will be measured in terms of nanograms per milliliter (ng/ml) and can range from zero to the thousands. A "normal" score depends on your age and risk factors, since PSA levels go up with age and even relatively low scores may signal trouble for those at higher risk. A 1996 *New England Journal of Medicine* article, for example, suggested that a score of 2 or more might signal cancer for Black men between the ages of forty and fifty. For White men of the same age, a score below 4 is considered "normal." Make sure your doctor is familiar with the way recommended levels change with age and race.

As with cholesterol and testosterone, free PSA—the amount that's not attached to protein—turns out to be a more precise indicator than total levels. The more free PSA you have, the less likely it is that you have cancer. "Generally speaking, if you have 25 percent or more free PSA, you have less than a 5 percent chance of having cancer," says Jerry Sullivan, MD, head of the Urology Department at Louisiana State University Medical School in New Orleans. "If your free PSA falls below 10 percent, there's a two-thirds chance that you have cancer."

Though doctors often tell you to abstain from ejaculation for two days before the test (ejaculation may cause your PSA levels to go up), some don't know, or don't let you know, that you should abstain from being anally penetrated for at least that long or longer. Even the digital rectal exam (see box on previous page) may affect PSA levels, which is why your doctor should take your blood for the PSA before he puts his finger inside you. A prostate biopsy can raise your PSA levels for up to four weeks. The effect of having your prostate pounded by a penis for half an hour, or longer if you're lucky, has yet to make the research agenda of the American Urological Association.

BPH Treatment

Unless BPH symptoms are so severe that they're interfering with daily life, "watchful waiting" is usually the treatment of choice. If you do want active intervention, treatment for BPH tends to divide into efforts to shrink the prostate, relax it, or surgically reduce or remove the part of it blocking the urethra.

Prostate shrinkers are medications that stop testosterone production, such as finasteride (Proscar, which you may remember from Chapter 5 as the baldness drug Propecia). If you're thinking your Propecia's a twofer that makes a PSA unnecessary, sorry: The daily dose required to retard baldness is too low to fix your swollen prostate. Finasteride results are unpredictable, and you usually have to use it for six months to see if it works. Extract of saw palmetto berries *(Serenoa repens)*, available from doctors and herbalists, seems in some trials to be as effective as finasteride, with fewer side effects. Other herbal therapies that may help include African plum *(Pygeum africanum)* and beta sitosterol, a substance isolated from corn and soybeans.

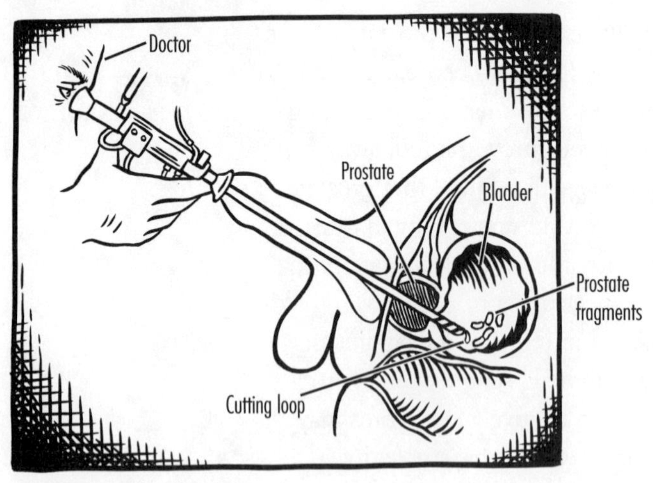

The TURP procedure for BPH

Prostate relaxers, better known as alpha-adrenergic blockers, relax the smooth muscle tissue of the prostate so that urine can flow more easily. Though many such drugs exist for treatment of high blood pressure, only three—terazosin (Hytrin), doxazosin (Cardura), and tamsulosin (Flomax)—are approved for BPH. If your prostate is small and you are still experiencing blockage, these drugs are probably more effective than finasteride.

Surgery, however, remains the most frequent treatment for BPH if medical therapy fails. At present there are at least ten different surgical methods employed to cut, burn, push, laser, or microwave away prostate tissue, all with an incomprehensible series of initials, many still in investigational stages, and some suited only to treating men with a certain size prostate.

In the United States, 90 percent of BPH operations are a procedure called TURP, or transurethral resection of the prostate. The surgeon inserts a long, thin rod with a circular loop of wire on the end down the urethra and into the bladder. A light at the end of the rod helps the doctor see, while the wire allows him or her to chip little sections off the prostate. An electrical current passed through the rod seals blood vessels closed. TURP usually means from one to five days in the hospital, a catheter in your penis for three days to allow you to pee, and complete recovery after about three weeks. For 75 percent of men, it will probably also mean retrograde ejaculation, meaning your semen shoots into your bladder (you pee it out later, and still feel your orgasm) rather than out of your penis. TURP may also involve more medically problematic complications such as incontinence (for between 1 and 2 percent of men), impotence (for 10 percent of men), and narrowing of the urethra (for 3 percent of men).

Prostate Cancer

With one in five men developing prostate cancer (a higher rate than breast cancer in women), scientists are still scrambling to figure out why one man's prostate develops a tumor while four others' don't. Prostate cancer rates are no higher for gay men than for straight ones, says Dr. Waters, though with overall rates so high, that may not be reassuring. Men who've had prostate cancer, some fatally, include a number of baby boomer icons: Dick Sargent (the first Darrin on *Bewitched*), Desert Storm commander Norman Schwarzkopf, publisher Michael Korda, junk bond trader Michael Milken, *Courtship of Eddie's Father* star Bill Bixby, writer Anatole Broyard, actor Sidney Poitier, and Washington, DC, mayor Marion Barry, to name a few. While genetics is one factor for prostate problems (see "Tests You Need," page 345), others seem to include diet (fatty foods are bad), body type (narrow-shouldered men may be at higher risk), and even location (cancer rates are highest in those parts of America that get the least sun, and lowest in the sunny South). One theory is that vitamin D, obtained from sunlight, is protective against prostate cancer. Researchers have fastened on that as one explanation for much higher rates of prostate cancer among Black Americans: Since dark skin absorbs sunlight differently, Black men produce less vitamin D. Others think that genes and diet may be the cause of the fact that Black men get prostate cancer 66 percent more frequently than White men do.

As with BPH, above, the digital rectal exam and a PSA are usually the first steps in detecting a problem. If either or both of those are irregular, the doctor will take a biopsy, using a rectal probe and an ultrasound monitor to see your prostate, and six tiny spring-loaded needles to take samples from it. The procedure isn't terribly comfortable—it apparently hurts more the more nervous you are, and at its worst some men describe it as something like being punched in the stomach—and it may be days before you're back in the mood for anal sex. Intestinal upset, a little blood from your rectum, and some in your cum or urine are also common for as long as a week afterward. As of this writing, doctors are experimenting with newer, more accurate biopsy techniques, including ultrasound technology and "serial biopsy," which increases the number of samples to twelve without significantly increasing the discomfort.

Trying to figure out what to do with the results of the standard prostate biopsy may be even more uncomfortable. Unlike breast or lung cancer, which shows up on an X ray or can clearly be detected by touch, prostate cancer may be much thinner, or more spread out. A biopsy is "like looking *with* a needle in a haystack," writes Patrick C. Walsh, MD, coauthor of the excellently written (but unfortunately titled) *The Prostate: A Guide for Men and the Women Who Love Them* (Warner Books, 1997). Cancers that are just on the surface of the gland, or those in parts of the prostate not sampled, may be missed by needle biopsies. Furthermore, getting a positive result does not make the doctors positive of anything. "As many as 30 percent of prostate cancers will not develop into anything life-threatening," says Dr. Waters, who says that considering your PSA score, how many of the six needle samples were cancerous, and something called a Gleason score—which rates how malignant the biopsied cells look under a microscope, on a scale from 2 to 10—is needed to decide on next steps. "If you have a Gleason score of 7 or above, further kinds of tests are clearly necessary to see how far the cancer's spread," says Waters. In addition to bone and CT scans, a test approved in 1998 by the FDA may represent a major step forward in prognosis. The test marks prostate cancer cells with a radioactive isotope that can be read by a special scanner, giving further and better information on the extent of the cancer's spread.

With so many variables, there's often room for ambiguity—and difference of opinion—about the proper course of treatment. "They wanted to operate on me the next day after seeing my PSA score," says Jim, fifty, a computer programmer in Los Angeles, "but with two months required for convalescence, I wasn't ready." After visiting a support group of prostate cancer survivors at the University of California, Los Angeles ("I heard a lot of bitterness there about doctors minimizing effects of surgery," he says), as well as cancer and radiation specialists, Jim decided he'd avoid surgery in favor of less invasive and less definitive methods: hormone-blocking therapies, and implantation of radioactive pellets (see "Prostate Cancer Treatments," next page). In the meanwhile, he worked with a nutritionist on a stringent diet (heavy on low-fat, high-protein sources such as fish and white-meat turkey, light on dairy products, and a total ban on red meat) that he claims brought his PSA level from 36 to 1.9. Urologists say they wouldn't chance a diet-alone approach with such high PSA levels. Jerry, forty-eight, a computer programmer, wouldn't, either; he just wanted his prostate out. "I was completely freaked out by the fear that I'd never have sex again," he confesses, "but the idea of cancer scared me more." Henry, eighty, a volunteer AIDS counselor and former advertising man from New York City, made a similar choice for himself. "Schmuck," he said to himself before having his prostate removed two years ago, "do you want to be worrying about this cancer again ten years from now?"

Prostate Cancer Treatments

What kind of treatment to pursue for prostate cancer depends on if, and how extensively, it's spread. If it's contained in the prostate, survival rates are promising—90 percent or higher over the next ten years. "I was told I had 'the best cancer to get,'" jokes Jerry. Prostate cancer grows slowly, and the older you are, the more slowly it grows, leading some doctors to call it a "pathologist's cancer": visible under the microscope, but often not in real life. "For older men or men with advanced HIV disease, prostate cancer may definitely be something you die *with* rather than die from," says Dr. Sullivan.

FOR CANCER THAT HAS SPREAD

If your cancer's spread to surrounding lymph nodes or beyond, what you want to risk depends on how long you expect to live and what quality of life you want. Cure is not yet possible for prostate cancer that's widely metastasized into the rest of the body, though treatments that "blockade" your testosterone production can ease bone pain and slow the cancer's growth. The less polite word for that treatment is castration, chemical or surgical, and although the doctor can use certain methods to keep your scrotum looking close to normal, it rarely feels that way. Hormone blockading makes you impotent, reduces your sexual desire, and will give you the hot flashes, personality changes, and weakened of bone density experienced by women in menopause.

Some men who've experienced it say that castration sounds more traumatic than it is. You will not, contrary to some rumors, get a high voice (or regrow a full head of hair). Estrogen, medroxyprogesterone (Provera), or megestrol (Megace) can help with some of the symptoms, but if you're sexually active, you may want to consider spot radiation, which eases the pain without forcing a loss in sexual function. The hard truth is that while hormone blockading can contain pain and the spread of the cancer, as of this writing there seems to be no difference in survival rates between men with advanced cancer who start hormone therapy early or late. Only certain kinds of prostate cancer respond at all to hormone therapy, and hormone therapy seems to change overall survival rate only in men with cancer that's minimally advanced beyond the prostate. Much as with AIDS before combination therapy, a patient's desire to do everything, and the drug companies' desire to sell everything, may be forcing people into early, though not so useful, courses of treatment. Men spend over $1.3 billion annually on hormone blockers, points out Dr. Walsh, without any evidence that the therapies they are using prolong life.

TREATMENT FOR LOCALIZED PROSTATE CANCER

What to do about prostate cancer that hasn't spread, much as with any serious medical decision, depends on how comfortable you are with uncertainty, how likely your condition is to progress (even with localized cancer, there are different stages), and how long you expect to live.

Watchful Waiting

Depending on your Gleason and PSA scores, the wait-and-see approach may be best, since treatment may be more trouble than the disease itself. "While a full third of men over fifty have small prostate tumors, only 10 percent of them develop into cancer that causes serious health problems," says Dr. Jerry Sullivan of Louisiana State University. "If you're over seventy or think you have less than ten years to live, treatment may not be for you." If you and your doctors (you should always get a second opinion) decide you want to treat, conventional therapies divide basically into what one irreverent prostate support group member refers to as "cut or fried": surgical removal of the prostate, or radiation therapies to zap it.

TURNING A GAY GAZE ON TALK ABOUT PROSTATE CANCER TREATMENTS

All the prostate cancer survivors interviewed for this book stress the importance of communicating with other patients and survivors, preferably *before* you go for treatment. Jerry, the computer programmer, mentions Us Too, the international support network of men with prostate cancer, as a "good group" to contact, while Jim found a support group at UCLA. Since neither the literature published on prostate treatments nor most urologists have a clue about what the removal of your prostate is going to do to your anal sex life, it can be especially helpful for gay men with prostate cancer to talk about their experiences with each other.

If you can't find a gay support group, consider starting your own. Jerry founded one in the New York area shortly after his diagnosis. Each week, seven or eight gay male prostate cancer survivors, their ages ranging from the late forties to eighty-six, meet at Jerry's Manhattan apartment. Jerry recounts one member's story of accidentally peeing on a sex partner—and the partner's unexpected sexual excitement over this unintended water sport. He's also taken to posting some of the support group's proceedings on the Web (www.mindspring.com/~jerryrh/prosstop.htm), which can be an excellent organizing tool for any gay man with prostate cancer and no support group. "Our attitude is that if nothing's off-limits in conversation, it's good for our health," he says.

Not talking may be a health hazard for straight and gay men alike. Us Too surveyed a thousand prostatectomy patients and two hundred urologists. Three in ten patients said their doctors did not discuss any quality-of-life issues, including physical side effects, prior to the operation. Fewer than half of the men surveyed said their doctors had addressed their emotional and psychological factors as well as physical ones. Meanwhile, 70 percent noticed a decline in their sex drive, and more than 75 percent reported erectile dysfunction following treatment. Ejaculation becomes impossible after the prostate is removed. "It took me a while to realize that though nothing came out, I could still climax internally," says Henry with a smile. "I'm the safest guy around to have sex with."

Radical Prostatectomy

Total surgical removal of the prostate is the most medically popular and most invasive option. The procedure lasts from ninety minutes to four hours and is usually followed by a hospital stay of three to seven days and time away from work of three to six weeks. Because the whole prostate is removed, so is much of the anxiety about prostate cancer spread, though side effects from the operation go well beyond downtime from work. Many surgeons inadvertently cut the nerve bundles on either side of the prostate, making erection impossible. Dr. Waters estimates that between 50 and 60 percent of prostatectomies are followed by some kind of hard-on problems, with younger men more likely to retain erectile function than older ones. Dr. Walsh, who pioneered a newer nerve-sparing surgery, estimates that with that approach, 90 percent of patients in their forties, 75 percent of men in their fifties, 60 percent of men in their sixties, and 25 percent of men in their seventies will stay potent. Viagra, the erectile dysfunction remedy that's the rage, helps 43 percent of those who are impotent from prostatectomies, and the erection injections sold under the name Caverject help even more (see page 172). You have a year or possibly two after the operation, however, before you will even know for sure whether you have impotence problems or not.

Nowhere in any of the massive amount of published literature is the question of anal pleasure after prostatectomy addressed, though gay survivors of radical prostatectomy say that it is radically diminished. Ejaculation, too, is changed without a prostate: You get the sensation but no output. Urination may happen more often than you'd like. All men experience a certain amount of incontinence after surgery—you have a catheter in your penis for about two to three weeks afterward—and some 3 percent experience permanent serious bladder control problems. Between 10 percent and 20 percent experience minor leakage from their penises, such as dripping when they cough, for the rest of their lives. Kegels (see page 41) can definitely help, both for speedier recovery and for long-term control. So can panty liners and a soft penile clamp, kind of like a U-shaped clothespin with a Velcro strap and a gel foam rubber bar. Not the greatest under tight jeans, but it could be a conversation starter.

In other countries, such as Sweden, radical prostatectomies are performed at rates much lower than in the United States. Still, American men with prostate cancer tend to live longer, making urologists insist that it's the most effective treatment for high-grade cancer, and best for all men with progressing cancer who expect to live more than ten years.

Radiation Therapy

This is done at a radiation therapy center, five days a week, for seven to eight weeks. The traditional approach is to zap the cancer from outside, shooting radiation through the skin, bladder, and rectum. "Basically, it fries the prostate," says Franklin C. Lowe, MD, of New York City's St. Luke's–Roosevelt Hospital. Unfortunately, it also cooks some local tissues: though the fifteen-minute procedure doesn't hurt, common aftereffects include local skin burning, burning during urination, rectal bleeding, brown-tinged semen, and diarrhea. Less erectile dysfunction occurs with radiation, though problems take longer to make themselves seen: Some patients report having hard-on difficulties as much as a year after the procedure. Others undergoing radiation complain of inflammation of the rectum, known as radiation proctitis, which doctors didn't warn them about. According to urologists, radiation is considered best for men expecting to live less than ten or fifteen years, or those who have other conditions that make surgery dangerous or impossible.

Newer radiation techniques are being done at academic centers, but will probably be more widely available shortly. These include:

• *Conformal 3D radiation therapy.* This zeroes in on the prostate using a computer, and allows for greater doses of radiation with less damage to the bladder and rectum. The process requires thirty to fifty CT scans of the patient's pelvis so that the computer can reconstruct the landscape, and you spend each of the ten-minute sessions with your bottom half in a special cast that keeps you from moving. If you were potent before you went in for treatment, you have an estimated 60 to 70 percent chance of staying that way. Ten percent of patients, however, experience either rectal or urethral narrowing, as well as some of the other side effects described with external radiation, above.

• *Interstitial brachytherapy (seed implant therapy).* In this one-day-and-one-night-at-the-hospital process, a hundred or more radioactive "seeds" are implanted in the prostate, using a transrectal ultrasound for guidance. Postprocedure discomfort can be greater than with the other two forms of radiation therapy, says Dr. Lowe, and unlike other radiation, it's most appropriate for early-stage cancer and men with smaller prostates. Urinary problems such as retention or cystitis are more common, and there's as much as a 20 percent chance of rectal bleeding. You are, however, more likely to stay potent—80 to 90 percent of men experience no erectile dysfunction after a year.

If the idea of deciding how to treat your cancer is making you crazy, take a deep breath. According to a massive 1997 analysis of more than sixty thousand patients, any treatment at all, including watchful waiting, yielded a survival rate of ten years for more than 90 percent of patients with low-grade cancer. With medium-grade cancer, three-quarters of men were alive ten years later, regardless of treatments. For high-grade cancer, medical intervention helps: Watchful waiting yielded a survival rate of only 45 percent, while radiation and prostatectomy yielded survival rates of 53 percent and 67 percent, respectively. As for those who question the value of life beyond the hard-on, remember Anatole Broyard's observation. "In my case," wrote the critic in his account of his prostate cancer, "after a brush with death, I feel that just to be alive is a permanent orgasm."

MEDICARE

Unfortunately, your cholesterol gets higher and your prostate gets bigger just as your wallet gets smaller. What kind of health care the most vulnerable are entitled to, and how that care is to be paid for, is a question that swirls continually around Medicare, the federal program to provide health insurance to the elderly and disabled. Some politicians have fought in recent years to raise the age at which you can begin collecting benefits from sixty-five to sixty-seven. Others have pushed for fifty-five. At the moment, Medicare covers most Americans who are sixty-five or over, or who are under sixty-five and have been receiving Social Security disability insurance (see box on page 423) for two years or more. The program, like the politics around it, is split into two: part A, which pays for hospitalizations, skilled nursing home care, and home health and hospice services, and part B, which pays for doctor's services and other outpatient care. If you want part B, you have to pay for it (about $44 a month in 1998).

Medicare provides generous benefits in some areas (up to 150 days of hospitalization, unlimited outpatient mental health visits, hospice care, and so on), though it asks recipients to meet deductibles and copayments. It has two areas, however, with no coverage whatsoever: home care of the help-with-chores variety and prescription drugs. Most old or disabled people need one or both of these, so private insurance companies offer Medicare supplemental policies to fill the gaps (called "Medigap" coverage). In most states, people on Medicare are offered a standard menu of ten different plans, known as plans A through J. Once again, since the private sector is involved, many insurers refuse coverage to those with preexisting medical conditions or disabilities (see "Limited Engagement: How Insurers Avoid You," page 318). Even the Medigap policies that cover prescription drugs (which only plans I and J do) limit coverage to a maximum of $3,000 annually. Since a condition such as AIDS can run up to $15,000 a year in pills, that's not going to do it. Check with a local aging, AIDS, or disability organization for help working the system and covering what you need.

If you do buy Medigap coverage, make sure you know what you're buying. Some companies won't tell you they're selling you "attained-age" policies, whose premiums increase as you age. "Community-rated" policies, such as those the American Association of Retired Persons (AARP) sells to its members, have fixed premiums. One way to do without Medigap coverage is to join the growing number of Medicare managed care plans, which now enroll more than 16 percent of Medicare participants. These plans, some of which charge you an extra premium, all offer lower copayments than Medicare, and free extras such as immunizations and checkups. Some also cover a limited amount of prescriptions. On the other hand, all the drawbacks of managed care, such as a narrow choice of doctors, restrictions on drugs, and difficulty finding specialists, may apply (see "Managing Managed Care," page 323). And increasingly, companies are discovering that the old birds weren't quite as ripe for the plucking as they'd hoped and are withdrawing from the market, leaving the least scrupulous providers to provide care to those most in need.

As with Medicaid, you also have extensive appeal rights on Medicare, including external review if you are enrolled in a Medicare HMO. If your health condition is serious, HMOs must review your appeal within seventy-two hours, and in all cases you can reappeal and have the decision sent to an objective third party, the Center for Health Dispute Resolution, though it may take as long as six months to see results. "Only 2 percent of people appeal their Medicare denials," says Joe Baker, associate director of the Medicare Rights Center (www.medicarerights.org) in New York City. "But of those who do, 70 percent get findings in their favor." So, are you appealing?

GIMME SHELTER

Doug Goldschmidt, who worked with housing developers prior to running groups for older gay men in New York City, explains that housing options for older people are generally aimed at three types: "the 'go-gos,' the 'slow-gos,' and the 'no-gos'." The "go-gos" are those of us who are ready to stop working but are not ready to significantly scale back our activities. Retirement communities for this group can feature homes that range from $100,000 to over

TURNING A GAY GAZE ON HOMES FOR THE ELDERLY

In senior centers, hospitals, and nursing homes, many are reliving the bad old days where homosexuality was a love that dare not speak its name. "I get calls from hospitals and aging organizations all the time," says Mary Jean Sanford of SAGE New York, "where people who work with the elderly will say, 'I think that so-and-so may be, um . . . we're concerned that they might be, uh . . .' And I'll say, 'You think they're homosexual and you want to know what to do about it?' 'Yes!' they'll say with huge relief. 'How did you know?'"

If the people in charge can't say the word *homosexual,* they're not going to be able to provide the kind of support you need as you grow old. And while all of us can suffer through a spaghetti lunch or short hospital stay where we have to hide our sexuality, that gets really tough for old gay folks at a home. A number of planners are working overtime on market research for retirement communities serving gay men and lesbians (our number-one preferred amenity is a gym, number two's a theater), but as of this writing plans for Our Town in San Francisco and Rainbow Gardens in Boulder, Colorado, remain on the drawing board and awaiting investors. One Florida retirement community, the Palms of Manasota (it's the name of the region, not a racy pun), is up and selling to gay men and lesbians, and it's down the road from the women-only clubhouse and pool of the Resort on Carefree Boulevard. Another retirement community friendly to gay men and lesbians is under construction in Ohio. Meanwhile, increasing numbers of us who have neither children nor the $600,000 retirement nest egg Merrill Lynch suggests for "married couples" used to living on $70,000 a year are waiting for answers about who's going to give us shelter when we're old.

RETIREMENT REQUIREMENT?

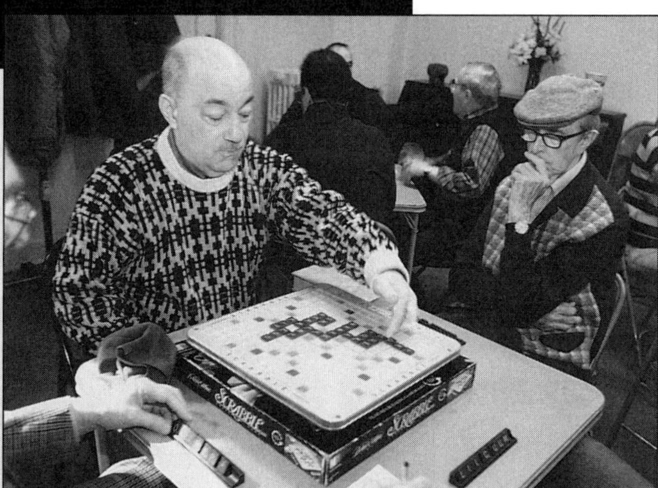

It is impossible for old age to be borne in extreme poverty, even by a wise man.
—Cicero

He is richest whose pleasures are cheapest.
—Henry David Thoreau

A shout out to all the preretirees in the house: What's the first thing you think of when you hear the letter S? The correct answer is not sex, apparently, but savings, according to Per Larson, guru of gay money matters and author of *Gay Money* (Dell, 1997). If you were among the many gay men who didn't get Larson's lessons early enough to recognize that the twenties was when a lot of us were supposed to be saving—who knew that waiting on tables was the most untaxable income you'd ever make in your life?—then the forties is make-or-break time, according to Larson. "After years of exploring the possibilities of being, we now define what we want to do," he notes. "Where once we struggled to minimize spending and maximize income, we now focus on building assets and minimizing liabilities." Of course, plenty of us didn't struggle to minimize spending in our earlier years, but that's a different story. We'll write *Gay Without Money.*

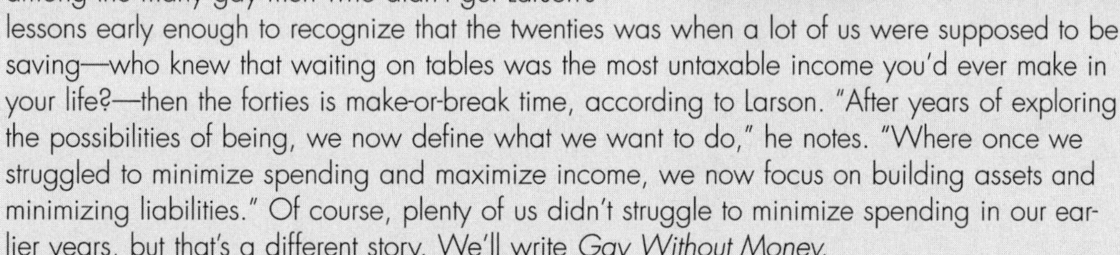

Self-direction—the ability to entertain and sustain yourself in a variety of inner ways—has been noted as a psychological retirement requirement for as long as there have been advice books on the subject. Larson adds a financial fillip, stressing that gay men would be wise—particularly as life gets longer and downsizing gets stronger—to develop a self-supervised, quasi-independent set of skills that allows you to maximize control of your life and your "work product." That doesn't necessarily mean starting your own business—*Gay Money* stresses the value of "intrapreneurship," a move within a company that allows you greater independence and mobility in the event that you hit the "lavender ceiling" or are downsized out entirely. If you're doing publications design and production, could you consolidate your operations to allow for the possibility of work from home? If you're a company stock analyst, can you adopt a "foretelling" or "catalyzing" role that would allow you both to consolidate your behind-the-throne-status and eventually to take some clients on the side?

In another reworking of what researcher Raymond Berger calls gay men's "crisis competency" and what Dr. Huskey calls "our natural fabulousness at aging," Larson sees gay men as particularly suited to the challenge of making our way toward independence. Not only do we have greater numbers of two-income-no-children families, but we've had to act on our feet, monitor our environment for changes, and think outside the confines of tradition for years now. Our practice at camouflage makes us good actors, a requirement for any independent businessperson. Why, we're positively made for entrepreneurship. "We have years of experience," Larson says, "spinning gold out of straw."

Numerous books, including Larson's, offer more specific advice on the money and plans you need to maintain your fiscal health. If you're ready to get to the level of budget worksheets and financial risk assessment, or need to know the difference between a Roth IRA and a regular one, how to insure a car for you and your partner, and all the rest of those financial matters that never seemed to matter until you realize you don't know what you need to about them, check out *J. K. Lasser's Gay Finances in a Straight World,* by Peter M. Berkery Jr. and Gregory A. Diggins (Macmillan, 1998), or *4 Steps to Financial Security for Lesbian and Gay Couples,* by Harold Lustig (Ballantine, 1999).

HOME IS WHERE THE HEALTH IS

"If someone goes into people's houses and helps them rearrange their lives a little, they can often get five years more there," says Dr. Huskey, who makes regular house calls to homebound elderly patients. Staying home while you're not feeling well may be difficult, but if you have an expert—a geriatric social worker, a gerontologist, or a geriatrician—meet with you and your caretaker, you may be able to get excellent advice on ways to stay healthy at home. Following are some strategies that can help.

FURNITURE REARRANGEMENT

Make sure your furniture's arranged in such a way that it gives you something to hold on to as you walk through, says Dr. Huskey. Objects that you use every day should be stored at waist level to minimize bending, slippery throw rugs should be replaced by carpeting taped down firmly from underneath, and you should have grab bars and security rails for tub, bedside, and toilet. For those whose sense of style is the last thing to go, these come in different colors.

ACCESSIBLE MEDICAL INFORMATION

Make sure all your medical information, including a list of all prescriptions you're taking, is available to you and to others. One in six seniors is prescribed inappropriate or unsafe medications, and nearly 17 percent of those wind up in the hospital as a result. Far greater numbers suffer confusion, fatigue, and other symptoms because their doctors have given them inappropriate drugs that take too long to clear from the body or interact badly with others. If you do fall sick, make sure people can tell what you've taken. "After seeing the patient, my first stops are the freezer, the refrigerator, the medicine cabinet, and the bedside table when I'm making a house call," says Huskey. Many cities have "vial of life" programs, where such lists are put into a special vial in the freezer or taped to the refrigerator, where emergency medical technicians know to look for them.

ASSISTIVE DEVICES

"Vast numbers of older people aren't taking advantage of the devices that there are to minimize isolation and increase self-reliance," says Jere Kelly, MD, a geriatrician at Northwestern University in Chicago. Among them: no-bend shoe horns; turning aids for faucets, stoves, and doorknobs; big-handled gardening tools; one-hand cutting boards; and touch-on, touch-off lamps. More sophisticated devices include automatic medicine dispensers, bathtub lifts, bubble or ripple mattresses designed to prevent bedsores, beds with bathing functions, disposable portable toilet systems for use while standing or lying down, and a huge variety of large-print products, magnifying lenses, and hearing aids. "Some of these may sound expensive," says Rosemary Bakker, president of ElderDesign, a company specializing in "therapeutic environ-

$1 million and offer amenities such as golf, swimming, reading groups at the clubhouse, and the like. "Slow-gos" need assisted-living residences, which are often more like hotels than houses, with private rooms or apartments but also meals and supportive care (such as maid service, help with chores, and some basic nursing) provided. "No-gos" among us usually move to skilled nursing facilities, better known as nursing homes, where residents get continuous care or help in caring for themselves. While some retirement communities span the continuum, others hope you'll forget about the long term when moving into their lovely facilities. Think twice before buying that condo with all those stairs down to the beach, because stares down to the beach may be all you're able to manage twenty years later.

Even if you've saved diligently, nursing homes—more like hospitals than homes, in spite

ments for an aging society" in New York City. "But not when compared to a $40,000-to-$80,000-a-year stay at a nursing home."

COMMUNICATION FROM AFAR

The portable alarm systems of the I've-fallen-and-I-can't-get-up variety, where you touch a small button worn around your neck or wrist to call for help, are only the beginning. Many cities have "early alert" programs, where mail carriers come inside and investigate if mail isn't being picked up as usual. Increasing numbers of states also have special relay systems that allow people with hearing or speech disabilities to type in their messages to an operator who translates to the other caller. Commercially available products include telephones that translate voice to text, have lights that flash as well as a ring, and voice-activated dialing. Computer software that translates text to voice and vice versa is quickly moving from science fiction to strangely affordable.

FREE OR REDUCED-FEE SERVICES

These can range from a meals-on-wheels program that delivers food to programs at local senior centers to programs that provide low-cost or free repairs to private homes. The local office on aging maintains a list of programs for people over sixty or sixty-five. Some of these are especially for people who are ill, and some aren't.

PRIVATE SUPPORT SERVICES

Some of these programs have to be paid for out of pocket, and some are covered by Medicaid and Medicare, though rarely adequately. "Getting reinforcements can make a huge difference if you or your caretaker is at the breaking point physically or psychologically," says Dr. Huskey, "though the best time to search out support is *before* you reach the breaking point." Possibilities include:

- *Day care programs.* These give the elderly a break from the usual caregiving, and offer a range of structured activities and a meal. Some offer medical treatment and weekend or evening care.
- *Home health care.* These services bring in aides to help with chores of daily living such as bathing, as well as more skilled aides to help with administering medications, wound care, and other services.
- *Visiting-nurse services.* For even more skilled care, including changing of bandages, infusions, injections, and basic diagnostic care.
- *Short-stay nursing home care.* Some providers will accept patients for short-term stays. If you're a caretaker arranging for this service, make sure to negotiate the length of stay before arrival. Some foster care agencies and homes may also take elderly people briefly.

of the name—are prohibitively expensive for all but the lavishly wealthy. Even Medicare pays only for a maximum of one hundred days. "The vast majority of the patients I've seen have been forced to rely on Medicaid [the health care program for the poor] to cover nursing home costs," says Dr. Huskey. "They require you to spend down every cent, liquidate every asset. And of course this is another place where married heterosexuals get privileges we don't, since a legally married partner can keep the family house and car while the other gets care. If you're two men together, you need to make sure you've done the necessary transferring before the bills start rolling in, because they will certainly go after your jointly owned house and car and whatever else you have."

If you or your partner is ill or infirm, a number of legal documents are necessary to ensure many of the basic rights granted without question to married couples (see box on page 422). More complicated is finding a way to undo the laws of the land, whose general discomfort about sex and the elderly is magnified when passed through the filter of homophobia and fear of AIDS. "I called ten assisted-living facilities to find a place for my nephew, who has AIDS," explains Bill Laing, a former psychology professor and creator of the gay-friendly Palms of Manasota retirement community in Florida. "All of them, when they heard he had AIDS, said they'd have to get back to me. None did."

Nursing homes, with their greater emphasis on rules and structure, are even greater offenders. "A nursing home is a home, and you are entitled to many of the same rights there as in a private residence," insists Dr. Huskey, "including the right to privacy, pursuit of sexual satisfaction, and the use of sexually explicit materials to get you or a partner sexually aroused." In spite of his insistence that hospitality begin at the nursing home, Huskey and other advocates for the elderly acknowledge that most old-age homes have yet to come into the modern era and give gay men and lesbians a gracious reception. Massachusetts entrepreneur Brenda Cole was an aide in a nursing home outside Boston when she heard a resident asking to be wheeled up to see another resident who lived on the fifth floor. "The nurses staunchly refused," says Cole. "They explained that the women had lived together for thirty years, that they were lesbians, and that the home didn't allow them to see each other."

Twenty-five years later, Cole went on to found Emerald City Residences, Inc., to plan and build senior housing alternatives friendly to lesbians and gay men in ten cities across the country. While conducting market research, Cole heard stories echoing her own observations and experiences. "One eighty-two-year-old gay man went to a nursing home short-term to recover from surgery, and was visited every day by his life partner and friends," she recalls. "He was so proud of his support system that he came out to the staff. Things changed immediately. He was no longer welcome to dine with the other residents, and his caregivers at the home started wearing rubber gloves." Men talking to SAGE and other organizations tell of being heavily sedated if they dare make sexual advances, of being separated from or not allowed to room with their life partners, and of being informed that homosexuality is something "we don't talk about here." The fact that many older gay men and lesbians already do not feel comfortable or safe speaking about their relationships, particularly in hospital settings they may not have seen since they were forced into electroshock therapy in their youth, only deepens their reluctance to file complaints or push for better treatment.

These and more general health reasons, such as the cardinal rule that you want to be around other sick people as little as you can when you're sick yourself, are among the reasons why geriatricians including Dr. Huskey advise you to stay in your own home for as long as possible (see box on page 362). The fantasy of moving into an old house with a bunch of friends is a good one, though as Cole points out, it pales once one of you breaks your hip. "We need to think about the what-ifs as the decades pass," she says, confident that when it comes time for the youngest baby boomers to move into nursing homes, there will be more choices. There are already a growing number of continuing-care communities, places that offer you smooth transitions from independent living to assisted living to nursing home care in one place. You offer them an entrance fee of between $20,000 and $40,000, and a hefty monthly payment. None of the 1,300 continuing-care communities in America is gay, but how long can that last? "All over the country we've started the evolution of all-gay or gay-supportive communities," says Ellen Ensig-Brodsky of the Pride Senior Network in New York, an organization dedicated to promoting services sensitive to gay, lesbian, bisexual, and transgender seniors in nursing homes and other facilities. "If we can build our own retirement and assisted-living facilities, the nursing homes and continuing care will follow. Then we need to turn our sights on the long-term care insurance needed to pay for it all."

Parenting Your Parents

It's been an eight-year ordeal, including a five-year nursing home epic. We've each spent upward of $100,000.

The best solution we found was an elderly assisted-housing program. It was hard to get them into it, and since my parents were fixed-income civil servants, we had to pay the rent. But they immediately bonded to other people in the home. My mother's been deaf her whole life, and always refused to even try a TDD. It was so liberating for her to be around others in the same situation. I called, and she answered the phone. She wrote, "I can't talk, we're going to a party." I cried, it was so beautiful.

I lost my business partner and closest friend to AIDS, and at a very young age. I've used caring for him as a guide for my parents. Losing dozens of friends does prepare you.

Think of it as a dry run for your own old age, or a cruel joke that finds you taking care of someone who never really understood you. It may be a chance to return love and support that made you who you are, or a Zen exercise in being present. Perhaps it's a way to put the terrible lessons you learned caring for friends with AIDS into practice, as if you needed any. However you conceive of it, taking care of a parent is one of the hallmarks of middle-to-old age. "The first time you change your mother's diaper, it really hits you," says Carl, fifty, an interior designer whose parents both became ill simultaneously. "She's become your child."

While gay men are less likely than our straight siblings to be caught in a so-called sandwich situation, simultaneously taking care of young children and elderly parents, there are other reasons why the parental boomerang comes home to gay baby boomers. "The fact that we don't have children of our own leaves other family members thinking we should be able to take up more of the slack," says Dr. Huskey. John, forty-one, now caring for his Alzheimer's-afflicted mother and a mentally retarded brother in Brooklyn, New York, says his caretaking position was in some ways the logical result of his being the favorite child. For Howard, forty-five, years of AIDS caretaking experience made him a natural in the family's eyes, and his own. "I couldn't not," he says. "My family didn't know how to operate in a hospital. They didn't know about entitlements like Medicaid, or how to set up a support group. I'd had lots of experience."

Many of the issues raised when taking on care for a parent—loss of freedom, loss of privacy, the exhuming of old familial conflicts, and feelings of powerlessness over a parent's decline—are the same for both gay and straight children. For gay men, though, some burdens may be heavier: Childhood wounds may be deeper, apartments in urban areas may be smaller, and we often lack traditional supports such as religious institutions. Depending on our parent's condition, having Mom or Dad move in may also mean revisiting parental disapproval of your lifestyle or lover. If you think you can balance the two, think again before opening the door.

"Looking back on it now, there were assumptions I made that in retrospect I must have been crazy to make," says John, who cooks for and feeds his mother and brother daily before sitting down to eat with his lover, Michael. "Michael's a social worker, and he's been great. But we thought we'd have more leeway with our lives, that we could maintain some social life, stay away overnight, or at least go to the movies. The reality is that she can't be left alone, ever, for a moment. It's been a tremendous strain on our relationship, on my career, on everything."

Responsible caregiving begins with an honest assessment of what you want to give as well as a realistic estimation of what you can provide. "I live in a studio apartment in the middle of the city with my boyfriend," says Ray, thirty-nine, a computer programmer whose mother's injuries after a fall prompted him to consider leaving his partner of five years to care for her. Ultimately Ray decided to help his mother find a place in a senior-citizen complex rather than disrupt his own life. Peter, fifty-one, who runs a mental health agency, almost lost his own mind traveling to Boston repeatedly to try to arrange his parents' care. "My father was just out of the hospital, my mother was extremely stressed, and the doctor was not communicating with either of them," he says. "They're from the generation that looks at doctors like deities and don't know that they're entitled to clearer explanations." After unsatisfactory meetings with the cardiologist, he contacted a local hospital and found a gerontologist at the local elder-care center who would see both mother and father. "Gerontology looks at old people holistically," he says, "understanding health problems as part of the aging process. And it was during the wonderful experience with that doctor that we discovered there was something called care coordination." For the year since, a trained social worker has accompanied his parents to the doctor and worked with them to get the answers they need to make life decisions. "For as much as $300 and as little as $90, she does all the things I can't do long distance," says Peter. "My mother has taken to calling her to talk about things, like how she kind of liked having some space to herself while my father was in the hospital. I love that." Peter and his lover, John, are now trying, with less success, to locate a care coordinator to help John's mother in Mississippi.

If you do decide to take in a parent, a number of things can help ease the stress. Claire Berman, author of *Caring for Yourself While Caring for Your Aging Parents* (Henry Holt, 1996), echoes a theme that runs through the literature on caregiving: "If we are to successfully manage the care of our parents," she writes, "we have to learn, first of all, to care for ourselves." Some other advice:

Get Support

"The first thing you need to do is join a support group," says John. Numerous organizations, both formal and informal, exist to help people cope with caregiving. Support groups are out there for those caring for people with specific illnesses, such as cancer, as well as general support for caregivers. Some gay-specific groups exist as well: New York has a support group for gay men and lesbians who care for people with Alzheimer's, for example.

Look into Day Care

John found a program for his mother that runs from 8:00 A.M. to 4:00 P.M., and says that without it he wouldn't be able to work at all. "If you think you can do it all yourself," he says, "it's a recipe for disaster. I feel better with this program because I know she's getting the kind of attention she needs."

Work with Siblings

Unresolved sibling conflicts often rear their head when a parent is ill, though siblings can also be a font of strength. "If I didn't have my brothers," said Carl, "I would have lost my business, I would have lost my mind, and I certainly would have gone broke." Even if there is an "in-charge" sibling, decisions regarding parent care are best made with the participation of everyone involved. Convene a family conference at which you decide on how to divide up work and expenses. "If you need help," advises Berman, "ask for it, and be specific." Practice sentences like "I'll have Dad stay for a month, but I need $300 to cover expenses." Send invoices. Be calm but unyielding.

Maintain Focus

Caring for an ill parent is not the time for resolving past conflicts, advises Berman, who says clarity of purpose is imperative to successful caregiving. "I did all my therapy in the eighties," agrees John. "These are not the circumstances under which I can be working out unfinished business. She's Mom and she's not Mom. I can't relate to her the way I related to her when she was whole."

Consider Your Lover

Think about your lover—before you no longer have one. "It got to the point where I'd wake up at five in the morning and hear Harold's mother calling for him," says Everett, fifty seven. "And she wouldn't listen to me or speak to me. It wasn't workable." In some cases, the fact that your partner doesn't have all that past history may make him see what to do more clearly. "George made it clear that he was there with me no matter what I wanted to do," says Peter, thirty-eight, whose mother arrived on their doorstep in a full-fledged nervous breakdown. "I just sat there in shock while he made all the doctor's arrangements, pulled strings to get appointments. A month later, when she wasn't getting better, he had us look into getting her a place to stay where she could get more support."

Be Resourceful

Try to maintain as much of your own life as possible, and use every source of help you can in that effort. "Rather than having them move in with any of us, my brothers and I each took a week to be with my mother while my father was in the hospital," says Carl. "That way the strain wasn't constant." Chapter 10 offers some other concrete tips on how to be a better caregiver.

Helping a parent as he or she falls apart may even leave you feeling a little more whole. Carl's account of his experience sounds like what Erikson might describe as a step toward finding integrity rather than despair, bringing him closer to his brothers and a renewed appreciation of his father's drive and stubbornness. "Instead of resenting my father's refusal to talk about my sexuality, I came to admire his sex drive," says Carl. "He got into trouble in the nursing home, trying to be a ladies' man. He was always introducing me to single women, trying to get me married, right up to the end." John, who had a very contentious relationship with his mother, says she now refers to Michael, his lover, as his husband. "That," he says with a smile, "is something she never would have done when she was intact."

A Political Agenda for the Ages

When I was little and people called me a dirty kike, I went to my parents, who could help me. When it turned out I was a fag, I couldn't go to them for help, so I went to gay liberation, which is a glorious part of my history. We had to say, "Gay is good," we had to work on believing it, and we had to stand up and say, "We're not going to take this shit anymore." Now we have to say, "Old is good," we have to believe it, and we have to stand up and say, "We're not going to take this shit anymore."

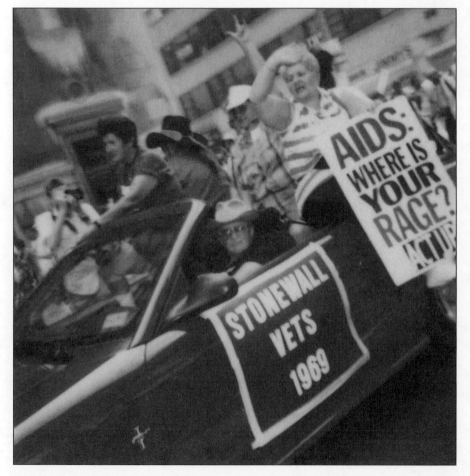

"A lot of issues important to all gay men and lesbians are left on the shoulders of old gay men and lesbians to deal with," says Del Martin, an inveterate political organizer and a member of Old Lesbians Organizing for Change. The statement, like the name of her organization, is bold enough for old ("Why euphemize?" asks Martin) gay men and lesbians to see without bifocals or distortion. That's the way she wants it. Martin, long a beacon of vision for old men and women, urges younger ones—like those in their sixties—to join the fray. "It's not complicated," she says. "Pay attention!" Among the important issues are the five listed below.

1. *Accessible health care.* "While a few executives may be getting multimillion-dollar golden

parachutes, the older Americans who are the first to go in a downsizing may be the last to get care," says Martin. In just the six years between 1988 and 1994, the proportion of retirees fifty-five and older who got health coverage from a prior employer fell 23 percent. Medicare, as discussed above, does not provide the prescription drug or home health care coverage needed to take up the slack.

2. *Accessible home care.* "There are eight thousand doctors in the District of Columbia," says Dr. Huskey. "You know how many have the balls or eggs to make house calls? Two. I see a lot of taxis available at lunch hour, and a lot of doctors who could afford to get in one and go see somebody. Meanwhile, you know how much it costs every time a homebound person has to get him or herself into the hospital for a routine treatment? Four hundred of your and my taxpayer dollars." Other forms of home care, such as aides to help with basic chores, are almost always the first things to go in local Medicare or Medicaid cuts. Only two states fund respite care, which allows caregivers to take a needed break from their ordeals. Day treatment programs are rarely covered sufficiently.

3. *Places to live.* "There are already more applicants for senior housing programs than there is housing," says George Neighbors Jr., Gray Panthers field director, "and more than one-third of old people in the United States are living in a poor or near-poor family." There are no assisted-living or "continuum-of-care" facilities for gay men or lesbians, and nursing homes, often abusive to all residents, even more frequently single out gay men and lesbians for punishment (see "Gimme Shelter," page 360).

4. *Social Security.* Old lesbians and gay men are just as divided as everybody else on how to revamp Social Security so that there's enough money for the boomer generation, but they all know that change has got to come. "You know what Social Security is right now?" asks Doug Kimmel, Ph.D., City University of New York professor and cofounder of SAGE New York. "Spousal benefits. And how about inheritance tax? Straight spouses pass significant amounts of property to each other tax-free, but we can't. Medicaid? Same bias. It's a nasty heterosexist system out there, and practically everything we do has some kind of problem as a result of the fact that the person we're sleeping with is not legally regarded as our next of kin."

5. *Ways to be counted.* "How many gay people over sixty-five are there?" asks Kate Seelman, Ph.D., director of the National Institute of Disability and Rehabilitation Research in Washington, DC. "We don't know, because the Census Bureau doesn't really ask." Del Martin says she's horrified by "all these intake forms we have to fill out that have no options besides single, married, and divorced. I know we can't all be open, but those of us who can, should—about both being gay and being old. You know how it's freeing to say you're gay? Well it's just as freeing to be out about being old."

6. *Employment and a living wage.* "Economics wasn't my best subject in college, but it doesn't take a Ph.D. to see this great economic boom of the nineties seems to have left most of us out," says Martin. "The Employment Non-Discrimination Act has to be a priority." Less than half of Americans are covered by employer-provided pensions, many are losing their jobs before Social Security benefits become available, and a staggering 24 percent of old Americans have an eighth-grade education or less. "When they talk about the budget surplus, that surplus is Social Security funds," says Martin. "Privatizing social security through individual retirement accounts and raising the age to sixty-seven isn't the route we favor. Taxing the biggest wage earners more heavily and raising workers' salaries could also raise revenues, and would let working people get some of the benefits now."

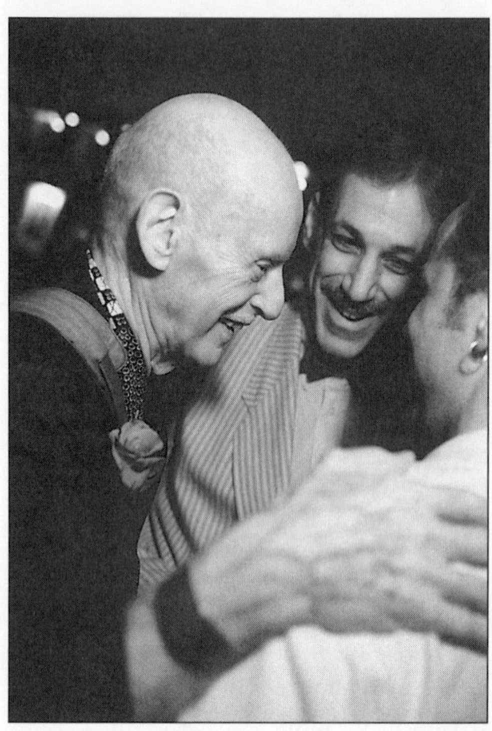

Sage Advice from Your Elders

1. Know People Your Own Age

"I introduce people into support groups, and sometimes I'll hear them say about people their own age, 'Oh, I wouldn't be in a room with those old farts,'" says SAGE New York's Phillip Piro. "But how else are you going to get comfortable with the issues?"

2. Know Someone Older

"That'll really give you perspective," says Piro.

3. Play

"I hate to say 'be creative,' because that sounds so demanding if you're not Picasso," says Columbia University's Dr. Kertzner. Perhaps a more inclusive way of putting it is what New York city psychoanalyst Ken Corbett, Ph.D., calls "the enjoyment of mental freedom," the ability to allow yourself to play without feeling constricted or judged (see Chapter 11). Never mind if you're not the best at it: What do you get lost in? Watercolors? Cards? Cooking? Make time for those things that absorb you so completely that time seems to stop.

4. Don't Watch Too Much Television

"I really just vegetated for years," says Arthur, seventy-two, a midlevel executive downsized out of his New York City job in the 1970s. "Get outside if you can. If you can't, go inside, into your spirit."

5. Get Real

"Don't feed the drama of aging," says Ram Dass in his *Conscious Aging* lecture. "Your denial of aging, or your milking of it by being so attached to it, are both getting in the way of realizing that who you are has no age. Who you are is in a body that has age, it's in a personality that is aging and changing, but you yourself aren't."

6. Explore (Your) Nature

Ram Dass puts it more baldly, advising that people "make friends with death." Find a community of people who aren't afraid to confront their deaths and grow inwardly, he suggests. "If you don't, then you've got books. . . . And tune back into nature more deeply so you can feel the natural cycles of which your body and personality are a part."

7. Be Out Somewhere

"I wasn't able to tell my daughter, because she would have told my ex-wife, who would have told my mother, who was still alive," says Mark, sixty-three, in Dallas. "But I so enjoy my work with Men of All Colors. I'm very proud." SAGE's Phillip Piro says that "being out everywhere can be too much" for many people he sees, but he urges everyone to "be out somewhere." We need to talk.

FURTHER READING

Beauvoir, Simone de. (1972) *The Coming of Age*. London: W. W. Norton & Co. A study of age and attitudes toward the elderly, through the ages.

Berger, Raymond. (1995) *Gay and Gray.* Binghamton, NY: Haworth Press. An update of the classic study of the issues surrounding gay aging.

Berman, Claire. (1996) *Caring for Yourself While Caring for Your Aging Parents*. New York: Henry Holt and Company. Not gay, but plenty timely if you need it.

Dass, Ram. (1992) *Conscious Aging: On the Nature of Change and Facing Death*. Boulder, CO: Sounds True. Two audiocassettes of lectures given at the Omega Institute by the brilliant bisexual Harvard professor turned spiritual sage.

D'Augelli, Anthony R., and Charlotte J. Patterson. (1995) *Lesbian, Gay and Bisexual Identities over the Lifespan: Psychological Perspectives*. New York: Oxford University Press. Academic but compelling series of articles on aging and identity.

Isensee, Rik. (1999) *Are You Ready? The Gay Men's Guide to Thriving at Midlife*. Los Angeles: Alyson Publications, Inc. Advice on how to age well from the author of *Love Between Men* and other popular advice books.

Larson, Per. (1997) *Gay Money*. New York: Dell Publishing.

Levinson, Daniel. (1978) *The Seasons of a Man's Life*. New York: Ballantine.

Lustig, Harold. (1999) *4 Steps to Financial Security for Lesbian and Gay Couples*. New York: Ballantine. Fiscal advice on everything from buying joint car insurance to planning for retirement.

Margolis, Simeon, and H. Ballentine Carter. (1998) "Prostate Disorders," in *The Johns Hopkins White Papers*. Baltimore, MD: Medletter Associates, Inc.

Sheehy, Gail. (1998) *Understanding Men's Passages: Discovering the New Map of Men's Lives*. New York: Random House.

Walsh, Patrick C., and Janet Farrar Worthington. (1997) *The Prostate: A Guide for Men and the Women Who Love Them*. New York: Warner Books, Inc. Don't hold the title against it—it's worth reading.

PART 3

MAJOR MEDICAL

CHAPTER 9

Are You Positive? Treating HIV

Coping Basics • Immune Basics • Monitoring Your Immune System • How Antiviral Drugs Work • Why Antivirals Fail • To Treat or Not to Treat? • Sticking With It • How to Know if Your Therapy's Working • What's Buggin' You: Opportunistic Infections and Malignancies • Wasting Away Again?

Everything I do, everything I've been able to do, has proceeded from acceptance of three words that came with my diagnosis ten years ago: I don't know.

I was at a party the other night where there was a palm reader. "Go over," everyone kept saying, but I was scared to death. Finally she looks at my hand and starts telling me what a strong lifeline I have, and I'm thinking, "You must not be very good." I told her about my diagnosis and she just looked at me and said, "So?"

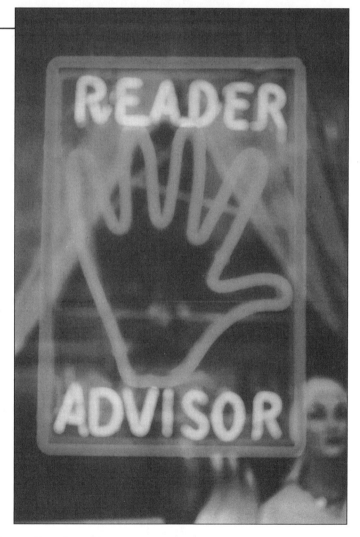

"I'm positive" has always seemed a strange turn of phrase with which to convey the news that you had HIV. As time goes by, the ironies have changed in tone, but not in essence. We have come a long, long way from the time when the only thing that seemed certain when you tested positive for HIV was that you were going to die from it. After nearly twenty years of psychological and pharmacological struggle against the epidemic, a combination of treatments now seems able to slow or even halt the progress of HIV. Anti-HIV drugs, known more simply as antivirals, have had a Lazarus effect on many, raising them from death's door. The infections that now account for more than 90 percent of HIV-related illnesses can be predicted, and in many cases prevented with additional medications.

Yet there is still so little to be sure of when you have HIV. No one knows exactly when to start the new drug "cocktails" that fight HIV, how long they will continue to work, or their cost to our internal organs. For some, their physical cost, the up-to-$15,000-a-year price tag, is already too high, leaving people scrambling to find other drugs to use or programs that will help them pay. The drugs that should prevent infections don't always work, and they've yet to find the pill to cure the hatred, fear, or indifference that most of America directs at people with HIV. "If I'm still getting diarrhea, should I stop? If I stop, will I get sick? If I get sick, will my family slam the door in my face? I'm already sick of my job, but can I find another one that gives me health insurance? What do I have to do for the luxury of a simple answer?" asks Benjamin, forty-two, a university employee in Washington, DC, intoning what might be called a mantra for the positive man.

Learning to accept uncertainty is one of the hardest parts of life with HIV. Believing that the uncertainty justifies skipping testing or treatment in favor of waiting and hoping is one of its biggest traps. Whether you've just found out you're HIV-positive or have been struggling with it through ten years and five antiviral drugs, your universe of choices is still expanding. You will often have to make decisions with little information, and the decision you make today may affect your ability to make other decisions in the future. "Do the best you can with the information available at the time, but make sure you consciously choose to do something," advises Pablo Colon, director of GMHC's Treatment Education and Advocacy Department. "Not making any decisions about treatment means the virus is going to make decisions for you, and that's not healthy."

In 1983, while hospital attendants were refusing to enter the rooms of "AIDS carriers" and social workers were refusing to touch their paperwork, a handful of gay men with AIDS gathered in Denver to imagine better forms of support and nourishment. First among the "Denver Principles" they agreed upon was the assertion that they were people with AIDS (PWAs), not victims of it. "AIDS undermines my health, but it doesn't undermine my personhood," Max Navarre, one of the founders of the PWA Coalition and an early GMHC board member, summed up later. Fifteen years and the deaths of all those PWAs who were at Denver later, it's a first principle worth remembering. Finding out you're positive raises all sorts of hopes and fears about life and death, being sick, your relationships, your sex life, your career, and just about everything else. Your diagnosis may depress you, awaken feelings you thought you'd gotten past about being gay, or galvanize you into doing things you'd long deferred. Even those who find the shock of HIV a call to action or a "gift" admit that it's a gift that keeps on giving you pause. "I think of it like a roommate that doesn't go away," says Rob, thirty-four, who says his diagnosis helped him to leave alcoholism and what he saw as meaningless restaurant work behind in favor of a sober and more fulfilling life as an HIV-prevention worker.

But beneath that slow and steady pressure on your immune system and your psyche, your humanity is intact. You are a person living with HIV. There are an estimated six hundred thousand to nine hundred thousand of you in the United States alone. Believe it or not, there's never been a better time to have HIV, because you have lots of options.

Coping Basics

Chapter 10 of this book, which talks about coping with illness, is something you should read even if you feel perfectly fine. It spells out four things that can be helpful when you've gotten a diagnosis:

1. *Support from friends, family, or other people with your condition*
2. *Health consciousness about how to take care of yourself through diet and exercise*
3. *Information*
4. *Treatment you trust (along with some kind of health insurance to pay for it)*

The chapter also sets out a general warning that goes double for HIV. For as many experts as there are out there on any illness, for all the newsletters and organizations and personal testimonials and pharmaceutical ads showing happy, healthy people rock-climbing or throwing javelins, there is no one pill or strategy for dealing with the virus. You can't pack all the best information about HIV and AIDS into an ad, a chapter, a book, or a shelf of books. New drugs are being developed, and new theories floated and shot down, faster than a chapter like this can go to press. Seeking up-to-date information—page 400 lists some good resources—is a must. So is realizing that there are always more opinions than right answers in AIDS medicine. Of the more than 50,000 people with HIV illness who have come through GMHC's doors for support in the last twenty years, there have probably been half as many strategies that people swear work to help them stay healthy.

There *is* a basic framework for understanding HIV and how to make decisions that are right for you. If you know you're HIV-positive and are well enough to talk, read, or listen, you're ahead of the game. The sooner you know you're infected, the sooner you can begin to form a strategy. Recognize that your mood, your bank balance, and your T-cell count (see "Immune Basics," page 381) may change as often as the cut of fashionable jeans. Mood swings are particularly common right after being diagnosed with HIV, and right after finding out that you have AIDS. Indulge in a period of depression if you must. And then get to work.

Do Tell? When and How to Disclose Your Illness

My father said three words: "I told you," and it wasn't just HIV he was talking about. He was thinking of all the arguments we'd had over the years about how being gay was sick, about how I wasn't healthy. That made me sick. And sad.

The firm was the last place I would have expected to get support, but the plan my boss and I came up with was a dream. For the first time since the holiday party, all the employees were called together. Company policy, my boss explained, was to let all employees with chronic health problems work for as long as they felt able. "Randy has AIDS," he said, "and he is still an employee in good standing." I can still see him sliding a list of hot-line numbers down the conference table and telling everyone to call if they had questions. It was deadly silent for a minute. Then my secretary leaned over and said, "Does this mean we have to be nice to you now?"

Whether it goes back to the days when hunter-gatherers were forced to leave their sick behind, or to more modern, produce-or-perish industrial-era thinking, there are long-standing cultural commands to keep your weakness secret. For men particularly, notions of masculinity, self-sufficiency, power, and health are all bound together. The Americans with Disabilities Act, which was enacted in 1990 and took effect in 1992, outlawed discrimination against the sick in the workplace or public spaces, but writing out people's desire to distance themselves from illness

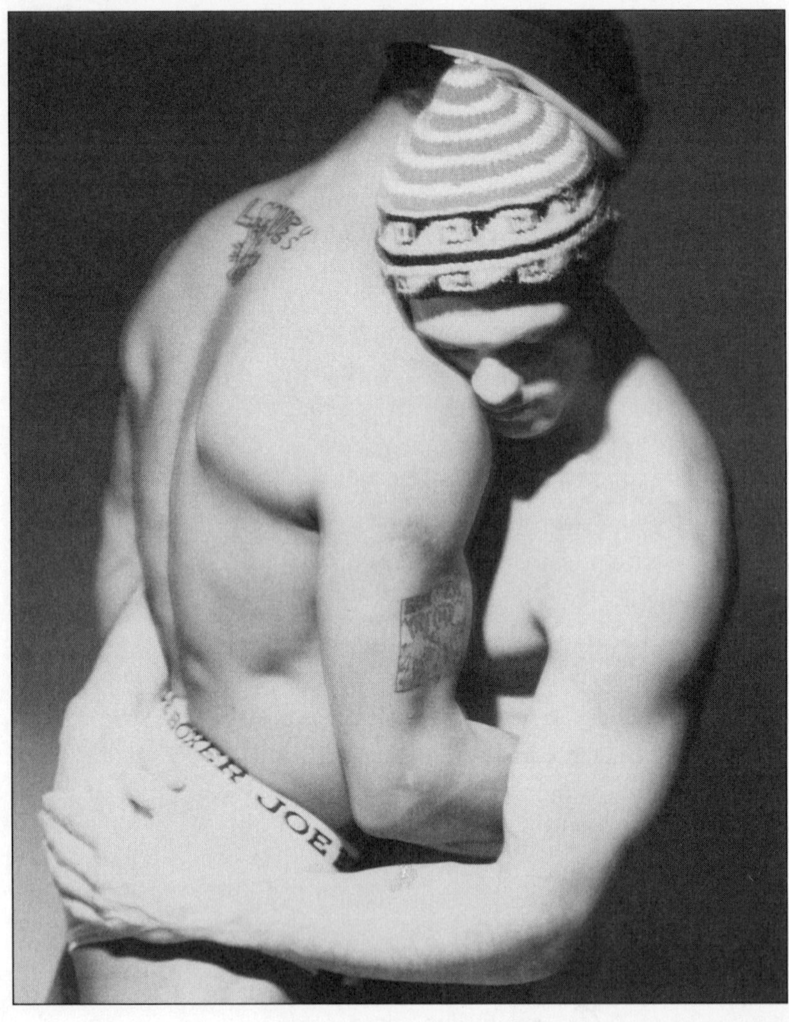

will take more than legal reform. Even though it's "your" illness, telling someone you have cancer or a potentially fatal heart condition can provoke a range of reactions about authority and weakness, dependence and expectations, that go well beyond a simple wish of sympathy.

Talking about HIV is even more complicated. Unlike other illnesses, HIV is tied to sex and drug use, things the world—and in many cases, we ourselves—would rather not discuss publicly. Like being gay, which in the public imagination is already linked with AIDS, some people see your HIV infection as a choice, and so blame you for what makes them uncomfortable. Many gay men describe the experience of disclosing that they have HIV as a kind of second coming out, resonant with all the same shame, confusion, and misunderstanding they experienced the first time around. "My brother reacted to the news by telling me I was a fag and deserved to die," says Randy, a former computer programmer. Unlike coming out as gay, disclosing your HIV status is something you have to do—or, at the very least, think of doing—with your sexual partner (see page 115 for a discussion of those special dynamics). And though people with HIV have done a lot of which we can all be proud, the thought that HIV is proper punishment for sex can be hard to shake. "I thought I was way beyond the AIDS-is-God's-punishment stuff," says Sam, forty-five. "But when I found out, all I could think was 'That's what I get for being such a slut.'"

You may have made bad choices, or acted in ways that hurt you or others, but no one deserves HIV as punishment for having sex. You can't control people's reactions, but you don't have to accept them as your own. As with coming out as gay, you may find unexpected dividends in coming clean about your HIV. "Before you do it, you're terrified, and maybe for good reason," says Randy. "My brother couldn't accept it, but so many others, including people who were sicker and in worse shape than me, have been open. When you talk with them, you can just feel the barriers come down, and the relief rush in."

Before you pick up the phone and tell everyone you know (strange as it may sound, that's a common coping impulse), ask yourself some telling questions.

THE QUESTION OF WHO

I've been on local news, written articles, am completely up front about my HIV in New York. But back home, I'm silent. I can't stand the idea of telling my mother.

I didn't want people in my field knowing, so I just told a few close friends. I told them they could tell whomever they needed to tell for their own sanity. At this point, I'm not sure who knows and who doesn't.

Communicating news of your HIV status makes you vulnerable. Thinking about whom you want to share the information with means thinking through the level of intimacy you wish to establish with someone, or reckoning with the one you have already. If you tell your aunt in Fargo and ask her not to share it, will she call other family members against your will? If you don't tell your roommate or lover, will he find out by looking in the medicine cabinet? Can you really make it to both doctor's appointments and work meetings without a word to your supervisor? Does that nice neighbor with the red ribbon really need to know, or will today's confidence become tomorrow's hottest gossip at the Ladies' Village Improvement Society?

One thing's certain: People talk about others who are positive. If you do tell only a few people, you may want to let them know whom else you've told, in case they too need someone with whom they can talk freely.

THE QUESTION OF WHEN

My mother called the day I got news of my HIV status. I didn't know whether to tell her I was gay or HIV-positive. I did both. She asked when I was coming home to Oklahoma, and I said I was going to stay in New York, where the treatment was better. Then she asked how they'd get the body back. That snapped me out of my woe-is-me attitude. I told her I'd have the body burned and shipped back to her in an envelope, and then I hung up. Later I sent her some information from GMHC.

There's no good time for bad news, but consider whether or not the person you want to tell is in a good position to deal with it. Are there major things going on in his or her life? Is there time to have a reasonable conversation, and a way to comfortably end a conversation if necessary? The seven-hour drive to the family reunion is probably not the best time to reveal to your folks that you have a terminal illness. Likewise, you won't want to announce your news five minutes before your flight leaves, leaving a family member or friend gasping at the gate.

THE QUESTION OF HOW

I know someone who has a dog named T cell. That way, she says, she'll always have at least one.

I have a friend who's always making jokes. "Well," he says, "I figure I might as well live it up in the year I have left." Or "I figured I should get myself photographed before I waste down to a skeleton." He kind of laughs, but I don't find it that funny.

Consider the way in which to disclose your status. By phone? In person? In a letter? Via tattoo on the arm or inner thigh? Each of these methods has its drawbacks and advantages. Remember, though, that the impact of hearing an HIV diagnosis can be intense for people even if it's *your* diagnosis. Be ready for further discussion. If you don't feel ready for it, you might consider whether you're ready to tell.

THE QUESTION OF WHY

I knew a guy who was closeted, and the way he dealt with his AIDS was the same, always covering up and denying. I don't want to be clutching at life that way, clinging to a fiction. I want to go through this transparent, open for and to the world. I hope to die that way, open to the world, and open for discussion.

So there I am, first night in Portugal, finding my way toward a bar listed in the gay guide, when a man jumps out of the shadows waving a hypodermic needle. "Give me all your money or I'll give you AIDS," he screams at me. I said, "I already have AIDS." "Give me your money or I'll give you AIDS!" he repeated. "No, really," I told him. "I already have AIDS. I take AZT and 3TC and . . ." He just turned and ran back into the alley.

What do you want from the people you tell? Recognizing your motives may help you plan your disclosure, or decide whether to do it. Consider what you stand to gain if the reaction is positive and what you stand to lose if the reaction is negative. Being clear about what you want, such as financial support, a place to talk through fears, or a more honest sexual interaction, may help you ask for it more clearly. If the person doesn't prove receptive, you can move on to someone who is. If the person you're telling flips out, remember that—just as with being gay—it says more about them than it does about you.

THE QUESTION OF WHAT

What makes people who are practically strangers, when they hear you're positive, ask, "How did that happen?" or "How'd you get it?" I always look at them and say, with great earnestness, "Perinatal transmission."

Telling someone about an illness may result in a slew of additional questions. Many of these—of the "How long?" "What next?" or "What can I do for you?" variety—can often be a way of directing the potentially overwhelming emotions of the situation. If there are questions that aren't helpful or which you find offensive—as in "Who infected you?" or "How could you do something so stupid in this day and age?"—you can say you don't feel comfortable answering,

TELLING QUESTIONS: HAVE YOU . . .

- Scheduled a good time and place to break your news? Give yourself plenty of time to have a discussion, and a place to get away afterward.
- Played out the actual disclosure in your head and prepared yourself for various reactions, positive and negative?
- Made sure you have a backup system, a person you can turn to for support, in case the person you're telling has a reaction you didn't expect?
- Gotten information (preferably published) and referrals ready? Things change so quickly with HIV that even doctors can't keep track. Handing someone information can be a way of saying that you want this person to educate him or herself, and can spare you from having to pretend to know things you don't.
- Stopped expecting miraculous transformations? People who were attentive to your needs prior to your illness will likely remain so afterward. People who were self-absorbed are also likely to stay that way.

or that it seems beside the point. Be prepared, though. "How'd you get it?" is one of the most common—if not the most charming—follow-ups.

Immune Basics

Syndrome—whether that's chronic fatigue syndrome, toxic shock syndrome, or acquired immune deficiency syndrome (AIDS)—is a term the medical profession gives to groups of symptoms, especially to those that don't seem to have any logical link. That AIDS is called AIDS today, long after we know what causes it and how it develops, reflects the dated nature and imprecision of the term (see box on next page). Focusing just on AIDS, one of the later stages of infection with the human immunodeficiency virus (HIV), is like taking your car in for new brakes after you've run into a wall. You may have to do it, and if you pay enough money and attention, you can probably repair the damage and keep it from happening again. It's more useful to try to figure out how to stay out of harm's way before damage is done. That means looking not only at how to keep HIV from getting into your body (see Chapter 2) but also at the early stages of what this slow-acting, fast-reproducing virus does once it's there.

From the moment it gets inside your body through blood or semen, HIV does what most living things (with the possible exception of some of this book's readers) want to do: procreate. In order to do so, the virus has to face down your immune system, the body's defense mechanism against organisms introduced from outside. Normally, the immune system protects against invaders—germs you breathe in, organisms in the food you eat, bacteria riding on a hand you shake or the tip of a penis you suck—by using an array of different cells and chemicals to prevent the new arrival from taking up residence in your body. Sometimes that happens without your being conscious of the process, and sometimes the effort required to neutralize an invader makes you sick. While it may seem that your immune system has failed you as your fever mounts or your glands swell, these are actually signs that it is hard at work. The pus around that splinter that got infected? It's also a sign of immunological effort, white blood cells building up as they do battle against the foreign object.

"White blood cells" is the catch-all name encompassing most of the active cells of the immune system. There are various types of white blood cells, each with a particular role to play in the complicated choreography of immune response. Lymphocytes are among the primary dancers in the company, with B and T cells among the most important. T cells float around our bodies looking for bugs or foreign invaders that aren't supposed to be there. Once a T cell identifies an invader, it may also send out signals to other immune-system cells, such as B cells, to come and help mount an attack. T4 cells, also known as CD4 or helper cells, are responsible for regulating the attack—they coordinate different actions of the various immune responses. T8 cells, also known as CD8 cells, come in two varieties: cytotoxic CD8 cells release substances to neutralize infected cells, and supressor CD8 cells tell the body when to stop the onslaught. Macrophages—the word means "big eaters"—scour the circulatory system, looking for dead cells or foreign material to consume. Once the body is able to figure out a successful way of containing a particular bug, memory cells "remember" the strategy for next time. That's why we don't get sick from the same strain of flu, or hepatitis A, twice, or why certain vaccines are able to provoke a low-level immune response that helps protect us forever against a more serious challenge. Naive cells—those not yet programmed for a particular illness—maintain your potential to battle future infection.

WHAT'S IN A NAME? AIDS

Coined before we even knew there was a virus that caused it, the term AIDS doesn't mean much anymore. It's more accurate than "gay-related immune deficiency" (GRID) or "gay cancer," which were among science's first suggestions. But if you're looking to describe the medical realities of living with HIV, including the long periods when things happening inside your body don't show themselves outside, the term "HIV disease" is much more meaningful. For government benefits, however, or entrance into a whole system of support structures created in the bad old days when most people found out they were sick by landing in the emergency room with an AIDS-related infection, the term "AIDS" remains highly important. Getting an AIDS diagnosis may mean you can get Social Security Disability Insurance and other benefits (see Chapter 10). If you have AIDS and virtually no money, you can get SSI, federal subsidies for the retired and disabled. Having AIDS sometimes means you can get into certain meal programs or local support groups that don't admit people with HIV disease, no matter how sick. Even if you get better, once you've had AIDS, you can often continue getting benefits.

If you are HIV-positive and have a CD4 count (also known as a T4 or T-cell count; see "Immune Basics") below 200, that means you have AIDS. Even if you don't have fewer than 200 CD4 cells, testing positive for HIV and having any one of twenty-four different conditions means you meet the government's definition of AIDS. Among the conditions the Centers for Disease Control and Prevention (CDC) consider "AIDS-defining" in men:

- Candidiasis of bronchi, trachea, or lungs
- Candidiasis, esophageal
- Coccidioidomycosis, disseminated or extrapulmonary
- Cryptococcosis, extrapulmonary
- Cryptosporidiosis, chronic intestinal (of more than one month's duration)
- Cytomegalovirus disease (other than liver, spleen, or nodes)
- *Cytomegalovirus retinitis* (with loss of vision)
- Encephalopathy, HIV-related
- Herpes simplex: chronic ulcer(s) (of more than one month's duration); or bronchitis, pneumonitis, or esophagitis
- Histoplasmosis, disseminated or extrapulmonary
- Isosporiasis, chronic intestinal (of more than one month's duration)
- Kaposi's sarcoma
- Lymphoma, Burkitt's (or equivalent term)
- Lymphoma, immunoblastic (or equivalent term)
- Lymphoma, primary, of brain
- *Mycobacterium avium* complex or *M. kansasii,* disseminated or extrapulmonary
- *Mycobacterium tuberculosis,* any site (pulmonary or extrapulmonary)
- *Mycobacterium,* other species or unidentified species, disseminated or extrapulmonary
- *Pneumocystis carinii* pneumonia
- Pneumonia, recurrent
- Progressive multifocal leukoencephalopathy
- Salmonella septicemia, recurrent
- Toxoplasmosis of brain
- Wasting syndrome due to HIV

GIVE PEACE A CHANCE? TURNING A GAY GAZE ON IMMUNE SYSTEM METAPHORS

Some people have found the militaristic discussion of HIV and the immune system—CD4 cells as generals, HIV as an invader that kills off the generals, and your body at war—unhelpful, symptomatic of Western medicine's obsession with doing battle rather than restoring balance. Better, they say, to recognize that your body, like the world itself, is made up of many elements, constantly interacting, living, dying, and reproducing. You may find it more useful to imagine your body as an ecosystem, with HIV as a toxic algae bloom. You may want to see your white blood cells as bouncers, firmly escorting the unruly customers that are opportunistic infections out the door. "I think of my immune system cells in French aprons and feather dusters, and HIV as a really sticky, awful form of dust," proclaims Sandy, thirty-seven.

If it works for you, go with it.

One method of attack is the creation of antibodies, proteins that interfere with the ability of the germ to cause infection. The standard HIV test really tests for antibodies, signs that your immune system has responded to the virus by producing these proteins to try to block it. It usually takes about three weeks for your body to produce enough antibodies to register on an HIV test, a point known as seroconversion. Antibodies play several roles, including marking foreign matter and infected cells for destruction by other parts of the immune system.

With all these tools at our disposal, why can't our bodies control HIV? Viruses in general have always been difficult to defeat, since many insert themselves in other cells in order to reproduce. HIV is among the most damaging of all, installing itself in the CD4 cells that coordinate the rest of the immune response. HIV gets inside the cell and alters the cell's genetic material (DNA), making the CD4 cell—once a mighty warrior in the battle against disease—into an HIV factory. Each infected CD4 cell produces hundreds of thousands of viral particles, known as virions, and then dies off. Each of those virions can go out and infect more CD4 cells, which then produce more virions. A person infected with HIV produces billions of new viral particles every day. This is known as the process of viral replication.

The more CD4 cells HIV kills off, the more vulnerable your immune system becomes to attacks from bacteria, fungi, parasites, and other viruses. It is often these germs and bugs—some of which may have been inside your body and controlled by your immune system since childhood—that make you sick in the course of HIV illness, not HIV itself. Because they take advantage of the opportunity provided by your weakened defenses, many of the most serious of these illnesses are known as opportunistic infections, or OIs.

As long as some CD4 cells remain, your body will attempt a powerful resistance to HIV, with the battle between the virus and your immune system continuing for years. For 95 percent or more of people, unless you use medication or some other form of immune system reinforcement, HIV wins: The number of CD4 cells you have gradually declines, the number of viral particles rises, and eventually you get sick.

Long Time Coming? HIV, AIDS, and How Long You Have

In a panic about your HIV test and the follow-up blood work? Worried that every traffic jam or moment of stress is costing you a CD4 cell while you wait for treatment? Saundra Johnson, an

GAME, SET, MATCH? TREATMENT FOR THE NEWLY INFECTED

HIV comes on strong. For anywhere between 50 and 90 percent of people, getting infected with HIV means getting sick within a matter of weeks and experiencing flulike symptoms, swollen glands, or a rash as your body struggles to recover from the onslaught of the virus. That mini health crisis, known as seroconversion illness or acute retroviral infection, may also signal a major opportunity.

People who have had HIV for a while often have years to consider whether to start combination therapies that work against HIV (see "To Treat or Not to Treat?" page 394). If you think you're in the first weeks or months of HIV infection, though, doctors suspect you might be able to act fast and use treatment to permanently change the course of disease. Without reinforcement, levels of HIV spike in those first few months, the virus inserting itself into T cells and then multiplying. The higher levels of HIV climb in those first few months, the more difficult they may be to lower when you confront the virus with medication later. Research jargon calls this the "set point" of the virus, the highest peak.

Reinforce your bodily defenses with medication early, say some doctors, and you may be able to keep that set point so low that the virus never really gets a foothold. The experiments are new, and have involved small numbers of men, but those who've participated have been able to keep their viral levels low for years. "My doctor won't say I'm cured," says Dieter, fifty-five, one of the men in a drug trial for the newly infected. "But he says I'm as close as anyone on the planet." Until there's longer-term data, this is more hope than fact; we don't yet know whether this approach will give people an edge that lasts, or just the privilege of an extra ten years of taking fairly toxic medications. It's this same idea, with even less hard data to back it up, that has some doctors prescribing the "morning-after" treatment known as PEP, postexposure prophylaxis (see box on page 73).

Still, early data look promising. If you're "lucky" enough to know that you've just been infected, talk to a doctor as soon as you can about the possibility of treatment.

educator in GMHC's Treatment Education and Advocacy department, says the best answer to the question of what to do now that you know you're HIV-positive may be to go home and chill out. "I had one guy in a workshop who was so tense he was going to blow a gasket," she says. "He was waving around his lab report and asking all these questions, but the information wasn't getting through because he was all twisted up. I had to tell him, 'Go home, relax, and let's talk later. You're not going to drop dead from HIV tomorrow. I can't tell you about your heart, nervous as you are, but the best treatment for tonight would be to rent a movie.'" Todd Yancey, MD, at the Bentley-Salick Center in New York City, says people will wait for years to get tested, and then panic the moment they get a positive result. "They'll say, 'I've got to do something, now!' I'll say, 'You waited for seven years to get the information, and it would be smart to wait awhile and think things through before doing anything.'"

How much time do you have? While researchers scramble to identify the genetic sequences that may definitively identify the few who will never progress to AIDS, or the medications that will allow you to keep asking "How long?" until prostate cancer or one of the other old-age illnesses gets you, the averages are pretty clear. Without any treatment, 50 percent of HIV-infected people progress to AIDS within ten years of infection, and about 75 percent reach AIDS after fifteen years. Younger men take longer to get sick ("younger" in this case means men under thirty), and some doctors suspect that cofactors such as sexually transmitted diseases and a history of using speed or cocaine may influence how fast you get AIDS or how long you survive after your first serious infection.

How often you get care, and how you pay for it, is definitely a factor in survival. More than 70 percent of leading American AIDS doctors surveyed by GMHC said that how a patient pays determines what treatment they receive. The preconceptions doctors have about how likely you are to make use of treatments also matter: Black and Latino men in America, for example, even those who see doctors as frequently as White men, receive substandard treatment both for HIV and to prevent infections associated with it.

Two terms are used commonly to describe the lucky ones who seem to beat the odds and survive, or thrive, with HIV. "Long-term survivor" usually refers to someone who's had AIDS and lived for significantly longer than the three years or so that used to be the average survival time after diagnosis. "Long-term nonprogressor" is the name given to people who have had HIV but no weakening of the immune system over many years. This latter category is rare, comprising only around 5 percent of people who are infected.

There's no name yet for people whose genetic makeup allows them to fight off HIV so completely that they don't even get infected after they've been exposed. Researchers have found some of these protective gene sequences, though, and are developing theories to explain them, including one that suggests that genetic resistance comes from being descended from survivors of Europe's plague epidemic in the Middle Ages. It's a White thing—they have yet to find the gene sequences that protect people of African or Latin American descent, though they have found evidence that as many as 20 percent of African-Americans may be genetically *more* likely to be infected.

Monitoring Your Immune System

I sit in all these groups with guys rattling off their numbers. Me, I try not to pay attention. I've had three T cells for the last five years.

I came back to work from the doctor and Patrick said, "How are you?" with that pregnant pause. In fact, I wasn't so good: My T cells had fallen to 120. "Patrick," I snapped, "you've got to find a way of asking me how I am that doesn't make it sound like you're getting ready to go to my fucking funeral. And don't tell me the story about the guy with three T cells who's survived for five years."

HIV's attack on your immune system is constant but covert. Most people with HIV don't look or feel sick for years, though that doesn't mean you should hang out and wait for pneumonia to send you to the emergency room. Start monitoring your immune system as soon as you know you're infected, and you can put the information to work against the virus, predicting the progress of your HIV disease and how you might halt it.

Learning to read your immune system means keeping up with a changing vocabulary of evaluation, since useful tests, and our understanding of them, are constantly being refined.

The first thing you want to do is establish a "baseline," a series of points that map out where you're starting from so that you can see if your immune system is changing. The blood, circulating through as many parts of your body as it does, provides important markers, not only of HIV and your immune system, but of the way organs such as your liver and spleen and pancreas are affected both by the virus and by the medications that control it. A series of blood tests is often the first step in detecting potential problems or determining how you're responding to the medications meant to prevent them.

While you'll learn more about lab reports as you go along, there are three markers that are particularly important. Think of them as the three cornerstones upon which you build a strategy for staying well.

Cornerstone #1: CD4-Cell (Also Known As T-Cell) Testing

WHY?

"CD4-cell levels are the best available way to assess the health of an HIV-positive person's immune system," says Dr. Yancey, "but as a hard-and-fast marker, they aren't reliable." Yancey is exacting, and CD4 levels are far from precise. "There's up to 30 percent variation depending on what lab you use, how much sleep you got the night before, your age, your gender, whether you have a cold, or even the time of day—CD4s are highest in the evening," says Yancey.

Nonetheless, the lower your CD4 count, the weaker your immune system, and the more likely you are to get sick. Most healthy people have a range of somewhere between 1,000 and 1,200 CD4 cells per cubic milliliter of blood, though again, it varies. Having fewer than 200 of these cells gives you an official AIDS diagnosis and risk of the AIDS-related pneumonia known as *Pneumocystis carinii* pneumonia (PCP). Having fewer than 100 means even greater vulnerability to a number of other infections (see "An Ounce of Prevention," page 410). Since the number of CD4 cells is so variable, it's more precise to look at the *percentage* T4 cells represent of the total number of T cells. This figure changes less from day to day or from lab to lab. "Thirty-five percent is normal, and 20 percent is the sign that your immune system's been 'compromised,' or seriously weakened," says Yancey.

HOW OFTEN?

"If you've just been diagnosed, a couple of CD4-cell tests spaced at least two weeks apart can be good to set a baseline," suggests GMHC's Saundra Johnson. People with a count higher than 500 should repeat the test every three to six months. People with fewer than 500 CD4 cells or less than 20 percent should test every three months. If you've just started anti-HIV treatment, get a test before, one a month after starting, and then another in three months. Getting blood drawn at the same time of day, and using the same lab, can help you compare results more accurately over time.

HOW MUCH?

Anywhere from $60 to $600, usually covered by private insurance, Medicare, or Medicaid.

Cornerstone #2: Viral Load Testing

WHY?

This is the technology that has helped revolutionize how you make treatment decisions about HIV. "Before, doctors would look at T-cell levels and symptoms and try to make smart guesses about what was in your future, but in essence we were in a reactive mode," says Dr. Yancey. "Now, by quantifying the virus, we can be proactive." There are two different kinds of viral load tests in common use, the branch DNA (bDNA) test and the polymerase chain reaction (PCR) test, and both are accurate. Counts from the PCR test are approximately twice that of the bDNA, but that has to do with the way they express results, not the total level of your virus. Charts usually refer to viral load as "HIV RNA."

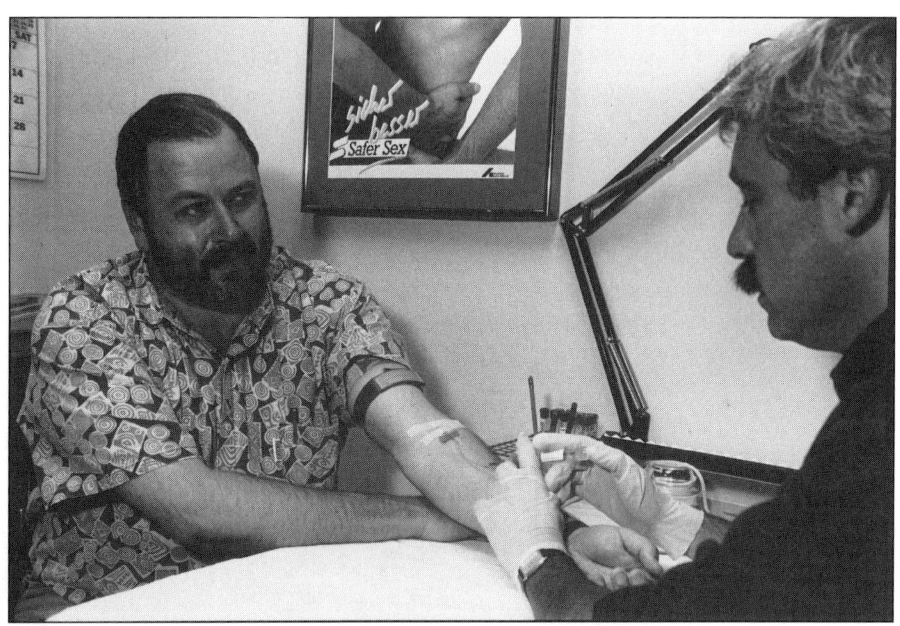

The higher the number of "copies" of virus in each cubic centimeter of blood, the greater your chances of getting sick and dying. "People with a thousand copies of HIV at baseline have an 8 percent chance of getting AIDS within five years," says Howard Grossman, MD, a New York City AIDS doctor. "People with a hundred thousand copies have a 62 percent chance of getting AIDS in the same period. Factor in CD4 counts, and you get an even better estimate."

As with CD4 cells, sharp changes in levels of virus are considered triggers for when you should start treatment for HIV, as well as for how you'll know if an existing treatment is working. We don't know how high a viral level can go. Over a million copies is not uncommon, though most doctors consider a viral load of over ten thousand copies to be too high for comfort.

The lowest number of copies that a test can detect depends on the test—the PCR can measure down to four hundred copies, the standard bDNA goes down to fifty, and several other "ultrasensitive" tests can go down to between twenty-five and fifty copies. Ask your doctor which one is best: If you're on medication and are responding well, you probably need the ultrasensitive. If you change doctors, see if your new one can use the same lab as the old one did to help with continuity of results.

HOW OFTEN?

If you've just been diagnosed, you want two viral load tests, spaced two to four weeks apart, to get a baseline, and then one every three months. If, as a result of a viral load test, you decide to start anti-HIV treatment, get a test right before, another four weeks after starting the drugs, and then another every three months.

HOW MUCH?

That depends on the test and the state, though private insurance and Medicaid usually pay for six viral load tests a year. Your doctor can file a medical-necessity form or call the insurance company if changes in your treatment require more than that. As of this writing, some insurers consider the ultrasensitive test too new to be covered.

Cornerstone #3: Symptoms

I was never much for doctors, but let me tell you, I really don't like going now. Just the smell of that office is enough to remind me that I'm infected, that I might be facing something serious, and that there may be nothing I can do about it.

After going to doctors who just looked at my blood work and told me what to do, I now work regularly with a naturopathic doctor who starts with a half-hour conversation about how I'm feeling and then draws my blood. It's a little more expensive, but for my peace of mind, it's well worth it.

The third essential way of tracking the health of your immune system is lower-tech, but highly important: Pay attention to your body. How are you sleeping, eating, digesting, and feeling? Do you have any infections? Diarrhea? Weight loss or weight gain? People in earlier stages of

CHARTING YOUR PROGRESS

It took me two years to learn not to schedule an appointment to get lab results back before an important meeting at work. Even if the news is good, my mood's likely to be thrown off.

Occasional changes in CD4 cells or viral load can be shocking, but they may not be reflective of much. "It's much better to look at two or three readings to see what's happening," says GMHC's Saundra Johnson. "And in our experience, if you get results back that look like they should belong to a different person, they probably do. Make sure you check the name at the top of every page, and if your last name's as common as mine, you better also check whatever other identifying numbers they use." Remember how often CD4 cells fluctuate, and look back at the circumstances of your test before you declare yourself cured or ready for intensive care. "Don't go the first day after having the flu and have your CD4 cells done," Johnson advises. "They take a while to bounce back." Even if you weren't sick or tired, balance how much weight you give a test result with a reality check. "How you're doing shouldn't be determined completely by 'Oh, my CD4 cells are up thirty,'" Johnson says. "Another question is, how are you feeling? With viral load tests, remember that those are big numbers, so a change from thirty thousand to sixty thousand is not a big change. From thirty thousand to five hundred thousand is big, or thirty thousand to a million is big."

Never base a treatment decision on a single result, agrees Dr. Grossman. "It's the trends you want to look for, not the individual tally." Some labs now chart T cells and viral load over time on the last sheet of their reports, though patients who see more than one doctor, or who are in a clinical trial, may be juggling two or three sets of reports. "There's a handy software program called Labtracker where you can punch in the results and make graphs," says Johnson, "or there's the method preferred by many people we see. Get a three-ring binder where you put all the lab results you get, in chronological order, and find a doctor or treatment advocate who can help you interpret the results."

TAKE A NUMBER: HOW VIRAL LOAD AND CD4 COUNTS RELATE TO EACH OTHER

David Ho, MD, one of the world's leading AIDS researchers, suggests understanding the interrelationship by thinking of AIDS as a train wreck waiting to happen. If you are HIV-infected, you're on the train. Your CD4 count tells you how close you are to the crash site (AIDS), and your viral load tells you how fast you are moving. The higher your CD4 count, the longer you have before you get sick. The lower your viral load, the slower the train is moving. Antiviral treatment can slow the train down by lowering the levels of your virus, and in some cases can even reverse it by restoring some of your immune system. Less metaphorically-minded men can look at the chart below, which considers CD4 counts and viral load and tells you something about how likely it is you're going to get AIDS over the next three years if you take no medication.

PERCENT OF PEOPLE WHO GET AIDS IN THREE YEARS IF NO MEDICATION IS USED

If your viral load is		And your CD4 (T-cell) count is				
PCR test	**bDNA test**	**Below 200**	**201–350**	**351–500**	**501–750**	**Above 750**
Below 1,500	Below 500	**	**	**	3.7	0
1,500–7,000	500–3,000	**	**	2.0	2.0	2.0
7,000–20,000	3,000–10,000	**	8.1	8.1	8.1	3.2
20,000–55,000	10,000–30,000	40.1	40.1	16.1	16.1	9.5
Above 55,000	Above 30,000	85.5	64.4	42.9	32.6	32.6

*** indicates lack of data*

Source: National Institutes of Health

HIV disease will often develop physical symptoms that aren't considered serious enough to be classified as AIDS but which may indicate that HIV is multiplying: skin rashes, fevers, night sweats, diarrhea, and lack of energy. Even if something's unrelated, get it treated, since you want to minimize any additional stress on your immune system.

"It's easy to ignore symptoms," says Howard, forty-one, an actor who says ten years of HIV have helped him make a habit of avoiding doctor's visits. "Who wants to be reminded that they're sick?" Giving your immune system the support and attention it deserves by getting that athlete's foot or rash treated can make the difference between an inconvenience and a major health episode. It can also help establish a relationship with a doctor. "It's about shifting the model from sick care to health care," adds GMHC's Johnson. "We always say you need to be in a partnership with your doctors, but how are you going to be in a partnership with them if they don't even know you? And how are you going to know if you like them unless you see them?"

Checkup Checklist

Blood pressure, cholesterol, testicular self-exams, and all those routine screenings and shots you may have ignored become even more important when you have HIV, so make sure you get all the tests appropriate for a man your age (see Chapters 7 and 8). Because a weak immune system opens your body to attack from new germs or those you've long held in check, the following can give you vital inside information.

What?	Why?	What next?
CMV test (that's cytomegalovirus). See information on herpes, page 142.	90% of gay men have been exposed already, though it's only a problem for people with severely weakened immune systems (see chart on page 412).	If you haven't been exposed, protected anal and oral sex can keep it that way.
Dental checkup	Oral symptoms, including white patches in the mouth known as thrush and recurring ulcers on the gums, are among the first symptoms of HIV illness. Also, HIV makes gum disease progress faster.	Every six months for a cleaning and exam. If insurance doesn't cover it, see if your local AIDS organization or teaching hospital has a clinic.
Eye exam	Infections including CMV, toxoplasmosis, PCP, and HIV itself can all show up first in the eye. Most can be stopped. See an ophthalmologist who knows about HIV.	If you have 200 or more CD4 cells, get an annual exam. Under 200, go every three months.
Herpes screening	Herpes can appear inside your throat or intestine when you have HIV, and take longer to go away.	Daily treatment with acyclovir (Zovirax) may help prevent frequent outbreaks.
Lean body mass test	Wasting is common with people with AIDS. You want to know how much you had to start.	Nutritional supplements, growth hormone, and testosterone are possible treatments (see "Wasting Away Again?" on page 411).
Measles and chicken pox	You can't safely get the vaccination for chicken pox. If you have under 200 CD4 cells, the measles vaccination isn't safe, either.	If you haven't already been vaccinated or infected, avoid anyone with chicken pox, shingles, or measles.
Nutritional basics	HIV and medications to stop it can change the way you metabolize food and the number of calories you need, and often cause chronic problems of the gut.	See Chapter 6 for more information on everything from eating to coping with chronic diarrhea.
Syphilis test	Syphilis progresses faster to its more damaging, central-nervous-system form in people with HIV.	Get tested yearly or more often if you're having sex, and get treatment if you're infected.
Testosterone workup	As many as 40% of men with advanced HIV don't have enough, leading to depression, low sex drive, and possibly wasting.	Testosterone shots can help, as can patches you can put on your scrotum or elsewhere. Check with your doctor about cycling on and off every three months or so to avoid testicular shriveling and other side effects.
Toxoplasmosis test	Rare burgers and soiled kitty litter expose some of us to this common parasite by adulthood, but with under 250 CD4 cells it can cause serious illness.	If you test negative for toxoplasmosis, stay away from rare meat. If you have a cat, get it tested, too. If it's positive, either get someone else to change the litter box or put on gloves and a dust mask to keep from getting toxo on your hands or in your lungs.

What?	Why?	What next?
Tuberculosis	If you've been exposed to TB in the past, HIV makes you much more likely to develop active disease. If you have active TB now, HIV makes you more likely to die from it. If you've never tested positive for TB before, get a PPD test. Make sure, though, that they give a few shots in the other arm to make sure your immune system is strong enough to respond to any outside invader. If your immune system's too weak, or if you show signs of past exposure you will need a chest X ray.	Testing twice a year. If you have active TB, treatment can help cure you and protect those close to you. If you've been exposed to TB in the past, preventative medications can keep you from developing it.
Vaccinations	Pneumovax, and if you haven't already been exposed, hepatitis A and hepatitis B vaccines can protect you from illnesses made worse by HIV.	See page 299 for a complete list of immunizations.

How Antiviral Drugs Work

Treatment for HIV is divided into two parts: the antiviral (also known as antiretroviral) drugs you take to fight the virus, and the medications you take to prevent or treat the infections that may emerge when HIV has weakened your immune system. Antiviral drugs are the ones you start first; if they can stop HIV from replicating, then the virus may never weaken your immune system enough for the others to be necessary. Medical convention says that one drug, or even two, does not a highly active antiretroviral therapy (HAART) make: HIV may become resistant to one or two drugs so quickly that you usually need a combination of at least three antiviral drugs working together (for more on resistance, see "Why Antivirals Fail," below). No matter what combination you take, your goal is the same: to get HIV so low that it's undetectable with an ultrasensitive viral load test, and to keep it that way.

What's in a winning combination? The names of the different classes of anti-HIV medications —protease inhibitors, non-nucleoside reverse transcriptase inhibitors (NNRTIs), and nucleoside analogues—take their names from where in HIV's reproductive cycle a drug takes effect. Current thinking is to use a combination of two nucleosides and one protease inhibitor or NNRTI to hit HIV coming and going, interfering with two different points of the virus's reproductive cycle. "I think of the immune system as a basketball game, with the nucleosides and the NNRTIs as the forwards and the protease inhibitors as the guards hanging back to get the virus if it makes a fast break toward the end of the replication cycle," says GMHC's Johnson. For those of us who find sports metaphors as hard to understand as the appeal of an evening at Hooters, think of the protease inhibitors as the divas who come in with white gloves and some extra-strength Endust after the house has already been cleaned. If that doesn't work for you, see the chart on the next page for a visual try.

The Life and Times of a Virus: Stages of HIV Reproduction

1. *HIV enters a CD4 cell*
2. *HIV stores its genetic information on single-stranded RNA instead of the double-stranded DNA found in most organisms. To replicate, HIV uses an enzyme known as reverse transcriptase to convert its RNA into DNA. This process is why HIV is known as a "retrovirus."*
3. *HIV DNA enters the nucleus of the CD4 cell and inserts itself into the cell's DNA. HIV DNA then instructs the cell to make many copies of the original virus.*
4. *New virus particles are assembled and leave the cell, ready to infect other CD4 cells.*

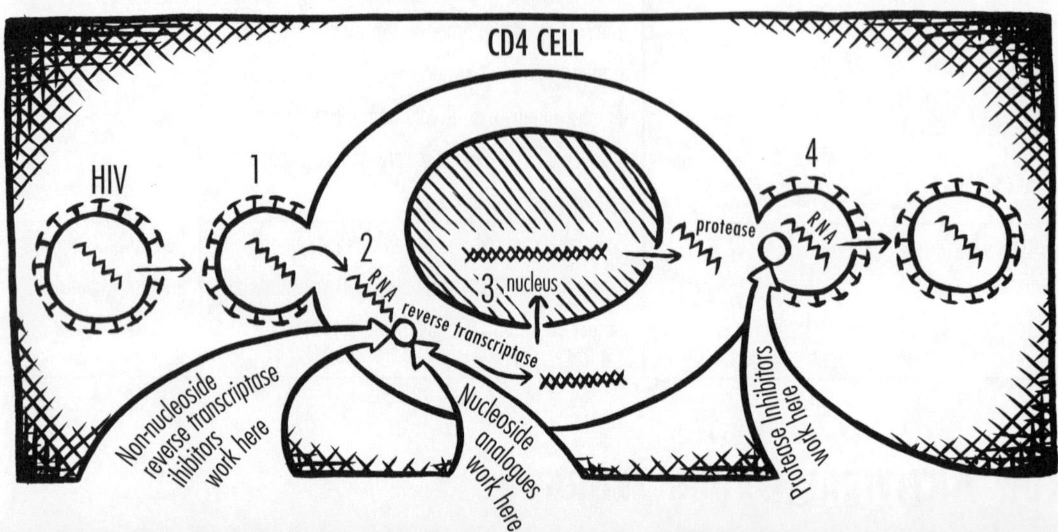

Non-nucleoside reverse transcriptase inhibitors	Nucleoside analogues	Protease inhibitors
The newest class of antiretroviral agents, non-nucleoside reverse transcriptase inhibitors (NNRTIs) stop HIV production by binding directly onto reverse transcriptase and preventing the conversion of RNA to DNA. These drugs are called non-nucleoside inhibitors because even though they work at the same stage as nucleoside analogues, they act in a completely different way.	They act by incorporating themselves into the DNA of the virus, thereby stopping the building process. The resulting DNA is incomplete and cannot create new virus.	Protease inhibitors work at the last stage of the virus reproduction cycle. They prevent HIV from being successfully assembled and released from the infected CD4 cell.

WHY ANTIVIRALS FAIL

All of the pleas and warnings to take a combination of anti-HIV drugs, to take them at the suggested times with or without the suggested foods, and not to skip a dose, no matter how sick or tired of it all you feel, stem from a single, basic fact: HIV is able to develop resistance to every antiviral drug available. Once the virus develops high levels of resistance to a drug, the drug doesn't work anymore. Worse, if resistance to one drug develops, then it may also cause resistance to other drugs in that class.

Understanding resistance means going back to the viral replication cycle, where HIV turned a healthy CD4 cell into a virus-producing factory. "I actually find it easiest to explain resistance by thinking of an underwear factory," says David Barr of the Forum for Collaborative

WINNING COMBINATIONS?

Federal guidelines suggest starting antiviral treatment with a combination of three or four antiviral medications. Choose one from column A and one from column B. Since guidelines change often, it's best to call (800) 448-0440 or check www.hivatis.org for the latest recommendations. All drugs, even those "strongly recommended," have potentially serious side effects (see chart on pages 398–399), and the medications in each section are listed in alphabetical order rather than order of preference.

	Column A	Column B
Strongly Recommended	Efavirenz (Sustiva) Indinavir (Crixivan) Nelfinavir (Viracept) Ritonavir (Norvir)+Saquinavir-SGC (Fortovase, soft-gel cap) or HGC (Invirase, hard-gel cap)	Stavudine (d4T)+Lamivudine (3TC) Stavudine(d4T) +Didanosine (ddI) Zidovudine (AZT)+Lamivudine (3TC) (sold together as Combivir) Zidovudine (AZT)+Didanosine (ddI)
Recommended as Alternative	Abacavir (ABC) Amprenavir (Agenerase) Delavirdine (Rescriptor) Nelfinavir +Saquinavir-SGC Ritonavir Saquinavir-SGC	Didanosine (ddI)+Lamivudine (3TC) Zidovudine (AZT)+Zalcitabine (ddC)
Insufficient Data	Hydroxyurea in combination with other antiretroviral drugs Ritonavir+Indinavir Ritonavir+Nelfinavir	
Not Recommended	Saquinavir-HGC (recommended only in combination with ritonavir)	Stavudine (d4T)+Zidovudine (AZT) Zalcitabine (ddC)+Lamivudine (3TC) Zalcitabine (ddC) + Stavudine (d4T) Zalcitabine (ddC)+Didanosine (ddI)

Research in Washington, DC. "In an underwear factory, you turn out thousands of pairs a day. Some of them come out wrong, irregular, because the high volume of production causes mistakes. The same thing happens in viral replication. So much virus is being produced that some of it is irregular." Whereas some of us find those discounted Calvin Klein boxer briefs irresistible, the irregular HIV virions, also known as "mutants," are distinctly undesirable. Your drugs don't work on some mutants, which then go about their business of infecting CD4 cells and reproducing. *All* of the virus made from CD4 cells they infect is then drug-resistant. While other, regular viruses are being killed off by the drugs you're taking, the mutants are happily gaining strength, until—in six months or less—they're so plentiful that your once-effective anti-HIV drugs are useless.

The higher the rate of replication while you are taking antiviral drugs, the greater the chance of developing resistance. "If you only made one pair of underwear a day, it would come out right and there would be no irregulars," explains Barr. If you can keep viral replication down below the level detectable by the ultrasensitive viral load test, the theory goes, the virus can't develop the momentum it needs to beat the drugs. If a drug dips to low levels because you missed a pill or threw the pills up before your body absorbed them, then viral replication—and the chance of resistance—increases.

To Treat or Not to Treat? Deciding Whether to Start Antiviral Therapy

My viral load has stayed steady for a while now, my CD4 cells are steady, and all I hear is "Get on the drugs, get on the drugs." What I need to hear is someone talking to me about the fact that I'm going to be taking twenty pills a day for the rest of my life, and am I really ready to do that? Frankly, I don't think so.

People say wait, but I say what for? To get weaker? To get sicker? I figure if I start out strong and keep it up, I'll have less to worry about later.

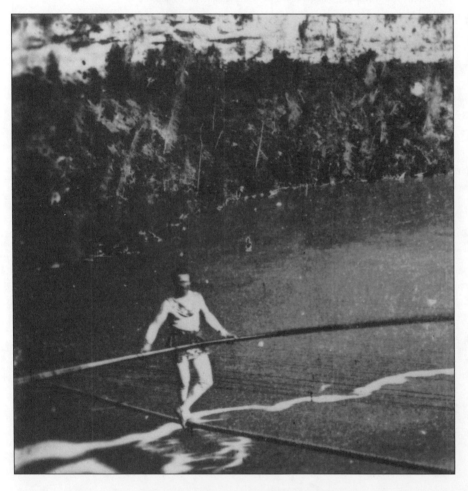

Deciding when to start antiviral therapy is one of the most confusing HIV treatment decisions there is. If you have symptoms of AIDS or advanced HIV illness, most Western doctors agree you should take anti-HIV drugs. If you have 500 or fewer CD4 cells, most guidelines recommend that you consider anti-HIV drugs. But for the thousands of people who have a low amount of HIV in their blood, no symptoms, and CD4-cell counts of 500 or more, the benefits of early treatment are less proven. "The medications still haven't been around long enough for us to know if starting earlier will really make you live longer," says David Barr, who's been on six different AIDS drugs himself at various points over the past twelve years. "And though we know that medications can reduce viral load, we don't know how long that reduction will last. If you start early, are you wasting an opportunity to get the benefit later?"

You may secretly long for someone to just tell you what to do, but it's an open question. "There's no right treatment decision," says Barr. "There's only the decision you think is right for you."

Making a choice that works for you means getting up-to-date information—not only about the available drugs and how to combine them, but also about the number of CD4 cells and HIV particles in your blood and whether they're rising or falling, whether the virus inside you is resistant to other drugs, and what the likelihood is that you are going to be able to take the drugs faithfully. You don't have to read everything that's ever been written about AIDS—even if you had eternal life, it would probably take all of it—but you do need to find information that's current and that presents things in ways you can understand. Learning a few basic common terms (see box on next page) can help. So can knowing a few good sources (see "Information Nation," page 400).

What do you have to lose by starting early? If treatment were as easy as popping a few aspirin, or as short-term as using a week's worth of antibiotics, virtually all doctors would probably treat. Anti-HIV medications, however, are a lifetime commitment: Once you start, you shouldn't stop. They can have side effects, which means that they may make you feel sick when before you were feeling fine. They almost always bring changes in your habits, ranging from popping pills and downing syrups throughout the day to spending hours on the toilet or going without food for nine of your eighteen waking hours. Most important, if your body doesn't tolerate the drug, or if you can't manage to do what you need to in order to use the medicine correctly, starting treatment can do more harm than good. Miss doses and HIV becomes resistant, meaning that what you do today could limit future options tomorrow, including your ability to use drugs that may be better, more potent, and easier to take.

On the other hand, you're more likely to tolerate the drug while your immune system is strong, and you may lower your viral load enough so that you never get sick.

HIV is mutating and perhaps becoming resistant whether you're on drugs or not. The longer you wait, the fewer options you may have. Several drug manufacturers have already come up with dosages that are easier to use. "For years, all we were doing was reacting," says Todd Yancey, MD, "trying to control the damage after it was already done, and prescribing the one drug we had, AZT, which didn't work well alone. Now there are lots of choices. I can't imagine, in a treatment-naive patient [see next page], that we couldn't find a treatment that was tolerable and would help."

With so much in flux, and antiviral drugs so hard on your body, many men in the gray zone have decided they'll use other choices. "They call it 'HIV treatment' or 'therapy,' but I think the same word they use for cancer drugs, 'chemotherapy,' sounds more appropriately scary," says Manuel, forty-two, who with 450 CD4 cells depends instead on a daily regime of immune-enhancing herbs, careful diet, regular exercise, and stress reduction. "I figure, why put something that harsh in my body before I absolutely have to? It's the people who took the medications they recommended in the 1980s who are having the most problems now. If I wait, maybe they'll come up with something better." Many people with HIV—including those on medications, and those who feel they can afford to wait—have found acupuncture, stress reduction, and nutrition useful as complementary approaches. Stress reduction, visualization, and other strategies may also help to stimulate the immune system (see page 314).

Scientists are still looking for ways to stimulate the immune system chemically. Though there have been many experimental compounds claiming to do that—"I have a GMHC list from 1986 that lists more than eighty," says Dr. Yancey—researchers have yet to find one that clearly restores immune function. Current candidates include interleukin-2, one of a number of cytokines, or chemical messengers, that stimulate the production of immune-system cells, and an immune-boosting vaccine (HIV-1 immunogen, brand name Remune) created by polio conqueror Jonas Salk. Use these to rebuild your T-cell stores even as antiviral combinations lower your viral load, the theory goes, and remission—the state where your immune system keeps whatever HIV is left in your body in check even after you stop the drugs—may move from myth to reality.

AIDS-SPEAK

GMHC's Department of Treatment Education can send you a comprehensive glossary of treatment terms, or you can find one at our Web site at www.gmhc.org. Meanwhile, here are ten common terms that sound like something other than what they are, and which may help you make your way through the wilderness of HIV information.

Adherence. It means stickiness, and in this case refers to your ability to stick to your medications. Given that you may need to take up to ten or twenty pills a day against HIV, not counting your vitamins and medicine to prevent infections, it ain't easy.

Breakthrough. This sounds good, but in AIDS-speak it actually refers to the moment when you develop an opportunistic infection, or an increase in viral load, even when you've been taking drugs to prevent those things.

Cross-resistance. Resistance is the ability of HIV to grow and multiply even in the presence of drugs that should kill it. Cross-resistance is when the same virus becomes resistant to drugs you haven't even taken yet.

Failure. This term refers not to you, but to your medication when it doesn't work to suppress the virus. That may or may not have anything to do with what you do (see *Adherence*, above).

HAART. Otherwise known as highly active antiretroviral therapy, a combination of three or more anti-HIV drugs. Wiseasses and realists call it *FAART*, "fairly active antiretroviral therapy."

Log. This is the technical term for exponential changes in viral load. A 3 log reduction means your virus went down 10^3, or dropped to a thousandth of what it had been. It's simpler, and just as effective, to talk in regular numbers and percentages, but AIDS experts rarely do. Here are a few to make it simpler:

- A "1.5 log reduction" is a 99 percent drop.
- A "1 log reduction" is a 90 percent drop.
- A ".5 log reduction" is a 66 percent drop.
- A ".3 log reduction" is a 50 percent drop.

Latently infected cells. These are the closet cases of the immune system, cells that have not yet been "activated" and so hide an inner secret: HIV infection.

Naive. You may object to being called so in real life. In HIV land, it's usually a good thing: If you're treatment-naive, it means you haven't tried any medications before, which often means you have more options (see *Cross-resistance*, above).

Prophylaxis. Refers to a course of drugs taken to prevent opportunistic infections related to AIDS. It's abbreviated *Px*.

Remission. More a theory than reality, this is the state when your immune system is strong enough to hold HIV at bay after antiviral drugs have brought HIV levels down and kept them that way for years. The hope is to couple antiviral therapy with some kind of immune-boosting approach, such as a vaccine, that will allow this kind of immune system reconstitution.

Retrovirus. This only sounds like an explanation for the seventies fashion craze. It's really a term for viruses such as HIV, which store genetic information in the form of RNA, rather than DNA, and then use an enzyme called reverse transcriptase to reproduce. Anti-HIV drugs are often called "antiretroviral therapy" or just "antiretrovirals."

Salvage therapy. In HIV, it means a treatment you try after another (or many others) has failed.

SAY WHEN? Once again, the federal guidelines change frequently. Here's an adaptation of what the Department of Health and Human Services says as of this writing about when to start treatment. Check the latest guideline updates on the Web at www.hivatis.org, call (800) 448-0440, or contact a large AIDS organization.

If you are	And your CD4 cells (T cells)/ viral load (HIV RNA) measures	Recommendation
Symptomatic (AIDS, thrush, unexplained fever)	Any value	Treat
Asymptomatic	CD4 cells<500, HIV RNA >10,000 (bDNA), or >20,000 (PCR)	Treat, if you really feel able to follow through on the therapy. Some doctors will wait if a patient's CD4 cells are between 350 and 500 and his viral load is less than 10,000.
Asymptomatic	CD4 cells >500 and HIV RNA <10,000 or (bDNA) <20,000 (PCR)	Many experts would delay therapy and observe, and some would start treatment.

Can I Get You a Cocktail? Choosing the Right Drugs

I resent it when people act like it's easy to take these drugs, or it's nothing, or AIDS is over. I'm an extremely regimented person, I do the same thing during the week and on the weekend, I'm an educated, organized person, and it's extremely hard. Your prescriptions don't run out at the same time, your refills expire, you can't let your guard down for a minute. Then there are the minor problems, like the intestinal symphonies that issue from somewhere deep inside you, usually in an important meeting. The more you try to suppress them, the louder they become. I mean, how long can you bear down?

Even if you follow the treatment guidelines above and one of the suggested combinations of medications (see page 393), that still leaves you with more than thirty possible combinations. The best tool for making sense of that tangle of options is a doctor with experience you can trust. "If a doctor takes a look at your lab work and dashes off a prescription without talking it through with you, either get more time with him or see if you can find another doctor," says Dr. Grossman. Dr. Yancey agrees, saying that a good doctor will try to make his thought process "transparent" for you, rather than delivering instructions. "If you were going to go and have an organ transplant, you'd expect more than a fifteen-minute meeting," he insists.

A little self-examination, and self-education, can probably make the choices simpler. Given that you're trying to choose a medication that will last a lifetime, you need to decide which of the many side effects and administration requirements seems easiest to bear. Norvir interacts badly with many other drugs and is taken with a high-fat, high-protein meal, so if you're on a bunch of other medications or have eaten macrobiotic for the last five years, it's probably not for you. Pancreatitis, a side effect of ddI, is made worse by alcohol consumption, so skip that drug if you're wedded to your happy hour. Crixivan has to be taken every eight hours and can't be absorbed by your body unless you eat little or nothing but low-fat, low-protein foods for two hours before and one hour after. If you're rolling through three time zones regularly or are already worried about losing weight, it's probably not the best choice.

"Deciding on a combination that works for you," says Paul Warren, treatment educator and counselor at GMHC, involves looking at how you feel about the medications as well as what they do for you and to you. "It's not a prescription, it's more like an arranged marriage," agrees Gerald, twenty-eight, who like many men held on to his prescriptions for a few weeks before getting them filled. Given your personality and circumstances, a particular choice may seem more attractive. Do you know where the public bathrooms are en route to work, so that you can make a quick stop in case of the diarrhea that is a normal Nelfinavir moment? Is it going to be easy for you to drink the eight glasses of water a day you need to keep from getting kidney stones from Crixivan? "Some people find it helpful, once they think they've found a workable combination, to do a trial run with Tic-Tacs or grapes and see what gets in the way of the schedule," says GMHC's Warren. "It's like those exercises they used to give to teenage girls thinking of having a baby, where they asked you to carry an egg around for three days to see how it really felt."

New technology, including tests of viral resistance (see box on page 409) as well as improvements in dosing, can also increase the chance that a medication will work and make it easier to take. These developments occur faster than most doctors who aren't AIDS specialists can track, so it may fall to you to familiarize yourself with what's happening out there.

COMMON ANTI-HIV DRUGS

Following is a list of current antiviral drugs, along with some of the most common side effects. Knowledge about drug action and interaction and available drugs themselves change often, so consult a doctor or a current source of information. Some good sources are found on page 400.

Many side effects pertain to whole classes of drugs. Protease inhibitors, for example, may interact badly with other kinds of drugs, and often cause redistribution of body fat (lipodystrophy), blood sugar problems (hypoglycemia and diabetes) and high cholesterol (triglycerides). Check with a knowledgeable doctor before beginning medication.

A note about names: the first class of anti-HIV drugs listed have three. The name in the first column is the nickname for the chemical compound, or the ingredients. The second name is the brand name. The third name is the generic name. It's absurdly confusing. Think of it this way. AZT is crushed peanuts, oil, and salt. Retrovir is Skippy. Zidovudine is peanut butter.

NAME	Brand Name/ Other Name	Class of Drug	Daily Dose (may change according to other drugs used)	Common side effects	Comments
Abacavir	Ziagen ABC	Nucleoside analog reverse transcriptase inhibitor (NARTI)	1 tablet, twice a day	Headache, fatigue, and in fewer than 5 percent of cases serious flulike allergy (fever, nausea, dizziness, vomiting, or shortness of breath).	Seek emergency care in case of allergy. If you've stopped because of allergic reaction, never take it again.
AZT	Retrovir, zidovudine	NARTI	1 tablet, twice a day (or two capsules, three times a day).	Headaches, nausea, anemia.	Take with food if you have stomach irritation.
AZT+3TC	Combivir		1 tablet, twice a day.	See entries for 3TC and AZT.	
ddC	Hivid zalcitabine	NARTI	1 tablet, three times a day, without food if possible.	Headache, fever, neuropathy (tingling in hands and feet), mouth sores, pancreatitis.	Drinking alcohol increases risk of pancreatitis. Acupuncture may help with neuropathy.

NAME	Brand Name/ Other Name	Class of Drug	Daily Dose (may change according to other drugs used)	Common side effects	Comments
ddI	Videx didanosine	NARTI	4 tablets on an empty stomach. Tablets are chewed or dissolved in water.	Pancreatitis, neuropathy headache, sleeplessness, diarrhea.	Drinking alcohol increases risk of pancreatitis. Acupuncture may help with neuropathy.
d4T	Zerit stavudine	NARTI	1 capsule, twice a day, with or without food.	Neuropathy, anemia, and, rarely, pancreatitis.	Drinking alcohol increases risk of pancreatitis. Acupuncture may help with neuropathy.
3TC	Epivir lamivudine	NARTI	1 tablet, twice a day.	Headache, nausea, fatigue, anemia.	
Delavirdine	Rescriptor	Non-nucleoside analog reverse transcriptase inhibitor (NNRTI)	4 tablets, three times a day.	Rash, headache, nausea.	If rash is severe, seek emergency care. Benadryl or cortisone cream may help with minor rash.
Efavirenz	Sustiva	NNRTI	3 tablets, once a day.	Dizziness, drowsiness, lack of concentration.	Take at night to avoid feeling side effects.
Nevirapine	Viramune	NNRTI	1 tablet, twice a day (start with 1 tablet a day for first two weeks), with or without food.	Fever, soreness, rash.	If rash is severe, seek emergency care. Benadryl or cortisone cream may help with minor rash; ask your doctor.
Amprenavir	Agenerase	Protease Inhibitor (PI)	8 capsules, twice a day.	Nausea, gas, headache, neuropathy, diarrhea.	
Indinavir	Crixivan	PI	2½ capsules, every 8 hours on an empty stomach or with a very light, non-fat snack.	Kidney stones, dry skin, chapped lips, headache, and nausea.	Drink eight glasses of water or more a day, especially before and after taking pills.
Nelfinavir	Viracept	PI	5 tablets, twice a day with food.	Diarrhea, numbness around mouth.	
Ritonavir	Norvir	PI	6 capsules, twice a day with full, high-protein meal, or six spoonfuls of syrup with same.	Diarrhea, nausea.	Capsules need to be refrigerated.
Saquinavir (SGC)	Fortovase (soft gel capsule)	PI	6 capsules, three times a day with food or within 2 hours of eating.	Diarrhea, nausea.	
Hydroxyurea	Hydrea HO		1 pill, twice a day.	Mild nausea, bone marrow suppression, hair loss.	Not yet recommended by federal guidelines due to lack of data.
adefovir dipivoxil	Preveon bis-POM PMEA			Nausea, diarrhea, elevated liver enzymes, depletion of carnitine.	Available to people already taking it, but the FDA has recommended against approval for wider use.

INFORMATION NATION

GMHC's Treatment Education and Advocacy department has a vast amount of information, including fact sheets and articles available on our Web site (www.gmhc.org) or by mail. If you don't know how to read a study critically, check out "Hope from Hype I," page 430, for some help with basic principles. *POZ* and *HIV Plus*, both magazines out of New York, offer user-friendly information in a glossy mag format, though there's a charge for individual subscriptions. Many not-for-profit organizations offer these magazines or other information free to people with AIDS. Their biases are free, too, so consult more than one.

Even if you get information, you may not be ready to digest it. "Many people do the ostrich thing for a while, and then move on to a more active involvement," says Dr. Yancey.

Newsletters	Web Sites	Organizations
These can be a little technical, but less so than the medical journals from which they draw much information. The name in parentheses is the publishing organization.	*These multiply as fast as the virus, and opinions of individuals are rarely checked for accuracy. Still, they're a great source of information and insight.*	*AIDS service organizations offer treatment information, educational seminars, fact sheets, and support. Again, GMHC can be reached through its Web site (www.gmhc.org) or by calling the hot line at (212) 807-6665. The four other largest AIDS organizations are listed in Appendix A, and you can call the national clearing house at (800) 458-5231 for additional listings. Other organizations of interest include:*
AIDS/HIV Treatment Directory (AmFar, New York City)	sci.med.aids *The* newsgroup for HIV-related discussion.	Buyer's clubs These not only sell alternative treatments, they educate people about them. Direct AIDS Alternative Information Resources in New York has a great info pack.
Notes from the Underground (People with AIDS Health Group, New York City)	www.aegis.com With over 17,000 articles, this is among the world's largest AIDS/HIV knowledge base.	Treatment education or advocacy organizations These include Critical Path AIDS Project in Philadelphia, Project Inform in San Francisco, and three organizations other than GMHC in New York: AIDS Treatment and Data Network; Treatment Action Group; and the National AIDS Treatment Advocacy Project.
Beta (San Francisco AIDS Foundation)	thebody.com An AIDS info clearinghouse.	*For more contact information about any organization listed in this chart, see Appendix A.*
PI Perspective (Project Inform)	www.hivatis.org The site for federal treatment guidelines on everything from HIV to opportunistic infections.	
SIDA Ahora (Informacion en Español, People with AIDS Health Group, New York City)	www.cdcnpin.org The CDC's page, including AIDS statistics, treatment guidelines, and a daily summary of news articles.	
Treatment Issues (GMHC)	www.medscape.com For doctors, but great for patients, with links to medical journals and presentations by clinicians.	
TAGline (Treatment Action Group)	hivinsite.uscf.edu A comprehensive HIV and AIDS information site.	
One privately published newsletter deserves special mention for excellence: AIDS Treatment News (1-800-TREAT12, aidsnews@aidsnews.org, www.aidsnews.org)		

Have You Reached a Verdict? Some Cases for Treating or Waiting: What Would You Do?

CASE #1: BILLY

Billy has suspected he was positive for about a year now, but he just found out for sure last week. He still hasn't told his boyfriend, Buck, about it. He went to the doctor and got his blood work back. He has 450 CD4 cells and his viral load is 25,000. The doctor says that these numbers are not great but aren't terrible, either. Billy feels fine physically, but mentally he's pretty upset. The doctor says that Billy needs to start treatment, and gives Billy some reading material about the drugs. Billy reads it at Starbucks over his favorite comfort drink—decaf mocha frappuccino—but then he throws the material away because he doesn't want Buck to see it. Should Billy start treatment?

Verdict: Yes, but not right now. His blood work indicates that his immune system is weakened, and his viral load shows he has a 16 percent chance of progressing to AIDS over the next three years (see "Take a Number," page 389). Still, it seems there are other priorities to deal with first. If he can't take the treatment information home, what is he going to do with those pill bottles? Figuring out how to tell Buck and deal with the drama (given that his name is Buck, it could be high drama) comes first. Unless Billy's drag name is Evelyn Wood, one speed-read over a frappuccino is just not enough. Is it dangerous for Billy to wait? Probably not. He has no symptoms, and hasn't even had a second set of blood tests yet. He should keep monitoring his immune system and begin to get things in order at home.

CASE #2: PETER

Peter has known about his HIV infection since 1989. He freaked out at first, but settled down and dealt with it, going to the doctor regularly and getting his blood work done fastidiously. He has 325 T cells and is proud that the number's been holding steady since 1991. He reads about HIV treatment, attends the treatment forums regularly at his local AIDS organization, and considers himself very knowledgeable about all this. He got a viral load count six months ago, and the count was 40,000, which alarmed both him and his doctor. At the time, Peter decided to wait a while before starting treatment. He had heard that new protease inhibitors were coming that were even better than those they have now, and he thought he would wait until one was available. Three months later, he got another viral load count of 40,000. Three months after that, his viral load was 92,000. Two months after that, it was up to 125,000. His CD4 cells haven't changed a bit, and he's still feeling fine. The doctor wants him to begin "meds" soon. Peter went home to think it over. Somehow, taking pills seems like giving in to the fact that he's sick, and that makes him both scared and angry. What should he do?

Verdict: In spite of his CD4 count, Peter's not a long-term nonprogressor. His viral load is climbing. Despite all his knowledge about HIV treatment, Peter has issues. He may feel angry or scared about the medicine and he was smart to wait until his therapeutic options were good, but now is probably the time to act. First, though, he needs to sort out his feelings so that once he does start, he will follow through and take his pills regularly.

CASE #3: PHILIP

Philip tested in 1998 because his boyfriend at the time made him do it. They had been together for three months, and the boyfriend was getting tested and told Philip that if he didn't get tested also, then the relationship was over. This guy was the first nice guy Philip had met in San Diego since arriving from Little Rock six months before, and Philip really liked him. The boyfriend tested negative. Philip tested positive, and three weeks later the boyfriend was gone. For Philip, the lesson was never to tell another guy he was positive, and to put the whole thing out of his mind. Lately, however, things aren't so good. Philip's lost weight, and he is tired all the time. He is getting scared. He remembers reading about new treatments for AIDS, but also has friends who look gorgeous, are HIV-positive, and don't take anything. He finally tells his best friend, Monica, about his HIV infection, and she gets him to her doctor. Philip finds out that his viral load is 325,000 and that his CD4 cells are 150. The doctor tells him that this is serious and recommends that Philip start therapy immediately. He gives Philip a bunch of prescriptions and sends him home. Philip has no health insurance, since the modeling agency didn't "do that" (the doctor saw him as a favor to Monica). What should he do?

Verdict: Treatment time. Philip's viral load is very high and his CD4 cells are seriously low. Because his CD4 count is under 200, he is already at risk for PCP, an AIDS-related pneumonia (see "What's Buggin' You," page 408). He needs to start taking medicine to prevent that before anything else. He needs to figure out what antiviral drugs to take, and a way to pay for tests and prescriptions. He needs to find a physician he can work with in the long term. Because he fits the official criteria for AIDS, he may be eligible for government benefits, or he can consider getting a job that will—after a waiting period—give him health insurance. Monica, who obviously has coping skills, may be able to help him get an appointment at the local AIDS organization, which in turn can help him get medical care and help him learn about HIV treatment. They can also offer a support group so that he can meet and talk with other people who have HIV.

Sticking with It

I didn't want to bring them home to my mother's house and have her ask me what the pill bottle was in the refrigerator. So I didn't.

I didn't feel sick before, but now, something that's supposed to keep me healthy is actually making me feel terrible.

I started getting numb from my knees down, and then I just went on strike. I told my doctor, "I am not taking this goddamn drug, end of story. So let's start with I'm not taking this and go from there." So I switched. Besides a little numbness around the mouth, I now have no side effects whatsoever.

"Ask a group of doctors how many of them have ever stopped a course of antibiotics before they were supposed to, and more than half of them raise their hands," says Dr. Yancey. That's about average: For all medications, no matter how serious the condition, only about 50 percent of people take their drugs as instructed. Now consider anti-HIV drugs, which often number twenty pills instead of one or two, have to be taken repeatedly with complicated dietary restrictions, and frequently make you feel worse rather than better. Given those issues, the idea that you're going to go through life without missing a dose is impossible. Things happen: You get stuck in traffic, you travel through a time zone (or five of them), you fall asleep, you leave your

KEEPING IT UP: HOW PEOPLE MANAGE THEIR MEDICATIONS

Every Sunday night I lay all my medications out for the week, and put them into one of those clear plastic pill containers with a compartment for each day. That way I can see when I'm going to run out and remember what I've taken.

Timing is everything for me. I know, when I brush my teeth in the morning, that I always follow that with my pills. When I come back from lunch at work, I always take my pills. When the news is on in the evening, I take my pills. For every medication, there's a corresponding event I do every day.

I get my medications by mail order, and the first thing I do is count out a week's worth and hide them away. That way, when I run out, I'm not really out.

My beeper is my buddy. It vibrates when it's time to take the drugs. When it goes off, I get busy.

For me, it's the afternoon dose that's the problem. I fall asleep watching TV. So now, every day I get my friend to call me at two-thirty, ring twice, and hang up.

I had to stop drinking. I mean, you're not supposed to drink on my pills anyway, but lots of people do. I couldn't. I'd wake up three hours past my dose.

The liquid tasted so bad I honestly thought I had to change—until I started chasing it with a spoonful of Skippy extra-chunky peanut butter, which was the only thing that took away the taste.

My boyfriend always was a nag, so now I get him to work for me. It's like judo—you redirect the energy that's already there.

pills in your boyfriend's apartment, or you're afraid to take them there in the first place. Sometimes you may feel too sick. Ask gay men why they didn't take their pills and the number-one response is "I forgot," with "I ran out" shortly behind. Dig a little deeper and they will, too, citing depression, the need for a "drug holiday," and other perfectly human responses.

In general, if it's been less than two hours since you missed a dose, you can usually take it anyway. You don't want to miss those doses—HIV resistance to some drugs can happen very rapidly. If it's been longer than two hours since you missed your dose, don't double up next time; just move on. If missing medication is a pattern, think about whether there's something you might be able to do, or someone you might be able to talk to, to help. "Of course, there are practical things you can do, like not staying out quite as late on Saturday night, keeping some extra pills in your office desk or gym locker, or getting a portable pill box," says GMHC's Paul Warren, "but often your emotional relationship to your medications has more effect on whether you can stick with the schedule. This is a lifelong commitment, and people aren't always happy with the marriage." Many organizations have treatment counselors who have practical tips on adherence to your medication schedule, as well as on how to coax more than a rushed, five-minute exchange of helpful information from your doctor. For more on doctor-patient dynamics, see Chapter 7.

If side effects are making you sick, check with other people with AIDS, your doctor, or a practitioner of complementary therapies to see if you can reduce them. Taking the amino acid glutamine and changing your diet may help control diarrhea, for example (see "On the Runs," page 256), while acupuncture might minimize the tingling and numbness in your legs. Sometimes your doctor will give you medicine to stop the side effects from your other medicine. It means more pills, but it may be worth it. When it comes to side effects from an effective antiviral regimen, it's usually better to fight than switch.

If you are having trouble, don't punish yourself, and don't stop for a few days and then start again. While stop-and-go treatment is being studied as a viable alternative for people with undetectable viral loads, we're not there yet, and deciding to stop without medical consultation could have seriously damaging repercussions. "The thing that makes me craziest is when people say, 'The side effects were so bad I could only do one dose a day this month,'" says Dr. Grossman. "The worst thing to hear is 'It was making me so sick that I took the weekend off.' Page your doctor if you're in trouble, and don't be a hero. This kind of problem happens all the time." If, for whatever reason, you need to stop taking an antiretroviral drug, it's usually better to stop taking all of them than to continue with only part of the combination. "Resistance is more likely to develop when there is an ineffective combination present than when there's no drug at all in your body," says Dr. Yancey.

Drug Dealings: Access to Medications

I went into Rite-Aid the other day and while I was waiting for my prescription, I asked them if I could use the bathroom. They said it wasn't open to the public. "I'm not the public," I said. "I'm a customer waiting for my drugs." They still said no, so I asked for the manager. "You mean to tell me you're serving people with AIDS in here and you aren't going to open up the bathroom?" I asked. "There are two choices. You can open the bathroom up, or I can contact every AIDS group in the area, including the one I work for, to complain." That bathroom was opened in two minutes, and it stayed open.

At up to $15,000 or more a year—and that's not counting drugs for opportunistic infections or lab tests or doctors' visits—you may not be able to afford any drugs at all. Access to care and drugs remains the biggest obstacle there is to getting treatment for HIV, particularly if you don't have Medicaid, Medicare, or private insurance. Even if you do, you may want to investigate the options that can help you get drugs, and perhaps health care, for less money, or improve the care you pay for.

A GOOD PHARMACY

Even at $5 a prescription, you may be shelling out $80 to $90 a month. Will your pharmacy fill two prescriptions at once to save you the copayment? Do they keep a few pills on hand to give you in case you run out? Are they friendly and prompt, or do you often find yourself at the mercy of an antagonistic, gum-cracking, teenage clock watcher? Your pharmacist is often the only one who knows all the drugs you're taking, and can advise you on bad interactions doctors might not catch. Mail-order pharmacies are also a possibility: They're usually cheaper, deliver to your door, and offer lots of additional information.

EXPANDED ACCESS PROGRAMS

AIDS activists fought successfully for the creation of these programs, which offer new drugs before they are approved for marketing but after studies have proven them safe. Expanded

CLINICAL TRIALS

In order to be sold in the United States, every drug must be tested for short-term safety, efficacy, and long-term efficacy and safety. For each of these three phases, companies run clinical trials, tests of a new medication where they provide the drug free in exchange for the right to monitor the recipient's bodily responses. If you go into a trial, you're helping AIDS research. If the drug works well, or if you've exhausted every other option, you may also be helping yourself. Many men enjoy the additional attention, the free medical care, and the feeling that they're on the cutting edge of care. Don't think, however, that a trial can substitute for the complete medical care you need. The research team is interested in their drug and its effects on you, but they are probably not going to spend hours figuring out how to cope with your flu or diarrhea.

Because researchers want to keep everything as carefully controlled as possible, trials have very rigid rules for who can and can't enter and what's expected of participants. Some ask for a two year commitment as well as hospital time, or lab tests, or monitoring and interviews with a doctor; others may last only a few months. Even if you qualify, make sure you talk through all the requirements carefully with a doctor and, ideally, with an AIDS advocate before you give your "informed consent." The AIDS Treatment and Data Network has an excellent brochure, "Should I Join an AIDS Drug Trial?" available for free via mail or through the Web (www.aidsinfonyc.org). The brochure summarizes some of the important questions. Among them:

- ***Will I get a drug or a placebo?*** If you're going in because you've failed on all other treatments, are you willing to risk getting a sugar pill, or a combination of a couple of existing drugs and a sugar pill?
- ***Will this "free" drug cost me?*** Some trials ask you or your insurance to pay for some lab tests or the screening tests you need to qualify.
- ***What do I have to stop doing or taking to participate in the trial?*** Alcohol? Another treatment? Any foods?
- ***If I get sick, will the trial doctors take care of or monitor me?*** How about after the trial is over? Sometimes they will, sometimes they won't.
- ***Is there a good treatment already available that might work for me?*** Some trials are held because a company wants in on the market, but it might be easier to go with what's already out there.
- ***How will I take the drug, and how often do I have to go for tests?***
- ***Will I get the drug for free after the trial is over?*** Sometimes you do, and sometimes you don't.

For a list of AIDS drug trials in your area, call the AIDS Clinical Trial Information Service (ACTIS) at (800) 874-2572, or check the Web at www.actis.org.

access is designed for patients for whom existing therapies aren't working. The drugs are usually free, but come with a different kind of cost: limited safety and efficacy data. You need a doctor to apply for you, and the drug company usually requires documentation about your condition and regular reports back from your physician. Some drugs, like the first protease inhibitors, were available only through a "lottery," but the subsequent outcry should have taught companies to have enough drugs on hand to run both clinical studies (see above) and expanded access programs.

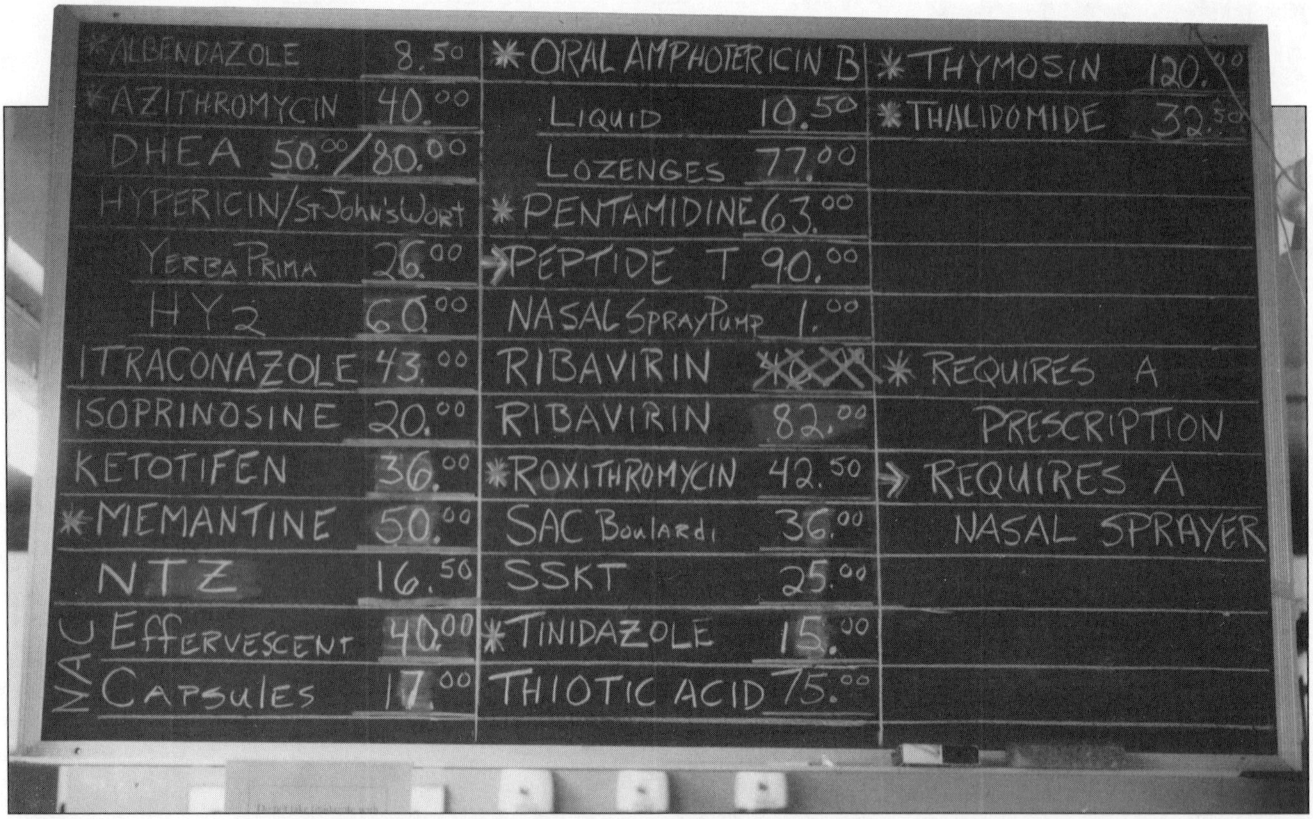

AIDS DRUG ASSISTANCE PROGRAMS

Commonly known as ADAP, these are state programs that offer free or low-cost medications to people with HIV who have too much money to qualify for Medicaid but don't have enough to afford the drugs. Some also offer help with basic medical care. What you get depends on where you live, though the AIDS Treatment and Data Network, which monitors ADAPs nationwide, estimates that a majority of programs now have waiting lists, budget crises, or sharp restrictions on who can get on AIDS drugs. Contact ATDN at (800) 734-7104 or www.aidsinfonyc.org for information on how to reach out to your local program.

BUYER'S CLUBS

Begun as underground organizations bringing unapproved AIDS drugs in from other countries, these have grown to be major sources of information and alternative therapies sold at cost or close to it. New York's PWA Health Group offers an excellent newsletter, *Notes from the Underground*, and there are buyer's clubs in Boston, Phoenix, San Francisco, and many other cities. For an online list, try www.aidsinfonyc.org.

How to Know if Your Therapy's Working

Since the goal of antiviral therapy is to reduce viral load to the lowest levels possible, viral load tests are the best marker of whether your treatment is working. A month after you start, you should see a dramatic decrease in your viral load. In three months, test again with the ultrasensitive test, throwing in a CD4 test, too. Viral load should be undetectable or close (see sidebar). Your CD4 may take a bit longer to go up. Even if they haven't, stick with it, and remember to ask yourself how you feel, not just how your numbers are. Do you have more energy? Have any symptoms cleared up? Keep monitoring your immune system and your feelings.

In general, a threefold reduction in your viral load while you're waiting to be undetectable is a sign that things are going well. In this case, size doesn't matter; that 300 percent change is as meaningful if you started with five thousand copies as it is if you had fifty thousand to start. Similarly, a threefold increase in viral load, no matter how small your total numbers, may be a warning sign that you need to rethink the drugs in your combination. Ultimately, though, you want your viral levels to be undetectable (see box below) using even the most sensitive test.

Among the signs that you may need to try some other drugs in your combination:

- Failure of your viral load to go down to undetectable levels within four to six months
- A rebound or reemergence of detectable virus after a period in which viral load was undetectable
- Any sustained increase in viral load of at least threefold from its lowest point
- Persistently declining CD4 counts

Development of a new opportunistic infection, strangely, may not be a sign of treatment failure. For some people it's actually a sign of immune health: Your body's renewed ability to fight means it's responding again to old infections. Hepatitis C, CMV, and MAC are all common infections to get as your CD4 cells rise and your immune system is "reactivated."

Though resistance is the most common cause for treatment failure, there are many different underlying causes. If you're missing doses or not following dietary guidelines, that's the likely reason for the problem, but even the most careful patients can experience treatment fail-

UNDETECTABLE . . . IN EVERY WAY? LOW VIRAL LOAD AND WHAT IT DOES AND DOESN'T MEAN

You hear it often in AIDS circles, and for those who've been around them for years, it's music to the ears: "So-and-so is undetectable." This only sounds like some kind of gay obsession with straight acting and straight appearing; it really means that your medication is working fine, and that viral load tests don't detect any virus in the blood. That's great news, because it suggests that the undetectable one is probably not going to get sick, or sicker.

Being undetectable, though, is not the same as being cured. Just as the naked eye can't see all the organisms in the body, the tests for viral load can't see all the virus in the body either. HIV isn't just in your blood; it is also in your lymph nodes, your testicles, and your brain. With a few exceptions, people who've stopped therapy have found their virus shooting up again. And as for those who think undetectable means you can't infect someone else or no longer need to have safer sex because there's no virus in your cum, let's repeat: HIV is in your testicles and in your brain.

ure. Your body may not be absorbing the drug—liver problems, or other drugs you're taking, may be keeping you from metabolizing medicine at proper levels. You may have used certain AIDS drugs in the past that make your virus able to resist the combination you're trying today.

Until recently, doctors couldn't even tell which drug was failing, leaving you to divine the cause from a collection of side effects and trial and error. Now, a number of doctors are using the genotype and phenotype tests (see box on page 409) to help determine which drugs to change.

If you and your doctor decide to try another combination without using a genotype or phenotype test, it's best to change all your drugs, or at least two of three. An exception to that rule is sometimes made if it's a side effect that's causing the problems and if you've begun to take the drug too recently to become resistant. Make sure you get a second viral load test before you decide a drug combination is ineffective, and talk over every change carefully with your doctor.

What's Buggin' You: Opportunistic Infections and Malignancies

"Opportunistic infections" (or OIs, in AIDS-speak) is the term given to all the infections associated with HIV that occur because of a weakened immune system. Opportunistic malignancies are the cancers that come with immune damage, including Kaposi's sarcoma (KS), non-Hodgkin's lymphoma, and squamous cell carcinoma of the anus.

The first and most important concept to understand about OIs is that they can develop in any of the many different systems in your body and can develop in several different bodily systems at the same time. Your immune system protects every part of you, and when it fails, every part can have problems. You can get tuberculosis in your eye, or PCP in your spleen. Staying very aware of symptoms and seeking prompt treatment for any and all of them is crucial when you start getting into the danger zone for opportunistic infections. So is learning the basic questions to ask about diagnostic tests, since a glance at the OI chart on page 412 will show you that fever, diarrhea, fatigue, and weight loss are symptoms of practically everything. Figuring out the cause of a symptom may mean a number of visits to additional doctors with expertise in treating your eyes, skin, gastrointestinal system, lungs, and nervous system, to name only a few.

The other important fact to remember is that between antiviral therapies and existing drugs, most OIs are preventable. Rates of many have dipped 75 percent or more since the debut of combination therapy, though that's no consolation if you're among the 25 percent who are still suffering. The variety of ailments, too, has been radically reduced. "At the moment, 90 percent of OIs are accounted for by only five different infections," says Dr. Yancey, "and for every single one of those there are preventive medications or a way to see the disease coming." Whether that will continue to be the case depends on how effective the antiviral drugs prove over the long term, and whether—as has happened before with AIDS—new infections become more common as people live longer. Opportunistic malignancies, unfortunately, have yet to be prevented, though rates of Kaposi's sarcoma have fallen with the use of combination therapy, and careful monitoring can lead to early detection and treatment of AIDS-related cancers.

WHAT'S YOUR TYPE? GENOTYPE AND PHENOTYPE TESTING

They're still experimental, but two kinds of tests—genotype and phenotype testing—may hold very important information about what drugs to start or what to switch to if your medication is failing. Because there are hundreds of mutated viruses in circulation, these tests try to see which ones are inside you and whether they make you resistant to medications. Why, particularly if you've never taken an antiviral, would you be resistant? Scientists have already documented partners passing drug-resistant virus to each other. One 1999 study estimated, for example, that 16 percent of the gay men newly infected with HIV in New York City and L.A. had a strain of the virus that was resistant to one or more HIV drugs. "Which means," says Dr. Yancey, "that a three-drug combination with AZT in it that would normally work beautifully would really only be a two-drug combination, which wouldn't work long-term. Three months down the road you'd probably discover that you'd become resistant to those drugs as well as the ones to which they have cross-resistance, which means you'd lose the option to use a number of available therapies."

If your medication isn't working, the genotype and phenotype tests may be able to provide a crucial piece of information: which one of your combination of drugs is faltering. "Here, too, we used to have to guess," says Dr. Yancey. "Now you can test." Neither test is foolproof, since they use the dominant virus in your blood. If there's another mutant in there, waiting to emerge once the dominant one is knocked off by drugs, you may be facing different resistance problems in the future.

HOW?

The phenotype test takes virus from your blood and "challenges" it with each of the available anti-HIV drugs. Where the HIV grows in spite of the drug, that's a drug that's not likely to be useful to you. The genotype test takes a sample of your virus, looks at its genetic sequence, and tries to match that with the genetic sequences of common mutants known to be resistant to different drugs. There are currently more than 250 of these and counting.

HOW OFTEN?

Though it's not approved, a few AIDS docs recommend a genotype or phenotype test once before starting treatment (to see if you're already resistant to any drugs). More recommend one of the tests if your current treatment seems unable to control HIV.

HOW MUCH?

At the moment, the genotype test costs $400, the phenotype test runs up to $800, and advocates are fighting with insurance companies to cover the costs.

Preventing OIs

The best way to deal with OIs is not to get them. One important way of avoiding opportunistic infections is to keep yourself healthy by eating right and staying away from things that can make you sick. These things are easy to say but hard to do. The fact that HIV makes living a "healthy lifestyle" more important does not make doing it any simpler.

No matter how healthily you live, you still need to protect yourself from OIs by monitoring your immune system and, if your CD4 count is low enough, by using preventative drugs. This isn't called "treatment" in AIDS-speak, it's called "prophylaxis." People may debate the whens and whys of antivirals, but there is good, long-term data on the effectiveness of prophylaxis, and clear information on when to start using it. In a field full of uncertainty, taking medication to prevent *Pneumocystis carinii* pneumonia, a common killer of people with AIDS, is perhaps the clearest, most effective treatment strategy there is. Yet many still die from the pneumonia, most because they tested too late or didn't monitor their CD4 cells. "Even if you're among the 17 percent of men who break through [get PCP in spite of taking the drugs to prevent it], you have a 70 percent chance of survival if you've been taking preventative medications," says Dr. Yancey. "If you haven't been taking them, your chances of making it are only a fifth as good."

ON THE REBOUND? WHAT ABOUT PROPHYLAXIS IF YOUR T CELLS CLIMB?

Many people with HIV whose T cells have been boosted by antiviral therapy ask the obvious question: Can we stop the other pill-popping now? Researchers remain divided about just how much true immune reconstitution is represented by an increase in CD4 cells caused by antiviral drugs, and whether you'll be safe or sorry if you stop the drugs you needed to prevent infections when your CD4 cells were low. Though it depends on the infection in question, federal guidelines recommend stopping prophylaxis after as many as six months of sustained CD4-cell increases. "In some cases, I'd recommend continuing to take prophylaxis for quite a while even if you have no symptoms," says Dr. Grossman, "particularly since the restoration of a very weak immune system may actually activate certain infections." Talk to your doctor before you stop. And for the latest information on federal recommendations, see www.hivatis.org.

Environmental Prophylaxis

Another way to prevent opportunistic infections is to avoid contact with the germs that cause them. Many times this isn't possible. Germs fly through the air, and they rest or grow on everything we touch, eat, and drink. You don't have to get rid of Rover (dogs don't get toxo), nor must you purge your purring precious so long as you don't touch any feline fecal matter (see "Pet Projects," in Chapter 12). Don't touch your baby nephew's fecal matter, either, or your boyfriend's (see "Fecal Foes," page 152). Whether you're going to be someone who turns his cheek to avoid a hello kiss is a style question, but that's not medically necessary unless the person greeting you is sick or has festering sores or something. "You need to find the difference between careful and crazy," says GMHC educator Saundra Johnson, who offers a few examples of things you can live without.

An Ounce of Prevention

Diagnosis and treatment of opportunistic infections can be complicated, particularly since many of their symptoms overlap, and the best drugs to treat them may depend on what drugs you've taken already. If you suspect you have an OI, get to a doctor immediately, and talk to

IMMUNE DADA: A WHIMSICAL LIST OF NO-NOS FOR THE UNDER-200-CD4-CELLS CROWD

- ***A field of pigeons.*** They carry cryptococcal meningitis. If you see them crowding in the piazza, walk on by.
- ***Soft cheeses.*** Fungal infections from soft cheeses grow. They carry *E. coli* and other bacteria, too.
- ***Still waters.*** They may run deep, but they breed encephalitis-carrying mosquitoes.
- ***Raw.*** Meat has toxo, eggs have salmonella, fish has parasites.
- ***The rocks.*** Ice comes from tap water, unless you made the cubes yourself with filtered water.
- ***Mouthful of pool.*** Or shower. If some water gets in your mouth, spit it out and don't panic. But don't open wide for it.

A more detailed discussion of food safety is included in Chapter 6, page 255.

an AIDS organization for the latest information on treatment. You should also read Chapter 10, "Coping with Illness."

The hope, though, is that you won't have to get many OIs, since you'll be taking medication to prevent them. Standards change, so make sure to check with current information sources (see page 400) for advice. As of this writing, the chart on the next page summarizes when to start.

WASTING AWAY AGAIN? BODILY CHANGES WHEN YOU HAVE HIV

I lost seventy pounds in sixty days. I told everyone I was on a diet.

I was eating like a horse, Häagen-Dazs ice cream with chocolate chips and cookies and malts in the morning and evening. But I just kept "wasting," a word I hate.

I got a call at my job at an AIDS organization. It was a foundation that fought world hunger. "We were wondering if you had someone who looked like he was starving to death we could photograph for an ad we're doing," the man said.

No image is more associated with AIDS than extreme weight loss and the frailty it causes. While many OIs cause diarrhea, lack of appetite, and weight loss, there's another syndrome—as yet unexplained—that causes pounds to drop from the outside of your body almost as fast as levels of HIV climb inside it. While some of those on antiviral therapy experience a redistribution of body weight (see box on page 251), those for whom the drugs aren't working, or those not on them, may experience a purer and more frightening loss. If you involuntarily lose more than one-tenth of your body weight, either with or without a fever and diarrhea, you may have wasting syndrome. Fat goes first, but if the wasting continues, you lose lean body mass your

If your CD4 count is	You should look out for	Best way to prevent it (in preferred order)	Common symptoms of active infection	Notes of interest
Over 500	Nothing special to worry about			Occasionally, Kaposi's sarcoma or lymphoma can occur in people with over 500 CD4 cells.
300–500	Candidiasis (oral thrush)	Topical treatment with creams or lozenges (troches) works better than preventive medicine	Creamy white patches in mouth or on tongue, pain or difficulty swallowing	Thrush in your mouth is not an AIDS-defining condition, but can signal a greater risk of PCP (see below).
	Kaposi's sarcoma (KS)	No prophylaxis at this time	Raised purple lesions	
	Non-Hodgkin's lymphoma	No prophylaxis known at this time	Swollen lymph nodes, fevers, weight loss, fatigue; lymphoma in the gut can cause rectal or abdominal pain and vomiting	If you have under 50 CD4 cells, or in other, rarer instances, you may also be at risk for lymphoma in the central nervous system.
	Tuberculosis	Isoniazid and vitamin B_6 for six months, or rifampin with pyrazinamide for two months. Test twice yearly to make sure you haven't been exposed.	Cough, weight loss, night sweats, fatigue, fever, swollen lymph nodes; TB can get in your lungs or elsewhere.	Don't use rifampin with protease inhibitors. Also, rifampin cuts your response to methadone, so you need to up your methadone dose if you're on both.
200–300 or less than 20% All of the above plus	*Pneumocystis carinii* pneumonia (PCP)	TMP/SMX (Bactrim), dapsone, primaquine, aerosolized pentamidine	Fever, dry cough, difficulty breathing, weight loss, night sweats, elevated liver enzymes	Because TMP/SMX is a sulfa drug, allergic reactions are common. One way of overcoming this reaction is to slowly build up your dose of TMP/SMX and desensitize yourself to the drug. This is effective for many people who otherwise find the drug intolerable.
Below 250 or 20% All of the above, plus	Toxoplasmosis (toxo)	Baseline test for antibodies, and if exposed, TMP/SMX or dapsone daily	Swelling of the brain (encephalitis), confusion, delusion, severe headaches, fever, seizure, paralysis on one side of the body. May also cause symptoms in lungs, heart, and eyes	
Below 75 or 5% All of the above, plus	Candidiasis (esophageal thrush)	Fluconazole possible, but not recommended; better to treat it as you get it	Like oral thrush, above, but with creamy white patches in throat, pain, and great difficulty swallowing	
	Cryptococcosis (cryptococcal disease)	None recommended	Meningitis, headache, fevers, fatigue, loss of appetite, confusion	
	Cryptosporidosis	None recommended	Diarrhea, abdominal cramping, nausea, vomiting, fatigue, gas, weight loss, loss of appetite, dehydration and electrolyte imbalances (sodium and potassium)	Avoiding tap water, swimming pools, and rimming (oral-anal sex) is the best prevention.
	Cytomegalovirus (CMV)	Oral ganciclovir possible, but since it's expensive, of variable effectiveness, and may make you unable to use it later for treatment, it's not usually recommended	Retinitis: blurry vision Esophagitis: pain in swallowing, ulcerations Colitis: fever, diarrhea, abdominal pain, wasting	
	Mycobacterium avium complex (MAC)	Clarithromycin, azithromycin, rifabutin; combination of last two may be more effective than either alone	Fever, night sweats, fatigue, diarrhea, weight loss, low platelets (thrombocytopenia), abdominal pain, enlarged lymph glands, enlarged liver, enlarged spleen	Test for TB before you start treatment, since you might need different drugs to treat it if you've been exposed to TB.

PROTEASE PAUNCH?

Gay men may be at a loss on how to stop new AIDS-related complications, but we waste no time in finding the dark humor in them. "Protease paunch" and "buffalo hump" are some of the popular names for an unpopular but undeniable tendency for people on antiviral therapy to develop fatty deposits around their middles and on the backs of their necks. While buffalo hump is rare, lipodystrophy syndrome (as this weight redistribution is sometimes known) may affect as many as 10 to 75 percent of people taking protease inhibitors. Even as your waist expands and fat accumulates around your trunk, your arms and legs are thinning and your face is wrinkling (giving you the dreaded "puppet face"). Some men have resorted to liposuction and plastic surgery to have the excess fat removed from their trunks and restored to their face and limbs, but accumulation of fat around your internal organs, high triglyceride and blood sugar levels, and reports of bone loss, all make this an issue that's more than skin deep. "I had a heart attack at thirty-seven," says Bill, an AIDS worker, and while that's rare, he's not the only one. Reports of diabetes, too, are not uncommon.

A number of men not on protease inhibitors have also developed the syndrome, leading preeminent New York City gastroenterologist Dr. Donald Kotler and others to wonder if it's related to the toxic effects of HIV medications—in particular those known as "NARTIs" (see page 398). One theory highlights the damage these drugs may cause to the mitochondria, sites of production in cells of a key source of energy involved in the breakdown of fat. The short summary offered by Dr. Kotler about the cause of the problem? "We don't yet know," he says simply.

In addition to testosterone (some anecdotal reports say putting a testosterone patch on the hump makes it go down), doctors are experimenting with the same human growth hormone that helps reverse wasting. The treatment has shown promise in reducing both bellies and backs, but it costs $18,000 for a three-month treatment—and often goes without insurance reimbursement for this "unapproved" use of the medication. Watching your cholesterol and blood sugar levels is definitely in order, as is watching the HIV treatment journals—as of this writing, many investigations of the phenomenon are under way.

body needs to metabolize food, propel itself across the room, and do everything else associated with daily life.

There is no prophylaxis for wasting, though a common attempt—stuffing yourself with fatty foods in an effort to protect against weight loss in the future—has not proved effective. "In the old days, we were so worried about people with HIV losing weight that we were telling everyone, 'Eat! Eat! Don't worry about it! Put mayonnaise on everything!'" says Fred Tripp, RD, CDN, of the Department of Nutrition and Food Studies at New York University. "But we weren't defending muscle mass, just body weight." Working out can help maintain lean muscle, though working with a doctor and nutritionist is equally important. Don't wait until you can see changes in the mirror or on the scale to get a lean body mass test (see page 251)—the weight may simply redistribute itself in ways you don't notice, and the more lean body mass you lose, the harder it is to get it back.

Ruling out other causes of weight loss, including the effects of various OIs, is one step in fighting wasting. Trying to improve your nutritional basics—increasing calories, stimulating appetite, and boosting internal processes that help digestion, absorption, and conversion of nutrients to muscle—is also important. Supercaloric nutritional shakes such as Ensure or Sustacal and the drug megestrol (Megace) can help increase your calorie load, though all do more to increase fat than to increase body mass. TPN, a liquid food substitute pumped into your veins, can also boost your weight, though it's much, much more expensive and not necessarily more effective than consuming the calories orally. Prescription drugs such as Marinol (or its organic equivalent, marijuana) can help boost appetite and reduce nausea, while the amino acid glutamine and soluble fiber can help to heal an irritated gut and decrease diarrhea (see "On the Runs," page 256).

Substances that enhance your body's ability to generate muscle are the best treatments there are for wasting. These include:

1. *Testosterone.* Sometimes prescribed to increase weight and muscle mass. Side effects of this steroid—including growth of the prostate, acne on your back, and testicle shrinkage—are just like those of illegal steroids (see "Vial Stuff," page 211). If you do pursue testosterone treatment, many doctors recommend either scrotal patches (applied to a shaved scrotum with a hair dryer) or twice-monthly injections in a doctor's office.

2. *Thalidomide.* Once banned for causing birth defects, it has shown some promise against wasting.

3. *Somatropin (Serostim).* This human growth hormone, a synthetic version of a hormone produced in your pituitary gland, can help build both lean body mass and weight. Unfortunately, it is hideously expensive, costing $200 to $250 a day for the several months minimum that you need it. The company that makes it, Serono Laboratories, Inc., has graciously capped

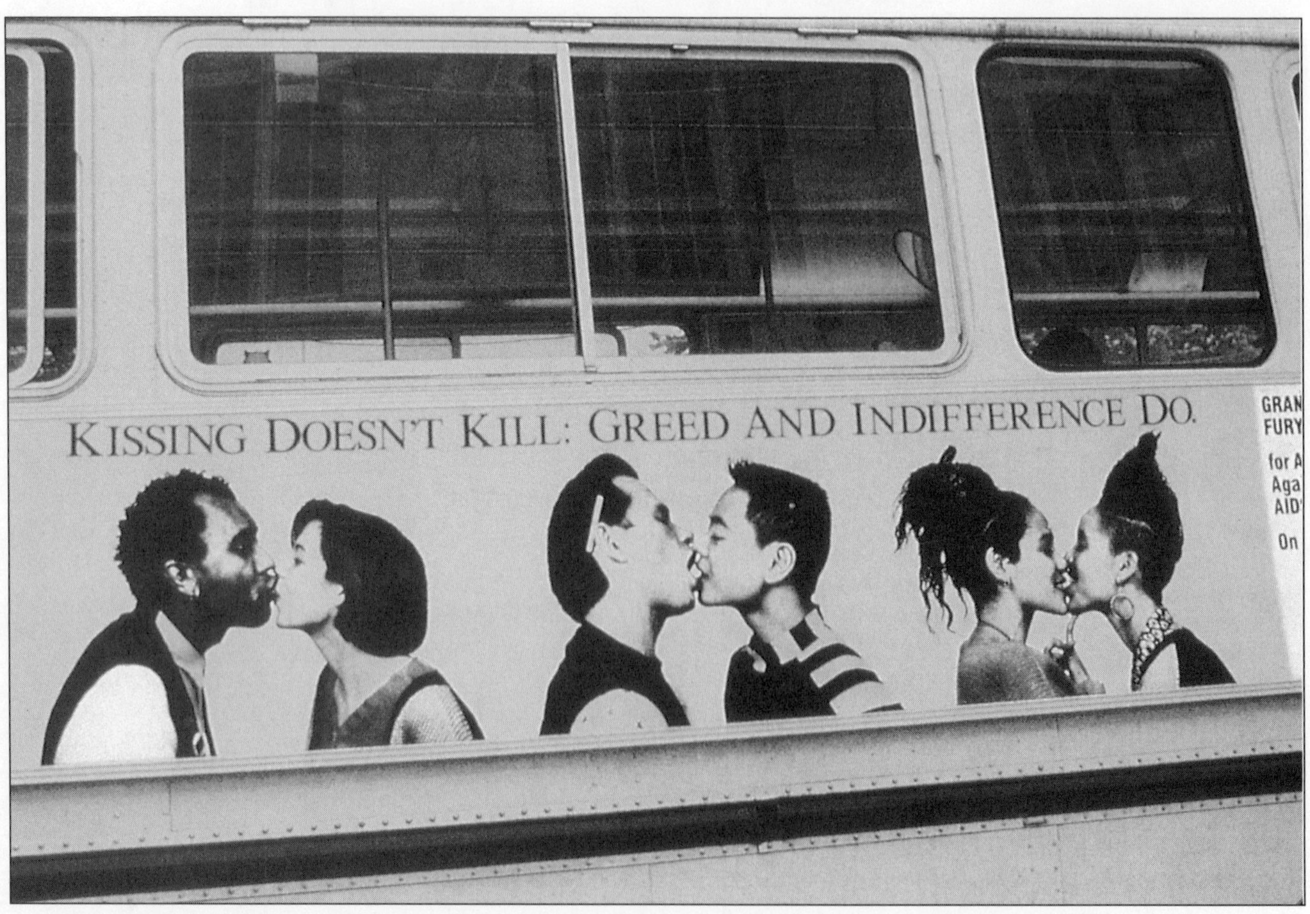

patient expenditures at a mere $36,000 a year, and offers a limited number of patients financial assistance. Medicaid, if you have it, may also cover the drug in your state.

The price tag of human growth hormone reveals another, less tangible form of decline that's been obscured by combination therapies: the wasting of the body politic. ACT UP continues, but at less than a tenth of its former size. Calls for universal health care and an affordable therapeutic vaccine are still heard, however faintly. But with so many people feeling better, and so much riding on the hope of pharmaceutical redemption, corporate actions that would have stuck in people's throats ten years ago, causing a convulsion of outrage, demonstrations, and headlines, are more frequently swallowed as an unpleasant matter of course. It's a symptom, perhaps, of a different syndrome than AIDS, the chronic fatigue that comes from two decades of trying to shout a cure out of the test tube and discovering one was never as close as anybody thought. Still, the decision by Serono Laboratories, Inc. to charge $36,000 a year for human growth hormone would have sent thousands of people with AIDS, and people who cared about them, to the barricades ten years ago. Today, most may find it's easier to rush to their pharmacy with the hope that changing their antiviral therapy will make them, at least, safe from HIV-related harm. That might be human nature. It's probably not human growth.

Here, too, wasting may lead to death. Access to health care, and affordable drugs, remains the biggest challenge facing men with AIDS and other chronic illnesses. New drugs have not closed old gaps: A 1998 survey of the urban poor in San Francisco, for example, found while 90 percent of middle-class people with HIV were on combination therapies, only 30 percent of the urban poor were getting them. Other cities report similarly dismal numbers. Reports from the 1999 Retrovirus Conference revealed that many people—as many as a third of those on combination therapy—may be experiencing rebounds in their HIV levels over the long run. Meanwhile, the promise of a card that gives every citizen the right to health care, or even the right to sue HMOs that mistreat them, grows ever distant, a quaint memory of the bad old days when good people knew that something must be done.

We still have the right to challenge companies who gouge the frailest, to march and fax and phone and fight for better access, and to vote people out of office who value campaign contributions over basic protections to our health. Swallow the pills you need, but work to change the system outside your body, too. Perhaps if those of us who are alive speak out, then the lives of the thousands who've died waiting for benefits or hospital rooms or doctors in overcrowded clinics won't seem so fundamentally, neglectfully, unspeakably wasted.

FURTHER READING

Current information is key when it comes to dealing with HIV, making the Internet and monthly publications some of the best reading (see "Information Nation," page 400). Still, there are a few books useful to the library of any person with HIV:

Bartlett, John G. (1998) *The Johns Hopkins Hospital 1998–1999 Guide to Medical Care of Patients with HIV Infection*. Baltimore: Williams and Wilkins. An exhaustive, clear, and relatively up-to-date reference on medical care for people with HIV.

Clum, Nathan. (1996). *Take Control: Living with HIV and AIDS*. Los Angeles: AIDS Project Los Angeles. California-based, but included a lot of useful practical information on everything from nutrition to benefits to insurance to finding a doctor to disclosing your status.

GMHC (1997). *Treatment Issues Treatment Glossary*. New York: Gay Men's Health Crisis. A guide through the land of medical babble, free to people with HIV. Also on GMHC's Web site, www.gmhc.org.

Kearney, Brian, and Project Inform. (1998) *The HIV Drug Book*. New York: Pocket Books. Everything you always wanted to know about HIV drugs, and quite a few other drugs, too.

Pinsky, Laura, and Paul Harding Douglas with Craig Metroka. (1992) *The Essential HIV Treatment Fact Book*. New York: Pocket Books. Dated in some ways (it's pre-protease), but so full of insight in others that it's a must-read.

CHAPTER 10

Coping with Illness

Dealing with Diagnosis • Emotional and Practical Support • Fiscal and Legal Support • Health Consciousness • Informed Choices • Treatment You Trust • Through the Medical Maze • Hospital-ity? • A Caregiver's Guide to Survival • Getting Better • Getting Worse

Sooner or later, your body will betray you. It can happen suddenly—you go to bed fine, and wake up at five in the morning with what feels like a knife in your heart—or gradually, as when you stop to rest at the third-floor landing and realize that six months ago you could run up five flights without even losing your breath. It may be more a feeling than a fact, a realization that the short-term back pain of today foreshadows a tomorrow of more constant pain, a time when you will cross the imaginary line that divides person and patient.

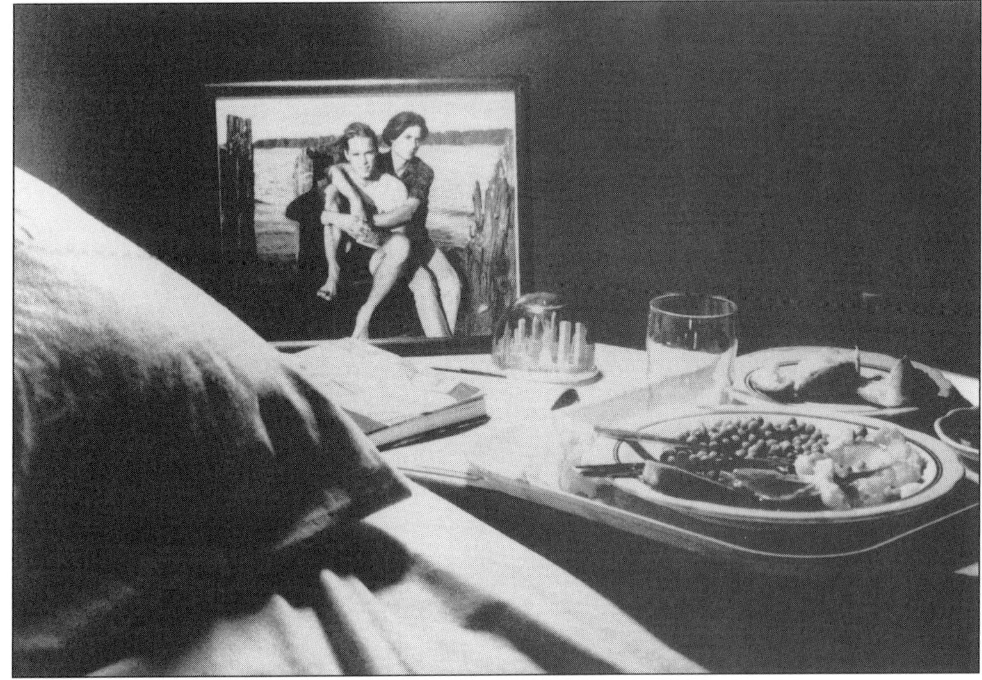

The healthy like to think of illness as something set apart. People coping with serious illnesses, though, find that the border between well and ill is poorly defined, something you cross often. While our health care system is designed to handle acute illness, rather than on-again, off-again struggles, the truth is when you've got your illness, you've still got just about everything: pleasure and pain, minor discomfort and extreme anguish, anxiety and moments of calm. And rather than just happening to people who are somehow broken or defective, says Michael Lipson, Ph.D., a New York City therapist, illness is "like childhood, something we all must go through." How strange, then, says Lipson, that "despite the thousands of us who have grappled with our own mortality, or had the ripples of a parent's or loved one's illness transform the way we see the world, our own sickness so often makes us feel singularly alone, diminished, or wrong."

DEALING WITH DIAGNOSIS

I got on the wrong train to go home, and got off at the wrong stop. I walked in front of oncoming traffic. I suddenly understood all those people who call the AIDS hot lines over and over and say, "I know all the facts, but I just need you to tell me again that I'll be all right."

It was intestinal cancer, heart attack, intestinal cancer again, prostate cancer, cataracts. And each time I was petrified for forty-eight hours and then asked the question: "What can I do to get this out of my body and go on living?" With all the people I've buried—a wife, a son, two partners, another son—I've never said, "I wish it had been me."

I just felt this overwhelming grief, like I was a child. I'd like to say it was more complicated than "Why me?" but that's what it was, the anger and the grief of "How could this have happened to me, who was supposedly so strong?"

My reaction to being told I was going to die was to go into immediate action: radiation, chemotherapy, change in diet. Like I was going to blow this cancer away, wham! I was in a clinical trial within the month. It was about a year later that I realized that even though my time was limited and I was very busy coping, I wasn't doing anything I loved.

Paul, an administrative assistant from Michigan, described his recent diagnosis with congestive heart failure as feeling "like something had exploded all over me." He arrived at the doctor with a gastrointestinal disturbance, he says, and walked out "with a Holter monitor, electrodes all over my chest, and the fear that I had five years to live." Virginia Woolf, in her 1930 essay "On Being Ill," says that illness puts you in an "undiscovered country," a world that has "changed its shape" in ways the healthy can barely comprehend.

How to survey that new landscape, its pitfalls and peculiar pleasures, cannot be charted in a chapter. Bookstore shelves are groaning with strategies for wellness: calls to political action, ways of reckoning with fear, strategies for spiritual development, and tips to deal with grief and feelings of dependence. Ways to deal with illness are as varied as the people who are sick.

For gay men, though, healing is often made harder by the fact that the conventional support systems—insurance companies, hospitals, families, religious congregations, even the Social Security Administration—often do not deem our life partners, or by extension our lives, worthy of recognition. In sickness, as in health, we are often forced to cobble together the supports we need as we go along. For twenty years, pushed largely by AIDS, we've tended each other, forced changes in the idea of the patient-doctor relationship and the drug-approval process, and made history. An estimated half of gay men in urban areas have cared for a friend or loved one with a terminal illness. Depending on the study, anywhere from 2 to 22 percent of us are facing down HIV infection, not to mention all the other illnesses—diabetes, heart disease, cancer—that affect men generally. The government keeps no statistics on the number of gay men who've died in the last twenty years. Our own address books and memorial service experiences tell us the toll has been excruciating.

Losses to AIDS have recently lightened, but the lessons are still with us. AIDS puts a magnifying glass to all the strains of sickness and the ways that society falls short in coping with them. Look through gay men's experience of the epidemic, and you'll learn a lot about illness generally. So if you've just woken up in the hospital, or had the doctor put a scary name to your nagging symptoms, take the deepest breath you can, and then—in the tradition of hundreds of thousands of other men (and the fullest, gayest sense of the term)—carry on. "I recommend the 'Oh, S.H.I.T.!' response to illness," says Paul, a volunteer AIDS hot line counselor who also works for the National Multiple Sclerosis Society. "As in Support, Health consciousness, Information, and Treatment you trust!"

Emotional and Practical Support

Marilyn is my sanity. I didn't tell my family until the operation was over, but Marilyn came at ten to six in the morning, took a car service over just to say, "Hi, love, I'll be here waiting for you when you come back." And she was.

George told me he had cancer, though he didn't say what kind. And I figured, okay, I've been there myself, so I can be there for him. He had some secrets—he's been with his lover for forty years, but people don't know they're gay—so mostly I just listened for what he wasn't able to say. That's what I've learned from all the caretaking: Listen for what isn't being said, and act accordingly.

Rosy, my dog, she was my therapist. Even in the hospital I got my Rosy visits. And my friend Ann, she would come in my hospital room, get my doctor on the phone, and talk about what to do for me.

Each of us has a mental structure, a set of assumptions and fantasies and skills we use to move through the world. Serious illness can strain that structure to the breaking point. "Whatever the chinks, wherever you feel weakest, I think that's where the water pours in," says Howard, forty-five, a New Jersey writer who's nursed more friends than he cares to count. "It's like you return to your baby self, the most exaggerated version of your neuroses." If you tend to feel, on down days, that no one's ever there for you, that's probably what you're going to feel when you need to stay an extra week in the hospital. If you feel as though you don't really deserve to get ahead in life, then sickness will seem a confirmation that you've gotten what you deserved. The strengths of your internal structure, too, the best and most resilient parts of your character, also appear more clearly under strain: hospitality under duress, humor under fire, an ability to persist and pursue. "I know one man, Raoul, who got KS lesions during college," says Marty, eighty, a former advertising man who's had treatment for two different kinds of cancer. "And he went to classes with the chemo pack on his back and the needle in his arm delivering the treatment. He went to classes with a needle in his arm! I got so much strength from talking to him and seeing that. How could I be any less strong when it came time for my own surgery?"

David Fleischer, a political trainer at the National Gay and Lesbian Task Force, suggests potential gay and lesbian candidates give themselves an acid test before they launch an election campaign, asking, "Do you have eight or nine people you can call on for help at ten at night?" Launching an effective campaign against your illness means asking a similar question. Whatever your various reactions to your illness—anger, depression, impatience with people who ask you how you're feeling, and terror that there won't be anyone to ask—lies a common truth: You can't get through it alone. The people you feel comfortable turning to for help may not be the same people you spent the most time with when you were well. "For most people with a serious illness, diagnosis is often followed by a period of social withdrawal and reevaluation," says Helene Kendler, a longtime coordinator of GMHC's buddy program. Cancel the party invitations if you want, but if you're expecting yourself (or your lover and yourself) to be all you need to get by, you probably need to think again. "Illness almost always takes longer and is more complicated than you think," says Kendler. "Even if you feel like you have someone to help you, that person's going to need help, too."

Given how much help gay men have needed in the last two decades, it's a shame how hard it can seem for some of us to ask for it. "For me, part of being gay has always been about *not* needing to turn to my family or anyone else for anything," says Scott, forty-five, from Tahoe, California. "I mean, you look at yourself early on and you find that the 'sickness' people make fun of is actually your sexuality, a part of yourself. You look to your family and find them unwilling to consider the details of your life. And that sets the tone. No matter what's going on, you say, 'I'm fine, I can handle it all myself, really. Don't bother me.'" Ken Pinhero, LCSW, clinical director of the Pacific Center for Human Growth in Berkeley, California, sees that self-reliance as natural compensation for "society's assumption that gay men are weak, predatory, flawed." When sickness or age rupture that image, says Pinhero, "it's common to feel guilty, or ashamed, like we weren't the men we'd told people we were."

The AIDS movement—with its emphasis on treating patients as people rather than victims—has reaffirmed our strength in the face of illness. But as AIDS has opened some discussions, it may have shut others down. Gay men sick with things other than AIDS find themselves strangely reluctant to talk about it, as if the magnitude of HIV has silenced any other suffering. "I made it a point to take my antibiotics at the same time as people taking protease inhibitors," says David, thirty-nine, who suffers from chronic fatigue, memory loss, and central nervous system damage associated with chronic Lyme disease. "I'd cover the pill bottle with my hand so no one could see that it wasn't an AIDS drug, but take my pills with a flourish. And then I realized I was a mess."

The slogan "All people with AIDS are innocent" applies to all people with illness; there's no shame in being sick. If asking for help is a skill you don't have yet, try getting support in a setting where that's expected. Some therapists are trained as medical crisis counselors, offering short-term support for the newly diagnosed, while many therapists have some general training in working with people who are ill. Cheaper, and perhaps even more powerful, is the support that comes from others who are going through the same things you are (see box on next page).

Fiscal and Legal Support

The "undiscovered country" of illness often includes oceans of paperwork and money worries. To keep from being washed away by anxiety, get as clear a sense as you can of your legal and fiscal resources. If you have benefits at work, stop by your human resources department and get another copy of your insurance information. If finances are not your strong suit, ask a

PATIENT POWER It is advice echoed by virtually every patient and provider with experience in healing: Find somebody else who's going through the same things you are. "One of the most effective ways to neutralize medical pessimism is to find someone who had the same problem you do and is now healed," writes holistic physician Andrew Weil, MD, in his best-selling *Spontaneous Healing* (Ballantine, 1996). Stanford University psychiatrist David Spiegel, MD, author of *Living Beyond Limits* (Times Books, 1993), has worked with breast cancer survivors to quantify that healing quality. In a study of eighty-six women with advanced cancer, randomly assigned to standard treatment alone or standard treatment plus weekly support groups, the women in support groups survived, on average, twice as long.

The American Self-help Clearing House, www.mentalhelp.net/selfhelp, keeps lists of statewide and national groups, and most disease-specific organizations such as the American Cancer Society or the National Multiple Sclerosis Society sponsor seminars or ongoing support programs. With the exception of AIDS organizations, though, few offer anything particularly gay. If you want to talk about your condition with other gay men, you may need to put a group together yourself. If you go regularly to a specialty clinic—an oncology center for cancer, for instance, or a renal clinic for kidney disease—you might ask your doctor if he or she has other gay patients who might be interested in forming a group. Hang a flyer on the clinic bulletin board, or contact your HMO's patient services office and request that the health plan publicize something for gay patients.

Benjamin Lipton, MSW, former director of GMHC's clinical services, has Crohn's disease, a chronic illness whose symptoms can include bloody diarrhea, cramping, and intestinal complications. When Lipton went to a sexuality seminar on the illness, though, he didn't hear the word gay mentioned even once. The Crohn's and Colitis Foundation of America let him include a flyer in their next mailing offering support groups for gay men. "The response was overwhelming," says Lipton. "It was the first opportunity we had to talk about ourselves. The work was well worth the reward." If you have Internet access, it may be easier still to find people with whom you can chat, and the freedom of anonymity. "Newsgroups for people with chronic illness are fantastic," says Lipton. "If there isn't one that addresses your problem from a gay perspective, then create one. You can be sure you're not going to be the first or last person looking for the same thing."

financially minded friend to help you review the details and fine print. Does your disability insurance kick in as soon as you stop working in your occupation, or only if you can't do work of any kind? Do you have life insurance that you could sell for money if you needed it (see "Your Money for Your Life," page 426)? Does the health insurance plan you chose when you were well include a lifetime cap on treatment or on medications? If you don't have any benefits to review, consider the options (see "Do You Get It?" page 321) and talk to someone at an AIDS organization or another patient advocacy or senior citizen group.

Straight couples may assume that the social recognition of their marriage can carry them through the hospital visitations, insurance scares, inheritance arguments, and difficult decisions that come with illness or the end of life. Not so gay men, more than one of whom has found himself stonewalled in the hospital waiting room, or watching as the home he thought he shared with his lover goes to homophobic Aunt Phyllis in Skokie. If you're ill, or even thinking that you might someday become ill, a handful of legal documents today can spare you—and your lover and friends—much anguish or pain tomorrow.

Below find six legal documents you need most, and six protections to which you're already entitled. Books such as *The Legal Guide for Lesbian and Gay Couples* (Nolo Press, 1996), *Death and Dignity* (W. W. Norton, 1994), or *Good Doctors, Good Patients* (NCM Publishing,

1994) offer samples of many of these, as do many "home attorney" software programs. If you're expecting conflict, though—you just know there will be catfights over that kidney-shaped coffee table, or your lover and your parents can already barely speak—consulting a flesh-and-blood lawyer is best. You can probably get the whole package for as little as $250, says Robert Bank, director of GMHC's Legal Department. Some gay community centers and AIDS organizations offer free or low-cost legal clinics.

Laws of Desire: Six legal documents you want

That was a horrible thing we did to him with the feeding tubes. It went on for eight months. He was semifetal, nonfunctioning. But we didn't know what he wanted, and once you start with lifesaving measures, you don't know when to stop.

1. A DNR. Also known as a do-not-resuscitate order, this document provides a yes-or-no answer to the question of whether you wish to be resuscitated by artificial means if your heart or lungs fail. If you're going into the hospital, the staff can provide you with one of these, and some insurers keep them on file for you in case you get taken to an emergency room where they don't know your preferences. Some refer to this as an "advance directive," though that term really applies to any of the first three items on this list.

2. Living will. Virtually all states let you create one of these, a document that spells out what you want to happen with your health care if you are in a terminal state or are unable to communicate. The question of whether they keep your heart or lungs going by artificial means (see "DNR," above) is one part of this, but living wills include a greater level of detail about

Laws of the Land: Six supports you already have

When I went to work the next day, they said there'd been a change. I thought they meant the schedule. No, they said, you're not needed in the dining room any longer. They stuck me in back washing pots. When I complained, they fired me completely.

1. The Americans with Disabilities Act (ADA). The bad news is, people in forty states can fire you for being a fag. The good news is, they can't fire you for being a sick fag. If you've been diagnosed with an illness that substantially limits a "major life activity," you're protected against being fired, denied promotion, passed over for a job, or being given a different benefits package because of your illness. Even if your employer *suspects* you have an impairment—such as when you get asked to leave your job at the restaurant because your lover has AIDS—you're protected from discrimination. You can't be denied service in public areas, or in a dentist's or doctor's office. It's all part of the federal law called the Americans with Disabilities Act, and it applies to all businesses with over fifteen employees. Homosexuality or bisexuality, right-wing rhetoric notwithstanding, is not considered a disability, and neither are problems connected to gender-identity disorder or illegal drugs. Asymptomatic HIV infection, HIV disease, and AIDS are all covered under the ADA.

Rather than a pink slip, what you can expect from your employer is "reasonable accommodation" if you request it formally. That doesn't mean your boss is going to spend half the company's annual earnings building a ramp out front for you. It does mean that you can ask for more flexible hours, time for a regular doctor's appointment, or modification of equipment to help you do your job better. Provided you disclose your disability through appropriate channels, rather than while chatting around the water cooler, you can also expect total confidentiality of your medical records, including storage of them separate from the rest of your personnel file.

2. The Family Medical Leave Act (FMLA). If you work somewhere that employs fifty or more workers within a seventy-five-mile radius, and you've worked 1,250 hours or more (25 hours a week, on average) in the past twelve months, the Family Medical Leave Act makes you eligible to take up to twelve weeks of unpaid leave if you get sick. Under the FMLA, you

(continued)

Laws of Desire: Six legal documents you want

(Living will, continued)

various situations. Do you want to be kept alive by a respirator? Do you want to be kept alive if you're so demented from Alzheimer's that you can no longer eat? If you're going to write a living will, be specific. One landmark study found that only 22 of 688 advance medical directives had instructions that were clear enough to guide medical care.

3. A health care agent or proxy (also known in some states as a durable power of attorney for health care) designates someone as a "health care proxy" to make your medical decisions for you in the event you can't. This is more flexible than a living will, since talking through the details of your condition as it progresses can allow your proxy to adapt the spirit of your wishes to the circumstances. Name an alternate, too; you never know.

All states allow either a living will, a health care proxy, or both. An estimated 85 percent of Americans, however, have neither, perhaps because we don't want to consider these painful possibilities. But remember, it won't be easier when you're seriously ill or in physical pain.

4. Power of attorney. This gives someone the right to sign your checks, access your personal information, cash in your investments, and the like. You can make authority broad or limited, and it can start before you're ill, or spring into effect when you become incapacitated. If the power of attorney is "durable," it stays in effect even if you're incapacitated. Some banks insist you have to use their forms for their accounts, though a lawyer can probably fashion an all-purpose document.

Laws of the Land: Six supports you already have

(FMLA, continued)

can also take that leave to care for your parents, your spouse (straight and legal only), or your children. Your employer still pays the same amount for your health insurance premium, and you get your old job or a similar one when you come back. If you're a "key employee," you may not be entitled to that protection.

To qualify for FMLA, you have to show your employer proof that you or your family member has "a serious health condition." Symptomatic HIV illness is one of the many conditions that qualify.

3. Social Security Disability Insurance (SSDI) is what people usually are referring to when they say they're getting "Social Security." It's a monthly payment, and you're eligible if you're disabled by illness or over 65, and if you paid Social Security taxes for at least ten years. The maximum payment is somewhere around $1,300 a month, and how much you get depends on how much you've paid in annually (it's that box that says "FICA" on your pay stub). The definition of disability for SSDI is a lot stricter than that used for the ADA: you need to be "unable to do any kind of work for which you are suited," and your disability has to be expected to last a year or result in your death, whichever comes first. Proving that involves providing a detailed account of every doctor you've seen for your disability, everywhere you've worked in recorded memory, as well as other supporting documentation (see "Paper Tiger," page 425). If your diagnosis has been "clinical" rather than based on a test result, the SSDI people may ask you to see one of their doctors. The application process takes three months minimum, and you won't get a check until six months after the start of your disability. If you have limited income and assets, SSI (below) may help while you wait. If your SSDI payments are small, SSI may also help supplement them.

If you get better, you can also go back to work for a trial period without losing your SSDI benefits (see "Get Back to Work," page 453).

4. SSI. Supplemental Security Income (SSI) is a federal program that offers additional money to disabled or retired people, and it uses the same definition of disability as SSDI above. Unlike with SSDI, you don't have to have paid taxes to get it, though you do have to be a U.S. citizen, have less than $2,000 in assets, and have limited or no income. Proving that means bringing bank statements, auto registration, rent receipts, tax returns, and anything else you can imagine that shows what you're worth. If your situation seems dire enough, the SSI worker can grant you emergency payments the very same day, or very quickly, on the presumption

(continued)

Laws of Desire: Six legal documents you want

5. Joint tenancy. This actually isn't a legal document, it's a concept you want included in such a document. If you own a car or property jointly with someone, make sure your agreement includes the key words "joint tenancy" and "rights of survivorship," to ensure that if either partner dies, the other will gain full use. If you're renting a house or apartment with your lover but have only one name on the lease, his death may also part you from your home; the landlord is under no obligation to put your name on the lease, and depending on where you live, you may have to go to court to win the right to stay.

6. Wills. If you die without a will, the vintage Barbie collection, the fifties-era turquoise appliances, and all the sequined gowns go to your next of kin, which in the eyes of the law include only blood relatives and legally married, heterosexual spouses. Your boyfriend doesn't count; neither do Scott, and Bob, and all the other friends who've supported you for the years you weren't speaking to your family. Since illness often draws together your biological and chosen families, your journey to the hereafter can be made smoother knowing that your mom got the silver and your partner got the rest, or vice versa. You need to draw up a will and appoint an executor, who receives a sum of money for presiding over the whole divvying-up process. Pick someone you think can handle all that responsibility as well as the pain of losing you.

One final note on legal documents: They're only as good as where you keep them. Make sure they're accessible to someone else besides you, and keep copies in multiple places with a note as to the location of the original. Don't put them in a safe deposit box unless someone else also has the key. If you change any of them, even a paragraph, consult a lawyer, since you often have to change the whole thing, throw away all old copies, and replace them with new ones.

Laws of the Land: Six supports you already have

(SSI, continued)

that you're disabled in the way your doctor says you are. An AIDS diagnosis, for example, often entitles you to presumptive payments. Those emergency payments will continue for six months, by which time your SSI application will presumably have been denied or accepted. If you're denied SSI, you still don't have to pay the money back.

In nineteen states you automatically get Medicaid, the health insurance for the poor, when you qualify for SSI. In the rest, you have to apply for coverage. As long as you have few or no assets, Medicaid is available to you whether you have a disabling illness or not (see Chapter 7).

5. Medicare. After two years on SSDI, you automatically become eligible for Medicare, the federal program that insures the disabled and those over 65 (see Chapter 8 for details). This may be good news or bad, since Medicare doesn't cover prescriptions, and group coverage you get from your employer (see the discussion of extended COBRA benefits, below) ends the day you qualify for Medicare. Check with a local AIDS or aging group to find out about what kind of supplementary insurance you might need and how to get it.

6. Extended COBRA benefits. When you leave some jobs, a law called COBRA allows you to get eighteen months of health insurance from your employer's group plan by paying their share of the premiums plus 2 percent in administrative costs. If you leave because you're disabled, you're allowed to extend that benefit to a total of twenty-nine months while you're waiting to qualify for Medicare. COBRA extension isn't automatic—you have to apply for it. When your SSDI is approved, you'll get a letter of confirmation. Send that "Notice of Award" to your employer or whoever is administering your health insurance, and ask for written confirmation that they received it and will grant you the eleven-month extension. They may or may not charge you up to 150 percent of the premium, rather than the 102 percent you have been paying. You have sixty days to do this. If it falls through the cracks, your coverage will, too.

As with all forms of public assistance and support, the rules change often and are significantly more complicated than the paragraphs above can capture. If you have any questions, check with a local patient advocacy group or the federal agency involved (see Appendix A for contact information). If you feel you've been denied benefits unfairly, appeal. If you feel you've been the victim of discrimination at your job, contact a local patient advocacy group or the Equal Employment Opportunities Commission (EEOC).

Paper Tiger: Being a Fierce, Effective Applicant for Government Benefits

If your government benefits office is a zoo, then at least be the tiger. While what you need may depend on how sick you are, there are some general principles that can help you get and keep federal support. *Take Control: Living with HIV and AIDS* (AIDS Project Los Angeles, 1996), an excellent (if California-based) guide for people with HIV, also offers some useful general hints, including the following:

APPLY IN PERSON

If you're well enough to do it, applying in person is usually faster, though you should call for an appointment before you go. If you're sick, ask them when the wait will be shortest. In general, the first Monday and last Friday of the month are crowded and should be avoided.

ASSEMBLE YOUR DOCUMENTS

Putting your documents together can take weeks, so get started. You should have a passport or a copy of your birth certificate certified with a raised seal or stamp (a photocopy is not good enough), a copy of your Social Security card, your driver's license if you have one, copies of your four most recent bank statements and pay stubs, a copy of your lease or rental agreement and receipts, and copies of your income tax returns for two years. If you don't have rent receipts, canceled checks work. If you don't have income tax returns, write down where you worked and what you made for the last two years.

If you don't have what you need, though, don't delay your application, adds Tom McCormack, author of the *AIDS Benefits Handbook* (Yale University Press, 1990). The wheels of government grind exceedingly slowly, and it's best to get things started and fill in the gaps as you go.

GET ORGANIZED

Make and file copies of every letter you send to a government agency, and file all letters you receive. Bring in personal documents such as passports or Social Security cards, rather than mailing them, and if they ask to keep them, get a receipt. Send your mail certified from the post office so you know it got there. Write down the name of everyone with whom you speak, the topic, and the date. All of this is a hassle, but you'll be glad you did it later.

KEEP IN TOUCH WITH YOUR CLAIMS AND SERVICE REPRESENTATIVES

Claims representatives help you before you get accepted for benefits, and service reps help with appealing decisions, changes in benefits, and changes of address. Make sure you know their names and phone numbers, and contact them regularly if things seem delayed.

ANSWER YOUR MAIL

The government usually gives you from ten to sixty days to answer, starting five days after they mail you something. So check often, and respond promptly.

APPEAL

Once again, the squeaky wheel gets the grease, especially if you squeak in the right way. If you're denied SSDI or SSI, you can appeal within sixty days. If the amount of money you get is changed, you can appeal that, too, though the deadline for this appeal may be as short as ten days. Get in touch with a benefits counselor and see if you can file a "waiver," which keeps your benefits from changing until your case is reviewed.

YOUR MONEY FOR YOUR LIFE: VIATICAL SETTLEMENTS AND WHAT THEY CAN DO FOR YOU

If finding somebody today to invest in the idea that you may die tomorrow sounds morbid, it can also be extremely useful. AIDS advocates and others who represent the terminally ill fought in the late 1980s for the right to "viaticate," or sell your life insurance policy to another person or company who gets the value of the policy when you die. In return, you get somewhere around a third to half as much money now, to use for those medical bills you can't pay or the business you want to start in the two years you have left. Do it wrong, though, and you may also wind up with major tax problems, loss of the government benefits you need to get continued care, and disreputable characters who take big commissions, legal fees, and other hidden costs. You have only one life to lose, and the insurance policy that covers it is often one of your biggest assets. Give yourself a reality check before waiting for a check from the investment company (or the little old lady in Omaha) who's bought your life span. Make sure you use a broker or purchaser licensed *in your state* (otherwise you may have to pay taxes out the wazoo and risk your confidentiality), and that you understand the thicket of restrictions and limitations. Don't get pressured into a hasty sale.

National Viator Representatives, (800) 932-0050 or www.nvrnvr.com, helps people find a buyer and wade through the legal confusion that accompanies the sale. They offer a great booklet called "Every Question You Need to Know Before Selling Your Life Insurance Policy." Also, talk to a local tax adviser or insurance expert, since the laws get hazy, particularly if your life expectancy is likely to be longer than two years.

HEALTH CONSCIOUSNESS

When I worked out before, it was mostly to see what was going on with Our Lady of Vapors in the back of the gym. This time I was much more serious, working with a couple of different trainers until I found one I really liked. After a while, I wasn't wasting away. I wasn't disappearing. I was rejuvenated!

If it were just my heart, just a question of the plumbing or the surgery, I'd get it fixed. But why is it so hard to get up in the morning to exercise or to take my medication? I have to ask myself: Do I want really want to live? What am I willing or not willing to do to be here? What's worth changing?

I read an article once by a woman who returned to smoking at something like age sixty-five. She said that even after years without cigarettes she'd felt irritable, like she was miss-

ing something she enjoyed, and that it wasn't her responsibility to put a pair of fresh, pink, unused lungs into the grave. That stuck with me. What makes you healthy may not be what makes you happy.

You don't have to look farther than the lifeless vegetables on your hospital cafeteria tray or the too-bright fluorescent light above the mirror in the bathroom to notice that things like nutrition and stress reduction aren't the strong suit of American medicine. With the Western tendency to treat the symptom rather than the system, staying healthy often means stepping outside the doctor's office and the frame of reference that simply asks whether or not you've taken your medicine today. "Most doctors I saw put habits like drinking or smoking in the 'comfort' category, like maybe you eat a quart of ice cream a day, but who cares," said GMHC board member Tonya Hall, who died of AIDS after a ten-year battle against both HIV and narrow-minded discussions of what it means to be healthy. "I used to think, 'I'm taking my medicine. So what if I wash it down with vodka?' It didn't really hit me till I landed in a hospital bed and a doctor told me, 'AIDS isn't killing you—drinking is.'"

Getting sick doesn't mean that you can never do anything "unhealthy" again. Diabetics may decide to have that cake anyway; some men with heart disease still light up. But if you tend toward declarations like "What does it matter anyhow?" try to stay as conscious of the choices you are actually making as you are of the feeling that illness has removed all sense of choice. "I had to learn that my doctor was a piece of the pie, my heart disease was a piece of the pie, my friends were a piece of the pie, my mood was a piece of the pie, but I needed to look at the whole pie," says thirty-seven-year-old Paul, who's recently gone back to school after receiving what he originally thought was a diagnosis of terminal illness. Often those individual pie pieces aren't easy to separate. Depression, which Paul had, turns out to be common after a number of health problems, from open-heart surgery to an AIDS diagnosis. Changes in diet, which Paul made, change the way your body responds to stress, drugs, and disease. Smoking and drinking can impact the progression of disease as well as their development in the first place. And a sense of connection with others—sexual, sensual, intellectual, and emotional—can all change your experience of illness. "I'd been to orthopedic surgeons who examined my disintegrating ankles and just talked about fusing them without talking about how that would make my knees disintegrate faster," says Harry, fifty-two, who's very clear that he regards his post-polio syndrome as a disability, not an illness. "I'd been to other doctors who blamed *me* for what they couldn't explain, or who thought I was hysterical, a hypochondriac. I finally found a doctor who listened, who got down on his hands and knees—rather than having me contort myself by pulling myself up on the table—so he could examine me. He believed what I told him and earnestly looked for a solution. That, in turn, restored some of my faith in doctors, and boosted my strength."

The words *heal* and *whole,* as Chapter 7 points out, come from the same root. If you've never considered the basics of nutrition, complementary treatments, mind-body techniques, or any of the rest of the practices used by the majority of the world's population, at least get some basic information. Chapters 5 through 7 talk about ways to treat your body right, or get someone to treat it for you. Chapter 11 talks of mental matters. Many reject the distinction. "People talk about learning the difference between your body and your soul, about how illness changes your body but not your essence. I don't see it like that right now," says Paul. "Fighting my illness takes all of me."

Informed Choices

I had months and months of terrible pain for scoliosis, spinal curvature. I tried everything: medications, acupuncture. Then I read an article about a gout medication that sounded promising. The doctor agreed to give me a shot. And the pain was gone. For months. Just like that.

There's a reason they give names to tropical storms. No matter how devastating, how torrential and all-encompassing, naming the turbulence provides people with a limit, a way to anticipate, to understand, and perhaps to master it. So too with illness. The old AIDS activist slogan "Knowledge is power" applies to many serious challenges to your health.

The Internet makes that search for information easier than it used to be. Again, if you don't have access, you may want to go to the library or find a friend who does. If you don't like computers, there are many books and national groups that offer information about virtually every illness. If you like talking instead, try patient advocacy groups, friends, or friends of friends. If you're too sick to do it, get someone else to try. "A week after getting hepatitis, I was paralyzed with Guillain-Barré syndrome, a disorder I'd never even heard of," says Lee, thirty-eight, in New York. "The doctors said it was rare, but within a month my friends had located five people, including a famous author, who'd had it. One friend interviewed someone who'd recovered and brought me the tape to listen to in the intensive care unit. Hearing about other people who'd managed to walk again gave me hope that I could, too."

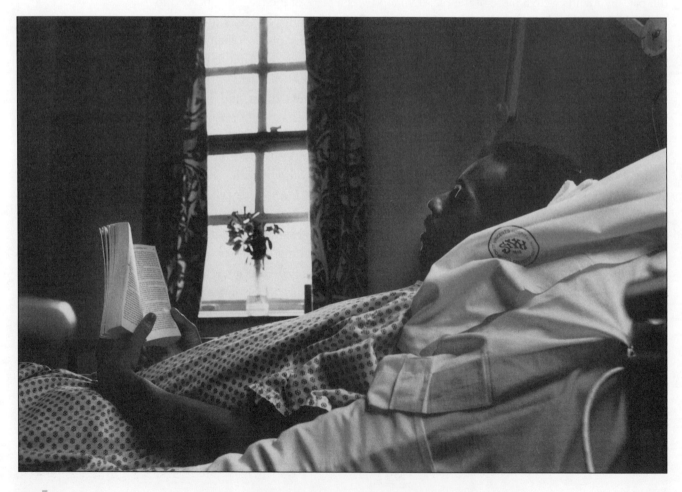

Information Nation

When you're ready, the information's there. Here's a chart that can help.

General health references	Internet sites	Newsletters
Health publishing is a growth market. A few books to look for: *The Physicians' Desk Reference* (Three Rivers Press, yearly) *The* reference guide to pharmacology, including information about side effects, dosage, and administration. Popularly known as the PDR. *The Merck Manual,* by Robert Berkow (Merck Research Labs, 1998) The self-diagnosis bible, it includes basic information about a range of diseases, in language you can understand. Good pictures, too. *The Men's Health and Wellness Guide,* by Charles Inlander and the staff of the People's Medical Society (Macmillan, 1998) This is one of several good guides to men's health, with alphabetic entries. *The Black Men's Guide to Good Health,* by James Reed, MD, Neil Shulman, MD, and Charlene Shucker (Perigee, 1994) Information about topics from high blood pressure and sickle cell disease to AIDS and substance abuse. *The Gay Men's Guide to Wellness,* by Robert E. Penn (Henry Holt, 1997) Like this book, focused on gay-specific health concerns.	*If you include newsgroups and Web sites, the information here is endless. Most of it is also unevaluated by professionals, so read carefully. A sampling of sites:* The Mayo Clinic www.mayo.edu No-nonsense advice from a leading medical clinic. Medline Plus www.nlm.nih.gov/medlineplus/ Medical articles from peer-reviewed publications, dictionaries, links, and more. Medscape www.medscape.com Internet browser Netscape's health site, with a particularly good AIDS section. *Men's Health* magazine www.menshealth.com The magazine's site, with dozens of answers for questions on health's light and lively side. Natural Medicine and Alternative Therapies www.amrta.org Lots of information and an extensive list of other related sites. Oncolink www.cancer.med.upenn.edu/ Extensive online database of cancer-related topics. Yahoo www.yahoo.com/health The search engine's general health site, with—not surprisingly—lots of links. End-of-life issues: www.islandnet.com/~deathnet/ Specializing in all aspects of death and dying.	*A host of newsletters take the latest scientific studies and turn them into language you can understand. Among the choices:* *Berkeley Wellness Letter* Subscriptions Department PO Box 420162 Palm Coast, FL 32142-0162 http://magazines.enews.com/magazines/ucbwl *Harvard Health Letter* PO Box 420300 Palm Coast, FL 32142-0300 *Johns Hopkins Wellness Letter* Box 1230, 3400 North Charles Street, Baltimore, MD 21218. www.jhu.edu/~newslett *Mayo Clinic Newsletter* For subscriptions call (800) 333-9038 www.mayo.edu/pub-rst/health/html *Health News* The consumer publication of the *New England Journal of Medicine* (800) 848-9155 *Tufts Health Letter* For subscriptions call (800) 274-7581 or use online subscription form at www.healthletter.tufts.edu

+ For information on HIV treatments, see Chapter 9.

Hope from Hype I: Reading Between the Lines of News Reports and Medical Studies

Online information about health is plentiful, fascinating, and often unreliable. "Studies show" is a line books throw around with abandon. Newspapers, inundated by press releases from PR consultants and patient coalitions that are fronts for drug companies, run stories of miracle treatments on page 1, and retractions on page 17. Remember the people who took laetrile for cancer? The man who got a baboon-marrow transplant for AIDS? Persistence in the pursuit of treatment may well help (see "Treatment You Trust," page 435). Those particular treatments, as it turned out, didn't.

Gathering information is easy, but gauging it is not. Next time you hear about a medical breakthrough, try to break down the story into parts that make it easier to separate hope from hype. As an example, consider the following fictionalized account:

> *Buenos Aires, September 15, 1999*—Researchers announced today that preliminary results from the study of a new cancer drug show that it may be possible to drastically reduce the spread of advanced prostate cancer among some men. The promising news was reported at a meeting convened by the University of the Americas in Argentina. Cancer researchers at the university, led by Dr. Manuel Fulano, said that twenty-one of twenty-five men, more than 75 percent of all those in whom the drug was tested, showed substantial decrease in the size of their prostate tumors over the course of a two-month period with no side effects whatsoever. Those taking the highest doses of the drug reported tumor shrinkage of 84 percent and diminished levels of cancer in surrounding areas. The drug, obecalp, the extract of a mountain plant that has been used for high blood pressure for some time now in the United States, is expected to be approved for marketing for cancer treatment by year's end.

This sounds, and may be, very promising. Now, rereading critically, consider some of the questions that are useful to ask in any report of breaking medical news:

WHO'S REVIEWED THE STUDY?

Unpublished studies, such as those announced at conferences, may or may not have gone through a peer-review process. In the research world, a researcher's work is only as good as his or her peers say it is. Until other researchers closely examine the data, a researcher is free to say whatever he or she wants. Peer review is required before a study can be published in certain medical journals, the most prominent of which include *AIDS, British Medical Journal, Journal of the American Medical Association, Journal of AIDS, The Lancet,* and *New England Journal of Medicine.*

Possible Hype Here: These data on obecalp were announced at a conference.

THE NUMBER OF PEOPLE INVOLVED, AND WHO THEY WERE

Also known as the size and nature of the sample. Numbers vary depending on the trial design, but generally speaking, the more the merrier. Trials with several hundred people, or studies of several thousand, usually tell you much more about a drug than studies with ten. Other things to think about in news reports are whether the patients were "randomized" (selected at random to receive the new drug or a different treatment) or drawn from a specific pool of volunteers who may or may not share your characteristics. A final calculation that's good to make is whether the report tells you how many people started the trial but dropped out at some point. Many reports ignore all the people who left because of side effects, which may mean you're not hearing the whole story.

Possible Hype Here: The sample size of the obecalp trial was only twenty-five people, and the drug was effective in only twenty-one men, with no information yet available about who they were or how many started the treatment.

THE LENGTH OF THE STUDY

Did the study continue long enough to provide the information you need to know? One of the reasons the AIDS drug AZT was wrongly considered effective as a solo treatment for HIV was that the trials stopped too soon for researchers to know its effect on survival.

Possible Hype Here: For treatment of a slowly progressing condition such as prostate cancer, two months may not be long enough to tell the whole story of obecalp.

WAS THE PRODUCT TESTED IN TEST TUBES, ON ANIMALS, OR ON PEOPLE?

Often the press carries reports on test tube breakthroughs, known as in vitro (in glass) experiments. In vivo (in live people) experiments are much more revealing. Gasoline kills hepatitis C in the test tube, but it's no miracle cure. Animal studies fall in between the two on the reliability spectrum.

Possible Hope Here: Obecalp was tested on people.

WHAT IS KNOWN ABOUT THE DRUG?

The Food and Drug Administration requires a drug to go through three phases of testing—for short-term safety, basic efficacy, and long-term safety and efficacy as compared to another drug or a sugar pill. The earlier the phase of testing, the longer it's going to take to see if it has any practical use for you.

Possible Hope Here: The fact that obecalp has been approved for blood pressure suggests that it has gone through these phases, perhaps in a different dose, and that there's likely to be information about it already. Try searching the World Wide Web or other computer databases—such as the National Library of Medicine's Medline database (www.nlm.nih.gov/medlineplus)—for more information about the drug. If you don't have access to these, consider calling a few treatment hot lines and/or patient advocacy groups for information.

SIDE EFFECTS

Only the last phase of drug testing searches for long-term side effects. Even once approved, any new drug carries risk.

Possible Hope Here: True, two months isn't long enough to know much. But the lack of any reported side effects, and the fact that obecalp is already approved for sale, suggests that it probably will not do any harm.

THE ALTERNATIVES

Does a decent drug already exist? Not all studies are designed for patients; some companies are just trying to capture a share of the market.

Possible Hope Here: Medications currently available do not permanently arrest advanced prostate cancer (see Chapter 8). Given the other options, obecalp sounds promising.

SKEPTIC STAPLES: THREE THINGS TO THINK ABOUT IN EVERY MEDICAL OR BEHAVIORAL STUDY

1. ***Is it cause and effect, or just association?*** Many studies note the association, also called correlation, between two things. That doesn't mean that one thing caused the other. "Assuming a causal direction leads you to incorrect conclusions," says Ilan Meyer, Ph.D., a researcher at Columbia University's School of Public Health. "The classic example used in textbooks is that A might cause B, B might cause A, or something else, C, may cause both." In other words, say a study finds, as one has, that gay men who help others are happier themselves. Is it helping others that causes those men to be happy? Or is it their happiness that makes them feel more like helping others? Or is it that they're rich, which causes them both to be happier than most other people and to have more time to help?

2. ***How many are they, really?*** You've read it countless times: "30 percent of the patients had marked improvement" or "in 80 percent of men tested." Look, though, to the numbers as well as the percentage. If only four people had a given disease in 1998, and four more people got it in 1999, the incidence of the disease increased 100 percent in a single year. That doesn't make it an epidemic.

3. ***Once is not enough.*** "Until the results of a study have been done over again somewhere else, take the results with a grain of salt," says Dr. Meyer. "Because of statistical methods, all studies typically accept a 5 percent chance that their results are wrong. When the same results are replicated by different studies, though, especially if using different methodologies, the chance for error shrinks to nearly nothing."

Resist the urge to leap for every new drug on the market. "If it's at all possible, I'd wait six months before trying a newly released drug or combination of drugs, since some side effects not caught by the approval process may take that long to emerge," says longtime *Treatment Issues* editor David Gilden. With thalidomide, the drug that caused birth defects in newborns, that process of discovery took at least nine months. And though the Food and Drug Administration has made the approval process more stringent since then, pressure from AIDS and other health care activists, and from the pharmaceutical industry, has speeded it up so much that some scientists on the FDA's own review board are now wondering if some drugs are approved too fast.

Inside Information: Examining Your Images of Sickness

My mind raced as soon as I got sick. I thought, "I shouldn't have gone on vacation. That's why this happened." Then I thought, "I can't tell my family. They'll just think it's my way of dealing with my depression, or of trying to get attention." I'm one of ten children.

The few people I have told, each time they ask me how I'm doing, I hear the pity in their voice and see myself as something pathetic.

Three years ago, when I was losing my sight, I was picking my dog. If I was going to go blind I was going to have the most beautiful golden retriever. That was my attitude: "If that happens to me, I'll get the most beautiful dog ever invented."

I was hospitalized frequently as a child and teenager for asthma. I was trapped in a respiration tent, and still remember the sound of my parents fighting with the medical staff, or the shock on my friends' faces. That's what I think of now when I think about getting sick.

What are you into? The question, so easily articulated on phone sex lines and in personal ads, is as important when you're thinking about illness. Each of us has "sick fantasies," ideas and feelings attached to the idea of being ill whose power is as intense, and as difficult to sort out, as those of our other fantasies. "You may have several contradictory ideas about your infection at the same time," advises *The Essential HIV Treatment Fact Book* (Pocket Books, 1992) in a brilliant discussion of the subject applicable to all illnesses. What you've seen as a child, reports in the media, the sick people you know, and what you imagine it means to be ill all come into play, note coauthors Laura Pinsky and Paul Douglas, and not all of them are pleasant.

If regular doctor's visits and medications are important to treatment, suggest Pinsky and Douglas, so is examining your fantasies of what it means to be sick. A number of leading authors and doctors, including Yale University surgeon Bernie Siegel, MD, have talked in different ways about bringing those dark fantasies to light, exploring the ways that people "participate" in their own disease process, and working to strengthen a patient's will to live. Among the exercises Dr. Siegel describes in *Love, Medicine, and Miracles* (Harper and Row, 1986) is "mapping the unconscious," asking patients to take crayons or markers and sketch images of themselves, their disease, their treatment, and their white blood cells. He also suggests you put into words a brief conscious history of yourself. What was happening before you got sick? What role does sickness play in your life and social relations? What did sickness change?

Dr. Siegel advises sick people not to feel guilty about their illnesses. The line between recognition of your role and guilt about it, however, can be as fine as any drawn by Dr. Siegel's crayon-wielding patients. Call it the "empowerment" backlash, the idea that since you participate in your illness, you're not thinking properly when you get sicker (see box on next page). In fact, rather than banishing your darkest thoughts, you might do better to explore them. "Think of it as steering into the skid," says Dr. Michael Lipson. "If you're struggling with a scenario where you lose power and are abandoned, go with it. Take it as far as you can. This person isn't going to come see you anymore? Okay, what then? You'll be alone in the hospital? Okay, what then? You're going to die? Okay, what then?" Often, says Lipson, "When you name the limit of your fear, you also reawaken your humor and your will."

Whether gay men are any more likely to succumb to these kinds of dark thoughts or defeat them is an open question. On the one hand, we already have had years of reinforcement for the notion that we are sick. On the other, we're no strangers to radical change, the kind that many healers say is needed if you want to get well. As with coming out, honoring your own priorities rather than the needs of those around you may be particularly important to healing yourself, however long you live. "If you want to figure out how to live well, start with self-healing," suggests Woodstock, New York, counselor Debby Ogg. She reels off a list of thirty-seven possibilities—everything from taking new risks in friendships to journal writing, creative dreaming to involvement with activism—while acknowledging that ambivalence is natural. "If you're among the many who didn't know exactly what they wanted before diagnosis," she says, "then these attempts to connect with yourself are going to be a little like trying on a coat or a hat: Does it fit? Is it comfortable? Does it make you look beautiful?" The desired outcome is a deep sense of comfort, not a cure. "Healing isn't always about beating death," she says. "Some of us make it through a particular illness, and some of us don't, and we're all going to die. It's about helping yourself thrive, really thrive, in the twenty minutes, or twenty weeks, or two hundred years you have left. Do you feel divided against yourself, or do you feel whole?"

Sugar is sweet . . .

The pleasures of placebos

Hypnotize patients, and they can cure their own warts, apparently sending CD4 cells to the trouble spot. Give some asthma patients harmless salt water inhalers and tell them they're filled with allergens, and they'll have life-threatening attacks. Give them the same inhaler and tell them it's a cure for asthma, and the wheezing will go away. Got an erection problem or blood pressure issues? For as many as 25 percent of us, a sugar pill we're told will help does, making our erections harder and our hearts relaxed.

We've come a long way from the time when doctors stocked jars of colored sugar pills with fake Latin names to give to patients. Perhaps too far. *Placebo,* which in Latin means "I shall please," has become a displeasing word to scientists and patients alike who've learned to skim studies for signs that a particular medicine is "no better than a sugar pill."

But what about when a sugar pill works? "A 25 percent increase in function is nothing to sneeze at," observes Don Freeman, MD, a psychiatrist and clinical instructor at the University of California, Los Angeles. Harvard University professor Anne Harrington, Ph.D., editor of *The Placebo Effect* (Harvard University Press, 1997), says that the effect has been shown on everything from tumors to pain relief, and has nothing to do with your personality, your new-age beliefs, or your intelligence. Rather, she says, determining factors include faith in your healer, and your belief in the authority of the system that surrounds you. Even rats experience placebo effects, becoming ill from certain injections long after the illness-causing agents have been removed from the syringes.

All of which makes it particularly important that you have confidence in your doctor's authority. Some doctors (or their stethoscopes, or their white coats) are placebos in their own right, which is why symptoms can abate as you enter the office. And while demand for any and all information you can find is the backbone of patient empowerment, information alone may not be enough. "There's an inherent conflict between two of our most sacred values in health care—honesty at all costs versus a commitment to the authority of healing," says Dr. Harrington. Finding a doctor you can trust, even in terms of what he may *not* tell you, is essential. And if you find yourself demanding exact explanations of the mechanism of action of a prescription, you may want to take a chill pill, if not a sugar one. A little bit of faith may be just what the doctor ordered.

. . . but you don't have to be

The negatives of positive thinking

The stories are endless. The woman whose tumor didn't grow after she got herself together. The man who started meditating and forced his AIDS into remission. As studies of mind-body links, spiritual practice, and self-empowerment have grown, they have begun to meld into a motto of the new millennium: "You have power over your illness." And yet, behind much talk of positive thinking, lurks the oppressive thought that you always have to be positive. "I think the demand for positive thinking can be dangerous," says Debby Ogg, herself a survivor of a "fatal" cancer and a counselor for others facing terminal illness. "I've never known a person who is constantly positive. Anger, fear, despair, or any of those so-called negative emotions are to be expected, felt, and expressed. What's harmful is emotion denied or repressed."

Asking "What's this illness for?" or exploring the connections between what you're experiencing now and what happened in the year or two before you got sick is smart. Punishing yourself for bad thoughts, inattentiveness to spiritual concerns, or unresolved emotional distress is not. "It's crazy to assert that you're at fault or haven't done something properly if you become ill," says New York City therapist Michael Lipson, Ph.D. "If illness and death are a failure, then every life ends in failure. There has to be a better model."

Similarly tricky is discussion of denial, the frequent target of twelve-step programs and self-help gurus. No, denial is not just a river in Egypt, and pretending you have nothing but a little cold when you really have a fever of 104 degrees is not so healthy. Making plans to travel across the world when you can't walk across the room may involve unnecessary, and exhausting, mental acrobatics for you and your caregivers. "It's different," says Dr. Lipson, "when a nurse who's drawing your blood wants you to discuss your death anxiety and you prefer to talk about the weather. That's a kind of avoidance, but it can be perfectly appropriate." Gregg, thirty-two, a video maker with AIDS from Chicago, puts it succinctly. "People ask me, being HIV positive, what keeps me going?" he says. "And I say, way too much coffee and a healthy amount of denial."

Treatment You Trust

You know how I used to score drugs? I would go across town at any hour of the day or night, walk into abandoned buildings, and dare anyone to stop me. That's the same energy I use now to find my treatments.

If I don't trust you, you can't take a splinter out of me.

I needed to replace my diabetes kit, but the doctor didn't call me back and her receptionist didn't know the basics. "Excuse me," I said, "you work for an endocrinologist, and people's lives depend on whether you understand these things." And then I found another doctor.

The staff at the hospital was great with Jeff. I just never saw the doctor. He would come by at five in the morning, wouldn't return my beeps. It got so that I was staking him out, waiting in the hallway outside his office so that I could find out what was happening with Jeff, what we should be thinking or doing.

Back in the 1980s, when AIDS seemed unstoppable, patient power took multiple forms. People traveled to Mexico to get ribavirin, rumored to boost the immune system. People grew Kombucha mushrooms in jars on their living room tables. Activists and doctors joined to mix chemicals and massive amounts of egg lecithin into a home version of the drug AL-721 in their basements. Patients smuggled in the anti–blood clot medication dextran sulfate from Japan, combed over pharmaceutical company study designs looking for the holes, and went to healing circles and macrobiotic cooking school. Most of these efforts didn't result in longer life that anyone could document. Many made people feel better about the life they had left.

Having treatment you trust is a must. No doctor is perfect, and the illness that altered your world so totally may not have changed his or hers as dramatically. But while researchers continue to look for the genetic links that show definitively why some people are long-term survivors of AIDS or cancer, some studies have already found that having a relationship with a doctor you can trust—and challenge—is one of the most important factors of survival. Other, less psychological considerations also apply. Research published in the *British Medical Journal* on rates of survival in 650 patients with colorectal cancer, for example, found that the skill of your surgeon is less a matter of degree and more a matter of life and death, causing survival rates to vary by as much as 30 percent. Long-term postoperative complications varied, too, from 0 percent for the best surgeons to 35 percent for the less skilled.

Choice is an increasingly scarce commodity in today's HMO-driven environment. If your insurer says you have none, or if your doctor says there's nothing else to try, consider complementary therapies (and perhaps a new doctor). Before the nausea makes you give up on chemotherapy, might dietary changes help in your situation? Acupuncture? Perhaps some of these approaches can keep you in treatment longer or make it more effective. "My philosophy is a variation on what the doctor's is supposed to be: Do no harm, and try everything," says Jim, fifty-eight, who says he's switched doctors and treatments four times in his battle with cancer.

Hope from Hype II: Making Sense of New or Alternative Treatments

He came back from the clinic $2,500 poorer and convinced that the ozone treatment was going to save him where drugs hadn't. For the first few months, he did seem better, but he kept going, and paying, even after his condition worsened. When he asked for written material to compare his progress to others', they said they didn't have any, but they did convince him that a prominent fashion designer was having the same treatment and had already bounced back. When I went to ask, they wouldn't allow me inside. He finally got so weak and confused that his parents had to send him to the clinic with his name and address pinned to his chest in case he got lost.

I ask four words before trying a new medicine: "Show me the data." I know you ain't gonna show me no money, so show me the data.

Some patients looking for new options search out clinical trials, carefully controlled experiments that test new treatments before they're publicly available (see "Drug Dealings: Access to Medications," page 404). Others look to older methods, alternative medical techniques articulated over centuries (see "Alternative and Complementary Medicine," in Chapter 7). Still others turn to treatments that are neither as controlled nor carefully developed: products marketed by healers, Western doctors, or others who swear they have found new ways to help. Some of these may work and some are scams, created by hucksters who recognize that serious illness is also serious business, with people paying just about anything in the hope that they'll keep on living.

If you're trying a treatment that's new but not in trials, the basic rules for finding health care go double: Try to talk to others who've done it, pay a preliminary visit to the provider, and make sure you tell your other doctors or healers what's up. If you need to go to a clinic, especially if you have to pay a lot or travel a long way, look for independent information about the facility before you commit. Watch out for the following warning signs that a treatment is more hype than hope:

THEY CLAIM THE TREATMENT CURES MANY DIFFERENT CONDITIONS

Be skeptical of claims that something is a panacea that has miraculous, cure-all effects. "The only thing that's miraculous," says David Gilden, long-time editor GMHC's *Treatment Issues*, "is usually the misrepresentation."

PROHIBITIVE PRICES

"Sky-high charges for a therapy that isn't going to be covered by insurance may be a warning," says Kevin Armington, MD, in Stony Brook, New York. Fly-by-night doctors want to make sure they're being well rewarded for their work before they have to take the money and run.

YOU ASK FOR LITERATURE, THEY GIVE YOU PEOPLE

If a practitioner can't refer you to anything whatsoever in writing, it's possible you've found the cutting edge. More likely you're being fleeced and he's getting a cut. "People who've been helped are fine," says Howard Grossman, MD, "but there should also be some printed information or, better yet, studies by an objective outside source." George Carter of the New York

City not-for-profit buyer's club Direct AIDS Alternative Information Resource (DAAIR) agrees. "Huge numbers of alternative therapies have had preliminary research done on them, and many other approaches have been discussed by buyer's clubs, newsletters, or other reputable sources of information," he says. "Since community organizations also have their biases, it's best to look at more than one source."

NO RIGHT TO TAKE THE PRODUCT OR INFORMATION ABOUT IT OUT OF THE OFFICE

Magic potions seem less magic in the cruel light of day, and when your friends or other doctors are looking it over. Also, if they won't tell you what you're taking—hiding behind the need to "keep it a secret until they get approval," or out of "fear of the FDA"—tell them you'll pass.

NO ALLOWANCE FOR OTHER TREATMENTS OR SUPPORTS

Be especially careful if the treatment provider is hostile to other doctors, your friends, or your family, or if you're asked to stop other treatments for your condition. Some people with AIDS, for example, have stopped PCP-prevention medications to pursue alternative approaches against the virus, and then gotten the preventable, but potentially deadly, pneumonia.

TAKE AN ORGANIZED APPROACH

"Try too many things at once, and you won't know if something's working or not," says Dr. Armington. Try to keep a log or record of how your feelings and physical symptoms change throughout the treatment.

Through the Medical Maze: Understanding Common Tests and Procedures

I'd lie in bed and listen to them talking about my CHF and ABG and multi-infarct this and CBC that and I'd think, "Where am I?"

If language marks the borders of shared experience, then getting sick is definitely foreign territory. It's not just your weak system that makes the vocabulary flying over your hospital bed sound like Greek to you—some of it *is* Greek or Latin, often abbreviated to make the classically precise terms faster to record. Skeptics may see it as a classic example of how a highly technical field such as medicine protects the authority of those who practice it by developing a jargon you can't follow. "It used to feel like when my parents would speak Spanish so that the kids wouldn't understand," says Jorge, forty-nine, whose repeated hospital stays have left him able to pick up a chart and read it with the speed of an ER technician.

In most large hospitals, your chart is no longer even at the foot of your bed, but rather at the nursing station. Soon "charts" will all be on computer, unreadable without the right kind of software. It's a symbolic as well as a physical transfer, showing how information flow is moving farther away from the patient even as information technology advances. Given those conditions, asking your health care team to act as translators is sensible. If you want a Berlitz-style guide to the medical babble, or if you manage to struggle to the desk to see your chart for yourself, here are a few abbreviations, prefixes, and suffixes that might prove helpful.

Say what? Making sense of your chart

What?	Where?	When?	Why?	Etc.
A.M.A. = against medical advice	Dexter = the right	a = before	ASHD = arteriosclerotic heart disease	c̄ = with
BMR = basal metabolic rate	ER = emergency room	aa = of each	CAD = coronary artery disease	s̄ = without
BP = blood pressure	GB = gallbladder	a.c. = before meals	CHD = coronary heart disease; or congenital heart disease	↑ = increase
BRP = bathroom privileges	GI = gastrointestinal	Ad. = to, up to	CHF = congestive heart failure	↓ = decrease
Bx = biopsy	GU = genitourinary	ADL = activities of daily living	COPD = chronic obstructive pulmonary disease	→ = leads to
CA = cancer	HOB = head of bed	ad lib = as needed, as desired	CVA = cerebrovascular accident	♂ = male
CBC = complete blood count	L = left	b.i.d. = twice a day	DM = diabetes mellitus	
CC = chief complaint	LLE = left lower extremity	dd in d = from day to day	febrile = fever	
Chol = cholesterol	LLQ = left lower quadrant	dur dolor = while pain lasts	Fx = fracture	
CNS = central nervous system	LUE = left upper extremity	emp = as directed	GL = glaucoma	
CSF = cerebrospinal fluid	LUQ = left upper quadrant	grad = by degrees	Hb or Hgb = hemoglobin	
CV = cardiovascular	O.D. = right eye	h.s. = at bedtime, before retiring	HHD = hypertensive heart disease	
CVP = central venous pressure	O.S. = left eye	ind = daily	IPPB = intermittent positive pressure breathing	
CXR = chest X ray	OOB = out of bed	m et n = morning and night	MI = myocardial infarction (heart attack)	
ECG or EKG = electrocardiogram	OPD = outpatient department	mor. dict. = in the manner directed	RHD = rheumatic heart disease	
EEG = electroencephalogram	OR = operating room	non rep; nr = do not repeat	SOB = shortness of breath	
FBS = fasting blood sugar	OU = both eyes	p.c. = after meals	*Useful prefixes and suffixes:*	
FH = family history	R = right	post-op = after the operation	-algia= pain	
GC = gonorrhea	RLQ = right lower quadrant	p.r.n. = as needed, as often as necessary	dys-= something wrong	
GTT = glucose tolerance test	RR = recovery room (or respiratory rate)	PTA = prior to admission	-emia= blood condition	
HCT = hematocrit	RUQ = right upper quadrant	q. = every	hyper-= high or elevated	
I&D = incision and drainage	SICU = surgical intensive care unit	q.h. = every hour (q.4h. is every four hours, q.8h. is every eight hours, etc.)	hypo-= low or insufficient	
I&O = intake and output (measure fluids going into and out of body)	sub Q = subcutaneous	q.i.d. = four times a day	-itis= inflammation	
LP = lumbar puncture		q.n.s. = quantity not sufficient	-megaly= enlargement	
ⓜ = murmur		q.o.d. = every other day	-oma= tumor	
PT = physical therapy		rep = repeat	-osis= abnormal increase or general disease	
RBC = red blood count		SOS = can repeat in emergency	-pathy= noninflammatory condition or disease	
RT = radiation therapy		stat = right away, immediately	-penia= deficiency	Sources: *Take This Book to the Hospital With You, The Complete Bedside Companion, The Essential HIV Treatment Fact Book.*
Rx = prescription		t.i.d. = three times a day	-plegia= paralysis	
S&S = signs and symptoms			-pnea= breathing	
TPR = temperature, pulse, and respiration			-sclerosis= hardening	
URI = upper respiratory infection				
VS = vital signs				
WBC = white blood cell count				

TESTING, TESTING, ONE, TWO, THREE . . . AND FOUR, AND FIVE, AND SIX . . .

The intern came over and started pushing and prodding him and sticking needles in him again, taking blood for the third time in an hour, asking the same questions someone had asked twice before. And I said to her, "Please—he's been on a gurney in the hall for twenty hours, he hasn't had a thing to eat, and he's scared. If you want to know what would make him feel better, can you please find him some food?" She was taken aback, but she came back with a tray.

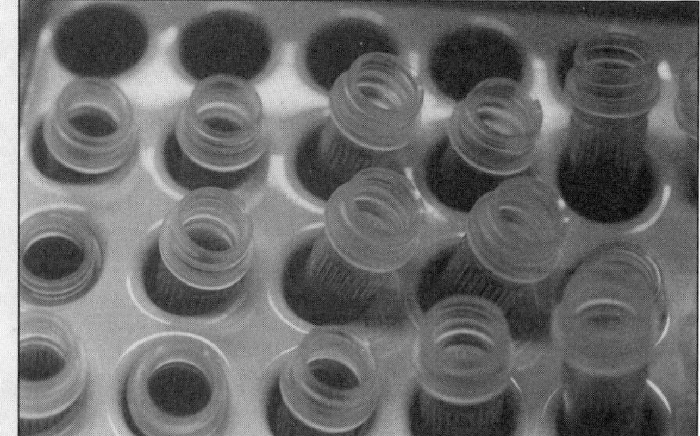

There are a few people who, delighted by the attentions of the doctors, develop Munchausen syndrome: a pattern of imaginary symptoms created to gain a doctor's attention and require ongoing tests and medical intervention. Most of us find the moment that the needle goes in to take blood, bone marrow, or spinal fluid distinctly less soothing. When it's our bodies and selves who are going in—to the MRI machine, or to the lab to give a stool sample—it's equally exhausting, an emblem of the endless self-examination illness seems to demand. For any but the simplest tests, it really helps to take someone with you; if they say it might be "a little painful," it'll probably hurt more. Your anxiety—and the added pain that comes from clenching your muscles or gritting your teeth the whole time—may also be somewhat relieved if you ask what Howard Grossman, MD, calls the five basic pretest questions.

1. What exactly does the procedure involve?
2. How long does it take, and is it painful?
3. What should I expect afterward? Will there be pain? Bleeding? Other side effects?
4. Is it covered by my insurance?
5. When will the results be back and who will give them to me?

Hospital-ity? Gay Stays and How to Make Them Better

This was a small-town hospital. They were horrified at the idea that someone other than a doctor would be actively involved in care. I kept calling doctors I trusted back in Washington and they'd say, "You could try this, you could try that," and the Michigan doctors would say, "No, no, this is our business, it's not your business, it won't help." But after weeks of that, I learned the secret, which was to say, "Well, would it do any harm?" And some of the things we tried began to work.

I'd had a bike accident and was taken to the emergency room with a fractured skull and a concussion. I was semiconscious, in shock, didn't know my name, address, or what day of the week it was. As the physician is stitching my head back up, a clipboard-wielding administrator comes over and starts asking me for detailed insurance information. After several questions I finally managed to slur, "Do you think we could do this another time?"

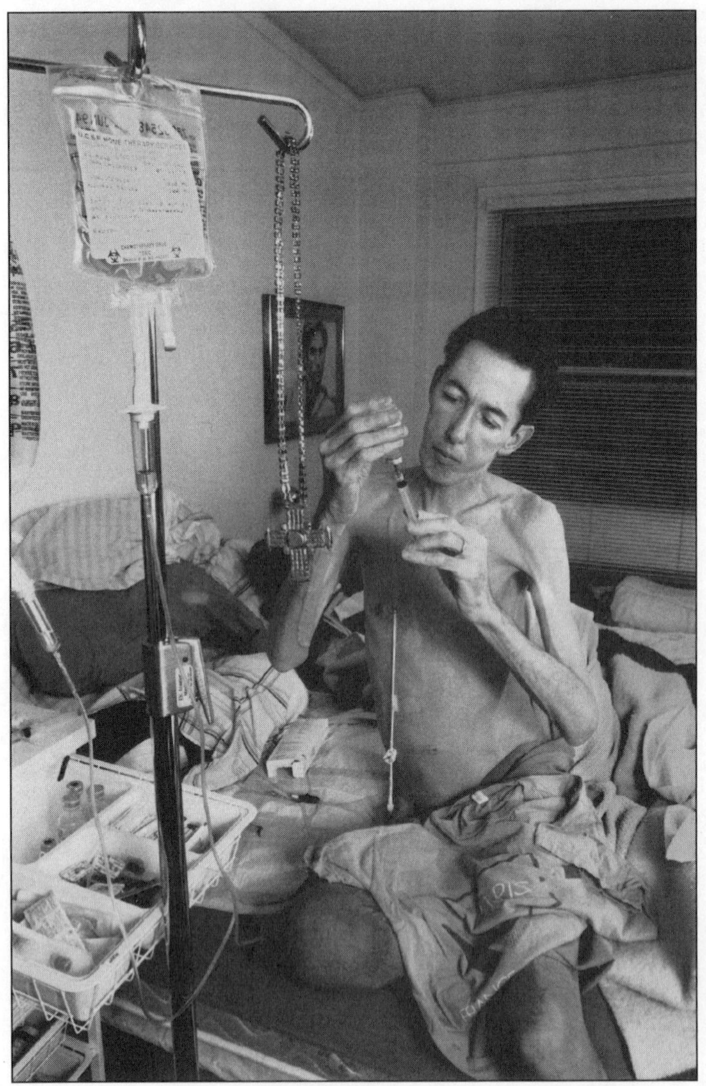

Hospital and *hospitality* come from the same linguistic root, but that's often where the similarity ends. Diagnosed with HIV in 1986, Robert, now thirty-four and a resident of Miami's South Beach, has been hospitalized nine times in four states. "I've dealt with everyone from the old warlord chief surgeon—he expects you to be *quiet*—to some very forward-thinking, cooperative doctors and nurses," he says. And while Robert praises the majority of medical personnel he's encountered as hardworking and well-intended, he's locked horns with more than a few. "I was passing a kidney stone and doing the textbook thing—rocking back and forth in extreme pain, not able to sit still—but the nurse didn't pick up on it," he says. "Instead, she kept telling me to get into bed and calm down. Finally I just screamed at her, 'If you're not going to help me, then just get out.' She fled."

The painful passage through a system that wants to calm and contain you, even when no one's sure exactly what's wrong, is in some ways a metaphor for hospitalization itself. While Robert eventually got rid of his stone and got out of the hospital (another nurse helped him diagnose and deal with his problem), he had to press for the attention he needed. Fighting calmly but persistently for what you need or, better yet, having someone else do that for you is the bottom-line rule for a hospitalization that is, if not hospitable, effective. "To whatever degree possible you need to be an active participant in your own care," says Lowell Levin, Ed.D., MPH, of Yale University. While it's healthiest to get out of there as soon as you are safely able —"Hospitals," deadpans Dr. Levin, "are no place for sick people"—your stay will be much more effective if you learn the rules.

The first question is whether the hospital to which you're going is right for you. Some doctors refer you to places where they can see you easily, or places where they know people, or places they have admitting privileges, rather than places that will suit you best. Some HMOs require that you go to certain hospitals, or give you a choice only if you fight. Make sure you're going someplace that has good care, not just easy access. Determine how experienced the hospital is in treating people with your condition. If you're going to have surgery, how many procedures has the surgeon done? Do they have experience with your condition or a special center used to treating it? Do they have useful information? Ask about the hospital's nosocomial (on-site) infection rates. Check into recovery rates and complications from the procedure you are having. Be calm, but as persistent as a kidney stone. Make sure, in case things get really bad and you can no longer make decisions, that you have legal supports in place to ensure they'll be made by someone you trust (see "Laws of Desire," in the chart on page 422).

Step 1: Getting in the Door

Most hospitalizations are not emergencies, and the best time to think about the admission process is *not* when an orderly slaps a dressing gown in your hand. "Once you've checked your clothing and put on the uniform of a patient, you're a part of a system rather than a person," says Michael A. Donio, director of projects for the People's Medical Society, a national, not-for-profit health care advocacy group based in Allentown, Pennsylvania. Possible time and tension savers include filling out the massive amounts of paperwork before you arrive at the hospital lobby, reading over the informed-consent forms so you know what you're signing, making sure you understand how phone and television service and room assignment work, and double-checking all arrangements by phone the day before your admission. As in dealing with other large bureaucracies (see "Paper Tiger," page 425), always take written notes of what's discussed, including the name and title of the staffer with whom you spoke.

Since all of this may seem too much to handle on top of your medical problem, involve a family member or close friend in the process. In fact, involve a family member or friend even if you *can* handle it all yourself. "From the first day, having an advocate to help you sends the message that you are not a helpless pawn of the system," says Donio, "and smooths the way to make your stay as simple as possible." The People's Medical Society, and many patients, suggest you run through the following checklist:

ARE YOU COVERED?

Are phones and TVs covered by insurance? How about stays beyond a certain point? If you're not insured, ask about admission via a free or low-cost program. If federal funds were used to build the hospital, then the facility is required by federal law to accommodate financially strapped patients, though physician's fees may not be covered.

A ROOM OF ONE'S OWN?

As a rule, insurers pay only a certain amount toward hospital room costs. Thus, if you want privacy, you may have to make up the difference—unless your doctor can justify the coverage. If you're low on outside support, semiprivate rooms may be okay, since a roommate can offer empathy and companionship.

TIME YOUR ARRIVAL

Does the hospital's billing period begin in the morning or in the afternoon? If you come on a Sunday, will anything happen until Monday? It may be cheaper to spend another night in your own bed, and then be admitted the next morning.

PLAN TO PRETEST

Spending a day waiting for tests that could have been done beforehand is exhausting and expensive. EKGs, MRIs, blood work, and other tests can be performed on an outpatient basis—and your doctor or insurance company can ask that it happen that way.

ASK ABOUT VISITORS' QUARTERS

Some hospitals offer visitors facilities for short-term stays, either in "co-op care" arrangements, where people can stay in your room, or at nearby locations. Reserve in advance.

WHERE'S THE BEEF?

Know when meals are served, especially dinner, and what the cutoff time is. If you're on a special diet, arrange for the preparation (and ask about any extra costs) in advance. Find out if nonhospital food is allowed, and if so, where on your floor it can be refrigerated and heated.

NAME A PROXY

Whether it's your lover, a family member, or a close friend, arrange for someone to make decisions and push your cause in case you can't. Check to make sure that legally documenting your proxy will also allow this person to be treated as a "family member" in terms of visitation.

MAKE A MEDICINE LIST

Tally up all your current medications (including any herbal and vitamin therapies) and leave copies with your proxy, with the attending physician (see "Learn the Players," below), and with the nurses' station. Bring the medications with you, too.

Step 2: Decor and More: Upping Your Comfort Level

START WITH PERSONAL EFFECTS

Must-brings should include all toiletries, a few sets of pajamas, and one set of clean clothes to wear on the day you get out. Slippers to wear as you're wheeled around for tests and the like will keep your feet warm. A pen and large-size Post-it notes are good, too, since you can stick notes up without marring that lovely Eisenhower-green wall behind the headboard of your bed. Limit sentimental items to a stuffed animal, a favorite issue of *Martha Stewart Living,* or some other things few are likely to want or you wouldn't miss if they got stolen. You may think you're finally going to read *War and Peace,* but you're not. Try a comic book, books on tape, or magazines instead.

PERSONALIZE YOUR SPACE

Flowers, photographs, and get-well cards add warmth to an otherwise sterile environment. They also send a message to hospital staffers: "People care about this patient, so treat him well." (If you're in the ICU, flowers aren't allowed, but you should be getting good treatment anyway.)

LEAVE THE ROLEX AT HOME

While you're away at chemotherapy or under the knife, rings, watches, cash, and other valuables can easily be misplaced—or stolen. Limit valuables to what's absolutely necessary, and be sure to label them with your name and room number.

BRING AN INEXPENSIVE WALKMAN AND EARPHONES

No matter how much you like your roommate, you probably don't need to hear him having the same conversation over and over with his visitors or phone pals. Your own repetitive conversations will be hard enough to bear. Also, sometimes they let you take music with you when they wheel you around on those long journeys for X rays and tests, which will help keep you from being bored out of your mind.

POST A VIP LIST

Write down important names and phone numbers, including those of key medical personnel, your proxy, family members, friends, an attorney, and the patient advocate, and place it in plain sight—either on the wall or on your nightstand. Have them put the name and number of your main caregiver on the outside of your chart at the nurses' station, too.

Step 3: Learn the Players

His fevers were so high they had to ice him down. The nurse would come in and stay with him and talk very gently, very simple conversations about where she liked to go swimming in the countryside. She would rub lotion on his legs and feet. She was doing her nurse's job, assessing his mental status, his alertness, but she did it in a way that was like a caring visit from someone who really knew what she was doing.

The doctor was such a great guy. He was relaxed. He'd sit down to talk to you, which is unusual. He'd make conversation, he talked about where he grew up. I'll never forget those conversations, because he was a human being. And by being that way, he made you feel like you were one, too, that you mattered.

Remembering that the staff of the hospital are human beings, and human beings with different functions, can make a big difference in your stay. Do you know the difference between an attending physician, a first-year resident, and a medical student? If not, bone up a little before you bed down. "Most patients enter a hospital not having a clue about its personnel or how they interact," says Paul Crockett, a Miami attorney and AIDS activist. "On top of the patient's health crisis comes an operational challenge: coping with the tangled web of doctors, RNs, nurse practitioners, LPNs, technicians, assistants, and cleaning people." Demanding a new IV bag from the orderly or begging the doctor for another pillow or blanket is a waste of the energy that is one of your most valuable resources.

Many books, including the People's Medical Society's *Take This Book to the Hospital with You* (People's Medical Society, 1997) and Rodger McFarlane's *The Complete Bedside Companion* (Simon and Schuster, 1998), offer an excellent who's who of the hospital and suggestions on how to deal with them. Here's a basic rundown:

ATTENDING PHYSICIAN

Every patient has an attending physician, a single doctor responsible for supervising all your care. This is usually, though not always, your doctor if you have one. The attending, or one of the two of them in a group practice, usually pays you a daily visit, and has overall responsibility for your case, including diagnosis, medications, treatments, referring specialists, and length of stay. Whatever changes in treatment are made, he or she will need to sign off, which is why you should if at all possible have someone you know and trust.

PHYSICIAN'S ASSISTANT (PA)

Doctors review and sign off on their orders, but PAs are often the ones ordering tests and medications. They're also around a lot more than doctors, and so are an excellent source of information on what's happening to you.

NURSE PRACTITIONERS (NPS)

Like physician's assistants, these nurses are trained and licensed to write prescriptions, order tests, and make complicated medical assessments under a doctor's supervision.

SOCIAL WORKERS

A vital and underpublicized resource, the hospital social worker may help you—and the caregiver you're driving crazy—get a little psychological perspective. More important, he or she also knows a lot about benefits and discharge planning. Make an appointment to say hello as soon as you get to the hospital, so you can build a relationship.

THE CHARGE NURSE

Each shift has one. The charge nurse, like nurses in general, is often around when doctors are not, knows the answers to many of your questions, and can do vital things such as see to it that you get your sleep medication or readjust the tube that's causing you pain.

REGISTERED NURSES (RNS)

Academically and clinically trained, they perform most of the hospital's basic medical treatments and procedures, including starting IVs or administering complicated medications. Nurses are overworked and under fire—they're being replaced by workers with fewer qualifications—so asking them several questions at once can save time and make a good impression.

LICENSED PRACTICAL NURSES (LPNS)

Less trained than RNs, but also trained in administering medications and injections.

NURSING DIRECTOR OR NURSE MANAGER

Responsible for overseeing the entire nursing staff, and someone *you* probably will see only if you're complaining your way up the organizational chart.

NURSES' AIDES

Those who bring the food, change the sheets, move the patient in the bed, and carry out other essential and undervalued tasks. They'll handle you more than anyone else, so be nice.

PATIENT ADVOCATES

Also known as "ombudspersons," they mediate disputes between patients and families and the hospital's staff. Definitely a good person to ask for if you have an unresolvable conflict or wish to file a complaint, though social workers and nurses are probably better day-to-day advocates for care.

ETHICS COMMITTEES

These are the people who make overall policy decisions about patient care, and they're the ones you go to when you have a conflict over an end-of-life decision. "They wanted to pull the plug on Patrick, and I knew that wasn't what he wanted," says Lawrence, sixty-eight. "So I went to the committee and said, 'I can't believe a Catholic hospital is thinking of ending this man's life, and with my connections, I'm going to make sure the bishop won't believe it, either.' You could have heard a pin drop in that room."

Step 4: Working the System

"A hospital is a strange institution, yet it's very much an institution," says David Rothman, MD, director of the Center for the Study of Society and Medicine at New York's Columbia College of Physicians and Surgeons. "It has its own schedule and mores, and runs according to those needs. Most of us don't wake up at 5 A.M. or eat dinner at 5 P.M. But in a hospital you do, because eating and sleeping coincide with the staff shifts." Knowing how to work from within the system can help you get out of it faster.

CONSIDER YOUR AUDIENCE

Visitors and patients often talk to staff, particularly anyone who isn't a doctor, as if they're idiots. They're too important for that kind of treatment, and if you treat them unprofessionally, they'll keep you out of the information loop. "Speak to people the same way you would if you were in the workplace with them," suggests Rodger McFarlane, author of *The Complete Bedside Companion*.

BE ASSERTIVE, NOT AGGRESSIVE

Advocating your cause does not mean being confrontational or adversarial. It means clarifying things so you *don't* become agitated and so you can avoid stressful confrontations. There are no stupid questions. There are stupid ways to ask them (see box on next page).

DEAL WITH YOUR ANGER

If you are mad at the person who infected you or the friend who comes and tells you how well he is doing, don't take it out on the staff. Talk with the hospital social worker, or address the anger at its source.

FEED THE NURSES

"They are the doctors' eyes and ears, can get to the bottom of a problem quickly, are always there, and make sure the physicians follow up," says Shed Boren, director of the AIDS program at Miami's Mercy Hospital. Treat them with respect. Be nice. Have your visitors bring them food and flowers, too. Know their names.

AVOID SECONDARY INFECTIONS

Every year two million people get infections in the hospital (known as nosocomial infections) they didn't come in with. Politely asking caregivers if they've washed their hands, awkward as it seems, can drive home the point that you're concerned. Staying well hydrated, avoiding unnecessary shaving cuts, getting enough sleep, and eating good food can all help you stay healthy.

SOCIALIZE

Forging alliances with other patients can provide good companionship, not to mention a wealth of dirt on how the hospital really runs. Who are the friendly nurses? What's the quickest way to expedite insurance claims? How much pain medication is *he* on? Where do *her* visitors go to eat?

CONSUME

"Historically, patients have been exactly that: patient, passive, and acted upon," says the People's Medical Society's Michael Donio. "But no matter how much you try to wrap medical services in the Hippocratic oath or Florence Nightingale rhetoric, they are still services." Approach your hospitalization like any good consumer: Know the product and assume you're entitled to good service. Included in the packet of information you signed, very likely, was the American Hospital Association's Patient's Bill of Rights, twelve points of service you can expect. The AHA document is worth reviewing. So is your treatment. If they want you to go for surgery or another complicated procedure, get a second opinion.

THE ART OF ADVOCACY (FOR PATIENTS AND CAREGIVERS)

We had one time when we took Bob to the hospital and they said his insurance wasn't good enough and I should take him home to die. I was crying. I felt like I was doing something wrong. But I said, "I'm a lawyer, you got federal money, and you have to treat us." It wasn't until I threatened lawsuits and got a patient advocate to call someone who called the president of the hospital that they relented, but the doctors were furious. Whenever they would come into the room after that, they brought a tape recorder, or someone who wouldn't say anything but would just stand there and write in little notebooks. Still, Bob survived.

Monitoring your own care, or having friends monitor it for you, is good medicine. "Don't assume that the medication on your IV pole is right, or that the test they're doing is appropriate," says GMHC's director of health care access, Susan Dooha. "Explain that you're nervous if it makes you feel better about asking for explanations. With less and less nursing staff, more and more people are receiving less and less care made with more and more mistakes." Similarly, if you're in pain or can feel something changing in your situation, let a staff person know, and keep letting them know until there is a resolution. Waiting more than five minutes in shit, piss, blood, or vomit is not okay.

If you do want to press for a change in anything from medication to room arrangements, be firm but not belligerent. "I think every family is sort of allowed to blow up in the ER or intensive care once a week or something—the staff can roll with that—but if that's your modus operandi, you're in trouble," advises Rodger McFarlane. "They won't punish the patient by not giving medicine or anything, but they will avoid the hell out of you, or give guarded answers to your questions."

Instead, explain you are just trying to be proactive and learn about the health care you or your loved one is receiving. Ration your requests—no nurse wants to be called in five times in an hour—and try to ask the right person and allow him or her time to act. If this doesn't produce the desired results, don't let the matter drop. Instead, talk with a supervisor (the head nurse, for example) or the patient advocate.

If the complaint involves health hazards, safety violations, or unprofessional or dangerous employees, there are more formal routes to be taken. Since all hospitals are state-licensed, the first step is to determine the appropriate agency or board to address with your concerns. (The People's Medical Society, at (610) 770-1670, can help you with complaints about doctors, nurses, or medical technicians.) Put your complaint in writing, including specifics, names and contact information for any witnesses, and copies of any documents that support your claim. If you don't hear back within a month, call and check on the status of your complaint. But remember: Consult an attorney now if you think you may later need to take the hospital to court.

JUST A LITTLE BIT LONGER?

After days or weeks tethered to a hospital bed, most people are focused on just one thing: going home. But as with hospital admissions, planning your discharge carefully can spare you lots of worry and expense. As soon as you are physically able, meet with the social worker to map out your posthospital strategy. This should include doctor's visits, prescriptions and other treatments, resolving insurance questions, applying for benefits and disability programs, and assessing nursing needs. "Find out from the doctors what the game plan is—what symptoms might arise, what problems you may encounter, and what to do in each case," says David S. Landay, author of *Be Prepared: The Complete Financial, Legal and Practical Guide for Living with a Life-Challenging Condition* (St. Martin's Press, 1998). "If they tell you that you may get a rash, you won't freak out if you get one. Rush out without thinking these things through, and you may be returning via ambulance to the emergency room. And never leave A.M.A. [against medical advice], without finding out whether that may jeopardize your insurance coverage."

If you feel you're being discharged too soon, protest. Also find out how much (if any) of your extended stay is covered by insurance, how to appeal if it's not, and what the turnaround time is to get reimbursed if you have to lay out cash. Medicaid has an appeals process that may let you stay longer, at least while they're hearing the appeal. Medicare has a medical-necessity clause allowing for adjusted lengths of stay, and should make some payments to the hospital, though not necessarily 100 percent.

A Caregiver's Guide to Survival

When Jon was dying, he put a sign up for visitors. It said: "This is not about you."

I asked my father, who was living in Florida at the time, to come to New York for the operation. We've never had a good relationship, but he was, after all, the physician I grew up listening to. When I came to, my father was there holding my hand and my boyfriend, Bobby, was just arriving. "Bobby," my father said in his doctor voice, "you must leave. Roberto is in a delicate state." The nursing staff agreed, and Bobby looked at him, furious. "I'll get you later," he said, storming out. Later turned out to be the next day. This time my father and uncle Hector were both there, and once again my father tells Bobby he shouldn't be there. Bobby raises his hands together over his head like Linda Blair in The Exorcist *and brings them down on my father's back, bringing him and my IV pole crashing down right into my fresh incision, thank you very much, and then runs out the door. My father gets up and runs into the hall after him, and a loud brawl ensues. The nurses and orderlies were buzzing for days.*

"Visitors in the hospital—family and friends—are like a lifeline, a bridge to home," says Darrell Greene, Ph.D., a New York City therapist. Alternatively, they can be the troubled waters, washing over you and forcing you to entertain them and protect them from your illness, your friends, or reality. If being ill, as Anna Freud suggests, causes us to regress to childlike behavior, the combination of illness and your parents can trigger some very old patterns. "I knew one man, when his family visited, he would be up and cheery and laughing," says Dr. Greene.

Tips for the Visitor	Tips for the Patient
Put the patient first. It takes a lot of energy to socialize when you feel lousy. Sometimes the patient may just want to sit quietly.	Designate a visit coordinator, and be as selective as you want about visitors. "My parents seemed helpless, but my friends made a schedule, just like it was work, so that I never had to be alone."
Time your visits. Check with the person coordinating visitors about what time is best, who else is coming, and what medical procedures are happening that day. Dropping by can be more exhausting than helpful.	Use communications technology. "They rented a pager, and whenever one person left, he passed the pager to the next visitor. That way, people didn't have to call *me* constantly for updates. They also made an e-mail tree, and someone sent out regular bulletins on that."
Pay attention to changes, and be ready to help. Step outside and check in with a nurse if you're concerned about a change. And if they come in, either step out for a minute or get out of the way.	Pay attention to changes. "I felt like I just had to keep entertaining them, talking and talking. But when I vomited over all their legs, I think they got the message."
Run out for errands. If the patient isn't up for company, turn the negative into a positive. Offer to run an errand, pay bills, or help with basic paperwork such as filling out insurance forms.	Sing out, Louise. "It's one of the good things about being sick: I get to ask people to do things. The truth is, I love having my hair washed. And it makes my friend David feel useful."
Don't just tend to the plants. Patients need lots of water (or juice, if you bring some), too. Help them stay hydrated, straighten the bedsheets when you can, fold and neaten.	Clean house from bed. "I just started clapping my hands when it got overwhelming, and saying, 'Okay, take the party outside, I need some quiet.'"
Give as well as take. If they've had many visitors, they're probably tired of talking about their condition. You can get that from the chart at the desk, or another friend. Try bringing some news from outside.	Dream, dream, dream. "I loved it when people came and read to me. I could doze, dream, or listen."

"Then, the moment they left, he would start to cry and say how upset he was about being sick." Nor are patients the only ones whose performances are strained in the hospital. "I've been with families or friends who pretend the patient isn't even in the room," says Greene. "They engage with each other, not the sick person."

Tips for the Serious Caregiver

The chemo was really throwing him for a loop. A nurse would come over right after and stay overnight, because he'd be so physically ill from it. He could never really stand to be sick in front of other people, even me. It was strange at first—this creepy home health care person would show up and he would ask me to leave. It made me feel odd, hurt.

When he realized they weren't going to find a cure in his lifetime, he moved to LA. He turned the tables in a way that was almost unforgivable, because part of the spoken and unspoken compact we entered into at the beginning of our relationship was that I would always be there for him, and he made it clear he wasn't going to be there for me. It was something he needed to do and was empowering for him in a way, to say, "I can do this by myself," but for me it was breaking the rules.

I called him from my friend Wendy's to see if he needed anything before I came. "See if he wants some chicken parmigiana," Wendy said. "Oh, no, really," he demurred. When I got there empty-handed, he was furious. "I thought you said you didn't want it!" I protested. "You've become so White," he said. "You know someone has to say no three times before it counts. And she's rich, too. I bet it was that boneless kind."

I am so lucky because when I grew up on the farm, the old people lived with us. There were foaling horses in the barn, people were having babies, we were caring for old people. It wasn't shrouded in psychology and mythology and religion and all. It was the most natural thing in the world.

The role of the caregiver, like that of the patient, is filled with fantasies, childhood impressions, media images, and conscious and unconscious fears about dependency. Investigating your fantasies about caregiving, complete with its imagined rewards and repulsions, can ease the burdens. The reality of caregiving, even as AIDS deaths slow, is that you probably won't be a stranger to the job: The number of households where one person is caring for another more than tripled—to 27.4 million—in the years from 1988 to 1998 alone. More people now rely on unpaid nonrelatives for care than on hired helpers like nurse's aides or companions. Since friendship and tenderness are two major gay strengths, and terminal illness is still a gay reality, gay men are especially likely to be changing bedpans or bandages.

Caregiving is an act of friendship and love, but it can come with plenty of pain. "It's no accident that the people who take care of you while you're ill are often not the same people whom you were closest to when you were well," says Hal Moskowitz, a longtime buddy at GMHC. "There's a lot of emotional baggage that needs to be unpacked, and if you or he can't handle it—if you're still trying to resolve issues you had with each other ten years ago—it can be too painful for both of you." Even if you've been nursing someone for a long time, the sense of pain at the situation may seem suddenly fresh. Horace, seventy-two, remembers the moment, after years of illness, when his lover, Chris, passed away, not to death, but into the unbreakable grasp of an Alzheimer's-like illness. "I came home from work one day and he was standing around looking afraid," he recalls. "I said, 'What are you doing?' and he didn't answer. My hair stood on end. It was like the invasion of the body snatchers, like a different person was there. And that's the person I took care of, nonstop, with diapers and all the rest, for the three years until he died."

Learning to be a witness to emotional reactions in yourself and in your "patient" is an important part of caretaking. For as many deep conversations as you may have, much will go unsaid. "Frank called me up in New York and said 'This is it, I'm ending it, get out here,'" recalls Howard, forty-four. "I spent $1,500 on a same-day plane ticket, risked my job by leaving abruptly. When I arrived in LA, Frank was there in the hospital room, looking cheerful. He said, 'I changed my mind.' And I thought, 'What am I going to say—"You mean I came all this way and you're not even going to die?"'"

Going all the way as a caregiver, whether that leads your patient to the other side of illness or into a face-to-face confrontation with mortality, takes particular practical skills. The best and most complete guide to them, *The Complete Bedside Companion* (Simon and Schuster, 1998), is an aptly titled bible of no-nonsense advice on caring for the seriously ill. The book is coauthored by former GMHC executive director and longtime caregiver, Rodger McFarlane, who has practiced what he's preached. Among the skills he names as important are the following:

LISTEN

Telling someone, "Don't die," or "You're fine, everything's fine," doesn't leave much room for the sick person to experience things. Often it's also not true. "The caregiver's biggest tool is listening, not making everything all right. Try to be comfortable hearing your patient and letting him know he can depend on you," says McFarlane.

HOLD YOUR ANGER (AND CHOOSE YOUR BATTLES WISELY)

"You will run into religious fanatics, total jerks, homophobes, racists, and sexists on the health care team, in your own family, and amongst your neighbors," says McFarlane. "What I ask myself is, will saying something right on the spot get the patient what he needs, or will it be less upsetting and more efficient to deal with it later? Sometimes you feel like you just *have* to say something immediately. With me, down South, it was the racial remarks, and every now and then a fag remark, that would get to me. But if I'm just asking an oncologist I'll never see again for an opinion on three chemo regimens, he can act like an asshole and prattle on about whatever he wants—and I'll take notes." If you do need to confront someone who's an integral part of the team, do so as calmly as you can.

HOLD *THEIR* ANGER

"Illness and death take place in the context of years of living," says McFarlane. "People have regrets and disappointments. And once you get sick, the balance of power is set against you. You're vulnerable, you've lost a piece of your identity—you've lost control of your bodily functions, for heaven's sake. And you're not free to express that anger to the medical team. You can't just scream at anyone, so caregivers get most of it, including the indirect stuff—needling remarks, passive aggression, indecisiveness. You have to learn two things. One is how to help sick people find appropriate expression for their righteous rage, and to work on those things they can change. The other is to be a safe target, to understand that they're not mad at *you*. If it's overwhelming, get the hell away, take a break. But remember that *they're* usually unable to get away, and how frustrating that is."

GIVE THE PATIENT RESPONSIBILITY

"Leave every piece of responsibility he can possibly handle himself right in his lap until he gives it back to you," advises McFarlane. "Grab the initiative anytime it's required, but certainly don't speak for him or tell him how he ought to feel. That's how we infantilize people. The Social Security check didn't come? Hand him the telephone. Especially if he's depressed."

KEEP THE INFORMATION FLOWING

"Being 'out of the loop' is one of the most frustrating parts of being in bed," says McFarlane. "If you're having a 'family conference' of care partners, include the patient if at all possible, or get back to him immediately with an update. If someone's feeling confused, break that up by explaining the next day's agenda clearly, in writing, and leaving it on the bedside table." If you're leaving someone who's confused or demented with someone (or in some place) that's unfamiliar, write a note explaining what's happening so that he or she can refer to it in an anxious moment. As for yourself, carry the nursing station number, the doctor's office number and pager number, and a short list of who's on what shifts with you at all times.

CARE FOR THE CAREGIVER

An estimated one-third of primary caregivers are sick themselves. Some 40 percent of people caring for the elderly are depressed. This is in part due to the dwindling availability of care for the old and sick, which leaves old or sick people caring for each other, and in part due to the fact that spending all that time in the hospital makes caregivers as vulnerable to infection and mood swings as the patients themselves. If you really want to help your patient, you'll show him or her how important things like getting enough water, rest, whole foods, and opportunities for psychic renewal really are by setting an example.

Care for the caregivers usually involves one of two strategies:

1. ***Take a break.*** A few states fund respite care, which offers temporary relief for caregivers who need a break from their duties. For the rest of us, relief is found by less formal means (see page 365, "Parenting Your Parents," for some tips). Practice asking friends or neighbors. Keep requests specific, like "Are you free to help on Tuesday nights?" rather than making general remarks about how much you could use help. Ask yourself, when there are four visitors coming, if you really need to be present. Mobilize everything at your disposal, spread the work around as much as humanly possible, and when you're off duty, stay off. Turn off the phone. Get someone to take you out for dinner. Meditate. However you like to recharge and reduce stress (see Chapter 11), do so with abandon. It'll help your patient if you help yourself.

2. ***Be completely present.*** Call it Zen and the art of caretaking. "What's most tiring is the split between where you want to be and where you have to be," says Michael Lipson. "When you manage to perform some focused tasks in a relaxed state, it can become enlivening rather than exhausting. If you're cleaning a wound and *just* cleaning the wound, completely attentive to that, you won't wear out." Of course, that's easier said than done. Awareness of the stages of attention—focusing, going off track, "waking up" to the fact that you've gone off, and refocusing—is itself something that requires practice. "Meditative and prayer traditions can be helpful in training yourself in some of the skills needed to turn caregiving into self-care," says Dr. Lipson. "Taking a break is great, but so is finding renewal in the act of caregiving itself And watch out for self-judging or chiding. The trap of thinking that your struggle is a failure is as dangerous for caregivers as is it is for patients."

PUSH FOR SYMPTOM CONTROL

"A very few people want to white-knuckle it through and suffer, but most don't get what they should," says McFarlane. "Preventing depression, sleep disorders, anxiety, diarrhea, nausea, bedsores, cramps, dehydration—that's all part of basic nursing care. All of those things can be effectively managed. Pain management? The only places that approach it systematically are major medical centers, cancer and AIDS centers, and hospices." Have the doctor start pain medication at the maximum dose and work downward, rather than the other way around. Chronic undertreatment of pain has been documented in numerous studies, particularly among patients who are dying or seem otherwise beyond treatment that will make them well. That includes drug users, who are given less pain relief. Whether homosexuals are "beyond treatment" in doctors' estimation hasn't been studied, though a staggering 85 percent of people with AIDS are estimated to receive inadequate treatment for pain.

RECOGNIZE THE LIMITS OF YOUR POWER

"I tell people to remember the mantra 'I am not the first person who has done this, and there has got to be a way to get through it,'" says McFarlane. "One man told me the only way to survive the guilt—because we all think terrible things, sitting there night after night praying in your heart that it will all just end, that it will stop—is to feel like you did everything in your power to protect them from unnecessary suffering and indignity."

GETTING BETTER

As soon as I found out I had HIV, I decided I didn't want to die alone. I immediately set out to find someone to die with, and I gotta tell you, my criteria were very loose. Once I found out I was going to live, the last person I wanted to live with was the person I'd chosen to die with.

"Once you've had your body betray you, you always have an eye out," says Debby Ogg. "It's hard to bring your body back to a pre-mortality state." It may be trickier still to bring back your old mind-set. "I always assumed I'd have two good years," says Dale, thirty-five, one of many men with AIDS experiencing the Lazarus effect new medications offer. "Now, instead of dying, I'm having to think: Does it matter that I never finished college? Do I need to rethink my attitude toward long-term relationships? What's a career ladder, anyway? I wasn't paying attention."

What Dale—and lots of other men—*are* paying is credit card bills, thousands of dollars of debt they thought they'd be dying their way out of. "You know the story of the person who goes out and buys a new Jeep Wrangler a month before they die? That was me," says Jerome, forty-four, from Phoenix, Arizona. "I always said I wanted to go out a million dollars in debt. Whoops." If you were more grasshopper than ant, spending everything you had in pursuit of decent medical care or a few last pleasures, you can take some solace in the fact that it made the most sense at the time. "Maximizing your liquid assets and mobilizing them in favor of retaining your mental and physical health is absolutely sensible when you're facing a terminal illness," says Tom Swift, an investment analyst and financial planner in San Francisco, himself living with HIV.

Swift says that the gay men he's helped back to sound fiscal health, who are admittedly on the better-off end of the spectrum, have an advantage that serves them well in the financial world: They're already well used to risk. In the emotional marketplace, too, your experiences with illness may bring new freedom from convention, and consequent rewards. "Almost dying sharpens your awareness," says Ogg. "That doesn't go away even if your illness does. You still have a sense of what's important, and of the shit you don't want to be bothered with anymore." The challenge is finding new ways of living with living, and new supports for your healthy self like those you had when you were sick. "Illness may have been an opportunity to be cared for in a way you hadn't been before," says Ogg. "The question is, how do you keep that once you get well?" In emotional matters, as in stock portfolios, experts suggest diversity. "Critically ill people get a level of care that can only be matched by a mother-infant situation," says Ogg. "No one adult can give another that kind of sustenance over the long term." Many AIDS organizations have begun to offer counseling and practical advice on coming back to life (see next page).

GET BACK TO WORK

A managing attorney in GMHC's legal department, Marla Hassner has counseled hundreds of chronically ill New Yorkers about going back on payroll. "Often," says Hassner, "the joys of better health come with new anxieties, from wondering what might happen if you relapse to worrying about whether old creditors will resurface and garnish your wages."

THE RÉSUMÉ GAP

"Don't lie on your résumé," says Hassner. "If you do, you can be fired at a later date." Instead, stay calm in your interview, and take heart from the fact that the prospective employer wanted to interview you despite your period of unemployment.

Hassner's clients use a variety of explanations to bridge the gap. "If you've done volunteer work, you may be able to say you've been consulting or doing special projects," she says. "You can say you took a personal leave, or even that you've been on disability but that you're feeling great now and can't wait to get back to work." You're not legally obligated to disclose either that you've been on disability or the nature of your illness, though if you're returning to the same employer, you may have to bring a bill of good health from your doctor.

THE PSYCHOLOGICAL BENEFITS OF WORK

"Many people aren't sure if they're feeling better because their disease is better, or because they don't have the stress of work," says Hassner. There is tremendous satisfaction in doing good work, but that needs to be balanced against other worries, such as how to cope with chronic diarrhea, or what happens if you get sick again.

THE BENEFITS YOU MAY LOSE

Income-based benefits, such as Medicaid and SSI, may be canceled if you earn more than the limit allowed in your state, though a law signed in late 1999 will make it easier to "buy in" to Medicaid (see page 326). If you've been disabled long enough to get SSDI, Medicare, or private disability insurance, there's yet another array of complicated regulations that can change from year to year and policy to policy, though 1999 law will make it easier for disabled people to go back to work without losing benefits. Because regulations are confusing, it's best to check with an advocate before plunging back into the job pool.

If you have a private long-term disability (LTD) insurance plan, these generally cut off some or all of your benefits if you return to work. Read your policy to see if you have a "residual" or "partial disability" provision to allow you to keep some benefits. Even if you don't go back, though, some plans will cut you off if they go to "recertify" you as disabled and discover you're healthy. Pay attention also to how often this recertification happens. If it's frequent, make sure to pay regular visits to your doctor, and have him document all health-related changes.

In some ways, illness and its remission leaves you simultaneously old and newly born. Confronted with a new "phase" of life, the skills you need are similar to those of men who are coming out, or coming into midlife (see "Adjusting for Age," page 336). The image you had of yourself may no longer match your new reality. But remember, after you get past the shock of living, how well your wisdom born of experience will serve you as you compete with others who haven't had your trial by fire.

Getting Worse: Death Do Us Part

My doctor tells me, "This is the new you." But when I look in the mirror and see how thin my face looks, or my ashy skin and caved-in chest, I don't like the "new me." I don't want the "new me." The old me is still inside, struggling to make peace.

I accepted I might go. I made plans, bought my own urn at an antique show. I wanted something really chic—that was my attitude. If you're really sick, death is your friend, not your enemy—that's a philosophy of mine. You can go down slugging, but don't get bitter.

Elisabeth Kübler-Ross, in the sixties, created what may now be the best-known model for death's approach: her five-phase theory of how people cope. But bargaining, acceptance, denial, and all the rest rarely happen in neat phases; rather, like sickness and health, they take place in a constantly shifting jumble of feelings and events. Nor do all of us end our lives surrounded by family and friends singing "Amazing Grace," or someone saying, "You can go now," as we move off into the white light. "Most deathbed scenes aren't pretty," says Rodger McFarlane. "The spiritual stuff is great if it works, but a lot of the Louise Hay tapes have cobwebs on them once someone's shitting themselves."

"Die in the morning, so that you don't have to die in the evening," suggests a Buddhist maxim. Finding a way to grapple with the moment is a personal choice, but it needn't begin only as your last living moment approaches. Whether you're dying at home or in the hospital, you don't get around much anymore once you're on your deathbed. If you can, as the Harvard-psychologist-turned-spiritual-teacher Ram Dass advises, "make friends with death" (see "Sage Advice from Your Elders," page 370), seeking out communities or books or teachers who are interested in that kind of internal exploration. If possible, do that while you're still in a friend-making mode, able to look into the options and your feelings, and able to talk them over. Are there what Catholic theologian Aristide Bruni called "incompletes" in your life: relationships that need to be changed, physical suffering that needs to be eased, spiritual questions that need answering?

Your doctors and loved ones may or may not be a help. Long after hospices have been shown to offer end-of-life patients more comfortable conditions, an estimated 88 percent of American deaths continue to take place in the hospital. Often that's no way to go. "Doctors as a group have been shown to have a strikingly higher level of discomfort with death than most professional groups," says New York City therapist Michael Lipson. "That's why they're doctors. They've chosen a field where everyone's forbidden to die." While issues such as whether pain relief should be a separate department or part of the anesthesiology unit may be discussed in medical school, most doctors' training includes little about empathic listening, ideas of mortality, or how to help people look at transitions. "The technological obsession with the body as a machine to be fixed, and accompanying talk of treatments and patients as 'failing,' probably do little to help," says Lipson, who leads trainings to help doctors to examine these issues. Resistance of this kind is among the reasons why an estimated half or more of doctors ignore do-not-resuscitate orders even when a specially designated nurse reminds them regularly of the existence of such documents.

Family and friends who will survive you may not be any more ready for your death than your doctor is. But what about the people on the other side? If you don't think there are people on the other side, what do you think is there? Really spending time with the idea of what's out there, beyond life, is important for you and for the people around you. Not having a sense of what there is to move on to, of what's next, is one of the things that keeps you hanging around long after you'd rather depart. "If there was no ground to land on," says Lipson, "ripe fruit might never fall."

Perhaps in protest of Western medicine's discomfort with the details of death (or Western religion's discomfort with the details of our lives), many gay men and other Americans have turned to New Age methods, including listening to people channeling spirits from beyond. The practice raises many eyebrows and questions about who speaks for and from the afterlife, and for how much money. But one particular bit of wisdom, relayed by "Emmanuel" and recounted by Ram Dass, stands out as hauntingly beautiful. "Tell them, Death is absolutely safe," he said. "It's like taking off a tight shoe."

FURTHER READING

Hampton, Paul. (1997) *HIV Law: A Survival Guide Through the Legal System for People Living with HIV*. New York: Crown Books. Like many books designed for those with specific illnesses, this one's useful for many a sick person or their caretakers.

Inlander, Charles, and Ed Weiner. (1997) *Take This Book to the Hospital with You*. Allentown, PA: People's Medical Society Books. A book about how to maintain some control in situations where little is normally found. Heavy on skepticism toward the medical establishment, and full of practical advice.

Kübler-Ross, Elisabeth. (1997) *On Death and Dying*. New York: Collier Books. A reprint of the 1969 classic. One of the most famous psychological studies of death, including explication of the now-famous "five stages" of reckoning as well as interviews and conversations.

Landay, David. (1998) *Be Prepared: The Essential Guide for Anyone or Any Family Member Coping with Serious Illness*. New York: St. Martin's Press. Like the title says, a manual for patient (and caregiver) empowerment.

Mace, Nancy L., and Peter V. Rabins. (1991) *The 36-Hour Day: A Family Guide to Caring for Persons with Alzheimer's Disease, Related Dementing Illnesses and Memory Loss in Later Life*. Baltimore: Johns Hopkins University Press. The bible of Alzheimer's care, but full of useful information for anyone taking care of somebody frail in mind or body.

McFarlane, Rodger, and Philip Bashe. (1998) *The Complete Bedside Companion: No-Nonsense Advice on Caring for the Seriously Ill*. New York: Simon and Schuster. Accessible language, clear analysis, and exhaustive detail on everything from making a bed with someone in it to cleaning up feces to using a suction catheter.

Quill, Timothy E. (1994) *Death and Dignity*. New York: W. W. Norton & Co. A doctor and former hospice director examines the ethical, legal, moral, and medical obstacles to comfortable death, and argues for a better model.

Rees, Alan M. (1998) *Consumer Health Information Source Book*. Phoenix: Oryx Press. Check your library for this useful list of support groups and information sources for virtually every illness. It's too expensive to buy, but definitely worth reviewing.

Siegel, Bernie S. (1986) *Love, Medicine, and Miracles*. New York: Harper & Row Publishers. The story of extraordinary patients by an extraordinary surgeon who has helped make thinking about illness as much a study of people as pathogens.

PART 4

BEYOND THE BODY

CHAPTER 11

Of Sound Mind

Changing Their Minds • Gay Bashing • Sanity and Where You Find It • Stressed to the Nines? • Cruising Mr. Sandman • Methods of Meditation • Therapy and You • Managed Care and Mental Health • Finding Dr. Right (Take II) • Depression and Anxiety • Psychotropic Medications • Suicide • Ending Therapy

I took my friend from Ireland to the local gay bar, one of those with tinsel everywhere and a lot of video screens showing Joan Rivers. "My God," he said, looking around. "This place looks like the inside of a hairdresser's mind."

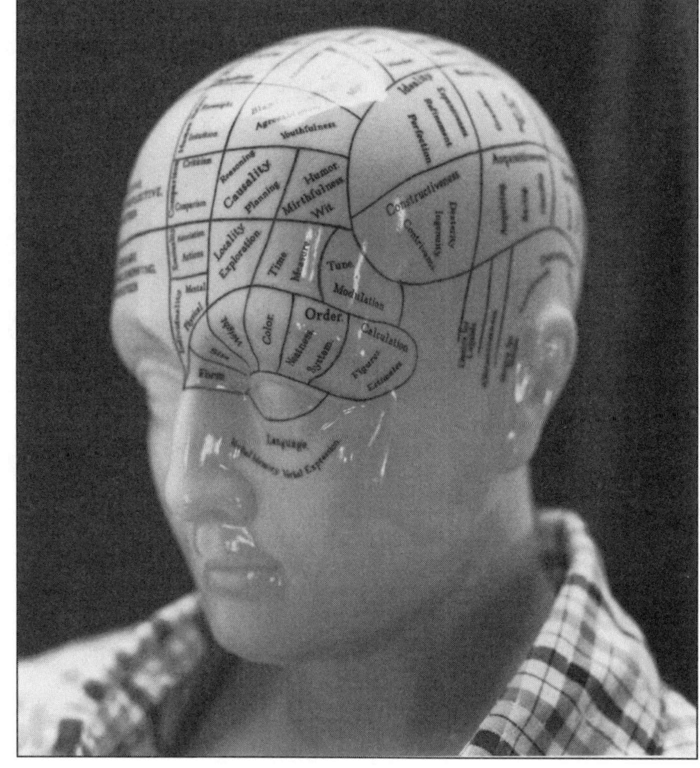

Trying to figure out just what a gay man's mind looks like—and what that might mean about gay behavior—has been a preoccupation of medical and social scientists for more than a century. "It's sick!" was the summary most of us heard from family and friends, though the words weren't theirs. Legal and medical authorities, long asked to look us over, have taken gay men's differences and seen them as symptoms. Men caught having sex with each other have been arrested; men wanting that sex have been judged guilty of arrested development. From the time psychiatrists came up with the word *homosexual* in the late 1800s, experts have labeled us "infantile," "overly attached to our mothers," "inverted," "narcissistic," or even "paranoid" and "homicidal."

The tools used to "fix" these problems have been even cruder than the analysis. In addition to the hormone treatments, prison sentences, and castrations inflicted on our bodies (see Chapter 7), doctors, priests, rabbis, and other counselors have also messed with our minds. Urging us to abstain from sex has been the most enduring treatment, and lobotomy the most disturbing, but history is full of others. "I was put in a mental hospital," recalls Mario, forty-seven, of his Texas childhood, "and given electric shocks until I told them I liked girls." Robert, thirty-seven, from New York, remembers that "the priest at our church said masturbating with other boys would send me to hell, but asked me to come in for special instruction, which included touching me." Joseph, twenty-two, had a more positive experience when his parents hauled him before a therapist in Santa Fe, New Mexico. "The therapist told my parents I was fine," he remembers. "He said the biggest problem was their need to change me."

CHANGING THEIR MINDS

Except for the five hundred or so psychiatrists who still try to set men straight using the destructive and absurdly named "reparative therapy," most in the field have recognized that it is the science that needed to change. Daunted by activists and our enduring love for men in spite of all the obstacles, the American Psychiatric Association decided in 1973 that being gay was not the same as being sick. Even seventy-five years ago, when medical treatment was more merciful than jail ("He's sick, he can't help it" was once a liberal position), gay men suspected that the problems were the doctors' rather than our own. Dr. R. W. Shufeldt, in a 1917 report, described his interview with a "loquacious, foul-mouthed and foul-minded fairy" who was "lost entirely to shame; believing himself designed by nature to play the very part he is playing in life." Historian George Chauncey, citing the incident above in his superb look back through the century, *Gay New York* (Basic Books, 1994), notes many such moments of "gay resistance," where gay men turned to health officials and justified love for other men as natural, ethical, and indisputable.

Most often, support for gay men's mental health has come not from men in white coats but those in dresses, leather jackets, or other outfits like our own (see Chapter 12). "Therapy? That was something White folks did," says Shelby, thirty-two, who says his own early sense of mental health came mostly from the group of Black "almost drag queens" he met at a pancake house in Jacksonville, Florida. "When I moved to New York and heard everyone talking about their psychiatrists, I felt like I needed support to deal with *that*."

While acknowledging that there are "common, clinical symptoms of depression and anxiety disorders," Laura Pinsky, MSW, director of Columbia University's Gay Health Advocacy Project, reminds us that "each of our personalities, our individuality, is the result of particular conflicts and their resolutions." The expectation that you'll be at a certain phase at a certain time, or that there's a single gauge of mental health, she warns, "often hides a conservative bias about what 'normal' really is." Instead of comparing yourself against someone else's standard—such as whether you have a boyfriend, how out you are at work, or how much money you make at your job—ask yourself how you negotiate conflict. Is your life moving? Are you stuck?

Ken Corbett, Ph.D., a psychologist who works extensively with gay men, suggests reframing the focus on mental illness to one on "mental freedom." For Corbett, that means freedom from the unconscious, "not being burdened by a conscience that's so severe or rigid that your sense of pleasure is inhibited." It also means freedom *of* the unconscious—being able to play, or follow your own fantasies or associations, without having outside expectations overwhelm your sense of self. There's a difference, in other words, between looking earnestly for a good gym or a boyfriend and obsessively searching for a workout or diet or partner to help you match some mythical idea of what Corbett calls the "good-enough gay." "All people live with different sets of standards," says Dr. Corbett. "There are the traditional ones: monogamy, social, and religious strictures. Then there's a whole other set of cultural ideals, which for us might

LABEL-CONSCIOUS: WHAT DOCTORS CALL YOU BEHIND YOUR BACK

The guidebook to contemporary psychiatric classification is called the *DSM* or, more formally, the *Diagnostic and Statistical Manual, 4th Edition* (American Psychiatric Press, 1994). This textbook, modified and reissued every few years in an astonishingly ugly array of colors, is the list of pigeonholes into which may be officially crammed every conceivable manifestation of "symptom," "disorder," "mental illness," "condition," or simple freak-out. Each one of these carries a five-digit number, a code you need to have next to your name before you get any insurance reimbursement for psychological treatment.

Gay communities and the *DSM* have had their problems with each other. In 1973, after a series of gay protests and political zaps, the American Psychiatric Association finally opted to remove homosexuality from the *DSM*, in effect deleting homosexuality from the list of mental illnesses. As with many legal amendments, the change on paper has not translated to complete reform in practice. While some psychiatrists accepted the depathologization of homosexuality as a responsible act of scientific reexamination, others saw it as a dishonest capitulation to political pressure. A small but vocal minority of psychiatrists continue to insist that gay is sick, forcing gay and gay-friendly doctors to waste precious time refuting them. The radical right's late-'90s multimillion-dollar ad campaign to publicize homosexuals who'd been "cured" helped rekindle the debate, and the APA moved in December 1998 to oppose any treatment that attempted to change a person's sexual orientation.

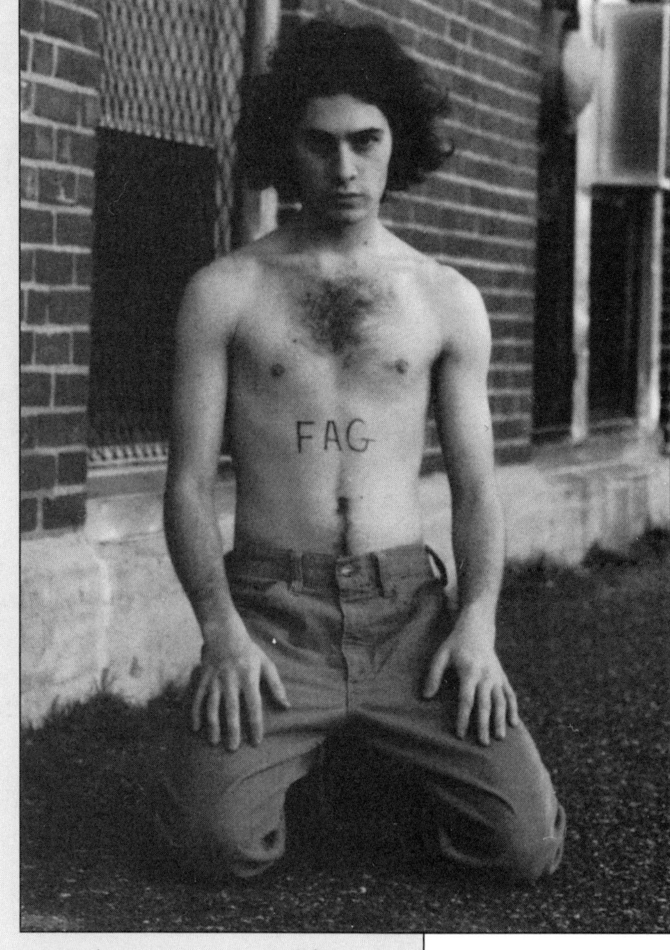

Some still find antigay prejudice between the covers of the *DSM*, however, and in the orientation of many psychiatrists. The new flash point is diagnosis with "gender identity disorder (GID)," a term instinctively understood by the many of us boys who preferred dolls to football, as well as by our tomboy sisters and transgendered individuals of all sexual orientations. Ken Corbett, Ph.D., is among those who see the diagnosis of gender-identity disorder as a kind of Trojan horse of homophobia, wherein girly boys and boyish girls are carted off to shrinks for diagnosis and "repair" based on some ill-examined idea of the "typical" boy or girl.

For transgendered adults, the whole debate over gender identity disorder includes a painful irony. While transgendered people don't want to be labeled "sick," that GID diagnosis is needed for insurance coverage of some of the expensive processes of gender reassignment, including hormone treatments. Insurance companies still balk at paying for genital reassignment surgery, even with a GID diagnosis. Some have suggested that this problem should be addressed by creating a medical—rather than psychiatric—diagnosis for a mind-body mismatch. This could emphasize to doctors, and perhaps to the world at large, that there are instances where it is people's anatomy—instead of their mind—that is in need of correction.

mean intense pressure about body image, about sex, about a range of things. As gay men, we're left to move back and forth. The important thing is not reaching some imaginary problem-free place, but looking at how you move through the contradictions."

Gay Bashing and Straight Hate

My friend and I were leaving the disco on Saturday and six or seven teenage boys stopped us. "Which one of you is the girl?" they asked. Before I knew it, I got slammed in the back with a baseball bat. We ran for three blocks as the kids chased us, throwing bottles and beer cans. It took me days to feel anything, and then I just felt rage and fear. On the one hand, it was "How dare he think he can walk up and slam me in the back just because I'm a gay guy." On the other, I realized if he'd slammed my head, I'd be dead.

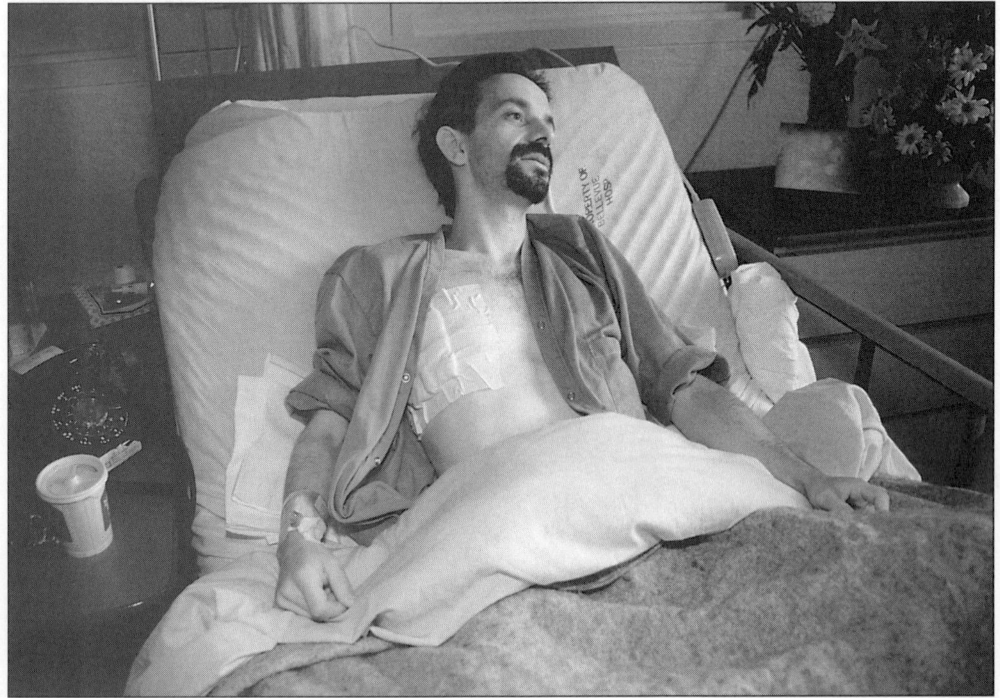

One psychological disorder that is deeply harmful to gay men, and very much in need of diagnosis, is that suffered by straight men who think that gay bashing (or raping women) is an appropriate response to their own anxieties. For too many straight men, "community building" has involved going to gay neighborhoods to beat down gay men and lesbians, often with sticks, baseball bats, or fists. Gay bashing, like gay visibility, is on the rise. While the Department of Justice reported double-digit decreases in violent crime nationally in 1997 and 1998, hate-motivated violence against gay people increased. Violence against gay men and lesbians in New York City rose more than 80 percent in 1998, with men in gay neighborhoods being clubbed, stabbed, beaten, thrown down subway stairs, or gouged with broken bottles as their attackers shouted antigay remarks. In Laramie, Wyoming, university freshman Matthew Shepard was pistol-whipped, burned, deprived of shoes and wallet, lashed to a fence in near-freezing weather, and left to die (he did) by two straight men he met in a bar. Months later, in Alabama, Billy Jack Gaiter was kidnapped by two men, bludgeoned to death, and then thrown on a pile of burning tires. In 1999, gay couple Gary Matson and Winfield Mowder were murdered in their California home; that same week, Pfc. Barry Winchell had his skull bashed in with a baseball bat by a fellow soldier after months of antigay harassment.

The fact that straight men bash lesbians too, often shouting "faggot" at the women or scrawling the word on their cars or windows, shows how much gender confusion lies at the dark heart of straight hate. Are gay men bashed because we raise the question, like those teens who took a baseball bat to the men in the account above, that boys and girls might not be as different as we think? Is it hatred of women, or homosexuality, that fuels the violence? Is there a way, in bashing back against that prejudice, that we can move from threatened victims—"I live in a gay neighborhood because I'm scared someone will hurt me otherwise"—to men who live a better model of community, one that stresses the strength, savvy, and humor of people who have moved beyond the law of the jungle?

The laws of the nation are little help. Less than half the states include gay men or lesbians in hate-crime legislation, the laws that impose penalties for threats, intimidation, name-calling, or physical and sexual assault based on identity. Forty-three states allow individuals to express straight bigotry by refusing to rent property to gay men and lesbians. The Supreme Court in 1998 found male-male sexual harassment to be illegal. In forty states, though, as well as in our nation's civil and military services, it's legal to fire a gay man or lesbian because of what we do in bed. Transgendered men and women—who are fatally stabbed, shot, beaten, and slashed in cities across America, have even less legal protection.

While most of the hate crimes you see on television are usually graffiti and vandalism directed toward property, the vast majority of violence against lesbians, gay men, and transgendered people is directed at our bodies, our flesh and blood. "I was waiting for a cab with some friends outside a gay club in Jacksonville, Florida," says Larry. "Suddenly a truck came wheeling around the corner, and three big White guys jumped out and hit me in the face with a pipe. You know how a split second can happen in slow motion? I remember seeing such a look of hate coming from them." Larry's friends managed to wrestle the weapon away from the attackers, who then got back in the truck and tried to run them down. The policeman who responded to a call for help was indifferent at best. It took two surgeries over seven days to repair the damage to Larry's face.

Like many men who've been gay-bashed, Larry suffered considerable psychological aftereffects from the attack. "I was afraid to go outside for a month," he says, "and didn't want anyone to touch me for three." He will never again go to a club unless he can park right in front. Although he went to his parents' home in Minnesota—where he found a support group for victims of violence—to recuperate, he says he felt obliged to downplay the fact that his attack was gay-related. "It's a pattern that's all too common," says Gary Norman, a hate-crime specialist at the Montrose Counseling Center in Houston, Texas. Common, too, is Larry's experience of indifference, or worse, from law enforcement. In 1997 a staggering 83 percent of antigay bias incidents reported took place within police precinct houses or jails. Shame about discussing such treatment, or reluctance to invite scrutiny of our sexual lives for any reason, can be its own kind of prison. "You can't assume that everyone is out at work. You can't assume their parents know that they're gay," says Norman. "Let's say you have to miss a few days at work, or you come home with bruises or a broken arm because you've been gay-bashed, and you're not out. It's awkward. These are things straight people, even those who've been mugged, often don't think twice about."

Sanity and Where You Find It

Most discussions of mental health are really discussions of illness, with people talking about therapy and treatment and problems instead of speaking about how they stay sane. Psycholog-

WHAT TO DO IF YOU'RE ASSAULTED

GET MEDICAL ATTENTION

Sometimes injuries that don't seem serious at first can get worse later. As soon as possible after the assault, see a doctor or go to a hospital even if you don't think you've been seriously injured, and bring a friend. "Head injuries often get overlooked," says Gary Norman. "Men say, 'I was pushed down and my head hit the concrete, but I'm okay.' There might be a concussion there. If you're punched or kicked, there may be internal bleeding or broken ribs. We tend to minimize our medical needs, especially if we're traumatized. Get yourself checked out, preferably by someone you can be open with about what happened."

DOCUMENT AND REPORT THE CRIME

Write down all the details as quickly as possible after reporting it. Photograph visible physical signs such as cuts, scrapes, bruises, torn clothing, and so on. Keep a list of the names of police officers, hospital workers, and court officials to whom you speak, and write down what they say. If you want the crime to be reported as a hate or bias crime, tell the police officer to note that on the report.

If you are attacked on the street, call 911. If you decide not to report a crime right after it happens, you can report the incident by going to the police station in the neighborhood where the crime occurred. If you file a police report, you may be eligible for financial compensation for damages. Always get a copy of the police report. If you need help reporting to the police, or if you want to talk to someone before reporting the incident, contact your local Anti-Violence Project. You can also call the New York City hot line at (212) 714-1141, which is available twenty-four hours a day.

TALK ABOUT WHAT HAS HAPPENED

Self-blame, isolation, hopelessness, or thoughts of suicide are all common. "The trauma of being physically assaulted for your sexuality is a life-altering experience," says Norman, "because the thing that 'caused' the violence, your sexuality, isn't going away." Try to talk with supportive friends, family members, or—and this can be especially helpful—other survivors.

You can find information about support groups, and supportive organizations, from the National Coalition of Anti-Violence Projects online at www.avp.org.

Adapted in part from information provided by New York City's Anti-Violence Project

ical journals, the *New York Times* noted in 1998, had published about forty-five thousand articles on depression, and fewer than five hundred on joy. For gay men particularly—who are four times as likely to see therapists as our straight counterparts, according to some studies, and often deal with stresses straight men often don't begin to imagine—therapy may seem the norm of health. Bad therapy, that is: A University of Washington study found a whopping 46 percent of gay men who were in therapy experienced their therapists as homophobic.

But what about the means, other than shrinkage, that we use to stay centered? Informal surveys find gay men using the same supports to stay happy as straight men, lesbians, and just about everyone else: relying on lovers, friends, family, and work. In interviews for this book, good friends were mentioned even before family, romantic interests, or sex—perhaps because they often tend to last longer than that trio (see Chapter 12) and because we make more time for them. "My brother and his wife have a whole set of complicated relations and private language with their two children," says Larry, thirty-two, an artist from Grosse Pointe, Michigan. "I have the same kind of enduring, complicated pleasures with my friends." Austin, twenty-eight years old, from San Antonio, agrees: "The best thing for me is just getting together with real friends on a lazy weekend, lying around the park or on somebody's roof and passing the time."

For some men, specific moments, more than specific characters, have delivered their most acute experiences of joy. Tracy, thirty-four-year-old clinical health psychologist, found his high note in his first performance with a gay men's chorus. "I'd come out recently, and there was a sea of thousands of faces, thousands of gay men clapping wildly and cheering," he remembers. "I don't cry easily, but I had to struggle to keep back tears." Charles, thirty-eight, from Houston, recalls seeing the PFLAG (Parents and Friends of Lesbians and Gays) contingent march by in his first big-city Gay Pride parade: "I'd just heard another story about a friend being tossed out of his house because of his sexual orientation," he remembers. "And I thought it was monumental that these people would not only celebrate their children's sexuality, but tell the world at large it was okay."

Stressed to the Nines?

Most of us begin to cope with stress from day one of our adolescent lives. Trying to keep from getting bashed or HIV-infected or thrown out of your job or sent out of your mind as you move back and forth between bars and baby-sitting and boyfriends and gym class and family gives gay men good practice in stress control, and good need for it. Stress is not necessarily distress; in moderate quantities, anxiety and pressure keep us motivated. "I'm at my best, my most productive and creative and energized, when things seem like just a little too much for me to handle," says Ramon, thirty-six, whose careers, like many a gay man's, have included cater waiter, freelance writer, actor, dancer, and other high-tension pursuits. Too much pressure, though, may cause what Steven Hobfoll, Ph.D., of the Applied Psychology Center at Kent State University in Kent, Ohio, calls the three emotional signs of overstress: anxiety, anger, and depression. On a physical level, too, stress takes its toll, and a variety of forms. "Stress usually hits you at your own weak link, which is determined by a combination of genetics and exposure," says Dr. Hobfoll. "If you're prone to colds, you'll get one with higher fever and more mucus when you're stressed. If you have HIV, stress may result in a drop in immune function." One pre-protease inhibitor study of ninety-three men with HIV in Florida and North Carolina found that men who had experienced one or more episodes of severe stress were twice as likely to develop symptoms as those who hadn't.

The Wisdom of the Body

Stress often makes itself felt in a particular body part or system, be it through tension headaches or a spastic colon. "Repeated research suggests that the stress you experience today may well manifest itself as next year's illness," says Sheldon Cohen, Ph.D., of Carnegie Mellon's Psychology Department, with stress increasing risk of many of the biggest threats to men's health: coronary artery disease, infectious diseases such as STDs, and autoimmune ailments, including AIDS. Physical symptoms of stress might just be your body's way of telling you that you need to wake up and skip the coffee. Among the common complaints:

• *Skin, Digestive, or Respiratory Problems.* The body's largest organs—your skin and large intestine—are among the quickest to reflect psychic distress. Asthma, too, can be triggered by stress.

• *Extreme appetite loss or gain.* Turning feelings into food, or denying yourself both, are common strategies for the overly stressed.

• *Trouble sleeping.* Insomnia's a common symptom, and there are special things to do to help (see "Cruising Mr. Sandman," page 468).

• *Headaches.* Tension, anyone? You can feel it in your temples, or behind your eyes.

• *Muscle pain or tightness.* Clench your nerves, and your back will often follow. Or your neck. Or your shoulders.

• *Heart racing, excessive sweating, worry about loss of control.* This can be a full-fledged panic attack (see "The Sixty-Second Shrink," page 489), but may also be a more moderate form of overstressing.

• *Feeling worn out or withdrawn.* When constant, these are also hallmarks of depression.

1, 3, 7, 9, HOW DO YOU KEEP FROM LOSING YOUR MIND?

Joy and perfection are fleeting by definition, but sanity and contentment may be maintained through more ongoing, enduring acts. Beyond the "sunsets" and "fireside chats" of personal-ad fame, the methods are many.

• Jack, forty-eight, publishing executive, Chapel Hill, North Carolina: "Writing in my journal nightly. It lets me focus on what's important, to ruminate on what's passed, and to plan for what's to come."

• Tim, twenty-nine, writer, Amherst, Massachusetts: "Sanity is sitting home on a Saturday night, alone (by choice, not by force), reading a book or a few back issues of *The New Yorker,* or even staring at the ceiling."

• Mark, forty-four, financial planner, Raleigh-Durham, North Carolina: "At six on a Sunday afternoon, when everybody else is leaving the beach, I get naked and ride the waves. The fading light invigorates me and I become beauty."

• Jamie, twenty-nine, food service worker, Birmingham, Alabama: "I find tremendous happiness when I sign that last check that pays the last bill for the month, and I know that the last $100 in my account is all mine, mine, mine to spend however I please."

• Refugio, thirty, graphics consultant, New York, New York: "I create different drag characters in the privacy of my own home. The latest is a pregnant nun character, sort of 'Agnes the Monster.'"

• Bradley, twenty-one, journalist, New York, New York: "Making out in bathrooms of bars, e-mailing with my dad, old boyfriends calling to say they're coming to town, and eating well, without skipping dessert."

• Dan, thirty-one, design consultant, San Francisco, California: "I make sure I have time to myself, time to be away from people. I walk a lot. Going to the gym and dancing help, too, and sex. Making my body feel good is the main thing."

• Ben, forty-seven, lawyer and entertainment producer, Worcester, Massachusetts: "Long bouts of aerobic activity, kissing, falling asleep, staying at hotels, being in new places with wide-open spaces or bodies of water. And of course, sunsets."

TURNING A GAY GAZE ON STRESS ASSESSMENT

One of the most common measures of stress and its effects is that developed by Drs. Thomas Holmes and Richard Rahe from the University of Washington. The good doctors looked at people's lives and assigned points corresponding to the stress level of forty-three major life events. Straight life events, that is: Absent from the list are things like coming out, having your HIV-positive lover's condom break, being homo for the holidays, getting the dildo stuck inside you, or trying to get a date when you're over forty-five. The emphasis of various events may seem off, too: If the death of a friend is only 37 points for straight people, it may be as serious for some of us as the death of a "spouse" (100 points).

Even so, the results of their study were striking. Scoring 150 points or more on the Holmes and Rahe scale in a year gave people a 50 percent likelihood of developing an illness in the next year. Score 300 or more, and you have a 90 percent chance of falling ill—assuming, of course, that you aren't taking steps to relax (see "Address the Stress," below).

For a full list, see www.teachhealth.com. A few highlights are below:

Stress Test: The Less, the Merrier

Death of a spouse: *100 points*
Marital separation: *65 points*
Jail term: *63 points*
Personal injury: *53 points*
Marriage: *50 points*
Fired from work: *47 points*
Retirement: *45 points*
Changes in family member's health: *44 points*
Sex difficulties: *39 points*
Change in financial status: *38 points*
Death of a close friend: *37 points*
Change to a different line of work: *36 points*
Change in number of marital arguments: *35 points*
Mortgage or loan over $10,000: *31 points*
Change in work responsibilities: *29 points*
Son or daughter leaving home: *29 points*
Trouble with in-laws: *29 points*
Outstanding achievement: *28 points*
Spouse begins or stops work: *26 points*
Starting or finishing school: *26 points*
Change in living conditions: *25 points*
Trouble with boss: *23 points*
Change in work hours, conditions: *20 points*
Change in residence: *20 points*
Change in social activities: *18 points*
Change in sleeping habits: *16 points*
Change in eating habits: *15 points*
Vacation: *13 points*
Christmas season: *12 points*
Minor violation of the law: *11 points*

From the "Social Readjustment Rating Scale," by Thomas Holmes and Richard Rahe, Journal of Psychoanalytic Research, 1967, vol II p. 214

Address the Stress

If stress is beating up on you, bash back. In addition to eating and sleeping well, get aerobic exercise (see Chapter 5), which breaks through anxiety like nothing else. Below find a number of other suggestions from therapists, experts at the National Institute of Mental Health, and great gay worriers.

SOCIALIZE, BUT BE CHOOSY

"People tend to isolate themselves under stress," says Dr. Hobfoll, "but play can be as important as, or more important than, work"—assuming, of course, that you play with people who make you feel good. "Avoiding toxic people—the mean, sarcastic, negative ones who make you feel hopeless—is one of the most basic and underused strategies of mental health," says San Francisco therapist Michael Bettinger, MSW.

FIND SUPPORT FOR YOUR GAY RELATIONSHIPS (AND NOTE THE PLURAL)

Gay men who are "experiencing discrimination from outside or who are punishing themselves from within are more likely to have stress turn into distress," says Ilan Meyer, Ph.D., a Columbia University researcher. His study of 741 gay men found that even a state of "vigilance"—looking at yourself with what Meyer calls "a third eye, wondering if someone's going to hurt or judge you for being gay"—contributes significantly to stress and depression. Find someplace to feel gay and good. Chapter 13 offers a few ways of starting.

MAKE A LIST

"I get so pressured, with so much to do, that I just stare at my computer feeling like I can't do anything," says Tim, a twenty-nine-year-old graphic designer. Prioritize and do the most important tasks first, checking them off your list as you complete them.

RATION YOUR WORRY TIME

"If I'm in the middle of a task, I see if I can consciously defer anxiety to later," says Peter, forty, a self-described "writer who worries too much." "I have time to worry and be distracted and feel terrible. I just do it after work." Some people schedule an hour or so to do nothing but worry, focusing on each anxiety, breaking it down into smaller problems, and taking it as far as they can toward solutions.

REDUCE PREDICTABLE SOURCES OF STRESS

"If you know that waiting at the dry cleaner before work is going to make you worry about being late, don't go then," suggests New York City therapist Michael Shernoff, MSW. "If rush-hour traffic makes you crazy, have a coffee after work and wait it out." Similarly, avoid the "maybes" and "possiblys" that keep you feeling obligated and on edge. Instead of "Maybe I'll be able to come by and help Dad clean the yard on Saturday," try "I can't do it this weekend."

ACCEPT WHAT YOU CAN'T CONTROL

If a problem is beyond your control and cannot be changed at the moment, don't keep coming back to it. Learn to accept what is—for now—until such time when you can change it.

BREATHE

Paying attention to your breath—how to slow it and deepen it—is one of the most useful worry relievers (see "Methods of Meditation," page 470). If at first you don't succeed, try again.

CRUISING MR. SANDMAN: INSOMNIA AND HOW TO HELP

> There is music here that gentlier lies, than tired eyelids upon tired eyes.
> *—Alfred, Lord Tennyson, "The Lotus-Eaters"*

> Sleep that knits up the ravell'd sleave of care.
> *—Shakespeare,* Macbeth

> After forty-eight hours, I'm pretty much sludge.
> *—John, age eighteen*

Get a bad night's sleep, and even the most sweet and dreamy of us gets tired and cantankerous. Get a bunch of bad nights, and you may feel like you're falling apart, or actually do it. Many major disasters of the last few decades—the *Challenger* explosion, the *Exxon Valdez* oil spill, Chernobyl, and the Three Mile Island meltdown—all were caused in part by errors due to someone's lack of sleep. Every twenty-four hours without sleep, researchers guesstimate, causes you to lose 25 percent of your awareness and mental function.

Insomnia itself isn't a disease, it's a symptom, says Sara Mosko, Ph.D., the director of the Sleep Disorders Center at St. Joseph Hospital in Orange, California. Medical causes of early waking or an inability to get to sleep can include asthma, heartburn, arthritis, "restless legs" syndrome, and sleep apnea, a predominantly male disorder that involves loud snoring, structural problems that restrict the flow of oxygen in the airway, and a consequent experience of waking up and falling asleep hundreds of times in a single night. Waking early is a particularly common symptom of depression or anxiety disorders. While serious sleeplessness should be treated by a doctor (sleep apnea, for example, may require going to a sleep clinic), a number of commonsense tactics can help you make it through the night.

- *Wind down.* Stimulants such as coffee and chocolate should be avoided anytime after noon, suggests Dr. Mosko. You also shouldn't do work, or have intense conversations, just before bed. "For at least half an hour before, forget anything more anxiety-provoking than a glass of warm milk," adds New York City therapist Michael Lipson, Ph.D. "Skip MTV and the evening news. Too many fast-moving edits and local tragedies set your mind racing."
- *The bed is for sleep (and sex) only.* Don't read or work in bed. You want to associate it only with sleep. If you wake in the middle of the night and can't fall asleep, get out of bed until you think you might be ready to try again. Spend no more than half an hour trying to get back to sleep and then get up and go elsewhere.
- *Stick to a schedule.* Try to go to bed and wake up at the same time, even on weekends. When you go to sleep late and then sleep in on the weekends, "your body is essentially living in two different time zones," says Dr. Mosko. Just when it gets used to one, you switch.
- *Exercise regularly.* Staying active decreases tension and helps you fall asleep. Don't exercise right before bed, however; it "activates" you.
- *Accept.* Accept occasional nights of less than optimal sleep rather than always struggling fiercely and uselessly against them. Once you're really upset and trying to force yourself to sleep, your body starts to associate bedtime with anxiety and reinforces the cycle.
- *Breathe deeply.* Slow, deep breaths relax us all (see "Methods of Meditation," below). See if you can let your body "breathe" you: Rather than forcing anything, just wait calmly until your belly and lungs fill up with air, and then release it slowly and wait again.
- *Say no to the nightcap.* Alcohol in the evening might seem like a good way to relax, but alcohol helps with only a shallow kind of sleep, and its sedation effect wears off.

If none of the above is working, try supplements such as melatonin (particularly useful for jet lag), over-the-counter sleeping pills, or prescription sleep medication as a short-term solution. Over the long run, prescription sleeping pills are often dependency-inducing, though they can help you gain some rest before you lose your mind.

If it's anxiety that wakes you, you may be able to break the spell through visualization. "Anxiety, even if it's prompted by others, is usually a series of selfish questions: 'What will *I* do?' 'What will happen if *I* . . . ,'" says Michael Lipson. "Try disrupting that by thinking about someone you don't know very well and imagining a series of wonderful things happening to him or her. Really follow the fantasy, picturing a series of pleasant occurrences—success at work, romantic pleasure, whatever seems appropriate. See if you get yourself on another wavelength, and back to calm."

Methods of Meditation

You're thirty minutes into Monday morning, the computers are down, Fifi went wee-wee on the Bukharan, your boss wants to write you up for the fact that he hasn't been happy in two years, and that message on your voice mail is not the hunk from the sauna, but a rep for the credit card whose limit you've exceeded. Need a break? Instead of reaching for the Xanax bottle or the tincture of Saint-John's-wort, why not draw on your internal reservoir of calm? Meditate.

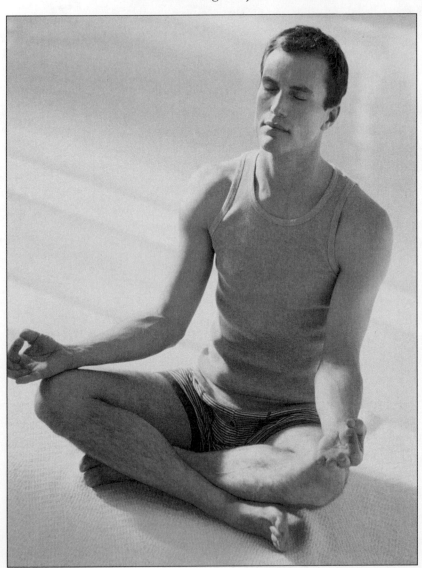

The Buddha said that there were eighty-four thousand ways of calming the spirit through meditation, making the muddied mind as clear as a glass of water. Most of these methods, like life itself, start with a breath, a renewed attention to the ins and outs of that "simple" process that brings life to our bodies and brains. Spiritual seekers throughout the ages have seen the breath as the doorway to the soul. Sufi mystics often use repeated forceful exhalation in their *zikrs,* the trance states where they join with God. Some Jews theorize that the unpronounceable name of God actually finds voice in the first cry of the newborn infant and the last breath of the dying man. There's the energy-releasing breath of fire of kundalini yoga, the trippy, vision-creating, holotropic breath work of post-LSD-era California, and the Tantric breath that aids orgasm without ejaculation (see Chapter 3). Even if you're more *Today* show than Tantric, your breath should probably still be the center of your relaxation strategy. "Lie down in a comfortable position," advises Art Ulene, MD, whose fitness advice became a series on the NBC morning talk show and the substance of his book *Really Fit, Really Fast* (Health Points, 1996).

"Take a long, slow inhalation through your nose, filling your abdomen and lungs. Then purse your lips and let the air slowly escape. Repeat the process, slowing your breathing with each breath until you find the pace that is most relaxing for you." Dr. Ulene recommends at least ten minutes a day of such relaxation.

Some people find it helpful to give their breath visual weight, to imagine it, for example, as steam they can see coming out of their noses toward their chests, and which they then breathe back in its entirety. Even so, holding that focus takes practice. So, for that matter, does breathing in for five counts, or out for seven, as many meditation disciplines recommend. To begin, unbutton your pants and allow your abdomen to fill slowly with air in what some practitioners call the "return-to-childhood" breath (see "Four Mind-Body Basics," page 219).

Mentally, most of us find our minds wandering during breathing or meditation, flashing to anxieties or preoccupations or distractions. Meditation literature often refers to this as "monkey mind," so named because of the way your thoughts jump and dangle like a monkey in a tree. You may feel like falling asleep, or find yourself racing with worries and associations. Rather than punishing or chiding yourself, simply note that you're thinking and let your focus return to your breath. A wonderful thing about your breathing is that, for as long as you're alive, it's always there to return to.

What else can you do as you meditate? Depends on whom you talk to. Below find four suggestions, from four different practitioners. You can start out with only five or ten minutes a day, or go right to half an hour. And if you're just starting, advises Jon Kabat-Zinn in his excellent guide to basic Buddhism and meditation, *Wherever You Go, There You Are* (Hyperion, 1995), don't talk about it with everyone. Take that time and spend it on a little extra meditation.

Breathe, Chant, and Think of Tahiti (but Quietly)

"For me, it's about turning off your self-talk," says Tom McDonald, Ph.D., psychologist and motivational speaker from Escondido, California. "You know, the talk that goes on in your head and that churns up emotions—happiness, sadness, anger? Quiet that chatter, and your body relaxes."

Dr. McDonald finds his quiet by closing the door and turning off the phone for a period each day. "I try for an hour," he says. "If your office is too crazy, then find a quiet room nearby. Breathing is important because it focuses attention on something immediate, so try counting your breath as it comes out, one, then in, two, et cetera. Then do muscle relaxation. Starting with your toes, tighten them for two or three seconds, then relax. Do the same with the arches of your feet, your ankles and calves, thighs and stomach and chest and arms, working your way up your body. Even scrunch up your face and then release the muscles.

"Finally, visualize something nice and calm—a beach on Tahiti—but not something that will stir up all your emotions again. Chant if you want—repeating the sound 'om' as you exhale is good. If you're in your workplace, do it quietly. You don't want to get thrown out."

The Lord on Line Two—Got a Minute?

"Meditation from my perspective is a way to wait upon the divine, to receive inspiration," says Lloyd George Tupper, DD, president of the Holmes Institute, a graduate school of consciousness studies based in Los Angeles. "There's a premise here, that our lives are part of something greater. By turning within and shutting down the human outside world, we can consciously reconnect with something we've become deafened to in the demands of everyday life.

"Instead of creative visualization," says Tupper, "I try to empty my mind so I can receive something. I lock the door, take the phone off the hook, fold my hands, and say, 'This moment of privilege is for me, to allow myself to be, as Emerson describes it, 'an inlet and an outlet to all that is divine.' I try to empty my mind of every circumstance, every event, person, memory, attitude, opinion, all judgment, and bask in the peace of this moment and be still.

"You can do that in sixty seconds—on an elevator, in the bathroom, at a stoplight. I've seen people doing it on airplanes—you can tell they're reconnecting. Close your eyes if it helps, and just sit there. You'd be amazed at what comes in."

Loving-Kindness

No one can buy love, but everyone can cultivate it, offers Sharon Salzberg, author of *Loving-Kindness: The Revolutionary Art of Happiness* (Shambhala Books, 1997). Her book, and the practice she leads at the Insight Meditation Society in Barre, Massachusetts, is an exercise in nurturing the seeds of loving-kindness within ourselves. Greatly condensed, the meditation begins with you sitting comfortably, reflecting on the goodness within you and formulating a wish. "Choose three or four phrases that capture what you most deeply wish for yourself," suggests Salzberg. "Make them simple. 'May I be free from danger,' or 'May I have physical happiness,' or 'May I be healthy.' Each phrase is a gift, and you should offer it to whatever version of yourself you can most easily picture as deserving." That may mean picturing yourself as a young child, or surrounded by friends or people who love you.

After you've done this for about ten minutes or so, change your focus to someone who has given or taught you much. This may be a great friend, or a teacher or benefactor. "Call this person to mind," suggests Salzberg, "perhaps by visualizing them or saying their name." Then repeat the same phrase you've been saying to yourself to them: "Just as I want to be happy, so may you be happy. May you be happy." If the phrase takes a different form with them, let it. After another ten minutes or so, switch again—this time to someone you feel neutral toward. Then move to someone you find difficult or who has caused you harm. "Try to recognize that just as you want to be happy, they want to be happy, though their ignorance keeps them from being able to do so," advises Salzberg. "If it's too threatening or difficult to say, 'May you be happy,' broaden it. Try 'May we be happy.'"

Conclude the meditation by wishing your phrase on the whole world, all beings, without division or exclusion or end. "The concepts of separateness that have dominated our lives have caused tremendous suffering," says Salzberg. "The goal is to experience a sense of unity with all others, to develop a sense of love so strong that the mind becomes like space, which cannot be tainted. If someone throws paint, it is not the air that changes color. It is only the walls, the barriers to space, that can be affected by the paint."

Turbulence at Thirty Thousand Feet? Bump with It

"Stress is holding on to something," offers John Thiels, doctoral candidate and teacher at the Cambridge Zen Center in Cambridge, Massachusetts. "The causes are not found in other people but in yourself. If you want to get rid of stress, then you have to let go of something. If you understand and believe in yourself, if you have a clear direction, then stress isn't a problem. If you don't have that clarity, then meditation practice is a way to find it.

"For me, the most important thing about Zen is direction: Why am I alive? No matter what situation confronts me, what would be helpful? Controlled breathing is very useful: I breathe in to a count of three, then out to a count of seven. Just doing this for five or ten minutes can help calm your body and mind. Repetitive physical movement is also good—walking, rowing, running—anything where your body, mind, and breath come together at least ten minutes every day. Ask yourself: 'What am I doing just now?' and pay attention to that action. Concentrate on now. During eating time, just eat; walking time, just walk. When the airplane is bumpy, just bump with it."

Therapy and You: Diving Inside

If you're feeling persistently down, or as though you're not making any progress in your life, then therapy in one of its many different forms may be a road out of the rut. Even if it's short-term—getting you over a painful breakup, out of an abusive relationship, into the job market, or in a better place about your sexual orientation—talking with a trained counselor can be liberating. "I think of therapists as community resources, not unlike clergy, local healers, or shamans," says Philip Spivey, Ph.D., a New York City psychologist with extensive experience working with gay men. "Whether you're in therapy with a group or one on one, it can be a means of making you whole, of getting to another, freer place." Michael Bettinger, the San Francisco therapist, agrees. "Gay men don't get much help with transitions," he says. "Dating, the end of our relationships, death of a lover, coming out: We're not taught how to cope with these things. The medical model says that therapy is something for people who are sick. The growth model recognizes that it can also help to provide a witness, a support that makes things easier."

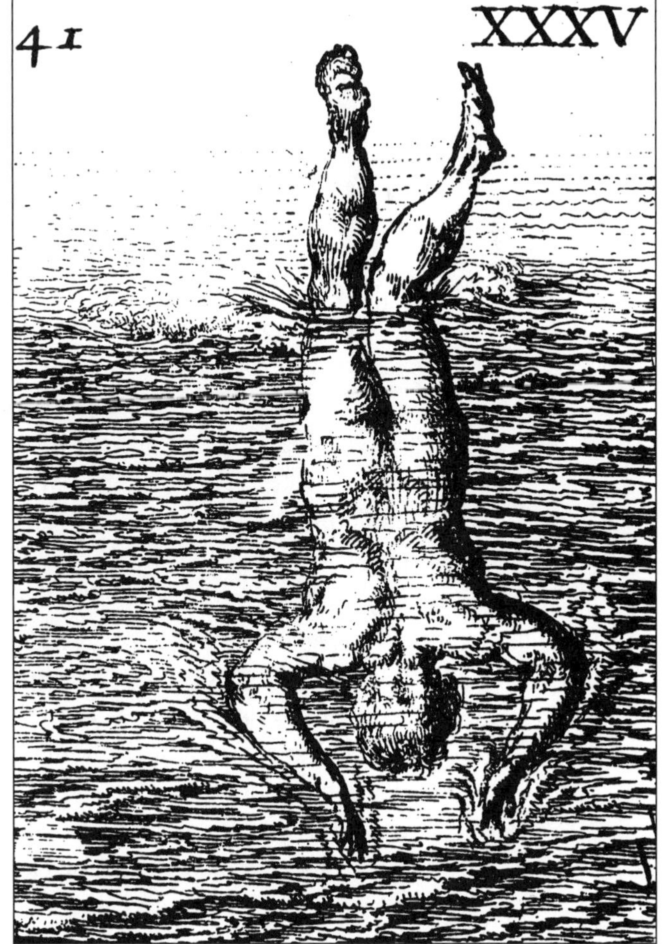

"Yes," jokes Columbia University's Laura Pinsky, "but does insurance recognize the growth model?" Though the exchange of money (and the undivided attention to which that money entitles you) is one of the things that distinguishes therapy from, say, a conversation with a friend, managed care has managed to drastically reduce the amount of money available for long-term psychological support. If you or a friend is in real psychological trouble, hospital emergency rooms offer psychiatric evaluation and crisis care. If you want ongoing care, you'll have to strike a balance between what you need and what your insurance will pay for. Among the options that may be more affordable are newly licensed therapists (who tend to charge less), group therapy with peer or professional support, and therapy with students still in training. If you can go during the day, rather than during the precious after-work hours, some therapists will also charge you less. It's a community resource, yes, but it's also a business.

MANAGED CARE AND MENTAL HEALTH

It's no accident that the number of prescriptions written has skyrocketed during the years that managed care plans have come to insure the vast majority of Americans with private health insurance. Ever mindful of ways to manage costs as well as care, many companies have adopted a take-a-pill-and-please-don't-call-me-in-the-morning approach whenever possible. Nowhere has cost control been more severe than in mental health services. While total health care spending fell by only 7 percent between 1988 and 1997, spending on mental health plunged by 54 percent. Two out of three insurance companies in America now limit the number of days you can spend in a hospital for mental health or substance abuse treatment. Half place sharp restrictions on the number of visits to a therapist's office or mental health clinic, often allowing a maximum of twenty a year. Fewer than one out of five will pay for the weekly visit that used to be thought of as standard psychotherapy when most of the therapists now practicing were in school.

The concept of limiting therapy, or at least taking a look at how you set goals and decide when to stop, is not entirely bad. "Nowhere else in medicine do you have treatment that goes on and on," says Steve Ball, CSW, a New York City therapist who left work with a managed care company to pursue practice as a private therapist in New York City. "It may not make sense to ration mental health care, but there are principles of so-called solution focus therapy that are useful. There's the 'miracle question,' for example. If you woke up tomorrow and your problem were miraculously gone, what's the first thing you'd do differently? How would you know if you were better? If ten was a miracle day and one was the worst possible, where are you now? What's the difference between a three and a five? Thinking these things through as clearly as you can may help you get a handle on what you're looking for, and how you'll gauge progress." Robert Cabaj, MD, a psychiatrist and associate professor at the University of California at San Francisco, agrees that a periodic check-in is crucial to deciding where you're going in therapy, and whether to continue.

The problem, warn Ball, Cabaj, and others, is that with managed care it's rarely you who's deciding. Even those managed care companies that say they allow up to twenty counseling sessions may only pay for one, or five, before requiring your therapist to file a detailed report justifying further treatment. Some actually demand that you take a medication—preferably an inexpensive one—in order to continue treatment. "They'll call and say, 'Doctor, why is this patient on Effexor? Are you aware that there is a medication that may be as effective and costs five times less?'" says Donald Freeman, MD, a clinical instructor in psychiatry at the University of California, Los Angeles. "And it's never an MD on the other end of the line." Even if your therapist is willing to do the work and accept the prescriptions required, the sense of the special, private bond between you and your therapist may be radically disrupted by the reports he or she is required to write. For companies that self-insure (see "Do You Get It? Insurance Sources and What You Should Know About Them," page 321), those reports, including details such as your sexual orientation and HIV status, may be accessible to your employer. "I always show my patients the reports I write, and try to provide as much relevant information as possible about the need for treatment without revealing any unnecessary detail," says Dr. Spivey. "I won't even give a zip code unless I have to."

If a managed care plan is paying for your therapy, suggests Michael Bettinger, make sure to ask your therapist a few questions:

- How many sessions do I get before you need to write a report requesting authorization to continue?
- Can I see the reports you submit?
- Will you continue to see me if the insurer denies the request? At what rate? Do you know how much of that is paid for by my policy, and how much I'll have to pay?
- Am I required to take any pills to continue treatment under the plan?

If you don't like the answers, it may be more your insurer's fault than the therapist's. "I decided to pay out of pocket for a private shrink," says Bill, forty-two, a public relations consultant from Pennsylvania. "I just didn't want my boss reading that I had questions about a relationship he didn't even know I was in."

Mind Fields: Forms and Practice of Therapy

In America, anyone who wants to can call herself or himself a therapist or counselor. And while more credentials do not necessarily mean more insight, certain people—counselors or social workers with a master's degree, psychologists with a doctorate, and medical doctors specializing in psychiatry—are often the only ones who have met licensing requirements that school them in professional codes of ethics. Among those ethics is the cardinal rule that no therapist should ever come on to you or have sex with you, and a confidentiality clause that makes it illegal for a licensed therapist to share anything you say with anyone (outside of your insurance company) unless you intend to do harm to yourself or someone else. Psychiatrists can prescribe medication and admit people into hospitals, which is something that no other therapist can legally do. Some insurance companies will reimburse only for licensed professionals, which is a good thing to know before you shell out the $95 that is the national average for a one-on-one therapy session.

There are literally hundreds of schools of psychotherapy, founded and refined by famous thinkers on the subject of the human mind. Though most therapists these days are eclectic, blending a variety of approaches, major differences often come down to a belief in how change is best achieved, and how long it takes. Should you be alone, or in a group? Hitting a phone book with a rubber hose to get out your frustrations, or free-associating on a couch with a therapist who sits supportively but silently behind you? Working with someone for six weeks on changing your behavior, or consulting a counselor for several years? Whatever your approach, says Laura Pinsky, a little self-diagnosis can go a long way in determining what kind of experience you're looking for in a doctor. "If you're struggling with substance abuse issues, I'd try to find someone who had insights and experience in dealing with that," she says. "If you're feeling intense guilt about your sexuality, make sure you have a therapist who really knows about sexuality and the coming-out process." And before you drag your depressed body to the library to decide if you need a Freudian or a Jungian, a Rogerian or a Rolfer, take heart in the fact that your psyche is not segmented as neatly as those disciplines. "If you start thinking and feeling differently, you're going to start acting differently," says California-based therapist Marny Hall, Ph.D. "If you start acting differently, you're going to start thinking and feeling differently. One approach quickly enters the terrain of others." The most important thing is to find someone you respond well to and see what happens.

In her classic consumer's guide for lesbians and gay men, *The Lavender Couch* (Alyson Publications, 1985), Dr. Hall goes on to divide therapeutic approaches into four different categories helpful in making sense of the tangle of options.

FEELING-BASED THERAPIES

Classic, lie-on-the-couch-and-talk psychoanalysis draws heavily on this model, as do a number of therapies that release memories and feelings through breathing and intense massage or other kinds of body work. Feeling therapies work to reveal feelings you weren't even aware of, and to explore the new insights and actions that can come from raising those feelings to consciousness. Central to almost all of these is the therapist's unwavering, nonjudgmental presence as you experience self-consciousness and conflict. Strong suspicions about the therapist's approval, or disapproval, or sexual interest in you or vice versa are common, and healing comes partly in recognizing how many of the perceptions of others come from within. "Having someone to bear witness to your life in an ongoing way—someone to tolerate your feelings no matter what they are—allows you to listen to yourself in ways you rarely get a chance to," says Justin Richardson, MD. Being trusting and honest enough to express whatever thoughts and feelings come up, no matter how off-the-wall, can help you get new insights faster.

THINKING THERAPIES

The best known of these is cognitive therapy, which attempts to look at self-defeating patterns of thought and substitute healthier ones. Replacing "I'm a terrible lover, I know I'll never get it up" with "I'm working on my erection problem, and I still give a mean blow job," is a crude example of this kind of therapy, which traces depression and helplessness to certain "automatic" thought patterns that make you feel negative about your past, present, or future. Often treatment is relatively short-term, occurring during fifteen or twenty sessions in a three-month period, and tries to help you recognize self-defeating thought patterns, marshal evidence to the contrary, and propose different explanations. As you go deeper, thinking therapies help you identify and disrupt certain essential assumptions about yourself and the world that may keep you paralyzed or pessimistic.

BEHAVIOR THERAPIES

These take a treat-the-symptom approach that helps you recognize and restructure your responses to certain powerful cues that cause you anxiety. "I believe we can write a psychology and never use the terms consciousness, mental states, mind, or imagery and the like," wrote the initiator of the behavior therapy movement, John Watson, in 1913. Biofeedback and relaxation exercises that help you get through a panic attack by deep breathing and lowering your body temperature (see "Alternative and Complementary Medicines," page 309) are examples of behavioral therapies that expose you to stressful or painful situations and show you a way through them. Aversion therapy, which includes strategies such as putting a smoker who wants to quit in an intensely unpleasant, smoke-filled, dark little closet, is also part of behavior therapy, and has been effective. Aversion therapy where gay men are shown sexy images at the same time as being made to smell ammonia or given drugs to nauseate us has not.

MEDICAL THERAPIES

People used to be reluctant to even call this therapy, since a common fear is that use of medications takes the control out of the hands of the consumer and places it firmly in the hands of the medical establishment. In fact, it doesn't need to be that way: Information readily available on the Web, in this chapter, and in numerous books offers detailed information about particular medications and how to minimize their side effects and maximize your choices. There have been a lot of gay graduates in psychiatry, and a lot of new discoveries in the last few decades. Rather than turning gay men into drooling messes or zombies happily accepting whatever Nurse Ratchet or Big Heterosexual Brother doles out, medication is being used by many who are fierce, out, and proud. For those who are seriously depressed, electroshock therapy may be another treatment that's gotten a bad rap (see next page).

Finding Dr. Right (Take II): Looking for a Therapist You Can Work With

In my family, men don't stop and ask for directions when they're driving. I think therapy helped me decide that I would rather be a person than a man.

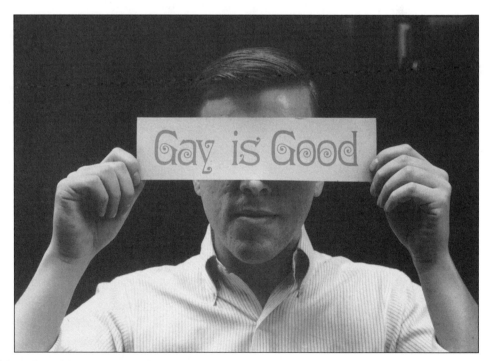

Finding a therapist means considering many of the same questions you asked yourself about finding a doctor (see "Finding Dr. Right," in Chapter 7). Do you want someone gay or straight? Male or female? Cold and clear, or warm and fuzzy?

As with finding other health care providers, the best source of referrals may be gay professional associations, health clinics, and friends. In the case of your therapist, though, your best friend's recommendation may not be appropriate. Anxious to preserve the only-for-you nature of the relationship that is the heart of therapy, many counselors will decline to see best friends or even close acquaintances. "Too much back and forth," says Dr. Hall.

SHOCK THERAPY: SHOCKINGLY EFFECTIVE?

Don't be shocked. Electroconvulsive treatment, or ECT, is the name now preferred by practitioners of this treatment for severe depression. Like the name, the convulsions are milder then they used to be, too. The fact that most of our knowledge of ECT comes from movies of the *One Flew Over the Cuckoo's Nest* variety, and that the cruder form of this therapy has been used aggressively and inappropriately in the past, hasn't helped its reputation. "Shock therapy was a weapon misused both by accident and by design," says UCLA's Dr. Freeman. "Today, I'd say without a doubt that it is the most underused somatic [nontalk] therapy in psychiatry today."

ECT is appropriate only for certain types of serious depression and mania, not for what Dr. Freeman calls "the dwindles," low-grade depression of the I'm-feeling-bad-at-work-and-wish-my-life-were-happier kind. Rather than undergoing bone-breaking, body-shaking convulsions, an ECT patient today goes under anesthesia and lies still as a small amount of electric current is passed through a part of the brain. No pain or discomfort is remembered. Since short-term memory loss can be one of the few side effects of ECT (you can lose the day before, and several hours after), you may not even remember the immediate lead-up, which may or may not be reassuring. If ECT is applied too often (more than three times a week), which it really shouldn't be, you may also experience "viscosity"—feeling as though you're moving through molasses, having trouble doing calculations in your head, and the like.

"For serious depression, though, there are a lot of upsides to this treatment," says New York City psychopharmacologist Ron Winchel, MD. While medications for severe depression generally have an effectiveness of between 65 and 75 percent, ECT gets a positive result as much as 80 percent of the time. It's fast, too: With the usual course of ECT treatment involving six to twelve sessions, most patients finish their ECT in the month it might take medication to start working (see "Psychotropic Medications," page 485). "I've watched patients rocket out of suicidal, determined-to-die depressions in as few as two sessions," says Dr. Freeman. "It's one of the most dramatic things I've seen in psychiatry."

The treatment should be used with great caution, if at all, in people with severe heart disease, or those who have seizures or seizure-causing brain tumors. If you're older or having immune-system problems, though, ECT may well be less intrusive than antidepressants, which may interact badly with other life-saving medications such as blood thinners and protease inhibitors. ECT is also good when you can't even rally the will to choke down food or a few pills, a not uncommon symptom of the seriously depressed. If doctors propose ECT, ask for details about how many times, whether they're planning on treating one side of the brain or both (treatments only to the right side of the brain are generally as effective and milder), and whether they're using the more modern ("square wave") machine that reduces side effects.

"If I fall into a delusional depression, I want ECT. Please tell them," says Dr. Winchel. "I have several patients who absolutely should have ECT, and who won't go near it because they're still imagining *The Snake Pit* or Elsa Lanchester on a bad-hair day. That's the image of ECT. The reality is a much prettier picture."

A basic gay-affirmative approach—one that recognizes some of the special challenges of being gay, but does not regard homosexuality as an illness to be cured or an oddity to be accommodated—is a basic requirement for any potential therapist. Particularly if you're working on sex, having to explain yourself or getting beyond the basic safer-sex lecture can feel like a burden (see "Dr. Love," page 184). If you're struggling with broader issues of how your sexuality interfaces with the rest of life (and we all should be, including straight people), how much explaining you want to do, and whether you do it with someone gay, is up to you. "Gay is only one of many things you are, and it may be related to only a small part of treatment," says San Francisco therapist Patrick Ennis, LCSW. "If you're the gay child of an alcoholic, the problem is likely to be that you're the child of an alcoholic, not that you're gay." Lorne Feldman, MA, a therapist and program director at New York City's Positive Health Project, says he prefers having a straight therapist. "I thought I'd like the shortcut to empathy that having a gay therapist would give, but I didn't," says Feldman. "I don't know if my therapist now is straight, but my assumption that he is makes me work harder. I do feel like I have to explain certain things. I also feel like the explanations let me listen to myself and give me a clearer picture of my own assumptions."

As for the idea that therapists themselves may be in therapy, that should reassure rather than repel. Sitting there and hearing all those personal things raises issues for therapists, not just for patients, and even those who have concluded their own therapeutic process are often under supervision with a more experienced colleague. "It's okay to ask if they're in supervision," says Feldman. "In a time when some studies find nearly half of gay men in therapy suspect their therapist is homophobic, it's important to think of yourself as a demanding and discerning consumer." Finding a therapist, in fact, may be less about the growth model or sickness model of mental health than about the shopping model. Tell a potential therapist right up front that you're going to try a few different therapists before you decide, and make sure you do so. Therapists like to know that you're a savvy shopper, not a passive patient. And if you ask, many therapists will also give you an initial session for free or a sharply reduced rate.

If you feel so depleted that you don't even have resistance to offer, don't worry. "Therapy has many junctures," Dr. Hall advises. "Just start with the first. Does talking to this person give you immediate relief? Does he or she seem open? At least trust your gut. As for the rest, you can always, and you should, reevaluate periodically." If you're lost for words, among the questions it might make sense to ask are:

- *Gay attitude.* Does the therapist think homosexuality is an illness? Have any gay patients? Have experience dealing with gay men with your complaints?
- *Orientation.* What is the therapist's training and approach? Is he or she licensed? Silent or vocal? Someone who uses touch, or keeps a distance? Does he or she give advice, or ask you to formulate your own? Therapists are often hybrids, but tend to divide into "way-back-whens" and "here-and-nows," says Dr. Hall. "Way-back-whens" use discussion of your past experiences, including childhood. "Here-and-nows" tend to focus on immediate problems and immediate solutions.
- *Time.* How often will the therapist see you? How long is each session? What's the policy on rescheduling, or on canceled appointments?
- *Costs.* Depending on the type of therapy and the therapist's training, fees can range from $35 for a group counseling session to upward of $125 for an individual psychiatry session. Is there a sliding scale? Will rates change if your financial circumstances worsen, or if your insurance refuses to cover continued treatment? Will your therapist take insurance coverage up front, or do you have to fork over the fee and wait for reimbursement?
- *Medications.* If the therapist isn't licensed to prescribe medication, is there a clinician the therapist works with who can? How familiar is the therapist himself or herself with the effects of these drugs and when they're needed?

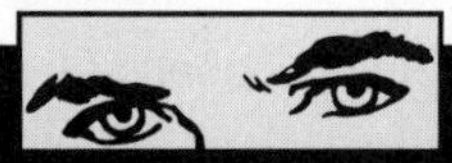

TURNING A GAY GAZE ON BEREAVEMENT

He died on Thanksgiving. The night after the funeral, I went to turn the light out in my room and it wouldn't go out. It would not turn off. I put in the video of our last Christmas vacation together, and when the video started the lights went out. I freaked out: puked, cried, fell into bed, huddled in the dark, watching that video of so much that was lost.

People bring a widow food and condolences after her husband's death, and for years afterward give her a muted respect. She's been through something. She's suffered and lost. The gay widower's place is much less certain, his past more shrouded in shame. "People don't say 'He lost his lover' with respect," says Henry, sixty, who's lost two. "It's almost a sad secret, something people whisper. It's one of the worst things about AIDS. Because going through all that, people don't wonder, 'How could he be so strong?' They wonder, 'Does he have it too?'" For those whose best friends have died, there may not even be a whispered acknowledgment of the connections severed by death, all the memories and shared moments that are lost.

The rituals we've used have helped. The memorial service, in all its variations, has been a salve to gay grief, particularly when it includes an opportunity for the audience to share, for all those widowed to speak. For all the awful stories of the lover made to sit silently on the "friends" side of the church while the family talked about Fred as a wonderful uncle, there are thousands more of problems solved creatively, of second services where friends and lovers told it the way they saw it, of ashes shared between family of birth and family of choice. And humor. "We were all gathered by the ocean, because Jorge had insisted that his ashes be thrown into the Atlantic," says Robert, forty-eight. "So Bob is wading out into the surf, and it's freezing, and all of a sudden Benny the Labrador retriever goes running in, and comes back covered with ash. And you know what dogs do when they're wet. *Shake-shake-shake,* and there were twelve queens shrieking, 'Eeee!' And it was like . . . 'Here's Jorge!'"

Grief doesn't end when a memorial is over. It doesn't end at all. "People say, 'Move on, get on with your life,' but really dealing with grief is about moving things over and opening up a space inside yourself to house the person you've lost," says Sandra Klein, MA, author of *Heavenly Hurts: Surviving AIDS-Related Deaths and Losses* (Baywood Publishing, 1998). As one of the first therapists to organize AIDS bereavement groups, Klein has a range of exercises to explore grief and defuse the fear that once you begin to feel it, it will destroy you. Among those she recommends is designating a time to grieve, setting a boundary (and a timer) that says, "In these twenty minutes I'll grieve, and if I'm not done, I'll come back later." That's for those of us who are afraid to open up our grief. For those who feel swallowed by it, Klein discusses many of the common reactions: the fear that having fun is disloyal to the deceased, the loss of all interest in the outside world, the telling and retelling of stories about the deceased, the cherishing of sorrow in the same way that you cherished the man who died. All of these, including bone-crushing despair, are normal.

"People who are not grieving say, 'Don't get depressed, organize.' Of course they're right," wrote Craig Lucas in Michael Shernoff's *Gay Widowers: Life After the Death of a Partner* (Haworth Press, 1998), a volume of essays by and about gay men who've loved and lost. Lucas's essay was written ten months after his lover's death. "I hope to be back in the ranks of the mentally balanced," he wrote. "But I do not believe I can get there without being here first. So here I am. This is my postcard from Grief. Don't write. Wish I weren't here."

Sad vs. SAD: The Diagnosis Name Game

Wave of Sorrow,
Do not drown me now:
I see the island
Still ahead somehow.
I see the island
And its sands are fair:
Wave of sorrow,
Take me there.
—*Langston Hughes, 1950*

Psychiatrists talk about depression as a central point from which to decide action, but there are a lot of gray areas—or rather, gray matters—in affairs of the mind. While figuring out whether you have a diagnosable disorder is important—"If you don't get the diagnosis right, you may not get the right treatment," warns Dr. Freeman—be cautious against pitting diagnosis against the weight of your own, and other human, experience. "Diagnostic codes started largely in response to the need to set standards for payments for certain kinds of treatments," says Dr. Freeman. "They've proven very useful for cost containment, but less useful for helping people. We've become so obsessed with diagnosis that we forget that there's a lot of human misery that falls outside of it that's still worth approaching." How you approach that misery depends on its character, and yours.

More and more studies of mood show that everyone has "mood cyclicity," times when you're up or down. There's little difference between the giddy, altered feeling you get from staying up all night and what a psychiatrist might diagnose as mild hypomania. The sadness that you move through after someone close to you dies, all too familiar to gay men (see previous page), may not be diagnosable depression; if you really are moving through the grief, rather than getting stuck in it, it's a healthy and necessary response. But it's still real sadness.

Having our moods cycle with seasons, too, from spring fever to the melancholy of fall, is also normal. But if you experience deep depression every fall or winter, you may not *be* sad so much as *have* it. Seasonal affective disorder (SAD) is a condition in which mood is connected with sunlight: the darker the season, the darker your mood. "There's a fine line between feeling whiny and confined in January and mild forms of SAD," says Dr. Freeman, "but even here in LA, where there's sun all the time, people suffer." Some people experience SAD when they move from a southern to a northern latitude, or when they move from an office with a window to one without. This is *not* demotion anxiety, but something significantly more enduring. "Generally, a diagnosis of SAD is made only after a patient has experienced seasonal depression for two years," says Norm Rosenthal, MD, senior researcher at the National Institute of Mental Health and author of *Winter Blues* (Guilford Press, 1998). Preferred treatment for the ailment is light, preferably a half hour or more in front of a light box. Though you can make one if you're handy, Dr. Rosenthal recommends you spend the couple of hundred dollars to order from an established company and spare yourself the power-tool anxiety. Stay about eighteen inches away (think makeup mirror, not interrogation room) and do it regularly each morning.

Depression and Anxiety

Everyone feels down, or anxious, or excited and jittery some of the time. The difference between an acceptable amount of any one of those moods and a diagnosable disorder is one of degree. Even diagnosable depressions have degrees. Dysthymia, for example, is a persistent low-grade depression where you can't seem to feel the same quality of passionate pleasure, excitement, or enthusiasm. "Everything's okay, but never wow!" says Dr. Winchel. A major depressive episode, by contrast, involves severe sadness, deep feelings of worthlessness, and extremely low levels of energy.

Early studies, many of which recruited gay men from bars, hospitals, or therapists' offices, found us to be more depressed than straight men. Later, more inclusive investigations tended to suggest another explanation: Bars can be depressing, and men who are in hospitals and therapists' offices need more care than those who aren't. "There is almost no credible, representative research comparing rates of depression and anxiety between gay and nongay men," says Robert Cabaj, MD, coauthor of *The Textbook of Homosexuality and Mental Health* (American Psychiatric Press, 1996). "What's clear is that, given the stresses we face, we're doing remarkably well."

The Three Major Mood Disorders

If you're not feeling so well, psychiatric diagnostic standards identify the symptoms of these three major mood disorders as follows:

DYSTHYMIA

It's pronounced "dys-THIGH-mee-a," and the diagnosis is made when your mood is depressed, most of the time, most days, for at least two years. Brief improvements are possible, but not for more than two months at a time. Also, at least two of the following symptoms must be persistently present: overeating or poor appetite, abnormal sleep (too much or too little), poor energy, poor self-esteem, trouble with concentration or making decisions, and hopeless feelings.

MAJOR DEPRESSIVE DISORDER

For you to be majorly depressed, you need to have some of the symptoms in the box on the next page. You need at least one from column A and three or more from column B, and you have to have each symptom for a minimum of two weeks before it "qualifies."

BIPOLAR DISORDER (MANIC-DEPRESSION)

The classic, movie form of mania has you feeling extreme euphoria or irritability followed by major depression (those are the two "poles" in question here). In reality, the episodes may be separated by years, or merge together so that you almost experience them simultaneously. The up periods may outnumber the down ones, or vice versa. Mania can be subtle and hard to diagnose. "For me it's like I can't finish an idea before another idea comes out," says Tom, twenty-nine, of his manic episodes. "I go to bed at two and wake up at five in the morning totally juiced. I painted my apartment in eighteen hours straight without stopping. But it all has an ugly edge: I get snappish, argumentative. I fight with service people. It's like I'm on a ride that's going so fast it's on the edge of being out of control." If this sounds vaguely like your friends on a Saturday night after a few lines of coke, there are definite similarities, except mania occurs without the powder, and you may not come down for days.

SYMPTOMS OF MAJOR DEPRESSION	
Column A (at least one of these)	**Column B (three or more of these)**
Persistent sadness Loss or very diminished capacity for interest, pleasure, or enthusiasm	Sleep problems (insomnia or increased sleep)
	Unexplained fatigue
	Poor concentration/memory/capacity to think
	Severe self-criticism, feelings of worthlessness
	Change in rate of activity: slowing down of mental and physical activity, or physical agitation
	Significant change in appetite/weight (decrease or increase)
	Frequent thoughts of life not being worthwhile, indifference to one's own death, or thoughts of suicide

Medication, therapy, or some combination of the two can help you move toward a more optimistic state of being. New generations of medication, in particular, have helped free people from the vise of depression without the debilitating side effects associated with many of the antidepressants of the past. For more on this new generation of drugs, read on.

Psychotropic Medications

You know, for fifty years I've been on testosterone shots; those helped me with sexual desire, but not with erections. It was not until this year, when I took Prozac, that the self-hate went away, and that's what really made the difference for me. I didn't even notice it was going, and then I realized, "I'm feeling good." Isn't that strange? It was the first time in sixty-seven years that I remembered feeling that good.

I refused to go on medication for a long time, for all kinds of reasons, the major one being an activist reason. I'm not going to take a pill to make me more manageable to the rest of the world so that they can feel better about sitting idly by while all my friends die. I'm going to be as crazy as I need to be to get through this.

It was experiments with LSD—in the lab, not the Haight—that were among the first to give researchers a sense of how certain drugs altered the function of the brain. If introducing this drug could cause hallucinations and strong feelings of reality in research subjects, the reasoning went, then perhaps the blunders of the brain—depression, anxiety, and psychosis—could also be chemically altered. Neuropharmacological lore says it was at a fifties cocktail party (a more common approach to mood altering) that two researchers in conversation stumbled onto the theory of how LSD worked by increasing levels of a chemical called serotonin to alter the mind's experience of mood and thought. Sometime around the same period, residents of a tuberculosis asylum in the South were given an experimental new TB medication that coincidentally boosted serotonin levels. Not only did it help their TB somewhat, but a few weeks later a number of them seemed a lot happier while they coughed. Presto—medical psychopharmacology was born.

Technology, and scientific understanding of the brain, have come a long way since the fifties. Today, science has identified serotonin and some five hundred other chemicals as neurotransmitters, substances that carry messages from one part of the brain to the other. With the exception of Viagra (see "Erection Solutions," in Chapter 4) and AIDS medications, many of the defining drugs of our era—the diet drug combo fen-phen, the "designer drug" Ecstasy, the antidepressant Prozac, the antianxiety drug Zoloft, and the rave party favorite LSD—are those that boost serotonin levels in the brain. Dozens of other medications work to increase or inhibit levels of serotonin, norepinephrine, and other neurotransmitters, combating depression, eating disorders, obsessive-compulsive disorders, and a range of other psychic problems.

At the same time, the embarrassment that keeps so many of us from medication suggests that no matter how far we've come in terms of high-tech brain scans, our minds may still retain images of the picture-perfect cheerleaders we were "supposed" to be. Of the estimated 17.6 million Americans suffering from depression, only one-third get treatment. "I've had a much harder time admitting I'm on an antidepressant than that I'm gay or have S/M fantasies," says John, thirty-five, who uses the norepinephrine and serotonin booster venlafaxine (Effexor) to cope with his anxiety and depression. "I feel so much better, but worry that I and everybody else can't be sure what's me and what's the drug." This Stepford-wife anxiety is echoed by Tom, thirty, a writer from Boston, who feared that going on antidepressants would render him a "happy droid."

Ron Winchel, MD, the New York City psychopharmacologist (that's what they call psychiatrists who know a lot about treating mental conditions that respond to medications), sees the resistance as another version of our failure to take a holistic approach to medicine. "The conventional view is that problems of the body should be treated purely through the body, and problems of the mind purely through the mind," says Winchel. "But in a scientific age when all activity—thinking a thought, buying a shirt, getting horny, accessorizing that outfit—can be shown to be mediated through certain physical transmissions in the brain, the mind-body split is no longer a viable distinction."

Nor, says Columbia University researcher and therapist Alex Carballo Dieguez, Ph.D., is it necessary to separate medication from other forms of psychotherapy, to believe that taking a pill means giving up on exploring the causes of your difficulties. "Medication may bring you to a level where you can *start* working on that kind of exploration," says Carballo Dieguez. "If you're so depressed that you're thinking of jumping out a window or have an anxiety attack every time you get out of bed, it can be hard to get anywhere in therapy." Just because you pay a visit to a psychiatrist doesn't mean every unhappiness and tension will, or should, be addressed by a pill. "Most depressed people can benefit from an initial psychiatric evaluation to find out if they have treatable depression," says Dr. Winchel. "In many cases, though, you'd do better to continue your work with a therapist, whether that's a psychiatrist or a different kind of counselor."

For all the fears of Prozac in the water supply, your doctor may actually be unlikely to prescribe it. Particularly if you're facing other kinds of illness (see "HIV, Depression, and Medications," page 488), internists and other doctors can wrongly attribute mental distress to your physical ills. Counselors or therapists who are not psychiatrists are often reluctant to recommend treating with psychotropic drugs. If one of them suggests you look into medication, you really should do so.

FINDING DR. RIGHT (TAKE III): PSYCHOPHARMACOLOGISTS AND HOW TO FIND THEM

Any medical doctor can prescribe medication, and this is often the easiest and least expensive route. "If you have a straightforward episode of major depression [see "Depression and Anxiety," page 482], there is about a 60 percent chance that any randomly selected antidepressant given in the proper dose will help," says Dr. Winchel. How best to adjust the dose, and figuring out ways to manage side effects, however, are questions some general practitioners are less comfortable answering. Even psychiatrists may be more or less familiar with nuances of medications depending on their training. "Psychopharmacologists are a little like caribou, herding primarily along the watering holes of large coastal cities," says Dr. Winchel. Happily, the same can be said of many gay men, though finding a gay psychopharmacologist in rural areas or midwestern states can prove difficult.

Organizations like the Gay and Lesbian Medical Association (www.glma.org) can help, and your doctor's understanding of sexual orientation is less important here than with a therapist. "So long as you feel like they respect you, will care if you no longer get a hard-on, and know about other side effects, it probably doesn't matter if they're gay," advises Winchel. If you have no idea how to start finding a psychopharmacologist, try calling the nearest large university-affiliated medical center and ask for the department of outpatient psychiatry. For certain conditions, such as obsessive-compulsive disorder or manic-depression, patient groups also maintain Web sites and clearinghouses for useful information.

Psychotropic Medications: How Long Do They Take?

I've been on Prozac, Klonopin, which is a benzo, Paxil, Zoloft, then off all that and on Effexor, Effexor with Wellbutrin to boost it, and then lithium with Wellbutrin, then lithium and Wellbutrin with desipramine, which is an older drug. And desipramine worked. There was a black and white change. I was still tired, but that gnawing anxiety that would send me crying as I walked down the street, it just went away. I've had occasions where I weakened the medication, and it came flooding back.

It was actually pretty simple—no side effects, little hassle, and a lot more days when I felt relaxed enough to engage with life. I was still myself, just more relaxed and optimistic.

One of the things to remember about psychotropic medications is that they aren't generally fast-acting enough to give you any kind of buzz or fast relief. While some anxious states can be relieved from the first dose, many antianxiety drugs can take three weeks or more to be fully felt, and the same is true for antidepressants. "In the MTV, digital age, we're not used to something taking six or eight weeks to evolve," says Dr. Freeman. "IV antibiotics can seem like a magic bullet against infection and leave you feeling better the next day, but this is more like planting a seed. You need to wait for a while for the result to appear, and it continues to grow." One University of Pennsylvania study divided those who didn't respond to Prozac after three weeks into two groups. Researchers doubled the dose for half the nonresponders, and left it the same for the others. At the end of another five weeks, both groups were experiencing the same amount of benefit. The moral? "Stick with it for at least three weeks," advises Dr. Freeman. "If you're feeling any benefit at all, stick with it for three more." If you're not feeling anything after a month and a half, you need a change.

CLEAN, SOBER, AND MEDICATED?

Those of us who have been addicted to alcohol or drugs can find something frighteningly familiar about the idea of taking a pill to make us feel better. In the old *Valley of the Dolls* days those fears were well-founded, though antidepressants today give you neither a buzz nor a habit. "Have you ever seen anybody selling Prozac on the street?" asks Dr. Winchel. Antianxiety medications can be a different story—if you've been addicted to alcohol, you may be particularly vulnerable to dependency on antianxiety drugs in the benzodiazepine family, so make sure you discuss the options with your doctor. If you do use benzos, try some of the slower-acting drugs such as clonazepam (Klonopin) and oxazepam (Serax) before the faster-acting diazepam (Valium) and alprazolam (Xanax). Buspirone (BuSpar) is a nonaddictive antianxiety pill with what Dr. Winchel calls "amazingly few side effects." The downside? "It's also not terribly effective in many people," says Winchel.

If you are in recovery and need to take antianxiety pills, take them consistently. Though it's counterintuitive, you're less likely to develop psychological dependence if you take pills on a regular, scheduled basis rather than if you just pop one when you want to feel better. It also takes lower doses of something like Valium to prevent a symptom than to treat one. And remember, so long as you're working closely with a doctor, taking prescribed medication may be a way to help you stay sober. "The self-prescribed drugs I used were to make myself blind to reality," says George, forty-two, who reluctantly began antianxiety drugs ten years after giving up alcohol and drugs. "The prescribed drugs help me deal with reality, to see it more clearly." Joe Amico, M.Div., executive director of the Pride Institute, a gay-specific drug and alcohol treatment center in Minnesota, estimates that as many as 80 percent of the men leaving treatment have found it useful to be on antidepressants. Both because they are prescribed medications and because they provide no discernible high, neither these patients nor professionals regard this as a "slip" from sobriety.

As for ending psychotropics, don't rush to do so the moment you feel better, and see a doctor before you stop. "An effective course of antidepressant treatment should generally run a minimum of nine to twelve months after you no longer have symptoms to avoid the risk of relapse," says New York City psychiatrist Beth Gery, MD. With the exception of sleeping pills and antianxiety medications, psychotropic drugs are not addictive, and even the dependency-inducing drugs vary widely in the amount of dependency they foster. Many psychotropics, though, can cause some physical symptoms if you stop abruptly, with the older tricyclic medications causing particularly severe, flulike symptoms. Even newer antidepressants often cause fogginess or some physical side effects. These are likely to be most severe in the week after you stop, but may continue for several more. In general, tapering your dose, the same way you started, is best (see "Side Effects of Psychotropic Medications," below).

Side Effects of Psychotropic Medications

Man's mind, as you know from trying to understand your boyfriend's or your own, is a complicated thing. And as it turns out, changing chemical activity in your brain to make yourself feel less depressed or anxious may also result in some less desirable changes. The sad truth is that anxiety, sex drive, and orgasm appear to use some of the same chemical transmitters in the brain, so getting rid of the bad may mean decreasing the good. The newer antidepressants, particularly those known as the selective serotonin reuptake inhibitors (SSRIs), can be tough on sex drive or orgasm. Picking your side effect, in fact, often determines which of many available antidepressants to try first. "Prozac, for example, tends to be somewhat stimulating, so it's good with someone whose depression makes them slow or lethargic," says Dr. Gery. "If someone has the agitated, anxiety-ridden variety of depression, another drug is better."

The two most important things to remember about side effects are that the most physically disruptive ones tend to get better, and that after a certain point it's better to switch than fight. "Generally, you tend to get all the side effects in the first three weeks, and all the benefits in the next three weeks," says UCLA's Dr. Freeman. "Here in LA, where people are very favorably inclined to natural methods and very side-effect-averse, I'll get calls at the first tremor or hint of nausea, with people saying, 'It's toxic! It's toxic!' So I start with the smallest possible dose, tell them to take it for three or four days until there are no side effects, then up the dose again and do the same."

For the record, few side effects associated with psychotropics are known to be dangerous. (If you get a rash or start wheezing, those could be signs of a serious allergic reaction, and you should get to a doctor.) Many, however—such as the sexual ones, which unfortunately prove among the longest-lasting—are seriously irritating.

A slow build to the therapeutic dose, the amount of a drug that makes you feel better, is designed to diminish side effects. A certain amount of adjustment up or down within that range is also common as you and your doctor work to find the point where the benefits are strongest and the adverse effects least noticeable. If you're finding the effects hard to get through, there are also other, more active ways of diminishing the downsides. A few possibilities:

- *Change the time of the day you take the medication.* Reasons to take a drug at a particular time are not always cast in stone. If a medication inhibits sleep when you take it at night, you may be able to shift it to morning. If something makes you feel nauseated for the first few hours, you might do better by sleeping through those effects. Discuss all such shifts with your doctor.
- *Use another medication or complementary treatment.* It may seem annoying, or expensive, to balance one pill or treatment with another, but it can help give a certain medication the opportunity to work. Using sleep medications to counter the sleep-inhibiting effect of another medication may work; so can combining two low doses of different antidepressants. Again, you can only do this with a doctor, which is why you want to see someone who knows what's up with side effects. The herbaceutical ginkgo biloba (see "How Does Your Garden Grow?" on page 317), the amino acid arginine, and the pharmaceutical sildenafil (Viagra) may all help with erection problems, while pilocarpine (Salagen) can help with dry mouth.
- *Change doctors.* Switching prescribing psychiatrists is easier than changing regular therapists, since your interactions with the former group of doctors tend much more toward "How does this pill make you feel, and how are you finding it?" than "Start at the beginning and tell me everything." If your doctor does not seem to care about consistently uncomfortable side effects, or has not discussed the problems with you to your satisfaction, consider changing.

HIV, Depression, and Medications

My psychiatrist gave me Halcion to sleep at night, and I'd wake up in the morning feeling fresh and rested. Then my regular doctor changed my HIV medication, and everything changed. I woke up feeling dazed, looked like a zombie. Within a week, I could hardly move.

Once I started antidepressants, I thought, What on earth did I think I was waiting for? This is so helpful.

For medicines to work, they need to be present enough in your blood to be effective, and not so present that they're toxic. The body maintains this balance by metabolizing all the medications you put in your body, often getting rid of the excess through the action of enzymes in the liver. While pharmaceutical drugs are tested individually to ensure correct levels of metabolism, things get more complicated when you mix them. Some HIV drugs and antidepressants, just like some recreational drugs and protease inhibitors (see "Drugs in Partyland," page 263), are a bad mix.

At issue is where in the liver the drugs are metabolized. Ritonavir (norvir), for example, inhibits several liver enzymes important for clearing many psychotropic drugs out of the body, including fluvoxamine (Luvox), nefazodone (Serzone), fluoxetine (Prozac), sertraline (Zoloft), carbamazepine (Tegretol), alprazolam (Xanax), triazolam (Halcion), and many others. Take one of these with ritonavir over time, even a short time, and you may experience intense buildup of the psychotropic, resulting in increased side effects, or worse. While some psychotropics can be metabolized through other pathways if one is whacked—"We've had some positive experiences using Serzone and anti-HIV drugs," says Dr. Freeman—coordination must be careful. If you have both a primary-care doctor and a prescribing psychiatrist, make sure they speak to each other whenever you change a medication. If you're using only a primary-care doctor, make sure he or she is familiar with the latest interaction data, and double-check with your pharmacist. "My doctor is so used to writing me out prescriptions that he wrote one out for sleeping pills without a thought," says Carlton, thirty-two, a policy analyst from Atlanta who's on a cocktail of five different HIV drugs. "It was the pharmacist who told me they have a potentially deadly interaction."

On the other hand, don't mistake depression—frequently experienced by people with HIV—as a necessary part of living with the virus. "Doctors often look at someone experiencing all the symptoms of depression—loss of appetite, lethargy, difficulty sleeping—and say it's the effect of the HIV," says Judith Rabkin, Ph.D., a Columbia University researcher who's done extensive research on depression and HIV-positive men. "It's not the virus, it's bad diagnosis. Even if the depression has a physical cause, such as low testosterone, it can be treated."

THE SIXTY-SECOND SHRINK

Looking for that final bit of bitchy ammo to fling at your boyfriend? Want to keep pace with your friends or your therapist? Although there are hundreds of diagnoses of mental problems, the most prevalent can be listed in a few major categories. Since new drugs—or new understanding of old ones—are frequent, check with a current information source or a doctor for the latest take on these conditions and medications.

Condition	Among the classes of medications used to treat it	Generic and brand names of some common medications	Common side effects
Mood disorders Depression is major, pervasive sadness; dysthymia is a prolonged, low-grade lack of pleasure (see "Depression and Anxiety," page 482).	Selective serotonin reuptake inhibitors (SSRIs)	Fluoxetine (Prozac) Paroxetine (Paxil) Sertraline (Zoloft) Fluvoxamine (Luvox)	Less severe side effects than other antidepressants. May include delayed orgasm, decreased libido, erection problems, agitation, headache, insomnia, sedation, weight loss, or weight gain. When stopping, fogginess and upset stomach—as well as mental upset—can be common if dose isn't tapered.
	Monoamine oxidase inhibitors (MAOIs)	Phenelzine (Nardil) Tranylcypromine (Parnate)	These effective medications may have serious side effects, including possibly fatal fluctuations in blood pressure if combined with the wrong drugs or food, particularly aged meats, wine, cheeses, and a number of other antidepressants.
	Tricyclics (TCAs)	Nortriptyline (Aventyl, Pamelor) Clomipramine (Anafranil) Desipramine (Norpramin, Pertofrane) Doxepin (Adapin, Sinequan) Imipramine (Tofranil) Protriptyline (Vivactil)	More side effects than the SSRIs and fewer than the MAOIs: dry mouth, constipation, nausea, sweating, light-headed feeling, sedation, and sexual side effects. Use with caution if heart disease is present. Tapering doses is a must when stopping, to avoid flulike symptoms.
	Miscellaneous	Venlafaxine (Effexor)	Delayed orgasm, decreased libido, erection problems (infrequent), agitation, insomnia, sedation, weight change, increased blood pressure.
		Nefazodone (Serzone)	Sedation, nausea.
		Trazodone (Desyrel)	Sedation, hard-ons.
		Bupropion (Wellbutrin)	Insomnia, edginess, decreased appetite, headache.
		Mirtazapine (Remeron)	Dry mouth, weight gain, constipation, drowsiness, dizziness.
Bipolar disorder In manic-depression, you may alternate between feeling superhigh and superlow. It's often hard to diagnose.	Mood stabilizers (antimanics)	Lithium (Eskalith)	Lithium is used to treat the manic phase of bipolar disorder; antidepressants, in combination with lithium, treat the depressive features. May be used in low doses, so side effects may be absent or mild. Possible side effects: increased urination, tremor, nausea, weight gain, poor coordination, sun sensitivity.
		Divalproex (Depakote)	Sedation, nausea, weight gain, liver toxicity.
		Carbamazepine (Tegretol)	Nausea, sedation, anemia.
		Gabapentin (Neurontin)	Usually well tolerated. Side effects include sedation and light-headedness.
		Lamotrigine (Lamictal)	Sedation, light-headedness, rash.

Condition	Among the classes of medications used to treat it	Generic and brand names of some common medications	Common side effects
Schizophrenia A general name for psychotic disorders that are marked by delusions, hallucinations, paranoia, withdrawal, and detachment. There is often a family history of the disease, which usually emerges between the ages of fifteen and thirty.	Antipsychotics	Risperidone (Risperdal) Olanzapine (Zyprexa) Clozapine (Clozaril)	Abdominal pain, agitation, dizziness, sexual dysfunction, sleep changes, vomiting, weight gain, and others.
Generalized anxiety disorders Can include a generalized, profound sense of worry about the details of life, or several specific worries, for a period of six months or more. Other, specific forms of anxiety disorder include those below.	Benzodiazepines	Temazepam (Restoril) Triazolam (Halcion) Alprazolam (Xanax) Chlordiazepoxide (Librium) Clonazepam (Klonopin) Clorazepate (Tranxene) Diazepam (Valium) Halazepam (Paxipam) Lorazepam (Ativan)	Short-term, the only significant side effect is too much sedation. When combined with alcohol, the alcohol is much more potent. Over time, effectiveness may diminish and dependency may develop. Tapering doses is often necessary when you stop. Failure to do so can result in seizures, anxiety, and insomnia.
	Miscellaneous	Buspirone (BuSpar)	Fewer than most, though may include tiredness, full-headed feeling.
Panic disorder Terror, helplessness, and heart-stopping, blood-chilling, absolute fear are all common features of panic attacks, which come out of the blue. Physical feelings may include light-headedness, palpitations, flushing, choking, churning stomach, and racing heart. Agoraphobia—fear of big open spaces, bridges, tunnels, lobbies, movie theaters, buses, subways, and any other public or crowded places from which escape might be difficult—is common.	Benzodiazepines Selective serotonin reuptake inhibitors (SSRIs) Monoamine oxidase inhibitors (MAOIs) Tricyclics	(see "Mood Disorders" and "Generalized Anxiety Disorders," in this chart)	Benzodiazepines work rapidly and effectively against anxiety, but there is a high risk of relapse when they are discontinued, and little data about their long-term effectiveness. Antidepressants take longer to work but have better long-lasting effects and make eventual successful discontinuation of medication more likely.
Obsessive-compulsive disorder (OCD) Do you wash your hands over and over again or vacuum the carpet multiple times in a day? Do you feel the need to go back and check to make sure the stove's off or the door's locked, not two or three times, but ten or fifteen? These are some common examples of obsessive-compulsive behaviors, which keep you repeating the same act or rehearsing the same worry over and over again. A special variety for gay men can take the form of HIV phobia, the persistent worry that you've been infected in extremely unlikely ways (paper cuts, walking on the steam room floor, etc.), repeat HIV testing, and constant doctor's visits.	SSRIs, possibly in combination with benzodiazepines	(see "Mood Disorders and Generalized Anxiety Disorders," in this chart)	*Source: Ron Winchel, MD*

Suicide

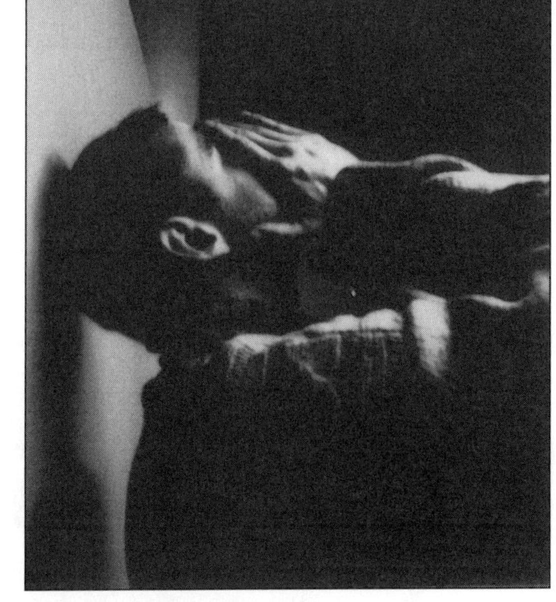

Last June, on Flag Day, I took fifty Fiorinals. All of my closest friends were dead, I couldn't get a decent job to save my life, and I was sleeping with someone who had a lover who was sexually dysfunctional and was only with me because he wanted to bust a nut with other men. He knew I was in trouble, since he had hidden the pills. But then he got up to pee and I found them and took them. All I remember from the emergency room is the doctor asking me why I had fifty Fiorinals to take, and me reciting the courage speech from The Wizard of Oz.

The guy we all worried about in college, the one who was totally depressed and mused aloud about the toxic potential of chemicals in the lab and refused to go to counseling even as his mood grew worse and worse, he never did it. But a few weeks later, another friend did actually kill himself. He was a sweet guy, no chip on his shoulder about anything, good grades, lots of friends. One day while on a trip with the glee club he started to babble crazy stuff. They brought him home to his parents, who made an appointment for him to see a shrink the next day. His father left him for a moment. He grabbed a big kitchen knife and plunged it into his chest.

An unimaginable prospect for many, suicide is a cherished option or a necessity for a few. Contrary to the myths, all kinds of people, with all kinds of coping skills, may decide to take their own lives. Though many more people try than succeed, an estimated 90 percent of people who kill themselves have a definable psychiatric syndrome. Gay adolescents make more suicide attempts than straight peers, though adult gay men don't seem to. For those who do, says Ron Winchel, MD, "suicide isn't a mystical experience or the careful conclusion of a reasoned discourse. It's an attempt to escape something unbearable that assumes no other solution. To the person with the hopeless melancholia of a suicidal depression, it's as logical as pulling your hand out of a flame."

Even if you're not deadly certain that you want to kill yourself, entertaining the notion can still be a warning sign. "Virtually everyone has some thought of suicide at some point in his life," says Herbert Hendin, MD, medical director of the American Society for Suicide Prevention in New York City. "If the thoughts don't seem fleeting, though, or if you're returning to them and filling in details about how you might do it, that's the danger zone."

If You're Feeling Suicidal

If you have thoughts of suicide, here are some of Dr. Hendin's suggestions:

GET TO A PROFESSIONAL

Seek professional help; use a friend to help you get it, if necessary. "Often, intense depression makes you feel unable to cope with anything, including self-care," says Dr. Hendin. "Getting a friend to go with you to a counselor, or to help you make a first call, can break the impasse." Don't just talk to the friend and leave it at that, though. "Even suicide hot lines, where there are trained counselors, may have a hard time assessing someone over the phone," says Dr. Hendin. "Going to see someone with a lot of experience working with suicidal depression—or better still, someone with experience in working with gay men with suicidal depression—is strongly advisable."

REMOVE THE MEANS

"The seriously depressed people who want to keep the gun in the house are those most likely to want to use it," says Dr. Hendin. If you have teased out ways you might commit suicide, try to get rid of the means, whether it's a gun or that extra bottle of sleeping pills you've been saving. Or get a friend to do it for you. Again, you may not be able to handle it alone.

If You're on the Receiving End of a Call for Help

"Sorting out the pain from life itself can be extremely difficult for suicidal people," says former GMHC coordinator of mental health services Maryann Kenney, "but they will often share some part of their confusion with a friend." If you're that friend, it's important to do a few things:

LISTEN QUIETLY AND CALMLY

"If someone's mentioning it to you, they're opening a line of communication you want to take advantage of," says Kenney. "Pay attention even to indirect comments, such as 'I should just give up' or 'This is no way to live.'" Rather than convincing them that they have much to be thankful for, see if you can ask them questions that determine their level of intent. "Ask them straight out if they're serious, if they have a plan, or the means to put it into practice," says Kenney. "In addition to offering a way to talk about the unspeakable, you'll be gathering information about how close to really doing it the person seems."

CALL FOR SUPPORT

A number of suicide prevention centers, including at least one in every state, maintain twenty-four-hour free hot lines (some are listed in Appendix A, page 581). Every hospital emergency room has a psychiatrist on call, as do many crisis intervention centers. If the threats of suicide seem at all real, no matter how vaguely articulated, really try to get the person help in evaluating their situation. If they won't call a trusted counselor—whether a local therapist or an AIDS or crisis hot line—you can.

TWO'S COMPANY

If you're in the room with someone you think is seriously suicidal, don't leave them alone, even for a minute, and get them to a hospital. Many suicide attempts can happen extremely quickly, and the suicidal person needs your presence. "It's like the pain of being alive is this impossibly heavy weight you're carrying, and you need somebody to carry it with you, because otherwise you're going to put it down," says Paul, forty-four, who attempted suicide twice in his twenties. "If someone tells you they have the means and the intention of killing themselves and you're not with them," says Kenney, "call 911 for them. Don't worry about offending or upsetting them; they're already upset." It's common to worry that you've betrayed your loved one by calling the police or alienated them with a long wait in a less-than-perfect hospital emergency room. "But this *is* an emergency," says Dr. Winchel. "And being dead is about as alienated as you can get."

Ending Therapy

If ending therapy seems to follow naturally after a discussion of suicide (see above), you're probably not ready to stop. The question of how to know when you're done with therapy is one of the toughest, notes Dr. Cabaj, who says "it's like how does an apple know when to drop from a tree?" Therapists, in general, can always see something else to work on, though they may not see their own investment as clearly. Just as you've invested feelings and attitudes and time in your doctor, he or she has an emotional—and financial—investment in you. "There's an old joke in medical school," says Dr. Freeman. "If you're the only knee specialist in town and someone comes in limping, you say, 'Take two aspirin and call me in the morning.' If there are four knee specialists in town, you say, 'Better do arthroscopy and physical therapy,' and who knows what else. It's a rare doctor who says, 'You know what? This problem seems bad to you now, but it will likely go away on its own. You don't need the kind of intervention I get paid the most for. Take an aspirin, have a massage. If it's still bad later, come back and we'll talk.'"

Even if you're sure therapy is crucial, a periodic check-in about whether you have met or maintained your goals is always in order. "If you start to think you're making a terrible mistake by leaving, or that you've failed in the therapist's eyes, that's a red flag that the therapist is overly invested in your continuing," says Dr. Hall. "You need to ask yourself what you're getting, and remember, you can always come back. Studies show that people who've had long-term therapy often go back three or four times in the course of their lives."

If you decide to end, most therapists advise a period of tapering down rather than the cold-turkey approach. "You know how they also say you get your greatest insight into yourself five minutes before the end of your therapy session? I had that experience as I was ending my five-year interaction with my therapist," says Benjamin, thirty-five, from Ann Arbor, Michigan. "The last three sessions were some of the most frank and insightful we'd had, and since we were ending, my therapist started revealing some things about himself and his feelings about our work together that I found totally surprising."

FURTHER READING

Corbett, Ken. (1999) "Homosexual Boyhood: Notes on Girlyboys," in *Sissies and Tomboys: Gender Noncomformity and Homosexual Childhood,* Matthew Rottnek, ed. New York: New York University Press. An academic exploration of some of the theoretical questions at the heart of the gender-identity question. For more on transgender issues, see Appendix B.

Hall, Marny. (1985) *The Lavender Couch: A Consumer's Guide to Psychotherapy for Lesbians and Gay Men.* Boston: Alyson Publications. The classic guide on finding a good therapist, pre–managed care but still timely.

Isay, Richard. (1996) *Becoming Gay.* New York: Pantheon. Thoughts on positive gay identity and the journeys we take to get there, from the doctor who helped psychoanalysis reframe its approach to gay development.

Jacoby Klein, Sandra. (1998) *Heavenly Hurts: Surviving AIDS-related Deaths and Losses*. Amityville: Baywood Publishing. Advice from one of the first therapists to begin AIDS bereavement groups.

Kabat-Zinn, Jon. (1995) *Wherever You Go, There You Are.* New York: Hyperion. One of the best books on the basics of Buddhist mindfulness, from the founder and director of the Stress Reduction Clinic at the University of Massachusetts Medical Center.

Norden, Michael. (1996) *Beyond Prozac: Brain-Toxic Lifestyles, Natural Antidotes, and New Generation Antidepressants.* San Francisco: HarperCollins. A discussion of various cures for the ills of modern living, including antidepressants, light boxes, sleep enhancers, stress reducers, and the "new" antidepressants.

Salzberg, Sharon. (1997) *Loving-Kindness: The Revolutionary Art of Happiness.* Boston: Shambhala Books. The loving-kindness meditation and many Buddhist basics, simply and beautifully explained.

Shernoff, Michael, ed. (1997) *Gay Widowers: Life After the Death of a Partner.* New York: The Harrington Park Press. Gay men who survived remember those who didn't, their own grieving process, and often, society's inability to respond.

CHAPTER 12

We Are Family: Friends, Long-Term Partners, and the Rest of the Clan

Friends over Time • Friend-Boyfriend Relations • Intimacy and You • Life Partners? • Dealing with Difference • Breaking Up Right • Domestic Violence • Family Ties • When Past Is Present: Incest • Parenting • Pet Projects

"Love makes a family!" read the sign that fluttered from the stage at the massive 1993 lesbian, gay, bisexual, and transgender march on Washington, DC. In an era when the concept of "family values" was being used to attack gay men, lesbians, single mothers, and anyone else who didn't fit the mom-dad-and-2.2-kids stereotype, it was a timely reminder, though probably news only to the White House, the Capitol, and some of the straight audience watching on TV. Most gay men and lesbians learn that lesson early, at the moment our families of origin step forward to support us, or when we choose to move away from them (or them from us) in search of people more able to accommodate our lives. Gay men and our friends have loved each other as family on our deathbeds and in regular beds, in living rooms and hospital rooms, throughout the life passages that so often—unlike the engagements and weddings and anniversaries and births of children and grandchildren of heterosexuals—pass unnoticed in any public way. That is changing, of course, with the marriage and "gayby boom" of the 1990s. Hallmark, though, hasn't noticed. And even most gay publications don't tend to run news of our commitment ceremonies, anniversaries, or adoptions.

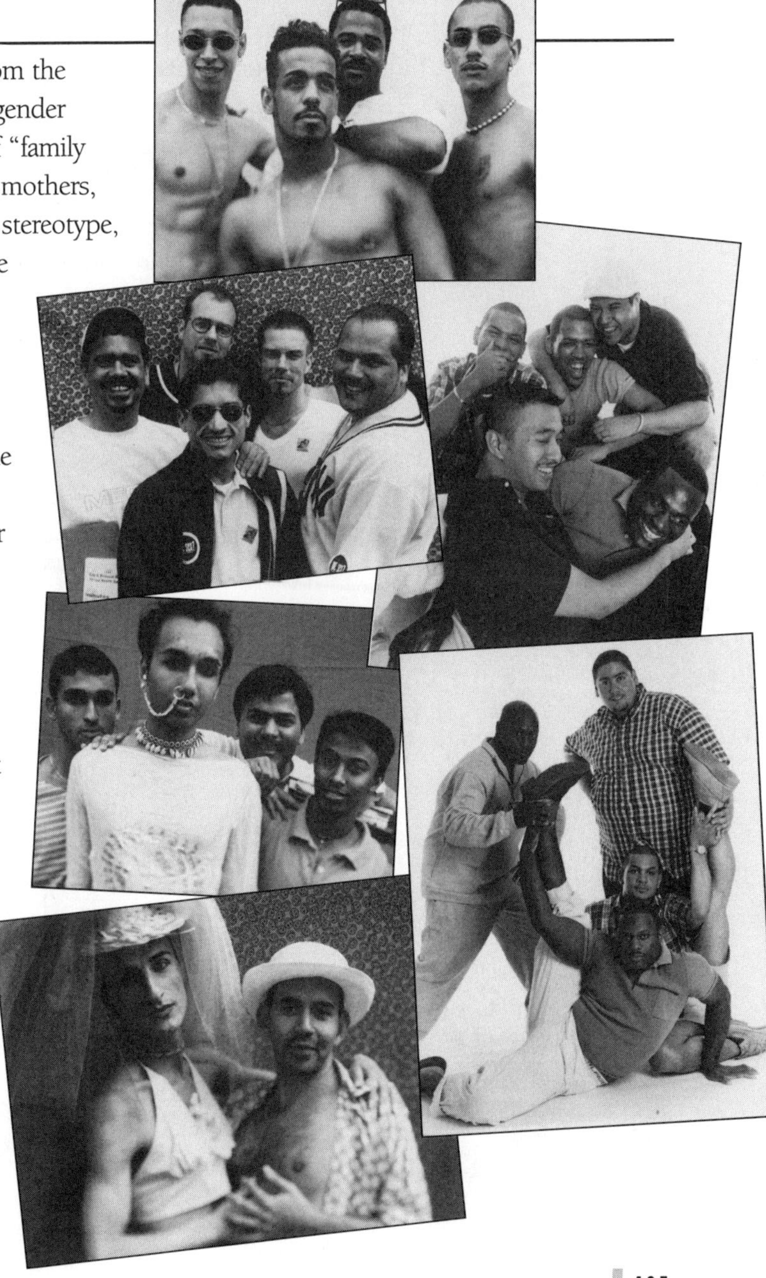

Still, you don't need framed wedding vows in the breakfast nook or a little one at home to have a family. For many gay men, the names we fill in on the "contact in case of emergency" form or enter into our wills are members of the groups that sociologist Martin Levine described as "remarkably stable networks" of friends where gay men feel "safe, comfortable and relaxed" over a period of years. Relaxed, at least, when a member of your dear "gay family" isn't working that last nerve only he or she knows just where to find.

Love does make a family. Yet love, as many of us know, is not enough to explain any important relationship. Many couples arrive in therapists' offices baffled about why they are having problems, since "we love each other so much." Parents who refuse to acknowledge our homosexuality often say it's because they "love us and don't want us to be unhappy." Spend a week at home, wherever and with whomever you make it, and you'll see that love and emotional support may make a family, but other things—what Levine identifies as "socialization, economic cooperation, social control, and sexual regulation"—are there, too. "My family? They're the people who know where I've been, including the bad places," says Jerry, fifty, who speaks to his family of origin in Idaho once a month or so but spends holidays and emotionally significant times with his New York friends. "There are the fun friends and the everything friends," agrees Tom, a publicist from Boston. "The everything friends are the inner circle, the ones I'll run out for at one in the morning or who can say, 'You know, you said you didn't want to do that anymore, and now you're doing it again.'"

FRIENDS OVER TIME: COULD THIS BE LOVE?

> Remember that who else but a bosom buddy will sit down and level
> Give you the devil, will sit down and tell you the truth?
> —*Jerry Herman, "Bosom Buddies," Mame*

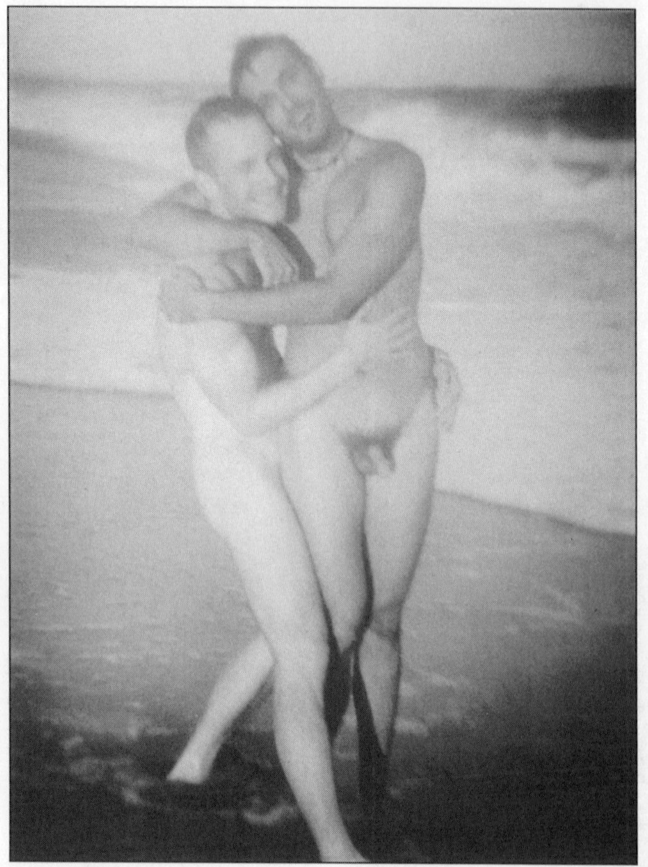

Theater fans still flush with pleasure remembering the duet "Bosom Buddies," originally belted out by two heterosexual women on the New York stage. As with so many of the camp classics favored by gay men across the ages (check out George Cukor's 1939 film *The Women*, and just *try* believing that the health spa isn't really a gay gym), the words in the mouths of babes and world-weary women alike seem also to be giving voice to words that gay men might say if the world allowed us to talk more freely. "Bosom Buddies" is a cherished tune to many of us whose truth-telling "sisters" come not from the womb, but from common experiences of coming out, going out, and hanging out over years and decades. If "sisters" sticks in your craw, call them your "girlfriends," your "brothers," your "posse," whatever. You know who they are. But do you give yourself credit for having stayed and struggled with them over the years? "Psychologists should really pay more attention to friendship," says Laura Pinsky, MSW, director of the Gay Health Advocacy Project at Columbia University. "Particularly since gay men and women are so much better at it than straight men tend to be."

Married to the Mob

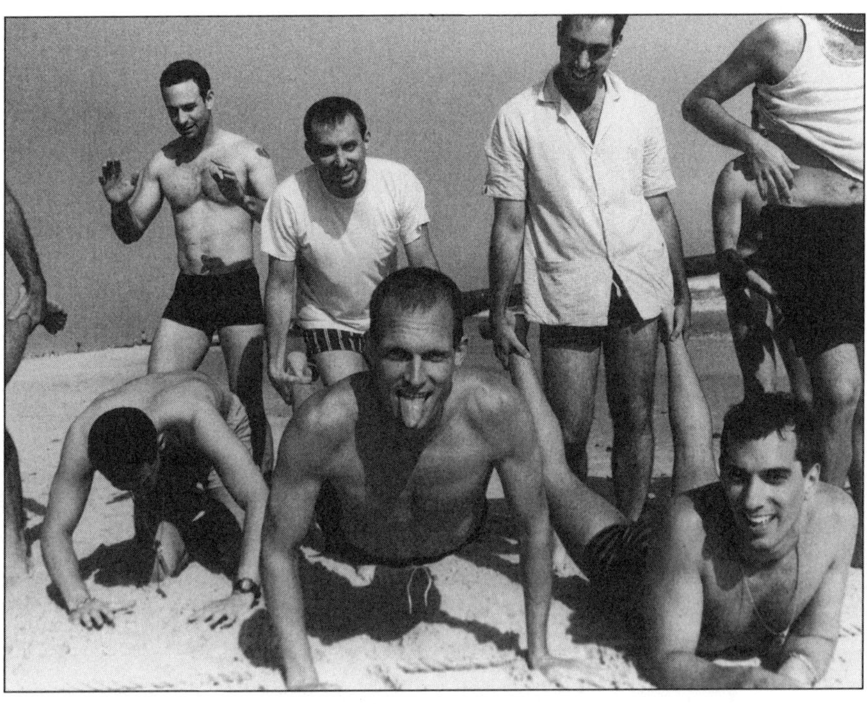

Every Valentine's Day we get together and watch horror movies. Fourth of July we have a picnic. We always celebrate our birthdays together. My birthday is right after Christmas, so I always go home to visit my family and leave right afterward so I can be with my friends for that. New Year's is a big deal for us. All seven of us have been together every New Year's for the last ten.

Don's an architect, and his boyfriend, Henry, is a psychologist. Shelby used to be in love with Don, but now it's he and I who spend the most time together. When Don's mother died, all of us went out to California for the service to be with him. Shelby lives in Henry's old apartment, and every Sunday for the last five years all of us have gotten together for what we call "family home evening," to watch videos and order in food. I used to choose the videos, until Don started complaining about my choices, which I thought was hostile, so I insisted he bring his own, which he'd started to do before I even asked. Last week's choice was abominable, I might add.

Everyone in our little group gets nervous when someone has a boyfriend, because it's like you suspect that he's going to leave the group, and that's what part of you thinks you should be doing. But now most of us have realized it's cyclical. When one of us complains about not having a boyfriend, the other will say, "Oh, please, next time you'll probably have one and some other of us won't."

Are you obsessed with the sweetness of wedding cake and the image of the couple on top? Why not stop to savor the flavor of what cultural studies professor Eve Sedgwick, Ph.D., calls the "nutty clusters," the complicated assortments of people and interconnections whose stories are often more intricate and interesting than the romance of a picture-perfect, classic couple. Sedgwick's analysis is drawn from readings of Charles Dickens and other Victorian literature, but as with much of her work, the lessons provide a framework for understanding the position of gay men at the dawn of the twenty-first century. Many of us in nutty clusters have, or have had, enduring, long-term relationships. But in these real-life fairy tales, romance is often just grist for the mill of memory and shared friendship, and happily ever after may mean living not only with the prince, but with all the other dwarves like yourself who have worked and cried and shared your life for years. "I like my boyfriends, but I think it's my friends who make me understand what it means to watch out for each other," says Neil, twenty-six years old, from Puerto Rico. "We keep a little black book at the top of the VCR at Judy and Louise's house, which is where we usually have sleepover parties. And whenever anyone says something particularly notable, we write it down, so that there's a record." Like many groups of friends, Neil's comes complete with favorite turns of phrase or private signals. "Like if you're talking to someone really boring at a party and you see one of your friends looking at you," says Neil, "you just casually rub the inside of your eye to say, 'I'm trapped.' Not necessarily for them to do anything. Just for them to know."

Lots of gay history is contained in such small gestures, or in the campy phrases only other friends of yours, or "friends of Dorothy," understand. Secret languages may sound sophomoric, but for many gay men they can also be about healing the high-school experience, replacing the burden of our secrets with the thrill of a private language shared by a small group to which we definitely belong. Richard Elovich, GMHC director of HIV prevention, sees the way groups of friends watch each other's lives as a powerful, underestimated force for gay male health. "Researchers seeking to improve productivity in American airplane factories in the 1920s discovered what they called the Hawthorn effect," he explains. "When they turned up the lights, people were more productive. Then they turned out the lights, and people were still more productive. Light, as it turned out, wasn't what made people do better: it was being watched, feeling like someone was paying attention. That's the role 'gay families' play for many of us."

John, thirty-nine, a comedian from Hawaii, describes his group of friends in ways that leave no doubt that though he's been single for years, he's definitely married—to the mob. "What's all this about 'family of choice'?" he asks. "We may have chosen in the first place, but boy, is *that* over. We're there like some strange group of relatives, together at holidays, weekends, special occasions, and day-to-day discussions of what we should eat, what so-and-so meant, or why one or another of us kept the other waiting. Even if some of us aren't getting along, we're together, for better or worse, in sickness or in health."

For sure. That's what family's for.

Friend-Boyfriend Relations

Well, when me and that man get to loving I tell you girls, I dig you but I just don't have time.

—Aretha Franklin, "Dr. Feelgood"

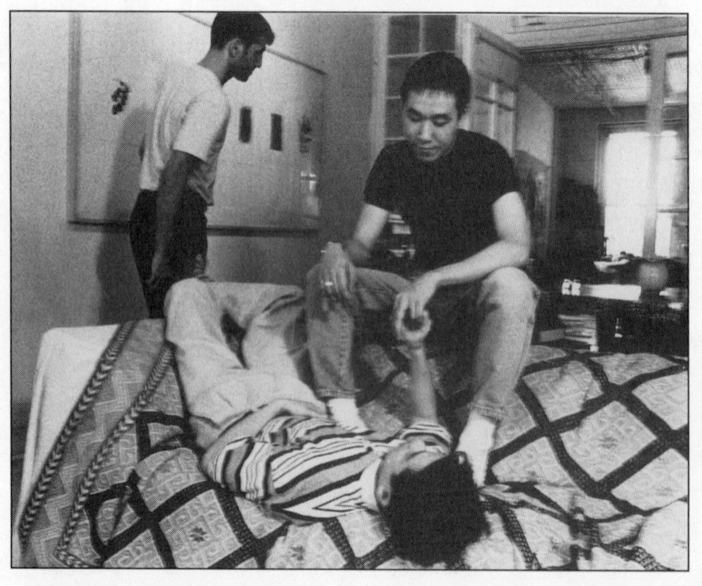

Deciding how or whether to blend friends and boyfriends is one of the perennial problems of being human. Straight couples may take "girls' nights out" or "bowling with the guys" as a matter of course, but what about when both of you want to be with the guys (or be the girls)? When do you spend time with your friends alone? For that matter, when do you spend time with your boyfriend alone, excluding the time in bed, to let emotional things develop? "I talk to a few friends every day, but I mean, those two would talk four, five, eight times a day," recalls Tony, twenty-nine, of his boyfriend, John, and John's best friend, Josh. "They were the lovers, really. I was the sex." Whether you even want your boyfriend to blend with your friends may vary from phase to phase of your life. "My friends and I talk a lot about finding a man who's 'portable,' whom you can take places without it being like, 'Oh, obviously I'm never going to be able to see anyone again as long as I'm with this person,'" says Tony. "At the same time, you want to know that you have a place that's boyfriend-free, where you can have some privacy."

How to blend friends and boyfriends successfully? Some tips from those who've tried:

If you're the one with the new boyfriend	If you're the friend
Coach him. "Before I introduced Tom to the guys, I made sure I took plenty of time to brief him," says Dean, twenty-nine, from St. Louis. "When he met them, he was able to honestly say, 'Dean has told me so much about you.' It helped ease the fears."	Support the new relationship. Unless he's involved with someone violent or harmful, give him some slack, advises Oak Park, Michigan, therapist Joe Korte. "Champion each other in trying new things, rather than slipping into a competitive, your-gain-is-my-loss mode."
Stand up to boyfriend bashing. "I had to ask several of my buddies to stop trashing Christian to me," says Mark, a forty-one-year-old dentist from Long Beach, California. "So what if he didn't know about gourmet food or classical music? He wasn't pretentious, which is what I found refreshing, and he was good to me."	Confront kissy face. "I can't stand being around two people who are cooey cooey smoochy smoochy all over each other," says Tim, twenty-nine. "Especially when I'm single. I told them, and they cut way back. We even all had a conversation about how their relationship had changed mine with Carl."
Two heads are better than one. "We refused to become 'glue sisters,' joined at the hip, and in the long run I think it helped us stay together," says Mark. "I know it helped my friends get used to him."	Stake your claim. "Until Ronny came along, Peter and I used to travel, hang out, everything. Suddenly it was like it never existed, so I asked Peter, 'Can we spend a week together, just the two of us, sometime?' Ronny was fine with it, much to my surprise. Peter and I had a great time, and I appreciated Ronny for being secure enough to step aside."
Easy on the criticism. "One of the most painful things about our relationship is the way that Mario criticizes my oldest and dearest friend," says Paolo, fifty-five. "He's 'unreliable,' he's 'inconsiderate,' even 'mentally ill.' It's not that it's not true. But what Mario doesn't realize is that Raoul is family, and that I could no more easily imagine life without him than without Mario."	Watch the "remember whens." "Sam loves to get together with all of us who went to college together to reminisce," says Larry, sixty-three. "But last time, after three hours of names he didn't know and reminiscences he didn't share, Sam's new boyfriend stormed out furious. 'You know what?' he shouted at Sam. 'Since you have so much to talk about, why don't you marry *them?*'"
Avoid cat's-away behavior. "When Don's boyfriend's out of town, suddenly he's available," says Roberto, twenty-two. "As if I don't notice that he's not returning my calls other times. How rude is that?"	Don't make him choose. "One friend in particular, one of my closer friends, is always leaving messages and inviting me to dinner without mentioning Jeff," says Ori, forty-two. "It's not helpful. He may not want to see him, but I wish he could leave it to me to be responsible about deciding when to go alone."

Intimacy and You

"How is so-and-so? Does he have a boyfriend?" goes the oft-repeated question. "Boyfriend?" comes the response. "You know he has an intimacy problem." Worse still is when you have that dialogue daily with yourself. "I feel this pressure," says Joseph, twenty-five, an administrative assistant in San Francisco. "It's like every time I meet someone attractive, I'm asking

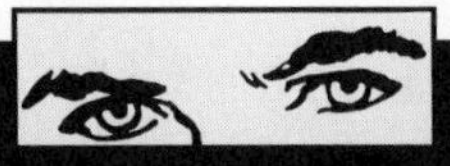

TURNING A GAY GAZE ON BITCHINESS

My best friend and I, we have this whole "ho'" routine going. He'll pull a quarter out of his pocket and I'll say, "Oh, is that your earnings from last night?"

We have names for everyone. I was seeing this guy named Terry Maymal, and he was hairy, so we called him Terry Mammal. This other one, Dimitri Halakitis, smoked, so we called him Dimitri Halitosis. The local gym, Better Bodies, we call Bitter Beauties. If you can't laugh at life, it laughs at you.

When people talk behind your back and you get worried, I don't think it's that you don't know what they are saying. I think it's that you know exactly what they're saying.

He is always such a bitch that we now call him Lady Miss C. And C does not stand for cute.

Cunty. Bitchy. Gay men tend to give their nastiest nature names that put the blame on women, but, darling, it has a lot more to do with you. Why gay men have made dishing an art form is open to more than one interpretation. Whether it's delightful or deadly probably depends on your mood. "There's the fun kind and the evil kind," says twenty-nine-year-old Tom. "Like when I called up my friend to tell him I'd broken up with Chester and he started in with the comments. I had to say, 'No, stop. Not this time. I'm not up to this.'"

At its worst, the bitter-queen routine can spring from self-defeat, an if-I-can't-be-happy-why-should-you-be kind of thing. At other times—and this is one place where gay men find a kinship with some women—it's a way of managing the pain of feeling powerless, an art form born of the knowledge that no matter what you do, you're still gonna be what you're gonna be. "At its most charitable, the bitchiness can be seen like an inoculation," says Philip Spivey, Ph.D., a New York psychologist who's worked with some of the most shade-prone youngsters at GMHC's young-adult program. "By cutting someone down to size, you make it so that when they go out into the world and hear those same things, it won't hurt so much." Still, says Dr. Spivey, most of the meanness is less therapeutic. "It's a pattern we learn in the schoolyard, from our fathers, wherever what I call 'gender betrayal' occurs," he says. "Gender betrayal is the lesson learned at a very early age that we need to fear other men rather than express love to them. And we give out what we get. If we get cruelty and humiliation and fear, that's what we deliver."

In GMHC's young-adult program, men practice what they call "shade reduction," reminding each other to ease off. It's an awareness not restricted to the young. Jeff, thirty-nine, a gay wag who can dish and diss with the best of them, when asked what advice he'd give about bitchiness to other gay men, pauses for a moment. "What do you mean, like how to do it?" he laughs. Then he reconsiders, hands flying for emphasis. "My closing-of-the-elevator-door advice? Use it sparingly, and don't let it use you." Spivey advises men he works with to try actively to counter familiar, negative patterns. "People say, 'I'll never find anyone to love, men are dogs,' this type of thing, and I ask them to think back to a couple of men in their lives they admired or trusted. Just as those men existed, there are others," he says. If you have yet to meet a man you admire, Dr. Spivey suggests a simpler exercise in the meantime. "Seriously consider who brings out the best in you, and who the worst. Then spend time with the people who bring out the best, whomever they are." In other words, there are times when C can stand not for *cunty,* but for *consciousness, calm,* and—oh, yes—*kindness.*

myself, 'Would *he* be a good boyfriend? Would *he?*' Underneath everything I do there's this refrain—'I don't have a boyfriend, so I must have a problem.'"

"Total intimacy—the state of being fully known—is a holy grail of the psyche," says Justin Richardson, MD, director of Columbia University's Center for Lesbian and Gay Health. "Even as we go on our search for total union, the fact that we are all individuals means we'll never quite find it." That doesn't mean you shouldn't look: "Striving for closeness and mutuality is one of the most—if not the most—gratifying pursuit of adult life," says Dr. Richardson. "But whether you have found 'the boyfriend' is not an effective yardstick of emotional health."

Measure instead how comfortable you are being known, in all your moods and feelings, by whomever you're spending time with. "If you say, 'I'm feeling really bad these days,' can that stay there for a while and be taken in by the person you're talking to, or is it a joke to be laughed away and *not* talked about?" asks Dr. Richardson. For all the talk of friends as good as gold and till death do us part, plenty of men feel like their friendships depend on things seeming golden, or on editing their bad parts so that no one sees them. Ironically, shadows are needed to give any picture definition. "If you aren't sure you feel known," suggests Dr. Richardson, "ask yourself what it is that you feel least comfortable revealing. Why is that you feel it's less desirable for *you* to reveal that part of yourself than when someone else does it?" What you're looking for is not someone who knows and understands everything—"that would be tyranny, not connection," says Richardson—but rather someone who allows you to feel comfortable enough to take risks and observe your own reactions. Did you smile when you said that sad thing? Do you feel scared after telling someone something personal? When do you feel like running away?

If this sounds less like a friend relationship than a shrink-to-patient one (see Chapter 11), Dr. Richardson admits to a belief in the healing, intimate nature of the psychotherapeutic bond. But you don't have to pay in order to play a therapeutic role for your friends, or have them play one for you. "Experiment with creating one authentic relationship, finding one person with whom you can strive to be honest and at times uncomfortable," suggests Richardson to those feeling intimacy-impaired. Be wary of the always-in-a-group-of friends pattern, or the weekend workshop that leaves you feeling really connected in the Sunday evening sharing circle and really at sea by Tuesday morning. "What you're looking for is a kind of consistency," says Dr. Richardson, "a length of contact with someone that allows you to follow your own process, or progress, like an unbroken thread."

And the next time someone asks if so-and-so has a boyfriend, there may be a different answer: "Not at the moment. But he seems well, and his friends are giving him good practice."

LIFE PARTNERS?

Love is not a feeling. Love is put to the test. One never says of pain, "That was not a real pain. It lasted for so short a time."

—*Ludwig Wittgenstein*

"Longtime companion" was the phrase used in obituaries to describe the partners of gay men who died before the *New York Times* would print the word *gay*. Today, when *lover* has appeared in the *Times* obituary section and *gay* appears regularly in headlines across the country, it

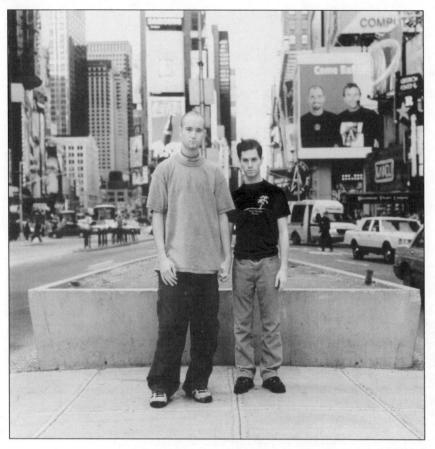

sounds especially out of sync with the times, though it's really only half wrong. *Companion* is too superficial for the deep love shared by men in a committed relationship. *Partner* sounds cold; *boyfriend,* trivial; *lover,* cheap. It is the *longtime* part of the equation—the changing way of loving and growing past old patterns into something new—that is the strongest test of love. Given that the number of famous living gay couples can be counted on one hand, longtime gay love is a work of heart rarely framed by the experiences of others. "I often hear that there are loads of long-term male couples. I don't know any," says Paul, a twenty-three-year-old student in Brooklyn, New York. "If I could get pregnant and settle down, I would. In the meanwhile, what I could use is some advice."

Couldn't we all? "When we were first together, we realized that much of the gay community viewed itself as a group of individuals, that everything seemed to be about cruising and singles," recalls Demian in Seattle, now entering his sixteenth year with his partner, Stevie. "We weren't doing that. What we needed help with was things like figuring out how to get insurance together for our apartment." And staying together. "If gay and lesbian couples had parents that remained married, we *might* have some idea of how to do it," says Demian. "But we're in a culture that seems to value serial monogamy, and have little skill in coping with stresses of work and culture. Gay men often don't even have the support of our parents. A lot of us have been divorced by them, too."

Demian and Steve did not go gently into singlehood. They responded instead by founding an organization, The Partners Task Force of Gay and Lesbian Couples, to provide others with some of the resources they couldn't find. Including a Web site (www.buddybuddy.com), booklets and videos with insights on same-sex coupling, lists of businesses that offer domestic partnership benefits, and lots of other resources, the Partners Task Force gets fan mail and requests for advice from gay men all over the world. "A *San Francisco Examiner* household-based poll found that a full 60 percent of gay men were in couples," says Demian, who has his doctorate in education and experience in conducting his own surveys for the task force. "Contrary to the stereotypes, the men surveyed by the *Examiner* were also more likely than lesbians to be in longer relationships." Committed as it is to countering the illusion of gay singlehood, many of the task force's 150 pages of resources are dedicated to this kind of information: essays, historical timelines, and photo galleries, as well as lots of support for the long-term goal of legalizing same-sex marriage (see "Get Me to the Church? Ways of Celebrating Your Commitment," on page 507).

"In the short run," says Daniel Garces, a therapist in Houston, Texas, "perhaps the best advice for couples is what Hendrix [Harville, the heterosexual couples counselor—not Jimi] calls a platinum rule of love: 'Do unto your lover as he would have you do unto him.'" That may mean buying Grape-Nuts even though you prefer Frosted Flakes, or making sure to keep the car clean even though you believe there are more important things to worry about. It may mean really stopping and thinking about your partner's sensitive points, the places where he needs help or the things that make him feel weak or insecure. What makes him feel cared about? How can you reach him on that level? "If he has an Achilles' heel, try to not use it to punish him," advises New York City therapist James Cassese. "Rather, see if you can protect that part of him, and take satisfaction in knowing that you won't go for his vulnerabilities in an argument."

Getting into his head, however, may require more work than you'd anticipated. You try to please him, and he freaks out. You need a shoulder to cry on, and he dispenses advice instead. You share something deeply important to you, and he greets it with monosyllables and turns on the television. It's all part of the challenge of the pretty little thing called love.

Change Is Gonna Come: Stages of Coupling

Stage theory is the fancy phrase for the idea, favored by psychologists and social scientists, that different phases describe the development of an individual, or a couple, over time. When it comes to gay men, these kinds of theories have often been used by psychologists to explain the way we're stuck, rather than the ways that we develop, but even broader-minded models may not capture your life's nuances. "Stage theory tends to assume that change is linear, that you finish one phase before starting another," says Barbara Warren, Psy.D., director of mental health services at New York City's Lesbian and Gay Community Services Center. "My suspicion is that it's less about evolving in one direction as cycling backward and forward, with a much less fixed time frame than most stage theories allow."

Still, if you and your partner think stage theory means the burning question of why Lorna Luft wasn't cast for the revival of *Cabaret,* it's probably useful to think about the ways in which change is gonna come. In the early 1980s, David McWhirter, MD, and Andrew Mattison, Ph.D., themselves a long-term couple, interviewed 156 gay men in loving relationships of one to thirty-seven years' duration. The book that resulted from this research, *The Male Couple* (Prentice-Hall, 1984), still cited as one of the best examinations of the phases of gay couplehood, outlines six stages:

• *Stage one: blending (the first year).* This is the "honeymoon" time, the lots-of-sex, lots-of-romance period where you feel that you're merging into one instead of two. You both long for each other and wonder when he'll call again, though you also are careful to stay "equal": spend equal time at each other's places, spend equal money, and so on. If striking that kind of balance scares you, or if you feel like you don't have enough to bring to the table, you may withdraw emotionally.

• *Stage two: nesting (second and third years).* Less sex, and more homemaking, are characteristics of this phase. Love may be blind for a while, but in this phase you look at his huge, kitsch reproduction of *The Last Supper* or the fact that he watches the news at 6:00 A.M. and think, 'I'm not sure I can live with that.' Sometimes you buy things together in this phase, and often you quarrel about what those things should be and how they should look. Differences in psychological tastes—what we are drawn to or put off by—also become an issue. When one of you wants to get back to the whispering-sweet-nothings of stage one, it's often with a new sweet someone who doesn't have so many opinions about your habits. In this stage, questions of jealousy and monogamy often arise.

• *Stage three: maintaining (years four and five).* The individuals "behind" the couple reappear: instead of just "we," there's you, him, and "we." Often you branch out, one of you doing some things without the other, taking on different responsibilities within the relationship and taking new risks outside of it. This is often the period when your family (or your partner's) draws close again, and when they get a realer sense of your relationship. It's also the time you tend to reveal your secrets, what you like and don't like about him or yourself. Sometimes the fear of being left is so strong and painful that you force the issue and leave yourself. Sometimes the conflict forces you to find ways to compromise to make the relationship stronger. This phase is when you need all the skills of conflict resolution you can muster (see "Fighting Fair," page 511).

• *Stage four: building (years six through ten).* If you've both made it this far, you have a greater sense of each other's dependability. Rituals whose regularity might have irritated you, such as eating at the same restaurant every Friday, may now seem solid, sweet, or at least something to accept. You know what he is going to say before he says it. As a result, you say less to each other and more to the outside world, often achieving greater financial stability, greater comfort in lifestyle, and increased productivity and independence. On the other hand, all that energy going outside the relationship can be threatening when one of you falls in love with someone else (that often happens in this stage), or when those arguments and their intense resolutions are replaced by neither of you even bothering to try to get into them.

• *Stage five: releasing (years eleven through twenty).* This often marks a big step: not the vows or "I love yous," but the merging of the bank accounts. In studies of gay men and lesbians, we tend to wait years longer than our sisters (that's our lesbian sisters) before we merge money. *Trust* is the word that summarizes this stage, with illusions and fantasies replaced by a sense of security about your current situation and a sense of loss about your potential. You're less worried about things disrupting the relationship and less worried about disrupting it yourself. For some, life gets boring: You're puttering around the house rather than reaching out to new friends, you sit through dinners with less to say, and you're probably (unless you got together at eighteen) beginning to face some of the questions of midlife, including the last-chance syndrome, which has you wondering if this is your last chance to find another partner or another life (see Chapter 8). Since nothing's wrong but you still feel restless, note McWhirter and Madison, "this stage appears to have more unpleasant features than some of the others."

• *Stage six: renewing (beyond year twenty).* This is the second honeymoon: a rejuvenation of the relationship with an emphasis on shared pleasures, tenderness, and a delight in looking back. Dissatisfactions in this stage tend to be more on the level of the individual than about the relationship: problems with aging, illness, and death of family or friends.

As with almost all research work on gay men, McWhirter and Mattison's work has been criticized for not being representative, although they never claimed it was. Few of the men they talked to were Black, three-quarters were called sissies growing up, and none of the couples was completely monogamous over time. It was also almost pre-AIDS, and the epidemic

THESE MAGIC MOMENTS

Stage theories such as McWhirter and Mattison's present carefully charted phases of development. Men who are together may remember them more as a series of distinct turning points.

- ***The your-friends-are-his-friends moment.*** "I knew things were fine when the next thing I knew, he and Duane and Charles were planning to go out on the Friday I was out of town on business."
- ***The visit-home moment.*** "He was the first man I'd brought home. I don't like the way I am with my family, or the way they are about my being gay, so it was a combination of exposing something intimate and embarrassing. Now I never go home without him."
- ***The monogamy moment.*** "When we had that talk, and decided to stay together through our differences, it felt so painful I couldn't sleep or eat. But I also think that was the discussion that has helped keep us together for fifteen years."
- ***The vacation-together moment.*** "We argued nonstop. All our control issues clashed. We had the discussion about opening our relationship in theory, and half an hour later I walked into the cabana to find him in our bed and a French surfer running out. When the vacation was over, so were we."
- ***The real-part-of-your-family moment.*** "My mother was going on about how she couldn't stand our wallpaper, and Henry just blew up at her. But she apologized, and they talked. It was gratifying, because it was like he was me."
- ***The debt-together moment.*** "Signing that big old loan for a house was more binding and serious than any vows. When Citibank says you're in it together, you're in it together, you know what I'm saying?"
- ***The I-can-take-care-of-you moment.*** "When my mother arrived on our doorstep in a state of nervous collapse, I thought I'd have one, too. Peter was wonderful, helping out and being kind and reminding me that all my life was not about my family's mental illness."
- ***The compromise moment.*** "I *so* did not want to move to that small town. There weren't good restaurants, there were no other Black people, I didn't like the house that much. But I did want to be with him. That's what primary relationship means to us: We come first and everything else is second."
- ***The public-acknowledgment moment.*** "Fifty of our friends and family raised their glasses and toasted our love together. My AIDS was a guest at the party, of course, but not too powerful of one. Then we left my parents and his sister in our house and went to a hotel, where the gay reservation agent gave us the honeymoon suite."
- ***The monogamy moment.*** Again. You only thought you had that conversation five years ago (see "Monogamy?" page 129).

has accelerated all kinds of developments even as it has shortened our lives. Still, it's a clear, comprehensive examination—and a view not seen too often—of the ways men make our lives together over a lifetime.

Harper Valley PDA? Public Displays of Affection

We were lying on the beach with our arms around each other. Now I admit Don was wearing one of those tacky thongs, but fashion don'ts are not against the law in Florida. A policeman came over and said to us, "You know, you can't do that here. This is a family beach." I thought, "If we'd been a man and a woman, that cop would have smiled at us and felt good." We got up and left.

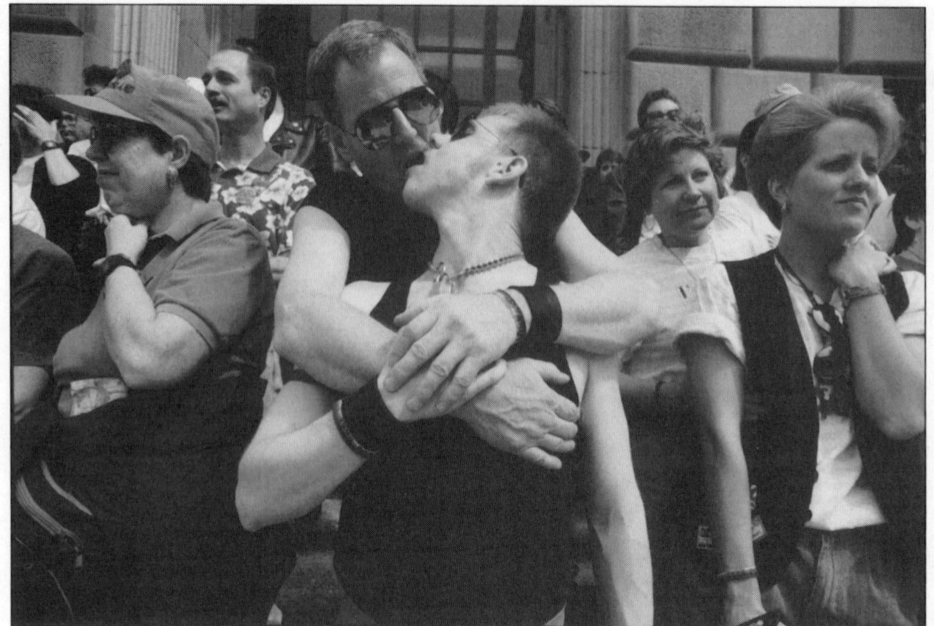

He took my hand the other day in the circus, but then when we went out and I put my arm around his shoulders, he froze. When it wasn't in the dark, it was a big deal.

Dateline *was doing a special on gay bashing, and the producer asked me and my boyfriend if we would stand on a busy street corner near campus and hold hands and kiss. I was wearing a hidden "hat-camera" and the producers were in a van nearby, watching everything. So David and I are standing there making out, and all these drunk college kids are streaming by and ignoring us. Finally one drunken guy stops. "Hey!" he slurs. "I want to tell you something." "What's that?" I said, stiffening. He got real close, jabbing his finger at us. "I just want to tell you," he shouted, "that I think it's great that you guys love each other like that!"*

Outside of four or five streets in gay America, slipping your hand lovingly into another man's means stepping into a zone where you may risk looks, nasty comments, or worse. While some Americans enjoy the idea that same-sex-loving men exist—"The tour buses now go by my building," says Martin, from Christopher Street in Manhattan, "so we made a sign that says 'Please Don't Feed the Queer'"—they're less enthusiastic about seeing that love made literal. "My father said he was fine with my being gay, so long as he never had to think about what we did in bed," recalls Adam, thirty-eight, the son of a ranch hand outside Tucson, Arizona. "It sounds reasonable until you realize that we're reminded of what heterosexuals do in bed every time we turn on the television or go to the movies or look at a billboard."

Some of us have decided that *PDA* should mean "please don't aggravate" the situation. You may be in a place where the small rainbow sticker on your car says enough. But thousands of us, and thousands who care about us, are choosing public displays of affection instead, deciding to take each other's hands on the streets, or in movie theaters, or in commitment ceremonies that make our love as lasting and honored (if not as legal) as the love of heterosexuals. "It was the first time our families had met," says Jerry, twenty-five, a restaurant maître d' who says his traditional black-tie-and-tails wedding festivities included a Hawaiian honeymoon and registering for china at the local Crate and Barrel.

If you're not into donning a tux or gown, there are other things you can do. "I'm so gay, I never realized that there was a whole wedding industry," recalls Ron, forty-five. "I mean, God forbid you shouldn't spend $500 on a cake." He and his lover, Roger, "surveyed the list of wedding requirements, took cake and flowers, and said, 'The hell with the rest of it.' We had people over to the garden, and read each other vows that we'd written. When I said I'd always love him, people cried. When I said I'd always make him late, they laughed. Then we all got drunk."

GET ME TO THE CHURCH? WAYS OF CELEBRATING YOUR COMMITMENT

- ***A private ceremony.*** "It's each other that needed to see and hear it," says Daniel, twenty-seven, an AIDS worker from Florida. "We wrote and read each other vows, and told each other how we wanted to grow old together, how we had never loved anyone like this. I think the fact that it was private made it more intense."
- ***An anniversary party.*** Deciding what your "anniversary" is may be the hard part. Stephen and Gerard count the first time they slept together, and marked twenty years with a church anniversary celebration. "This wasn't a commitment ceremony," says Stephen, "We were committed. This was about getting the Episcopal Church to say we recognize these two people are in a loving, supportive union and want to celebrate that."
- ***A housewarming party.*** This can be a light touch, marking a new stage without being a party that says you'll never part. "We added an element of surprise," say Peter and Bill in Lake Forest, Illinois. "Whatever the temperature was that day—you know, seventy-five degrees, eighty-two—you were supposed to dress like that's what year it was."
- ***Rings.*** "We haven't had a wedding," says Ronald, forty-five, "but we went to Zion National Park and saw some rings in one of those stands that sells rocks by the road. I said, 'Oh, we should get these,' and he said, 'Are we really ready for that?' But we were. And we've worn them, ever since. They show the world something about our connection, and the black shiny stone is just gay enough so that we don't have to feel like we're passing as straight."
- ***A shared ritual with other couples.*** This can be as flexible as you want, from a steps-of-the-Supreme-Court mass wedding protest to a less political exploration. "We decided to go to a weeklong couples workshop on the Big Island of Hawaii," says Dan, fifty, a jewelry salesman from Columbus, Ohio. "All of the couples were given an egg and asked to nurture it the same way we nurtured our relationship. Eric and I went to a secluded beach and laid the egg in a hollow, which we then sprinkled with flowers from our leis. The waves began to splash on us as the water filled the hollow, and slowly rolled the egg and the flowers out to the ocean. Holding hands, we felt that our love and relationship were now inextricably bound up with the sea, surf, and all of nature."

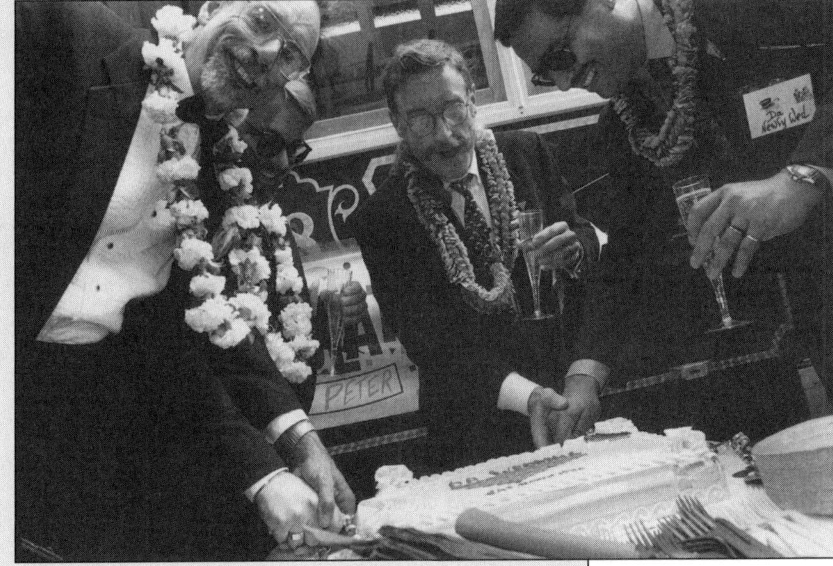

- ***An engagement.*** This strange heterosexual custom, a kind of marriage without formal bonds, suits some gay men perfectly. "Tim and I knew that we wanted to be partners for life, but we just weren't ready to move in together," says Ron, a thirty-three-year-old psychologist from Minneapolis. "He came up with the idea of becoming engaged. At first I thought it was hokey, but after a few days I really warmed to the idea. We printed up invitations and invited all of our friends and family to watch us swap rings."

GET ME TO THE CHURCH? WAYS OF CELEBRATING YOUR COMMITMENT (CONT.)

- *Wedding bells.* This can be as complicated as you want it, complete with seating charts, judges, rabbis, priests, and family. "We had a judge read from the vows that Christian priests used to celebrate same-sex marriages in the eleventh century," says Ron in San Francisco. "Roger's parents came, and we placed a special pane of glass in our bedroom window with an insignia for partnership." For George and Joe, from the Bronx, it was "chili dogs at the beach, thirty friends, and one of the sunniest, happiest days of our life."

Whether the ceremony need be a family affair is right up there with what you'll wear as one of the big questions. Forget the heterosexual worries, like which set of parents pays. The question is, will they come? "My mother kept asking why we felt the need to do this," says Stephen. "It was only after I got annoyed and asked, 'Why did you and Dad get married? Why did you want my sister to get married?' that she went quiet." At least she showed up. "Troy's father, who always asks what 'we're' going to do and when 'we're' going to buy a house, still doesn't know his son is gay," explains Perry, twenty-five, a fundraiser from New Jersey. "I know it's going to come around and bite the family in the ass, because his mother and sister came to the wedding and posed in all the pictures and videos and everything. They told the father they were going to a Broadway show. And now, every time I'm over for dinner, which is often, his mother grabs the glass of wine out of my hand and says, 'Watch yourself, you talk too much.'"

With so much trouble, wouldn't it be easier to skip the family frenzy? "If you're out to your family, I'd advise inviting them," says Ron, whose parents declined to attend. "If they don't come, that's their decision. If you don't invite them, you're closing a door on a part of your life that is one of the most important parts there is."

Same-Sex Marriage and the Law

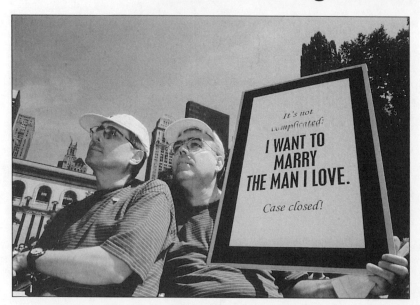

People diverge, calling it "the most important legal battle facing gay men and lesbians today" (Lambda Legal Defense lawyer Evan Wolfson), the victory we need to achieve so that we can "throw a party and close down the gay rights movement for good" (author Andrew Sullivan), and a terrible case of "mad vow disease" (comedian Kate Clinton). Most gay men want the right to be recognized for our love, commitment, and responsibility to each other in the same way that straight people are. Others insist that basic privileges such as health coverage should be available to all people, whether or not we're partnered.

Lawmakers ignore us all. Same-sex marriage isn't legal anywhere, and some thirty states have now passed laws refusing to recognize same-sex marriages. Several have even passed constitutional amendments denying same-sex couples legal recognition, attempting to put the question beyond a future challenge from the courts. Only Vermont, in a ruling the practical implications of which have yet to be worked out as of this writing, has ruled that committed gay and lesbian couples are entitled to similar privileges as heterosexual spouses.

What's at stake, besides the most basic acceptance by society of our love as valid and worthy of honoring? A sampling of the legal power of heterosexual marriage includes:

- *Decision making in the event of a health care crisis.* If you're not able to make your own decisions, your straight spouse can make them for you without special paperwork (see box on page 422); your gay spouse can't.
- *Inheritance.* Straight spouses usually get a minimum amount even if there's no will. Gay partners get zip.
- *No testimony in court.* Married straight people can't be forced to testify against each other, and can have "privileged" conversation (regarded as private) under the law.
- *Prison visits.* If he goes to jail, a wife usually gets to visit. A gay partner (unless he lives in a domestic-partner city and has registered) usually doesn't.
- *Tax breaks and burdens.* Married, two-income straight couples can be taxed higher than two-income gay couples (their combined income hits the higher bracket faster), and can only deduct half the capital losses in a bad year. However, married straight couples don't have to pay taxes on the health insurance benefits they get through one partner's work (and they get them). Straight people can also deduct alimony payments, which we also rarely get (see next item).
- *Divorce settlements.* Courts routinely divide up assets among straight married couples in the event of a breakup. We're left to the rare gay palimony case.
- *Social security.* Pensions and Social Security payments often go to a surviving spouse if his or her partner dies. Straight spouse, that is.
- *Compensation for victimization.* If a third party kills your straight spouse, either on purpose or through negligence, you can often sue. If someone bashes your lover's head in, you get nothing but heartache.
- *Bankruptcy protection.* If a straight married man files for bankruptcy, his wife's share of the property is often not vulnerable to creditors. If he dies owing money, creditors get nothing and the wife gets the property.
- *Green cards.* The spouse of a straight American can live and work as a permanent resident. Gay men were only recently allowed to come into the country officially, and have no standing as spouses under U.S. law.
- *Time off.* The Family and Medical Leave Act requires most employers with fifty or more employees to give you twelve unpaid weeks of leave every year to care for your seriously ill (straight) spouse (see "Laws of the Land," in the box on page 422).

Dealing with Difference

I just have one question: Could you sleep with the television on all night?

I don't believe in color blindness. In any interracial relationships I've been in, which is pretty much all of them, we bring the question to the fore. Sometimes it's a joke, like he'll say, "I don't know what restaurant to go to. I'm just a passive, inscrutable Asian, so why don't you decide?" But the much more serious thing is I feel myself seeing things through his eyes. Like, do all the rest of these men realize they're in an all-White room? Are they ever in a situation where there are one or two of them and a big group of someone else?

When they're obvious—he's sixty, you're twenty; he's White, you're Black; he's a blue-jean-wearing, guitar-playing hippie, and your idea of a good time is hanging out in Bloomingdale's on Black Friday—at least the fact that you have differences may be more discussed. "Some research has shown that gay couples with distinct differences, particularly an age difference of more than fifteen years, have a better time because they're not competing for the same things," says Manhattan psychotherapist Michael Shernoff. Still, one way or another, being with another man long-term means facing the moment when the distance across the table suddenly seems as wide as the Grand Canyon, or experiencing the mystification that comes when you simply can't understand how he can do what he does. Sometimes it's big questions, such as who wants a kid or what kind of information is appropriate to share with your friends. Often, though, it's the small things that provoke the strongest reactions. "How could he chew that way?" "What on earth could possibly be so hard about replacing the toilet paper roll after using the last square?" "Why does he always decide to brush his teeth after we both have our coats on to go out the door?"

COUPLES OF MIXED HIV STATUS ✚

I think that's one of the things that make your lover your lover: You show yourself to him, in all your hateful forms. I used to use my HIV against him. "How do you know how it feels to have your T-cells drop by forty percent?" Now, I try to be more even-tempered, but it's hard. HIV is a constant reminder for us both of the ways our lives are different.

Uncertainty is a strain on relationships, but it's one of the most comfortable places to remain when one of you is positive. "It's safer being hazy," says Mark, an attorney from Tennessee, whose lover, Jed, is positive. "We'll talk about the drugs, the doctor's appointments. But about the future? We want to be together, and that's all we know for sure." Robert Remien, Ph.D., principal investigator in a study of male couples of mixed antibody status at the HIV Center for Clinical and Behavioral Studies at the New York Psychiatric Institute, warns that insulating yourself from conversations about HIV can inhibit as well as protect. "Some of the challenges couples face, like communicating regularly about their lives, get complicated when you draw a line around a certain psychological area and hang up an imaginary 'Do Not Enter' sign," says Dr. Remien.

Ray Smith, director of Dr. Remien's Couples Project, says the advent of protease inhibitors "means the ground has shifted in new ways underneath couples of different HIV status" (see "Getting Better," page 452). Ongoing stresses include sex—the HIV-negative partner is often willing to take more risks, says Dr. Remien, while the HIV-positive partner may feel strange even about openmouthed kissing—as well as the difficulty of planning for a future. "We married when Fred was really sick, and I wanted him to go into the hospital knowing that he had the love of a good man," says Ralph, forty-five. "Six months later his viral load was undetectable, which was a wedding gift I still don't know whether to trust." The fact that the positive one in the relationship may have stopped work earlier, or may be anxious to achieve certain things before he goes, can also make setting priorities more complicated.

What to do? "Beyond some basics, like not nagging your partner about his health or medications or using your HIV status as a wall he can't get over, around, or under, it returns to the same old thing," says Michael Shernoff, himself involved in a "serodiscordant" relationship. "Communication, with a special attention to what it feels like to ask, or be asked, for help." If you need help to do *that,* consider a support group, either alone or together—they exist for both positive and negative men in many cities—as well as couples counseling (see "Dr. Love," in Chapter 4) or therapy.

Straight men and women—or at least straight women, since they're the one buying most of the self-help books—can always fall back on the *Men Are from Mars, Women Are from Venus* type of explanation. But what about two men living together? In a world where being male is supposed to mean being in control and needing no help, figuring out how to be dependent (and not "codependent," unable to see yourself as anything but a giant response to his insatiable needs) is a struggle with no guideposts. What would it mean for you to have to rely on another man emotionally? Financially? How can you find ways to talk rather than act? "'Silence equals death' applies to relationships, not just AIDS," warns Beverly Hills, California, therapist Ken Howard. "The solutions can be different for every couple, but the important thing is to learn how to communicate." Talking it through, no matter how excruciating, is the key to staying together.

Among other romance-enhancers gay men say they've found helpful: socializing with other gay couples, cherishing people who like both of you, and avoiding second-guessing. "If he says he'll make dinner for you, relax into it rather than rushing in and making suggestions about how *you* would make the sauce," suggests Dan, sixty-five. "If you ask him what road he wants to take to get home and he chooses the expressway, don't then wonder aloud if the back way would be better."

Fighting Fair

No matter how many nice tips you take on how to stay loving, bitter arguments are going to be part of the process of getting closer. "Even the best of relationships take work, not in the sense of drudgery, but in the need to constantly revisit issues and find out what's new, what's changed," says Dr. Remien. "If you feel choked and then act to clear away the weeds, that's probably healthy. If you're not growing or struggling, that's probably not." Michael Shernoff adds a salty postscript. "Judging by most of the men I see in my practice," he says, "if you can't fight, you can't fuck."

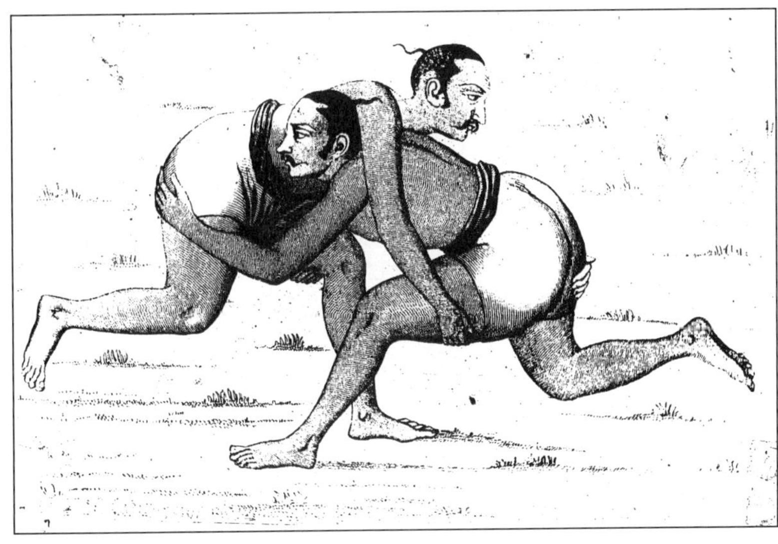

If you and your partner are doing more of the former than the latter, you should probably take some time to rekindle the romance (see "Relight My Fire," page 130). But often, no matter how much you may rub your sticks together, no sparks fly until there's been a difficult discussion to clear the air. Equip yourself with the rules of combat that can make fighting constructive rather than a bloodbath.

FIVE MODES TO AVOID IN AN ARGUMENT

The Escape Artist

This is the guy who runs out of the car during the argument, or storms out of the house without saying where he's going and comes back four hours (and as often as not, a drink or a quick sexual encounter) later. Calling a time-out (see "Weapons of War," below) is one thing, but leaving without a word leaves your partner stuck in the middle of a conversation, and is big-time manipulation. The more sophisticated version of this, adds Houston therapist Daniel Garces, is the psychological escape artist, who balks at the first sign of trouble and decides that "this is too much work and it shouldn't be." It should be. It is. Deal.

The Fixer

The fixer greets news of emotional distress with an action plan, ticking off what his spouse should do and then feeling surprised and hurt when his spouse, in turn ticked off, explodes. "There are lots of times when 'I'm so sorry, that sounds terrible' is better than concrete suggestions," says Shernoff. "It's usually best not to offer advice until he asks you for it. Or at least ask yourself if coming up with solutions is really a way of wiping away some discomfort of your own."

The Scorekeeper

"Yes, I know you did the laundry today. Did you know I walked the dog, and bought groceries and cleaned up?" This kind of tit-for-tat record keeping is particularly prominent in

WEAPONS OF WAR: MEN TALK ABOUT THE TOOLS THEY USE TO FIGHT THE GOOD FIGHT

- ***Try a letter.*** "We write each other notes that say things we just can't say out loud, like apologies. Then we can talk about them."
- ***Don't sleep on it.*** "We never go to bed angry. If it takes three hours to get calmer, it takes three hours, but you're not going to get sleep anyway if you're so twirled up you can't stand the idea of being next to him."
- ***No parent cracks.*** "Never, ever compare your lover to his parents. Even if you have a psychology degree, which I happen to."
- ***No ex-boyfriend talk.*** "The worst thing about hearing things like 'Your ex-boyfriend was right, you *are* uptight' is that he usually got the information from you."
- ***No threats about jumping ship.*** "Neither of us is allowed to drop a bomb and run away, threaten to run away, or say 'We'd be better off apart' unless we're really ready to go there."
- ***"I-statements" only.*** "You have to use statements that keep the focus on how you feel, not on what you think of him." As in "I felt completely disrespected when you were flirting with that blond boy in front of all of our friends." Not as in: "I hope you know that you have a serious problem and if I were you I'd start looking at that before you find yourself with lots of pretty boys to flirt with and no boyfriend to put up with all your abusive shit."
- ***You go, then I will.*** "Lots of therapists recommend this one, and it works for us. He talks for ten minutes and you just listen, without responding to those accusations that make you want to scream. Then you switch. Twenty minutes later, we're both a lot more lighthearted."
- ***Take a time-out.*** "I played sports in college, and it worked there. Either one of us can call it, and we stop the conversation for a little while and spend some time apart. Not hours, just enough to cool down. The person who calls the time-out has to reopen the conversation."
- ***Never say never.*** *Never* and *always* are banned, and exaggerating is strongly discouraged. "Saying 'You never want to go out, and I'd rather gouge my own eyes out than sit here watching another hour of hospital drama on TV' is overwhelming. If things stay specific—like 'I was really hoping to have dinner with Martin and Adam tonight, and feel like we haven't been out in a long time'—that's more manageable."

"codependent" relationships, where accusations and rebuttals provide some of the main energy of exchange. What can make scorekeeping all the more damaging, points out author Craig Nelson in *Finding True Love in a Man-Eat-Man World* (Dell, 1996), is that he gives you points only for things he thinks are hard for you. Even if you're sweating bullets trying to figure out how to assemble the new entertainment center, if that's your "job" in the relationship, you get no points.

"The real point," says Russell Park, Ph.D., a therapist in Columbia, California, "is figuring out a new way of looking at the work you do for the relationship." If you find yourself complaining silently about how much you do and how little you get, or bouncing immediately from attacked to attacker ("Yeah? Well, you haven't paid a bill in five months, so no wonder you have time to complain"), try to get out of victim or persecutor mode and in touch with the idea of service. "Each of us works in different ways to maintain our relationships," says Park. "Try to appreciate that, rather than wasting time resenting it."

The Placator

"Whatever you want, honey" is often a way of silencing discussion, warns Shernoff. The placator establishes a false peace, or caves in to his partner's demands but secretly resists. The seeds of resentment grow silently until they burst forth, often in the form of a breakup.

The Terminator

This man is dangerous to fight with, because he uses his personal knowledge of weak points to go for the jugular and destroy his opponent—you. Men in terminator mode say terrible things their partners remember long after the fight in question has passed, often to do with ex-lovers or parents.

Breaking Up Right

There was never an explosion. You know how milk boils up and overflows the saucepan? You don't notice it, but somehow a limit has been passed.

He mailed me an envelope full of dead cockroaches. He called up my friends and told them I'd beaten him. I started to think he was stalking me.

Maybe it's the old-time gay activist in me, but many of my closest friends are ex-lovers. That's how we made friends in the seventies. We slept together, and if it didn't work out, we stayed in touch. I feel like I've given them something important. I don't want to waste that.

Legalizing gay marriage is a struggle, but it seems easy to imagine gay divorce. That so many gay men (a majority of us, by many surveys) have been able to trade "Let's Call the Whole Thing Off" for a sweeter song—"Sexual Healing," say, or "Let's Stay Together"—is amazing when you figure how much tension the world, our parents, the fear of violence, and the realities of discrimination add to the ordinary stresses that come from living as two. "Think of the role models we have for male coupling," says New York City psychologist Philip Spivey, Ph.D. "Holmes and Watson. Laurel and Hardy. Abbott and Costello. Actually, Laurel and Hardy spent time in bed together on film, but they were also always beating each other on the head."

Absurdly, Batman and Robin and Bert and Ernie are probably the best mainstream media examples of fulfilled domestic partners, but if they're gay, they're not out about it. What is out in the open is how often people—including sometimes ourselves—expect gay men's relationships to founder. "Straight and gay people frequently ask me, 'Are you and Sidney still together?'" says Dr. Spivey. "I mean, what kind of funky stuff is that? Who asks straight men that question? Much rarer is for someone to say, 'How great, you guys have made it for twelve years.'"

Also rarely discussed are the mechanisms for making up. "It takes an enormous amount of work to go from mad at your partner to unmad," says Martin McElhiney, Ph.D., a psychologist in New York City. "It's hard to account for that process, for the move from the point where your teeth are clenched with anger to the point where you can touch each other or ask each other a question and feel caring rather than frustration."

Sometimes there *are* irreconcilable differences (see "Domestic Violence," below). Sometimes a little help is all that's needed. "We made a deal that if we were ever in trouble, we'd see a counselor," says Paul, twenty-nine, "and we did, and it helped." If you do decide to break up, talking is crucial even during separation. "It is usually the failure to talk—the keeping of a secret—that sows the seed for a breakup in the first place," says Shernoff. "Even if your 'secret' is just that you're no longer happy, you should air it," he says. "It gives you both a chance at resolution."

If you do think you've reached the end, *how* things end may determine how you feel and what your rebound period is like. Ambivalence, notes Eric Marcus in *The Male Couple's Guide* (HarperCollins, 1992), is natural: Even if you think you want to get out of your relationship, you're likely to be nagged by good arguments for staying in. Try not to play out that ambivalence at the expense of your partner. Usually one of you wants to end it before the other does. Marcus turns to author Diane Vaughan and her book *Uncoupling* (Oxford University Press, 1988) for warnings about ways that disguising your true feelings can make painful breakups even more agonizing.

Central to all of the "wrong ways" to break up flagged by Vaughan is a failure to be honest about what you want to do. Dishonesty takes many forms. There's "shifting the burden," where you make him so unhappy that he has no choice but to "decide" to leave. There's "the fatal mistake," where you seize on some error he made as an unforgivable breach, and then claim that his behavior provoked the breakup. There's "the disappearing act," where you vanish psychologically or physically, and "rule breaking," where you violate some basic, agreed-upon code of conduct and provoke a split.

The right way to end a relationship, say Vaughan, Marcus, Shernoff, and many other students of human relationships, is to take responsibility for your own desire to separate, and be honest and direct. And remember the rules of fighting fair (see page 511) here. You both may be replaying the conversation for months to come.

Domestic Violence

Stephen and I are in our kitchen, cooking dinner. The music is on, the windows are open, and we're chatting. "Patrick, will you cut the carrots?" "Sure," I say. "How do you want them?" "Oh, any way," he answers. I continue talking and dancing as I move on to the tomatoes, but suddenly he's angry. "Oh, honestly, look at these," he shouts. "These are no good."

When he sweeps them off the cutting board, I get mad, too. "Come on, why'd you do that?" "Don't tell me to come on," he screams. Within forty-five seconds, I've been pushed up against the wall, punched in the ribs, hit with a fist in the side of the head, and struck in the face and chest. By my lover. I run out of the room, terrified and confused, and he continues cooking. A while later he comes into the bathroom where, shirtless and shaking, I'm washing my face and neck. "Let me see," he says, gently taking my chin in his hand and eyeing my cut lip. I start to cry. "Oh, my darling. How can I do this to you? I love you so much," he says, hugging and rocking me as I cry. "You've got to help me, Patrick. I don't like hitting you."

What little research there has been reveals that gay men are battered by our partners at approximately the same rate that straight women are abused by theirs. In San Francisco, when they surveyed gay men walking by, men reported violence in one relationship in four. "Gay men are far more likely to be assaulted and injured in their homes by our lovers than we are to be bashed by a stranger on the street," says Greg Merrill, director of client services at San Francisco's Community United Against Violence. Yet instead of organized efforts to stop the problem, says Patrick Letellier, coauthor of *Men Who Beat the Men Who Love Them* (Harrington Park Press, 1991) and the battered man in the story above, there have often been assumptions and myths: that men who are beaten stay because they like it, that one man battering another is an equal fight, that men together "do that," or that domestic violence is limited to some specific group or type of gay man (bodybuilders, leathermen, men of color, low-income gay men, men who frequent bars, and so on).

What is domestic abuse? It's choosing to use some form of violence and manipulation to control a partner. Abusers may use psychological abuse (such as yelling, excessive jealousy, intimidation, or making threats), physical abuse (hitting, slapping, choking, kicking, using weapons), sexual abuse (rape, forced sex with others, refusing to practice safer sex), economic abuse (keeping a partner from getting or holding a job, demanding a partner's money, controlling his finances), or the destruction of property (smashing household items, destroying or selling valuables). It might be that your partner threatens to out you about your sexual orientation or your HIV status to your family or boss. Men who are being abused almost always experience some combination of the methods above, with the actual physical violence—often provoked by what seems like irrational jealousy or infraction of some "rule"—passing in episodes so quick they can seem surreal. Intense reconciliation, complete with the pleasures of being soothed and held, may go on for days.

For those who are being abused, says Letellier, what's most important may be to realize what domestic violence is *not*. "Domestic violence is not a 'sign of passion,'" says Letellier. "It's not about one man losing control of himself or having a 'hot temper.' Domestic violence is not caused by alcohol or drugs, or the stress of HIV. Most important, if you're being battered, it's not caused by you, you don't deserve it, and you can't prevent it."

"Lots of us have the illusion that it's going to get better," says Gerardo Montemayor, victim advocacy coordinator for the Anti-Violence Project of Horizons Community Services in Chicago. "But it's almost always like a snowflake rolling down a mountain. It doesn't stop. It usually gets bigger and more dangerous."

If your partner is abusing you, say experts, there are two things to remember: You can escape, and you don't have to face it alone. "Domestic violence laws may or may not be useful to you," says Montemayor, "since whether the court recognizes gay relationships as 'domestic'

STEPS TOWARD LEAVING AN ABUSIVE PARTNER

1. ***Name the abuse.*** It may be hard to admit that someone you love can be so destructive and hurtful. Start by telling yourself.
2. ***Talk to someone you trust.*** "The secrecy that surrounds battering can make you feel crazy," says Letellier. "Break that isolation."
3. ***Make your physical and emotional safety your top priority.*** "If he can't reach you, he can't harm you, at least physically," says Letellier. Before the next incident, think about a safe place you can flee to and how you will get there.
4. ***Have a bag packed.*** "Pack a bag with a change of clothes, a supply of meds, some money, train fare, a spare set of keys, copies of important papers, and anything else you may need in an emergency," says Diane Dolan-Soto, CSW, of New York City's Gay & Lesbian Anti-Violence Project. "If possible, leave the bag at a friend's house. If something really erupts with a partner, that's not the time to be roaming around the apartment packing."
5. ***Seek help from a domestic violence agency.*** "Though set up primarily for straight women, these agencies are increasingly available to gay men," says Letellier. Calling before the next incident is best. "It's important to know before a crisis that you have options," adds Dolan-Soto. "You'll feel less trapped."
6. ***Consider calling the police.*** As painful and frightening as it may be to appeal to the authorities, assault is illegal. If you're afraid of or in the middle of a violent episode, the police can help you get your things or yourself out of your apartment. In New York City, every precinct has an officer trained in dealing with straight and gay domestic violence. Police in Chicago, Columbus, Denver, Boston, and other cities have all been trained in responding to same-sex domestic violence. Of course, no matter where you are, your treatment depends on the individual officers who come.
7. ***It's not about forgiveness.*** Either after an incident, or after you've left, your partner may find you and beg you to let things get back to "normal." "Seek help alone," says Gerardo Montemayor. "It's not a couples counseling kind of issue. It's an issue of the abuser having a problem with power and control and needing help." As a survivor, Letellier says he had to make himself rules, like "Avoid eye contact. Never speak to him. If you run, run toward help," and rehearse them. Making your own short list of rules, and reviewing them regularly before you see him, can help you stay safe.

varies from state and state." The vast majority of battered women's shelters are not equipped to handle gay men, says Letellier, and are more likely to offer you a referral to a homeless shelter or a voucher for a hotel room than a bed. Still, programs to help gay men who are being battered are now found in cities such as Tucson, Seattle, and Minneapolis as well as in the gay urban centers of New York, San Francisco, Boston, and elsewhere.

FAMILY TIES

I hate that expression, "family of choice." My family is my family, and my friends are like family, but I don't want to choose one over the other. Why should I? There's a whole history there I want to honor and be part of, not leave behind to live in a gay ghetto where everyone acts like they were born twenty-five and White.

My mother spent the last money we had on a pair of boots. I remember picking change out of the pockets of old suitcases to try to get enough to get a meal. And sure enough, Joey spends too much, too. He'll take our paychecks, and before I know it, I'll be broke and lecturing him.

I said to Ken in exasperation, "If I find it, can I punch you?" Then I realized that's what my father always said when I couldn't find things.

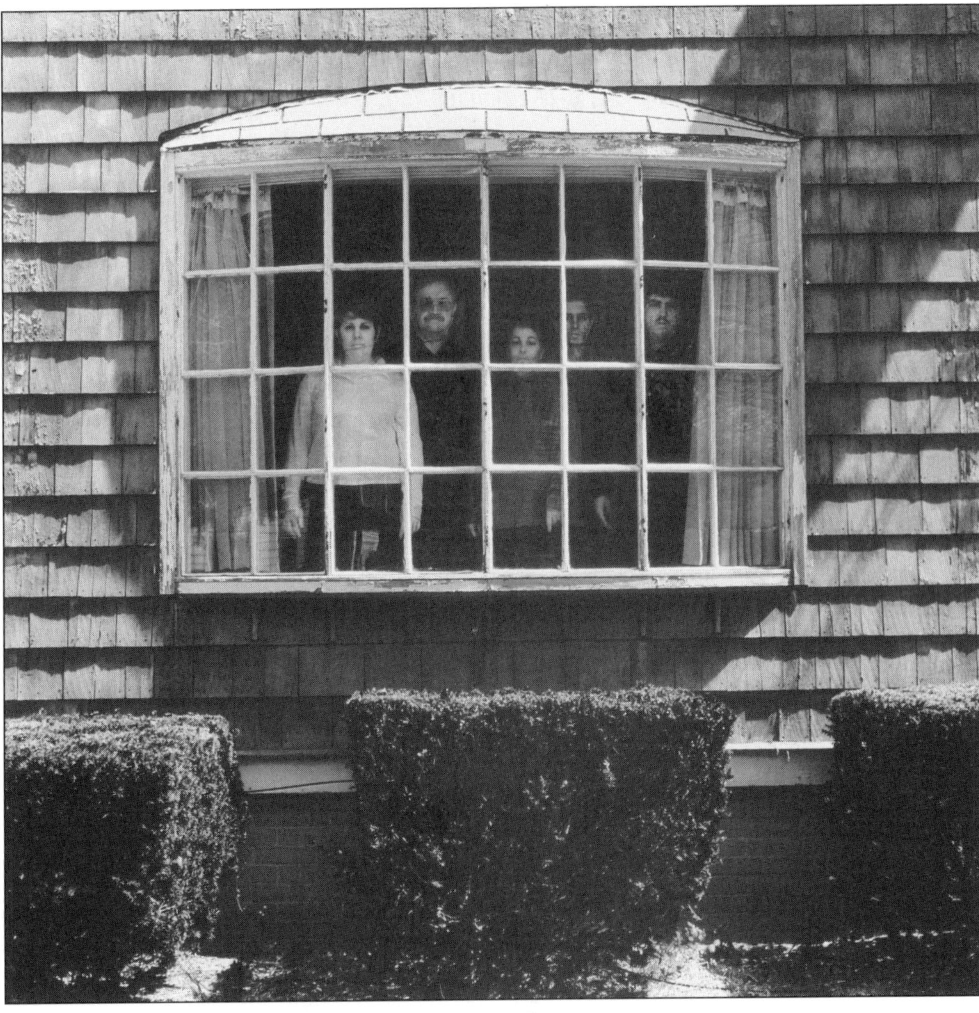

Whether or not you see your family twice a decade, twice a month, or daily, they're with you. And as often as not, looking over at your lover, you may find that somehow, miraculously, they're with him, too. "It's very common to be attracted to people who carry some of the traits, positive and negative, of the people who took care of us as children," says Michigan therapist Joe Kort. "That's the beauty of relationships, that they offer an opportunity to carry on unfinished business we had with a mother, a father, a grandparent, an aunt, uncle, rabbi, priest—and to resolve it happily." If you're lucky. Or you can find yourself in the doomed-to-repeat-history mode, reproducing certain patterns without getting beyond them to something better. "I went from a house where I had an angry, alcoholic father who refused to speak about the fact that I was gay to a house where I had an angry, alcoholic partner who refused to speak about the fact that *he* was," says Paul, fifty-five, a school administrator. "It took me a while to say, 'Wait a minute: This isn't just happening by coincidence.'"

The Parent Rap: Talking Through His Past

Even if you never meet his parents, you should talk about them. And not just about the coming-out questions that are often first-date kind of conversation. "Parents are a window to his soul," says Michael Shernoff. "Particularly in dealings with a romantic partner, where his parents were probably the biggest model he had." Make time with your partner to discuss:

Money. How much was there of it? How did his parents look at debt? Savings? Rich people? Poor people?
Expressions of strong emotion. Were there many in the house? Anger? Affection? How did he feel about them? What role did he play?
Caring for others. Were his parents warm or cold? What's his favorite childhood memory?
Change. Was there a lot, or a little? Was he happy with that or not?
Competition. Were there brothers and sisters competing for attention? How about one parent or another? Did he feel like he got some? None? From whom?
Socializing. Did his parents have parties? Did they like them? Friends? Did they like them?

Oh, and one important piece of advice. Be very careful before you criticize someone's parents, since you're really talking about part of him. "It's just like when someone harshes on your boyfriend," says John, nineteen. "It's one thing if *you* do it. It's a totally different thing if someone else does."

Homo for the Holidays? Bringing Him Back to Mom and Dad

I was at the Thanksgiving table with David's family, and everyone seemed to be enjoying themselves. The phone rang. "It's Sharon Portnoy," said David's sister. "Oh," I said, thinking I would be making a Jewish joke, "does she have a complaint?" No one laughed. It turns out that she was David's father's former mistress. She had more than one complaint.

My mother is very protective: "This one's just after your money." "That one puts you down." But she loved Dennis, because she could see that he was on my side, and that it gave him satisfaction for me to succeed. She would always invite him for dinner, talk to him in confidence about things like what would happen if I was left all alone. And when he saw my mother getting too emotional, he would direct the conversation to a better place.

George's mother took us out to eat at some fancy WASP restaurant for graduation, I think because she was so delighted to be getting rid of me. "So, John, what will you be doing next year?" For once I was uncharacteristically silent, and George spoke. "John's moving to California with me, Mother." She had a stroke internally, I know, but there was only the tiniest quiver of the teacup, which she put down gently. "You didn't tell me that, dear," she said. "Oh," said George's sister, "what a lovely view."

IF YOUR PARENTS DON'T KNOW YOU'RE GAY

Introducing partners and parents is a staple of sitcoms and most guides to gay coupling. If your parents don't know you're gay, a certain amount of awkwardness for you (and your lover) is probably unavoidable. It'll be worse, though, if you've told them misleading things before they got there. "The secret is to stick to the truth as much as possible, so when the time comes to tell the whole truth, it's more a matter of what you didn't say than trying to explain half-truths," advises Eric Marcus in his clear discussion of the issue in *The Male Couple's Guide.* Don't add imaginary friends to your vacations or explain away the one double bed because he sleeps "at his girlfriend's." And remember, even if *you're* used to the fact that you're closeted at home, your boyfriend may be reeling.

FOR PARENTS WHO KNOW ABOUT YOUR SEXUALITY

Even if they "know about you," meeting your partner may be a double-edged sword. On the one hand, it's often a huge relief for them to meet a real person, rather than the demonic pervert they're imagining (even if he is a demonic pervert, he's probably better than they imagined). On the other, it's a stranger, a gay stranger, in the house, sitting on the couch, forcing them to imagine—yuck—that the meaning of your sexuality is not just that you are free to baby-sit the nephews at a moment's notice or that you'll always come "home" because you don't have another family. Furthermore, there may be other relatives or friends around who'll want to know who he is, and that means explanations. "My family was fine until we ran into the neighbors, when they froze," says David, forty-two, from Wellfleet, Massachusetts. "Pat was just standing there, waiting to be introduced, while they pretended he didn't exist." In many groups, one member of the family may give voice to the hostile undercurrent experienced by everyone. "Sam's parents couldn't have been nicer, but his brother was a real asshole, making all these comments about 'crackers' and such," says Herb, thirty-four. "I'm not sure if he was more upset that I was his big brother's homosexual boyfriend or that I was White. After he left, we all had a nice visit."

IF THE FOLKS COME TO YOU

Confusion is as common as outright anger or hostility. Particularly in the moment they are forced to confront what author Craig Nelson refers to as "THE BED." "They gulped and stammered and ten minutes later they were out the door," says Monte, thirty-five, of his parents' entry into the small apartment he shares with his lover, Arnold, in New York City. "They called later and kept repeating, 'We love you to death.' We decided there was some AIDS anxiety there." Even if there's no obvious discomfort, there may be silence. "From the moment they come to our house, my parents stop asking any questions about our life," says Robert, forty-five. "I think they're afraid, somehow, that anything they say will lead to a discussion of anal sex. Like 'Oh, you like this candlestick? I had it up your son's ass just before you arrived."

Gauging successful family visits depends on what you mean by success. "It's been a gradual thing with us," says Ken, forty-four, of visits home to Ohio with his lover, Dave. "My family life isn't any more satisfying for me than it was before I met Dave. But I do remember the moment that I was able to be more worried about him than I was about my family's reaction. That was a milestone. And having him see my family has definitely helped him understand why I respond to certain things the way I do."

Before you visit the folks, talking with your partner and deciding how you want to handle issues such as being put in the room with twin beds, or next to the homophobic uncle at dinner, is a must. So is making sure that there's a time during the visit, even if it's a walk around the block, where you and your partner can be alone. Retreat is sweet.

If you wish to help your parents understand, the amazing and amazingly effective PFLAG (Parents and Friends of Lesbians and Gays) has chapters in 256 cities across the world and a range of publications including "Is Homosexuality a Sin?" (no), "Why Is My Child Gay?" (it's not their "fault"), and "Can We Understand?" (the answer, one hopes, is yes). They also have reading lists and contingents in Gay Pride marches and lots of nice parents who made their way through their resistance to the point where they could accept and support their children.

When Past Is Present: Incest

My father turned to me, looking hurt. "But I'm not your father," he said. "I'm your lover."

Brookline, Massachusetts, therapist Mike Lew, M.Ed., has a term for the soft, modulated tones often used by survivors of childhood sexual abuse: "The Voice." For gay men, whose early sexuality is often acted out in silence anyway, the whispers of sexual abuse—particularly at the hands or body of a male relative—are sometimes hard to distinguish from those of desire. "I never thought about it until my therapist began to press me," says Brian, thirty-two. "I mean, I knew the sex I wanted was supposed to be kept secret. I knew I enjoyed it. I also knew, at a certain point, that I had to start lying to avoid him, making up excuses so he couldn't get to me. I mentioned it to my mother, years later. She said the same kind of thing had happened to her, to her sisters, to my uncle, to half the family." For Brian, whose sex was with an older cousin, the lines seemed vague, but even sex with fathers or brothers might have had its pleasures. "That doesn't make them less abusive," says Mike Lew, who is the author of *Victims No Longer: Men Recovering from Incest and Other Sexual Child Abuse* (HarperCollins, 1990). "Just more confusing."

Assessing the effects of incest is complicated by the fact that it often happens before, or just as, we're learning what it means to be gay. "Male survivors of sexual childhood abuse, especially if they were older when the abuse happened, tend to blame themselves more," says Lew. "As men, we're supposed to be strong, tough problem solvers, not victims." Further complicating men's memories of incest is the fact that fear and arousal are close relatives, and that many men—including rape victims—respond to both with erections. If your incest experience included a component of pleasure, denying that enjoyment tends to drive it further into the realm of guilt and shame. "It's fine to ask yourself what may have felt good," says Lew. "It may help you to get at what you didn't want, the things you don't want to repeat." Remember also that, no matter how much you feel you wanted it, you were a boy, and being young made you vulnerable to people who abused your age to control you and take you over. "You can laugh at the idea of the child within, but for men recovering from sexual abuse it's powerful to look at images of themselves as children, and to heal those images," says Lew. Some male survivors find it helpful to carry around photos of themselves as boys, or write letters to themselves as children, supporting themselves in ways they didn't get supported when they were young.

Lew steers clear of debates about what age or what degree of closeness in your family makes sexual contact abusive, preferring to define incest "in terms of abuse of power and its effects." Often those effects are varied and, like the abuse itself, go to the core of what it means to be loved, to be vulnerable, to feel valued, to have a voice. Depression, feelings of wanting lots of sex with strangers, feelings of not wanting sex at all, fear of being "known," and suicidal feelings are all common among survivors of child abuse.

My mother walked into the bathroom as her brother was pulling me down to his groin by the hair. She looked, walked out of the room, and never said a word. I remember that silence at the dinner table as more painful than what my uncle did.

It's no accident that the national recovery network for incest survivors is called VOICES in Action, says Lew. If you're beginning recovery, the most important thing you can do is replace "The Voice" with your voice, an authentic expression of what you remember and what you're afraid of. Tell someone, anyone. Breaking the silence may also break old patterns, bringing up new feelings and fears. If you have a partner or close friends, it's important that you let them know what's going on and that you tell them as clearly as you comfortably can. Though your own reactions can be as varied as the weather, says Lew, strong emotions are common. "It's often a roller-coaster ride, but it won't last," says Lew. "If you feel yourself going up and down or in and out of various moods, remember that in the long run you're going forward." Your partner, too—if you have one—will likely be in for a rocky ride. "This involves getting through the effects of intense harm that's been done to you," say Lew. "You can't expect that it's going to be business as usual." Among the common reactions:

If you're coming to terms with having been abused, you may feel:	If you're the partner of someone who's been abused, you may want to remember:
Withdrawn. You may find yourself spending more time alone, feeling isolated, or checking out. As much as you can, communicate what's going on to your partner. He's not a mind reader. He didn't live your life.	It's temporary. For you, as for him, things may have to feel worse before they feel better.
Moody. People exploring recovery may feel great one day, despairing the next.	You didn't cause his feelings, and you're not responsible for alleviating them.
Confrontational. "Confrontation is not the goal of recovery," says Lew, "though it can be an important tool." There are all kinds of ways to confront the people who abused you or who stood by: fantasy letters, guided role playing, or actual encounters. VOICES in Action has a pamphlet, "How to Confront Your Perpetrator: Dead or Alive," that offers advice. Don't rush into it, reserve the right to change your mind, and don't go to the place the abuse occurred or be alone with the perpetrator.	His anger's not at you. If he has to blame someone for what happened to him and isn't yet ready to deal with who abused him, that someone may be you. Again, you can accept his right to be angry without accepting that you caused it.
Needy. "As memories of childhood return, so do childish urges," says Lew. These can make you playful, or clingy, or whiny. Sometimes your focus on your recovery can mean a lack of focus on the needs of the people around you.	Support him when you can. Support his efforts to get healthy outside of your relationship, through therapy or in a group. And take care of yourself—you can't help if you allow yourself to be victimized by him.
Sexually charged. Incest involves sex, power, and control. So does recovery. You may often feel really interested in sex one minute, and repulsed the next, or interested in getting off but not at all in kissing. Remember that part of recovery involves grappling with conflicted, damaged sexuality.	Hold your boundaries. Recovery from incest is about testing boundaries, making them healthier. The clearer you can stay with your own boundaries, the better you'll both be. You never have to do something you don't want to do, even if he says it's to help him.

How you find support while going through this process is up to you, though you shouldn't expect to do it in isolation. Particularly powerful is sharing your experiences in a group of survivors, especially male or gay male survivors. Whether that's a peer group or one with a trained facilitator depends on your local resources, though Lew says having a facilitator can make the difference between "a survivor group that's just victims huddling together and one where people are trying to grow and change and adapt." If you have a therapist you trust, even if he or she is not an incest expert, seriously consider staying in that relationship. If going behind closed doors and lying on a couch with an adult triggers bad memories, find another method.

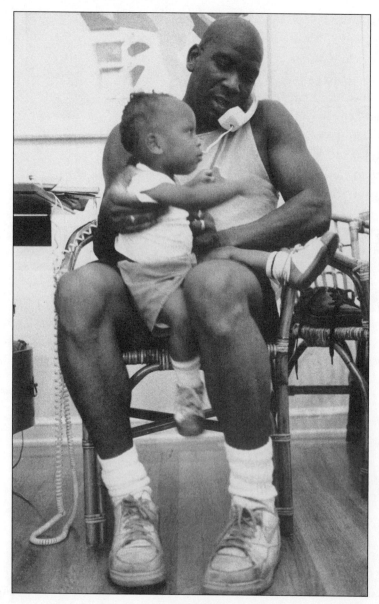

Parenting

When I go to the moms' house and Reese throws himself down the hallway shouting, "Daddy!" and flies into my arms, that is really joyful for me.

You hear a lot of people say, "Well, you know, I'd like to be a parent but I'm not ready yet." Well, I don't think I'm ready yet and I've been doing it for two years. I think that's what being a parent is about—the ability to commit to do the best you can with what you have and pray to God that it's enough.

When I went to look at apartments and told people it was for me and my nephew, they looked at me strangely. "You're gay and you want an apartment for you and your nephew?" It's been challenging. Once, though I couldn't prove it, when they heard I worked for Gay Men's Health Crisis, all of a sudden the apartment wasn't available.

I just went to a shower that was a gay father's shower. The gay mother's shower will happen later, but I don't know the women. There was my friend sitting in the center of a pile of presents unwrapping little pajamas with clocks and airplanes on them and all these men going, "Ooh!"

There's a reason there have been hundreds of books on parenting, with ten or more published on gay and lesbian parenting in the last decade alone. People in America often get more preparation and education about getting a driver's license than having a child, and no matter how prepared you are, raising children raises issues. For gay men and lesbians who are parents, that probably goes double. "Acting as a parent, I find myself confronting ambivalence about being gay I never even suspected I had," says Donald, thirty-seven. "I was with my son in the shower, and he reached over and grabbed my penis and asked me about it. It was totally innocent, but I felt this wave of fright, like somehow someone would think I was interested in a seven-year-old doing that. And that was followed by a wave of sadness, because I knew that feeling of shame came from outside me, from the society that says I'm not worthy of loving a vulnerable child without hurting him."

All of the studies attest, over and over again, that children of gay and lesbian parents are as normal as any other children, no more likely to be unhappy, or gay, than children of straight parents. And while many of us have thrown the babies out with the backwaters, leaving our small towns for an urban life that includes more partying than parenting, there are also an estimated five million or more gay and lesbian parents. Most of those parents came out after being married and having children, though that's changing as men come out younger and are more willing to fight for their right to parent. "I have always resented the idea that two men, no matter how loving, could never produce a child, and yet are discouraged from pursuing adoption," says Marco, thirty-three, a public relations executive who adopted.

For some men, parenting is as strong an urge as partnering. "I've always been a caretaker," says Duane, thirty-two, who is raising his sister's child, Rashid. "When my sister had Rashid, she was twelve, and six years later I asked her if she was ready for me to take him, because I was. And I'm not on my own with him. I have lots of friends who may not feel up to the commitment but who are fascinated by it in small doses. It's extraordinary to me how many gay men, especially Black gay men I know, are raising kids."

Paths to Parenthood

As I got older, into my teen years, I found my gayness and my parental desires growing. Now I realize that had I been a girl, I would have been pregnant by the time I was sixteen—that's how strong my desire for sex and raising children were. Leaving my teens tempered my 24-hour need for sex, but did little to curb my desire to be a father. I sabotaged so many relationships by asking on the second date (sometimes the first), "Would you like to have children with me?" I call this technique "HOW TO SEND A GAY MAN RUNNING." With no partner in sight, and the promise I made to myself at sixteen closing in on me (that I would have children by the time I was twenty-five), I poised myself to act.

Josh, a twenty-five-year-old self-described "gym rat" and father of an adopted baby boy, posted the above words on the Gay Family Values home page (www.geocities.com/wallstreet/8794) to encourage other prospective fathers. The Internet, and cities across the country, are bursting with stories of gay men finding ways to have children in their lives. One simple way is to help take care of the children in your "F of O," which is counselor-speak for family of origin. If that's not possible, or if you want to create a new F of O, there are many paths to parenthood.

DONOR DADS

These are men who give their semen, either in person or through a doctor, to a woman. In most donor arrangements, the donor signs away his legal claim to parenthood but may have some kind of agreement that allows him to see the child on a regular basis. If you donate sperm to someone known to you, though, particularly if you are not doing it through a sperm bank, doctor's office, or some other "official" intermediary, keep in mind that you are entering a legal gray zone and an emotional minefield. "Halfway through the pregnancy it became clear that we didn't understand each other as well as we thought we did," says Patrick, thirty-six. "All I really wanted, in writing, was some guarantee that I'd get to see the baby once a week or so. The mothers felt like I was trying to take away their baby, and was going to endanger their right for the nonbiological mother to adopt. It got to the point where the three of us would be arguing on the phone, with the pregnant mother—a good friend—crying and saying she would have had an abortion if it wasn't too late."

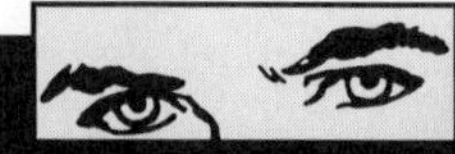

TURNING A GAY GAZE ON FAMILY LAW

What and who can make a family, including basics such as adoption rights, vary from state by state, or even county by county. Florida and New Hampshire ban adoptions by gay men and lesbians. Many other states allow second-parent adoptions, meaning that the partner of a gay man or a lesbian can also sign on to become a legally recognized parent. Regardless of specifics, the range of papers gay parents need to substitute for the taken-for-granted parental rights of married heterosexuals is considerable. "I always carry a paper with me documenting that I can take my daughter out of school, and another that says I can make health care decisions for her," says Jerry, forty-two.

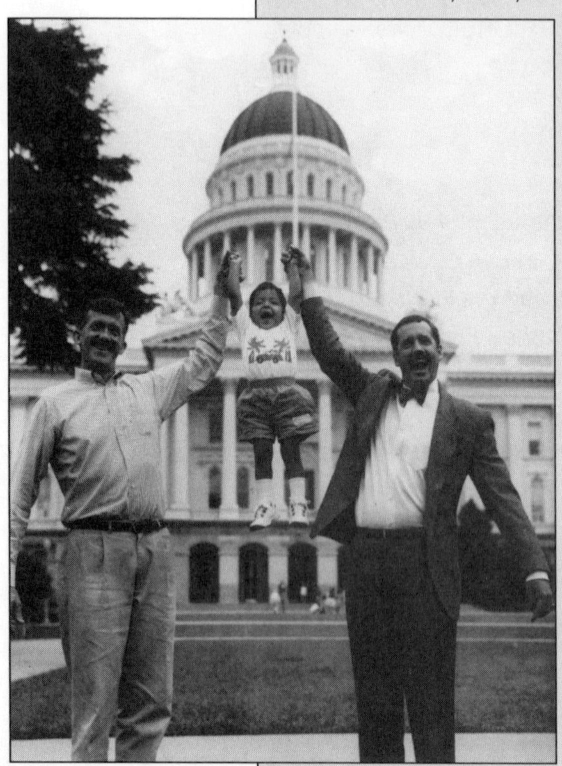

As with most places where gay sex meets the law, the law is inadequate. For biological fathers, even those who have agreed to donate sperm to a lesbian couple and have an ongoing relation with the child, the law tends to recognize only two categories: parent or nothing at all. The gay and lesbian community was split in the 1990s when a gay sperm donor who had an ongoing relationship with "his" little girl and the mothers who raised her sued the women when they wanted to stop his visits. In a series of rulings and appeals, the courts went back and forth on what rights, if any, a gay sperm donor had to see the child. Even rulings in favor of the gay man were a loss for the broader gay community, since the court's argument—that biological parents had rights, while nonbiological parents had none—cut the heart out of many same-sex parenting arrangements. Similar dismissal of the nonbiological parent is found when two gay men or two lesbians break up and the child's biological parent refuses to allow the one who is not the legal parent to have any rights of visitation. "I could handle breaking up with Josh, because he lied to me and I didn't want to see him anymore," says Eric, forty, a singer from Illinois. "But the fact that I couldn't see my son anymore, that I had absolutely no rights to continue my relationship with a boy I'd spent four years helping to raise, seemed to make my life feel like a lie."

A number of legal scholars have challenged the biological bias of the law, and argued for categories more reflective of gay and lesbian realities. Legal scholar Nancy Polikoff has argued for law that recognizes the people providing the care as the parents and sets biology aside. New York City law professor Fred Bernstein has added a gay male voice to the donor discussion, arguing for the creation of a category known as "involved donor" and a law flexible enough to uphold what many lesbians and gay men say they want in the first place: an arrangement where the donor does not assert the rights of a parent, and where the mothers are bound to stick by whatever original agreement they made regarding contact with the child.

Many couples and triples and quadruples who make up gay families have found it useful to write out coparenting agreements, documents that plan things such as visitation, custody, and support in the present, and in the event of future disagreement. These documents help everybody confront uncomfortable questions before they're really uncomfortable, but they may have little or no binding legal power. For now, when it comes to the courts, love doesn't make a family: Biology and what the court deems "in the best interest of the child" do. Which makes it essential that gay men thinking of parenting do two things that straight fathers rarely do: carefully examine their intentions, and consult an experienced lawyer.

Though you can conceivably go to court to press for more access to the child, the law is a blunt instrument, and gay and lesbian families can be delicate networks. Far better for everyone, says April Martin, Ph.D., author of *The Lesbian and Gay Guide to Parenting* (HarperCollins, 1993), is to be very clear about your intentions before going into a known-donor arrangement, and to recognize that any access you have is built on trust. "If you want to be a parent, be a parent," suggests Martin. "If you want to be a donor, assume that you have no legal claim whatsoever and that everything that happens depends on the discretion of the mothers. Ask yourselves the hard questions before conception: Is it going to be okay with you if the mothers don't want you to see the child? Are you going to feel bad if you can't bring your own mother by? Are you going to want your friends to know that you're the father? How will the women feel about that?" Perhaps the most important question is how easy it is to discuss conflict with the mothers, since some may be inevitable. "No matter what you agree about, a child is an enormous fact and everything changes," says Bill, a donor dad who loves seeing "his" boy once a week.

ADOPTION

There are different ways to adopt a child, and assuming you live in one of the forty-eight states where adoption by a gay man is not illegal, money is one of the main things that divides one from the other. If you have little or no money to spend on the process of adoption, then you're restricted to public agencies, which tend to have greater numbers of older children, groups of brothers and sisters, or newborns removed from their parents' care due to abuse or neglect. Many of these are children of color, and a lot have special needs, ranging from a little finger that doesn't work to something as serious as HIV, drug dependency, or developmental problems. If you are White and thinking of adopting through the public system, check your state's policies regarding "transocial" (meaning cross-race) adoptions. Other adoption options include using private agencies, working out an independent agreement with a birth mother, or working through an international agency. All come with costs from $5,000 to $50,000, extensive evaluation of your suitability as a parent, and the requirement that the adoption be approved in court.

New York and California have laws prohibiting discrimination in adoption on the basis of sexual orientation, but elsewhere (or even there) how comfortable your local public adoption system feels with you as a gay parent depends on the county you're in and the individual social worker assigned to your case. Gay couples often have an easier time adopting if one of them applies as a single parent, and it's generally easier for us to get children with special needs. "It's of course ironic that the same bureaucracies that feel that lesbians and gays are not suitable parents are quick to place with us the children who require the most highly skilled parenting of all," says Dr. Martin.

SURROGACY

Paying a woman to have a child for you may be the most expensive route of all. Ethical debates about this have only intensified with recent technological advances, which have allowed men to do things like take an egg from a White, Harvard-educated friend, fertilize it in the test tube, and implant it in the body of a less educated or economically privileged woman of color. On the one hand, people argue, this kind of procedure reduces the emotional attachment of the mother to the child she's carrying. Women who act as surrogates go into it with their eyes open and often with a conscious desire to help a childless couple. On the other hand, it can sound an awful lot like exploiting the wombs of the underprivileged, or leaving a very heavy suitcase for the Black porter to carry—for nine months.

Even without cross-racial, egg-of-a-stranger complications, surrogacy arrangements come with significant emotional baggage and expense, including legal and medical fees and an additional payment to the mother of $10,000 or more beyond her medical expenses. It is, however, possible, and a number of gay male couples have achieved it happily.

Parent Rap II: If You're Thinking of Raising a Child

"What we've created for parenting should be a model for mainstream heterosexual society," says Dr. Martin. "Going to 'considering parenting' workshops, seeing counselors, doing self-examination processes, looking at our conflict resolution skills—ours is the most planned parenthood in the world." Or it can be. In addition to the obvious, giant questions of who you are going to parent with and how you're going to afford it, here are some other things worth thinking about:

YOUR EXPERIENCE

Have you spent time with the children already in your family, or a foster child? Try to. Many states have foster-to-adopt programs, which allow you to take a foster child with the expectation that he or she will become available for legal adoption.

YOUR FRIENDS

"I feel like it keeps happening to me, where you call up a good friend to talk and all of a sudden they've put the two-year-old on the line. I love two-year-olds in small doses. I just don't want to talk to them on the phone," complains Dean, fifty-five. But Bill in San Francisco, himself a recent "involved donor," sees the demands of child care as a challenge that separates out the social wheat from the chaff. "The friends who always wanted me to be taking care of them, when Roy came along, I couldn't spread myself that far," he says. "Actually, it was a combination of Roy and the fact that I was taking care of a friend who was sick. But I felt that if they couldn't make the transition to helping *me* for a while, I was willing to let them go."

For gay men who don't have a supportive extended family, and particularly for single fathers (yes, you *can* do it), your support network is probably the most crucial element. "I ask potential single parents if they're sure they have five friends whom they can ask to be there at three in the morning," says Dr. Martin. "Be sure to use them, and the phone, frequently."

YOUR LOVER

Even if you're a donor dad with limited involvement, don't imagine that your partner's feelings aren't going to be important. "Hans had a better chance of adopting as a single parent, so I spent days hiding my stuff and being absent when they were doing home inspections," recalls Ed, thirty-two. "And then I thought, 'No, this is too much for me.' Hans wanted a child more than I did, and I left." Adoption agencies often prefer to list you as a single parent, though Dr. Martin advises against hiding anything from a social worker doing a home study. As for your lover, "it's unrealistic to think that a child is going to be only one person's preoccupation," says Dr. Martin. "It's a huge commitment, a love affair. Not sharing doesn't work with a dog, so it's definitely not going to work with a child."

HIV-POSITIVE FATHERHOOD ✚

One of the greatest sadnesses in being diagnosed HIV-positive for me was that I realized I wouldn't have kids, biological kids, of my own.

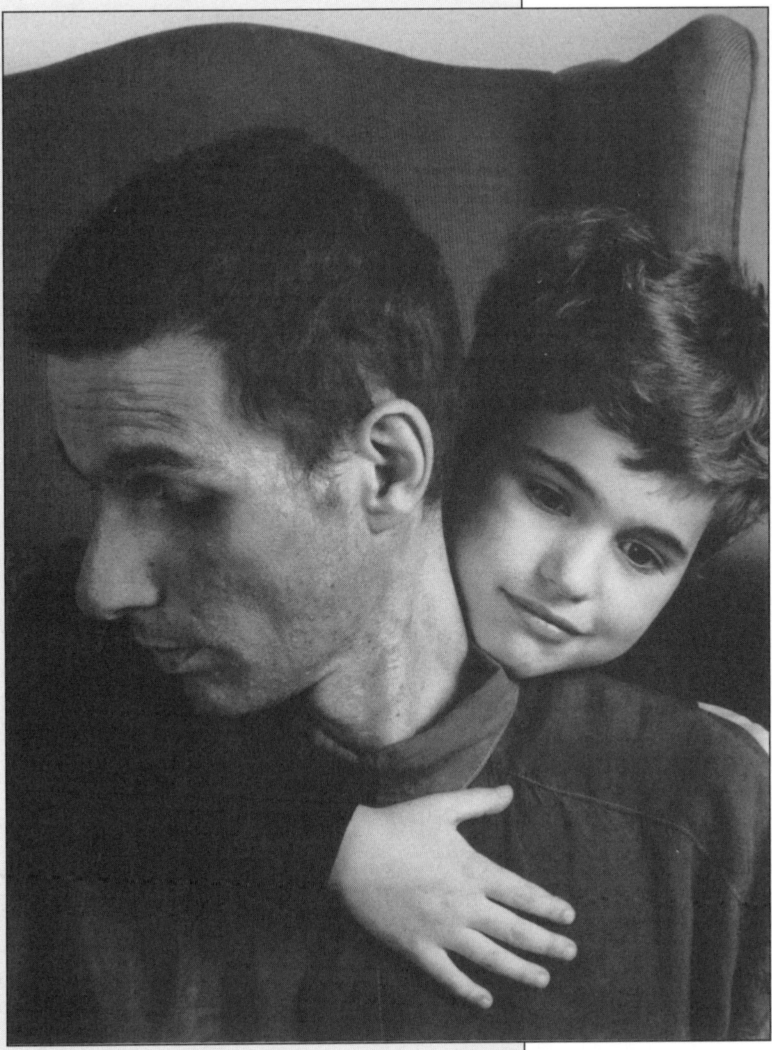

We felt that our child would be a lasting part of our legacy as a couple, though the agency would only let one of us be the adoptive parent. I went to Russia to adopt Nikolai. Alan only lived for two years afterward, so Nikki only has the vaguest memories of him. Yet for me, raising Nikki is part of my lasting connection to Alan.

More than a thousand men have traveled with mothers-to-be to a clinic in the San Paolo Hospital in Milan, where doctors in the ob-gyn clinic use a special centrifuge and heating process they claim can separate out the HIV-infected seminal fluid from the sperm itself. Until this highly experimental sperm-washing procedure has been studied more closely, though (the clinic's only published study involved just twenty-nine inseminations, and though all ten of the children born were HIV-negative, that could just be regular odds), being HIV-positive means confronting the fact that biologically fathering a child puts the mother, and perhaps your child, at considerable risk. Adoption is a far better option; while agencies require a medical checkup, says Dr. Martin, being positive is not in and of itself grounds for refusal. You do need to ask yourself about your support system, since becoming sick while being a parent can subject you, and your child, to incredible strains.

YOUR PRECONCEPTIONS ABOUT SEXUALITY

"He likes to get into a frock and has a female alter ego and knows show tunes from beginning to end and he's only four and half," says Bill. "And it makes me scratch my head. I have to constantly back up along the way and say, 'How would I feel about him being gay?' Is it my fault? I don't want him to be picked on in school. Then again, I don't especially want him to be a straight asshole, and if he's gay, he's certainly picked the right family to be born into, because we love him a bunch and we always will."

YOUR CONFLICT-RESOLUTION SKILLS

The painful truth is that no two gay men, however much we love each other, can produce a child. Having flashes of resentment toward the additional people required to have one, such as the social worker doing the home study or the lesbian mother with whom you're raising the child, is natural. So is clashing with your coparent, or your partner if he's not one, about decisions from name to baby-sitting to school to vacation. "There's no such thing as conflict-free child rearing," says Dr. Martin. "Part of parenting is getting very clear about how easy you find it to talk with everyone involved, *before* you reach the have-your-lawyer-talk-to-my-lawyer stage."

Especially important, says Dr. Martin and many gay parents, is a commitment to continuing your family bonds in the event of a breakup. "The world is so uncomfortable with gay families that it quickly conspires to redraw family lines when you break up," says Dr. Martin. "The law doesn't require you to continue to include your partner in raising your children. Your own family may urge you to cut him out. You may hate him and feel like you never want to see him. But your child has come to know the family based on the way you started out, and you can't violate those intentions without hurting your child."

YOUR SENSE OF HUMOR

"I picked a donor who was under six feet tall, and I have a son who is likely to be six foot seven," laughs Dr. Martin. "There's an old Jewish proverb that applies to parenting: 'If you want to give God a good laugh, tell him your plans.'" You may be focusing now on the few piddling things you can control. Good parenting, though, means good sense about how constantly your relationship with your child is going to change.

Sharing the Experience

No matter what route you take toward caring for a child, talking with other gay men who have done it in your area is the greatest help. More than forty groups nationwide, including groups for wanna-be dads and gay men who already are parents, are now operating nationwide. Family Pride Coalition (www.familypride.org) features online and print newsletters on gay, lesbian, bisexual, and transgender parenting issues, lists of parenting groups all over the world, and a straight-spouse support network for people currently or formerly married to gay, lesbian, bisexual, or transgendered partners. The Coalition's exhaustive lists of legal and adoption options are a resource must for anybody considering caring for a little one.

The most important resources, however, are internal. "Parenting is a little like taking religious vows, a kind of loving service in the interest of others," says Dr. Martin. "That kind of commitment has to be there."

PET PROJECTS

Truffle is a foot fetishist. He rubs up against the boots of every guy who comes in here. I don't know where he got that. Certainly not from me.

Sam and Wallace are something we take care of together, a place where affection goes—not toward your partner, but redirected toward other beings. There's an excitement when you come home and find a mini collectivity. The dogs create a kind of "there" there—a home out of what would otherwise be a couple's pad.

They're daddy's boys. They keep me grounded. Hershey's a good family dog, very loving and protective. The Dalmatian, Dalton, is younger and is just beginning to calm down—as much as Dalmatians can calm down! They help keep me focused on what's important in life. My friends say, "Come out and party, girl," and I say, "I will if you get up in the morning and walk my boys."

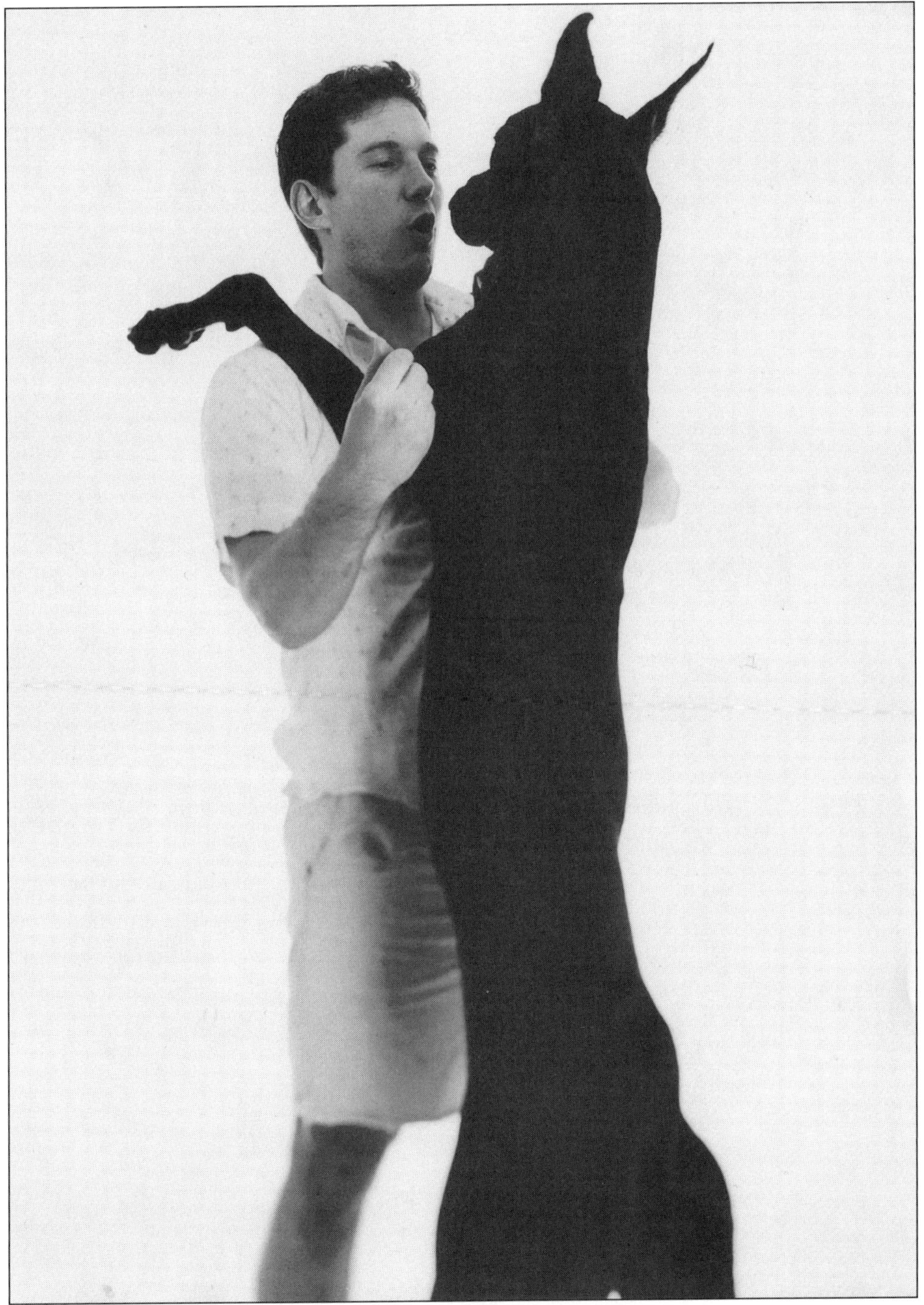

If love makes a family, pets are definitely in. And until adoption is easier or men can get pregnant, lots of us have four-legged or two-winged friends who are constant reminders of the power of caring and unconditional love. "I like that Henrietta's waiting at the door when I come home," says David, thirty-five, a San Francisco actor and accountant, of his tabby. "I inherited her from my ex-lover who died. Some of him lives on in her."

Whether your cat is your comfort, your pooch your pal, or your cockatoo your best critic, caring for a small creature who's always there to greet you may be as good for your body as it is for your soul. A UCLA survey of a thousand elderly people found that pet owners reported fewer medical visits than those without pets. Numerous studies have found that stroking a pet lowers blood pressure, slows the heart rate, and promotes relaxation. A Cambridge University study took people without pets

PET PEEVES: PROTECTING AGAINST ANIMAL-BORNE ILLNESS ✚

Though the vast majority of illness comes from other humans, there are health risks to owning pets. Turtles and birds are among the riskier pets for people who have weakened immune systems: Turtle feces carry salmonella, and birds have psittacosis (parrot fever), Mycobacterium Avium Complex (MAC), and other ailments carried by their droppings or the dust in their cages. A few safety precautions, though, can help pet owners stay problem free.

- ***Get your cat a toxo test.*** If your cat hasn't been exposed to the common parasite *Toxoplasma gondii* (most of us, and most of them, have), don't let him or her hunt in the wild. Raw meat, including mouse flesh, tends to carry the parasite. So does the fecal matter of those who eat raw meat, so if your cat's infected and someone else can easily empty the litter box, have them do so—into a plastic bag closed with a twist tie.
- ***Gloves and masks.*** If you're on litter box cleanup duty, wear gloves and maybe even one of those little dust masks. Likewise, handling Fido is fine, but you want several layers of plastic between you and his feces. You should even wear gloves when cleaning the fish tank, and gloves and a dust mask when changing the bird cage.
- ***Bites and scratches.*** All bites, including human ones, carry a high risk of infection. Cat scratches carry a bacterium that can cause lesions that look like Kaposi's sarcoma in people who have HIV, and swollen lymph nodes, joint pain, and fever that looks like seroconversion illness (see page 303) in people who don't.
- ***Lose the licking.*** Puppy love is wonderful. Face licking is not. Who knows where that cute little mouth has been?

If your illness is making it hard for you to care for your pet, you may be able to get help. There are at least a dozen animal service organizations around the country that offer people with HIV information and help with dogs, cats, and other important creatures in your life. Pet Owners with AIDS Resource Service (POWARS) in New York, (212) 246-6307, and Pets Are Wonderful Support (PAWS) in Los Angeles, (213) 876-PAWS, keep lists of others around the country.

and gave them a cat, a dog, or nothing at all. All those with pets reported that their health improved. Dog owners, who walked the most, fared best.

Not reported on, but proven time and again in the laboratory of real life, is how much dog walking can do to break the ice in areas where gay men congregate. "I've had people ask to borrow Lucy to meet people," says Bob, whose bulldog often rubs noses with Jack Russells, shar-peis, and other breeds of the moment on Manhattan's Eighth Avenue (known paradoxically as the "catwalk," though that's on account of its two-legged traffic).

FURTHER READING

Berzon, Betty. (1988) *Permanent Partners: Building Gay and Lesbian Relationships That Last*. New York: NAL/Dutton. Couples counseling advice from a veteran therapist and student of gay and lesbian relationships.

Island, David, and Patrick Letellier. (1991) *Men Who Beat the Men Who Love Them*. New York: Harrington Park Press. Personal stories and practical analysis of the dynamics of gay domestic violence and how to disrupt them.

Lew, Mike. (1990) *Victims No Longer: Men Recovering From Incest and Other Sexual Child Abuse*. New York: HarperCollins. Firsthand accounts and insights about surviving abuse from a leading therapist in the field.

Marcus, Eric. (1992) *The Male Couple's Guide: Finding a Man, Making a Home, Building a Life*. New York: HarperPerennial. Sound advice on all that the title suggests.

Martin, April. (1993) *The Lesbian and Gay Parenting Handbook: Creating and Raising Our Families*. New York: HarperPerennial. Parenting tips, legal analysis, and advice for the gay nation.

Martinac, Paula. (1998) *The Lesbian and Gay Book of Friendship, Love and Marriage*. New York: Broadway Books. A guide to marriage, divorce, parenting, and politics, well researched and clearly written.

Nelson, Craig. (1996) *Finding True Love in a Man-Eat-Man World: The Intelligent Guide to Gay Dating, Romance, and Eternal Love*. New York: Dell Publishing. Don't be fooled by the title. Lots of good advice here for men looking for love (as well as laughs).

Weston, Kath. (1991) *Families We Choose*. New York: Columbia University Press. Family, as the many interviews and analysis contained here reveal, is a many-splendored thing.

CHAPTER 13

Spirituality and Community

Gay Spirit • Waking It Up • Cultivating Your Spirituality • Heal the Church! • Homospirituality • AIDS and Spirituality • Community • As If

Almost everybody has had a spiritual experience at one time or another. Maybe it was a romance that made your heart swell with love for every living creature, or a death that put you in touch with the pain of mortality and a sense of loss you didn't think you could bear. Maybe you found a pair of leopard-skin pumps at a flea market that felt like a gift from God, or took a walk, just one, where suddenly you and a bird and the tree it perched on all seemed part of a single consciousness at harmony with itself. Whatever your experiences of spirit—that mysterious sense of connection with something beyond the merely physical or personal or temporal or man-made—your spiritual life is not exactly like anybody else's. "You cannot overhear God speaking to someone else," noted philosopher Ludwig Wittgenstein. There's no one way to do spirituality.

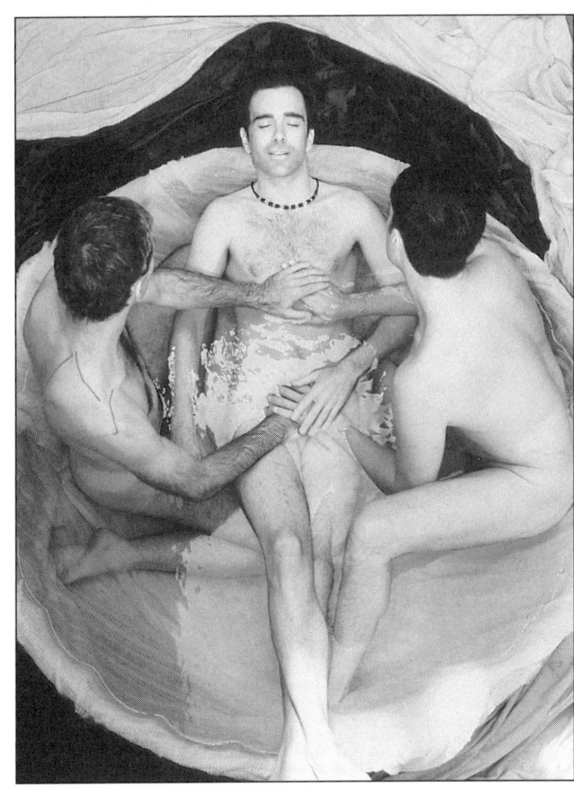

For many gay men, the question more often is whether there's any way to do it at all. "I feel more embarrassed talking to my gay friends about God than to my church friends about being gay," says George, twenty-nine. "I guess you could say it's a kind of closet. But my gay friends are so impatient. If I invite them to come to church, they just smile or brush me off."

Gay Spirit

If many gay men have left the talk of God to someone else, most of us felt like we were fired before we quit. For too many, our first experience of spiritual awakening was waking up to the fact that somehow, rather than the healing and togetherness promised by the church, synagogue, or mosque, we were feeling the pain of judgment, mockery, or exclusion. "For many years I described myself as having left the Church, but I understand now that I misspoke," wrote Fenton Johnson in *Wrestling with the Angel* (Riverhead Books, 1995), a collection of essays about faith and religion by gay men. "These days I say more accurately: 'The Church left me.'" Lots of gay men have found their way back to spiritual observance, traditional or otherwise, but we got there by boring through the antigay prejudice that is, unfortunately, a rock on which so many traditional religious institutions are built (see "Heal the Church!" page 541).

If you're not sure where the search for your own spirit might begin, start with a look in the mirror. What else but gay spirit has allowed so many of us to find each other, to shake off what society has said is wrong and embrace our desire and love for other men? It's spirit that has helped gay men care for each other when doctors and nurses were afraid to come into the room, to march in pride and commitment to each other, to form new religious organizations and political organizations and help older ones find more tolerant paths. Creativity, fierce humor in the face of opposition, love of beauty and irony, and the voices of divas singing out as if to God—that's all gay spirit. The vastly smaller number of fights in gay bars than in straight ones (let's not count cattiness)—that's gay spirit. David Nimmons, author of a forthcoming study of the hearts and habits of gay men, finds gay spirit in the vastly greater number of gay men than straight men who volunteer in community organizations, and in our ability to find a sexuality that is tolerant of difference. Health activist and writer Eric Rotes finds it in the men touching and dancing and swaying as one at a circuit party (that's also Ecstasy, but that's in Chapter 6). The large numbers of gay men in the priesthood, the church choirmasters and the organists, the sensitive Jews in the yeshivas, and the radical faeries in the communes—that's gay spirit. It may not be necessarily simple, pretty, drug-free, or fully self-affirming. But it sure is strong. "I was raised as a Black Southern Baptist in Mississippi," says Lidell Jackson, a forty-six-year-old community activist in New York. "I really did like and appreciate that experience. Since then, I've reexamined the conditioning I received. Some stuff I've kept, such as honesty and respect for other people's identities. Stuff about homosexuality and religion and how awful White people are—I've rethought all that jazz. Any piece of it that makes no sense, I've discarded."

Churchgoing is among the things Lidell has left behind. "My spirituality nowadays manifests itself in my behavior, in my respect for other people's existence, and my desire to help create a society that sees us all," he says. For thirty-seven-year-old Stevie, who moved from New York to a farm in Tennessee, spirituality has evolved to something "less like church, a special occasion, and more like my daily life. Working in the garden is a ritual. I've developed this spirituality of being in touch with the plants and knowing how to care for them. I've also learned follow-through, which was not a real strong point for me before. You can't just plant seeds and walk away. You have to water them and weed them and harvest them."

Watering and weeding and harvesting, picking out what doesn't work for you, nurturing what is alive, and feeling connection to some greater system such as the earth and the other people who walk it—that's gay spirit. It's human spirit. And in spite of all those who preach to the contrary, you don't have to be unambivalent in order to experience it, or pass your life in some state of Mother Teresa–like goodness. "It's so easy to think, 'I don't belong to a church or a synagogue, I don't have crystals or a garden or a boyfriend or even the possibility of really great sex, so how can I possibly have a spiritual experience?'" says Don, age forty-four. "But the more I talk to people, the more I realize that any time I practice the qualities the great religions espouse—love, kindness, forgiveness, devotion, service—I'm living my own version."

As it turns out, the processes that are good for the soul may also help the body. Though it's hard to pin down cause and effect, studies have demonstrated that when the spirit is willing, the flesh is strong. Gay men who are out of the closet, for example, have been shown in many studies to have less physical and mental distress. A recent Duke University study of nearly four thousand men and women found a distinct association between regular religious activities and lower blood pressure in people sixty-five and over. A similar report by Israeli investigators suggested that living in a supportive religious environment, a belief in God, and frequent prayer reduced stress and enhanced overall well-being. In *Healing Words* (HarperPaperbacks, 1993), Larry Dossey, MD, reviews numerous studies indicating a definite, though somewhat inexplicable, association between prayer and healing. Prayer in these studies—and the definition of prayer varies vastly from person to person, which is one of the things that makes the results difficult to evaluate—speeded recovery time from wounds, heart attacks, headaches, anxiety, and anesthesia. Prayer also seemed to affect "independent" or "autonomous" bodily functions, shrinking tumors and regulating hemoglobin levels. "Remarkably," writes Dossey of this body of not-quite-scientific knowledge, "the effects of prayer did not depend on whether the praying person was in the presence of the organism being prayed for."

Waking It Up

"A Great Energy Inside Myself": Walker's Story

"My family wasn't religious, but I went to a Christian-based high school in Richmond, Virginia. I liked Christianity. I was raised with Christmas, and I loved the story. The messages of love were the ones that got me the highest. The messages of exclusion—that if you don't accept Christ as your personal savior, you won't get into the Kingdom of Heaven—I couldn't relate to.

"In college, I had a strong yearning for spirituality, but I didn't know how to pursue it, other than praying when I really needed help. After college, while I was on tour as an actor, a woman in the company had a nervous breakdown. Witnessing her anguish, the natural question was, 'What's to prevent me from going there?' I plunged into self-inquiry, so much so that I began to live in fear. I confided in my friend Karen, who very lovingly listened, and then she started to tell me about meditation and a yoga she practiced. Not just hatha yoga, the movements, but yoga as union with divine consciousness, or our own personal inner divinity.

"Karen brought me a pamphlet about siddha yoga meditation and a mantra card. The card had a picture of a teacher, Swami Muktananda, and said something like, 'The mantra has a living force all its own. It vibrates with consciousness. Such a mantra has the power to give you liberation by cutting through all the knots of your karma.'

"When I read those words, 'cutting through all the knots of your karma,' it was as if something inside me released. I didn't know what those 'knots of karma' were, exactly, but I felt a profound relief. It's hard to describe, but it felt like a release not only of old anxieties and fears I'd been holding on to my whole life but a release of a great energy inside myself—a profound *whhshhhh,* a strong cosmic wind blowing through me. That's what I identify for myself as the moment of spiritual awakening.

"I've heard that the moment of awakening is unique for every person. For some people it may be dramatic. For some people it may be a subtle shift. But you know something has happened because the quality of your life has a lightness to it, and you may be more able to access love within you for other people and yourself."

Cultivating Your Spirituality

I remember when I was little, I was so unhappy, and I'd go on these walks and talk to God. It was never really a question for me of whether I believed. For one thing, I'd been indoctrinated at such an early age. But once I realized I was homosexual, and homosexuality put me on the outs with God, I did a lot of things that were outside. I stole. I outsmarted everyone, but being smarter than everyone only made me feel more alone and despairing. It wasn't until I bottomed out — until my ego was so exhausted that I literally couldn't think of another solution to try—that my relationship changed from asking God for things and being afraid of punishment to something internal, transformational.

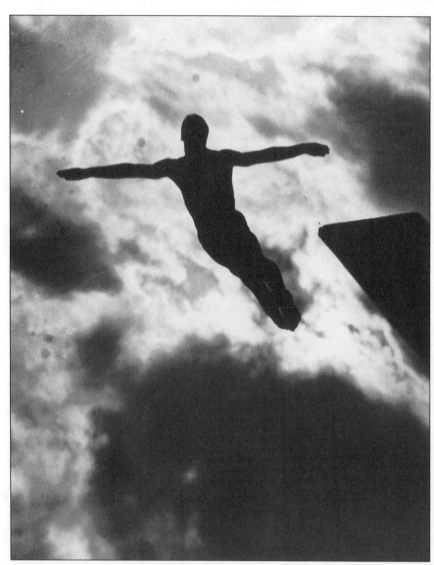

My boyfriend got involved with a whole spiritual quest, and we would always have arguments. He started going to church, which I hated because I had grown up Christian and hated the oppression and the history of the church. He went to a "gay-friendly" Methodist church. I went and walked out, it made me so angry. Later, when the minister asked Mark pointedly when he was going to get married, he left too, and started to search around for something that meant something to him. He read about Native American religions, Santería, got involved in the radical faeries. I would have arguments with him, saying I thought this was crap, that it meant nothing to me. I did get involved with drugs, and the drugs I chose—mostly K and crystal—would take me to these places where I had what I would have to say were spiritual experiences. I would pass out and have visions of either dying or being part of the universe and being very outside of my body. And while I was doing this unstructured, unsustainable thing, I witnessed Mark getting more centered through having a group of people where he could have a discussion about religion. It seemed to help him focus and gave him a community, which I felt I was lacking. So now, I've been trying to keep a more open mind, and I've been learning to pray.

The Bible didn't tell the whole story. It's not just rich men, as the Good Book says, that have a hard time finding their way into heaven. Given how little time there seems to be for reflection in many of our lives, it may actually seem easier for the richer among us to approach the subject, though whether you think of spiritual time as a luxury or a necessity depends on you. "I had taken every cent I had to travel to India, and was supposed to say this phrase given to me by my teacher a hundred and fifty thousand times," says Jyoti, fifty, a therapist in Half Moon Bay, California. "I was in this little windowless basement where there were a hundred and fifty thousand beans, and each time I moved a bean I was supposed to say the mantra. And I was thinking, 'What am I doing here? Why have I spent every cent I have to come to this little room in India and count beans? I'm from Texas. This isn't my tradition.' And suddenly, about fifty thousand beans into it, the mantra just went completely out of my mind. I couldn't remember it. So I just said to myself, 'Well, that's it. I've come all this way, I've wasted my time. My God.' And I said one of the Hindi words for God, '*Ram*.' And the whole mantra—I'm not supposed to say it aloud, but it was something like '*Ramapadanapayam*'—popped out of my mouth. One second later, I couldn't remember it. So I said '*Ram*' again. And the whole mantra popped out of my mouth. A hundred thousand beans later, I had my lesson. You can put your anxieties first, or your questions or doubts first, or God first. You choose. But whatever you put in that first chair, things line up behind it."

You don't have to go to India, church, or the bottom of your bank balance to find some way of cultivating a sense of spiritual well-being. You don't have to get rid of all uncertainty, either, or maintain a single spiritual focus. It's common to follow more than one path in the course of a lifetime, or to dabble in conviction and then dart out. "I remember I was in this born-again youth group," laughs Alan, who now describes long sessions of water sports as the time he feels closest to God. "So there I am, three hundred pounds and gay as a goose and going on with everyone else about Jesus and sin. I scared myself." In some ways, coming out—the constant process of finding ways to express the entirety of your gay self—is a search for spirit. Gay people, the Episcopal priest Malcolm Boyd told writer Mark Thompson in *Gay Soul* (HarperSanFrancisco, 1995), have not been able to "bullshit the process. We understand soul better because we've had to in order to survive." How do we do it? "Some gay people have survived by lying and not looking at reality," Boyd says. "They have become twisted and engaged in a self-destructive process. But for the gay person who is not self-destructive and who is striving to be whole and be healed, it's necessary to embrace the soul and deal with everything that's found there."

Some of what the soul contains is curiosity. Episcopalians turn to Catholicism, or vice versa. So many Jews turn to Buddhism that people in Buddhist retreats (when they're allowed to talk) now refer to themselves as "Buddhish" or "Jewbus." Christians turn pagan, pagans turn pious, many prefer yoga and spirituality of a more free-form variety, and if the interviews for this book are any gauge, lots of the transformations start as you grow older. You may begin to investigate affairs of the soul because you're drawn by a charismatic speaker, led to spirituality by a partner, or traumatized by his death. "I think I started because I would sit at Ronald's family dinner table and think, 'What are they all talking about?'" says Gabriel, age thirty-seven. "Ronald was a little horrified. For him, religion had all these bad childhood associations. For me, it was a piece of my heritage I didn't know anything about. From history I moved to practice. The God of my fathers wasn't something that was foisted on me, or which I was asked to blindly accept. He or she was something to engage."

Think of on-again-off-again approaches to spiritual development as a necessary clearing of past blockages, a kind of spiritual detoxifying. "I think the most important thing for gay men is to clean away baggage from the past," says the Rev. Michael Delaney, who left the Roman Catholic Church to become an Episcopal priest. "Whatever your denomination or upbringing, whatever they told you about who God was or wasn't—once all of that is cleared away, then you look inside yourself to see the most positive and energizing side of life. And that's your spiritual side."

How to Begin? Ten Tips

1. *Listen to your life.* "Remember that a vital religious faith is not a commodity," says the Rev. Peter Laarman of Judson Memorial Church in New York City. "It's not something anyone can acquire just like that. It's a question of wanting to live more truly and deeply. Discovering what steps to take always begins with listening to your life. I think many gay men find it difficult to listen to their lives when they are younger and engage in the fevered dance of finding intimacy and getting enough sex—a fevered dance I strongly encourage everyone to enjoy, by the way. It's usually when gay men get a little older that the search for life wisdom begins in earnest, and it's then that taking a more religious path becomes a realistic option." The Rev. Michael Delaney says the journey can begin by drawing on life-affirming moments that can help set the course for deeper spirituality. "Take whatever moves you: standing on the deck of a boat and watching the wind fill the sails, dancing, or seeing a particularly splendid sunset, and find yourself in that. Capture that moment and 'frame' it for future reference. That's a start."

2. *Look within.* "Close your eyes, count to ten, click your heels, and say, 'There's no place like home, there's no place like home, there's no place like home,'" advises C.B., a radical faerie from Brooklyn—and he's only half joking. "Spirituality starts within. It's about breathing, about coming into your body and awakening to the love and truth. It's about being alive in the moment."

3. *Connect with nature.* "I spend time at the ocean, even if it's a city beach," says Chris, a musician. "It's like where two worlds meet." Muslim mystics, the Sufis, hear God's voice in the calls of the birds; Native American rituals pay attention to earth, sky, the four directions, and the animals. "For the first time, I'm developing a sense of other creatures," says John, twenty-nine, a Legal Aid lawyer from Oregon who's working on a greater awareness of other living things, two- and four-legged. "I was driving the other day and I thought, 'I'm going to see a deer.' I knew that there were deer in the woods and I felt their presence. A year ago I would have thought I was loopy. Now I wonder if coincidences aren't something greater. It's just a matter of how you look at it."

4. *Find kindred spirits.* "A piece of the spiritual journey is one-on-one, and a piece of it is communal," says Atlanta-based therapist and bodyworker John Ballew. "Finding kindred spirits is important. It doesn't have to be the ideal spiritual community, but it's important to find a place that can be home base. It might be a church, but it might also have something to do with art, music, dance, or touch."

5. *Talk about it.* "So often I find that gay men think their spiritual yearnings or impulses would not be considered 'cool,'" says the Rev. Edward Townley, a Unity minister in Chicago. "The minute you express them, you'll be amazed at the number of people in the gay community who are very concerned and focused on spiritual issues and possibilities."

6. Go slow if you want to. "Spirituality isn't like a pill that you take," says Edward, thirty-five, baptized as a child in the African Methodist Episcopal Zion Church, schooled by Quakers, and influenced as an adult by his Japanese mother's Buddhist practices. "It's not like putting on a shirt and then 'Ah!'—you have it. It's something that you are, it's how you go. And it's something you should take slowly and gently and chart your own way. Don't worry about what other people think."

7. Do soul work, however you define it. "I'm a firm believer in psychotherapy," says Roberto, whose spiritual search began in a counselor's office. "Go within yourself and search for who you are, whatever that means to you."

8. Reach out. "If you feel there isn't enough spirituality in your life, do something to help someone else," suggests C.B. "Reach out. Give some money to charity, or volunteer. Do something tangible. Because when you create a bond with another person and go beyond what you're supposed to do, just because of the inspiration of your heart, God hears that and responds."

9. Practice. "Even if you don't believe in God or in a deity, even if spirituality is just an opportunity for you to connect with your own deepest self, spending a period in daily meditation and prayer can help," counsels Howard, a thirty-nine-year-old resident of New York's Staten Island. "For people who are just starting out, be realistic. You know, two minutes a day. That's a great accomplishment and can help you move on in your life." John, the Oregonian, says he's coming back to what he remembers as "the things the Jesus freaks in junior high were always saying, the idea that you should walk prayerfully, talk prayerfully, act with consciousness." Chris made up his own chant, which he recites while he runs at the gym: "I say, 'I am part of the earth now, and the earth protects me.'"

10. Try an intensive retreat. Sometimes the sheer force of habit that runs your life makes it impossible to institute or even envision any changes in your life. One way to jump-start your spiritual journey is to sign up for a weekend or weeklong retreat. Away from the distractions and daily demands of home, in some beautiful natural environment under the leadership of skilled facilitators, you might experiment with different forms of spiritual practice and discover some tools you can bring home (see next page).

A Second Coming Out: John's Story

"In college I was talking with my friend Darrell about my difficulty with women. He said he didn't have that problem because he was going to become a Jesuit priest. That threw me into a spiritual crisis. I felt the emptiness of my life. Darrell had this juicy spiritual life, while I felt I had no spiritual commitment at all in mine. All I did was pray to God to make me straight. I got no answer, so I felt we had nothing to say to each other.

"A few years later I was doing volunteer work at a crisis hot line in Lafayette, Indiana, working the midnight shift. One night I found myself counseling a distraught grad student who was sitting in the dorm holding a butcher knife to his stomach because he remembered a priest telling him it would be better for homosexuals to kill themselves than live a life of sin. I tried to be helpful, but I was primarily aware of how much his story was my own. I talked to him for three hours that night. Afterward, I remember getting on my knees and praying, 'Okay, God, what the fuck is going on?' It was the most honest prayer in my life. God's response to me was a mystical experience of love and grace that put all questions about orientation behind me. My life was transformed.

RETREAT!

People who practice various forms of spiritual exploration will often plan to do a retreat at least every year or two, to reinvigorate their daily routine with intensive practice under the guidance of helpful teachers. Levels of intensity vary, from nonstop weekend workshops to weeklong silent retreats. Levels of cost vary, too—from a thousand dollars a day to virtually nothing at all. Even if brief or free, spiritual retreats can create an impact that lasts for months or years.

If you do pursue an intensive workshop or retreat, make sure part of the advice you get is how to go about integrating it into your daily life. "I used to be a weekend workshop junkie," says Steve, thirty-five. "But every time I came back, my life felt like a downer, so much less intense, that I started putting energy toward more regular practice instead." Be especially conscious of transitions, and those in your life who haven't been where you have. Asking your boyfriend to call you by your new Sanskrit name, gushing endlessly about the new masturbation stroke you learned at your Tantric massage workshop, or carrying your vow of fasting forward an extra week after you get home may not do as much for your partner's spirit as for yours. Explain by example instead, and remember that even spiritual teachers are unlikely to be able to keep up their discipline every day without ongoing support from others. That's why God, or rather those interested in God, made monasteries—which are among the places you may want to retreat to. A list of possibilities is below.

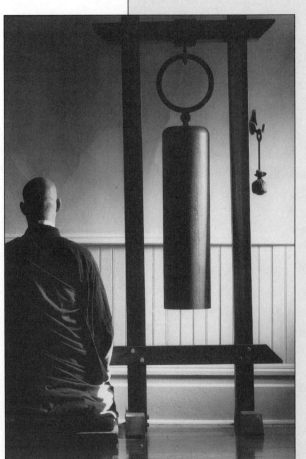

MONASTERIES

So long as you observe the rules of the house, many monasteries—Christian, Buddhist, and otherwise—make provisions for guests to stay for limited periods, individually or in groups. Your sexuality is usually not an issue, because they generally don't want to deal with it, whatever it is.

NEW AGE RETREAT CENTERS

New Age centers have been created all over the country to offer workshops in every conceivable form of spiritual pursuit, from feng shui to the enneagram to fasting to African drumming. Esalen (Highway 1, Big Sur, CA 93920, www.esalen.org), on the California coast at Big Sur, is the granddaddy of all New Age retreat centers. The Omega Institute (260 Lake Drive, Rhinebeck, NY 12572, www.omega-inst.org), in upstate New York, is one of many spin-offs. Some of the work at these may be geared to gay men, though most will probably be mixed. It's okay to ask before you go.

NONDENOMINATIONAL GAY RETREATS

Nondenominational retreats specifically devoted to gay spirituality are increasing in number. Since 1986, the New Mexico Foundation for Human Enrichment (PO Box 807, Albuquerque, NM 87103) has sponsored the New Mexico Lesbian and Gay Spirituality Conference, usually held Labor Day weekend. Through workshops and communal living, the conference creates a space for gay men and lesbians to explore their "sacredness" together. Gay Spirit Visions, an Atlanta-based organization (PO Box 339, Decatur, GA 30031, gayspirit.home.mindspring.com), has produced a conference for gay men each September for more than a decade at a retreat center in rural North Carolina. Its mission is to create space where gay men feel "safe in exploring our spiritual gifts and can work to heal the wounds that have prevented us from expressing ourselves more openly and fully." Both of these conferences offer workshops, rituals, and the opportunity to live with other gay men for three or four days. Amanacer (PO Box 767, Leona Valley, CA 93551), a retreat center in Southern California built specifically for gay men and lesbians, opened in 1998 with the intention of offering year-round programs that include special retreats for AIDS caregivers, people who are coming out, and those involved in twelve-step programs.

BODYWORK

Body Electric, the Oakland, California–based massage school (6527A Telegraph Ave., Oakland, CA 94609-1113, www.bodyelectric.org), offers a number of weeklong courses in erotic massage as a healing practice each summer at a retreat center near the Russian River, outside San Francisco. Other, shorter Body Electric retreats take place across the country. These retreats are often structured around rituals designed to heal the split between spirituality and sexuality. Related gatherings called Light Touch Retreats that combine yoga, movement, breath work, and meditation are produced by a group in Vancouver called Men in Touch (120-1857 West Fourth Avenue, Vancouver, BC Canada V6J 1M4, www.web.net/~sequoia).

RADICAL FAERIES

Radical Faerie gatherings (see "Earth to Gay Men: Pagan Passions," page 552) provide a much more informal, less structured experience than the kinds of retreats just mentioned. They're usually less expensive to attend and considerably more rustic, emphasizing tent camping and communal cooking. Short Mountain Sanctuary in Tennessee hosts two major gatherings each year, one at Beltane (May Day) and another at Harvest (in the fall). The Billy Club, a network of northern California faeries, throws at least four gatherings a year. Other faerie-owned sanctuaries such as Wolf Creek in Oregon, Ida in Tennessee, Zuni Mountain Sanctuary in New Mexico, and Destiny in Vermont also schedule special events that invite old friends and curious newcomers to visit. Information about all of them can be found in *RFD* magazine (PO Box 68, Liberty, TN 37095).

"The next day I found out about Lutherans Concerned, a social justice and support organization for gay and lesbian Lutherans that met just a few miles from my house. There I found other people who didn't share my belief that I would have to become heterosexual to be happy and healthy. I found the kind of community that was healing for me after going through a lot of isolation and hiding. That was my second coming out. Around the same time I fell in love for the first time. We would pray, then fuck, sleep all night, get up, fuck, go to Mass. It was very powerful. Sex and spirit have never been so connected for me."

HEAL THE CHURCH!

I don't belong to a gay congregation, and I don't think I'd want to. I see enough gay people. I like being with people old and straight enough to be my grandfather. But four of us, all gay and lesbian, wanted to pursue Jewish studies, and the rabbi met with us every week. We had an adult bar mitzvah together, and threw a big party afterward. It was the only time my lover's parents ever met my family, and the first time in twenty years that my grandmother left her house in the retirement community to come and visit.

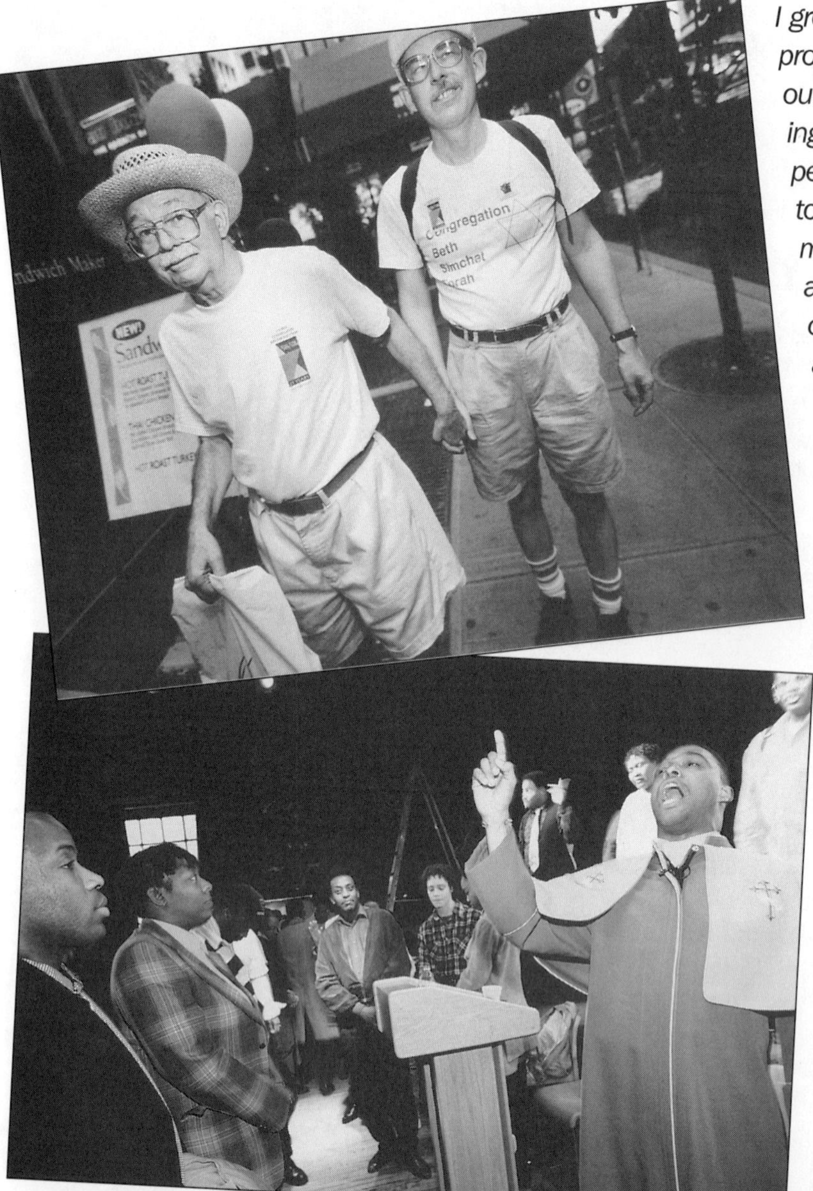

I grew up Catholic and gay, and that was never a problem for me. I never felt a necessity to take out an ad about my sexuality in the paper. Walking around hand in hand and all that is fine, but people of my age never did it. The fact that I go to Dignity, the gay Catholic organization, is a big move forward for me—it's probably the biggest advance I ever made. I went one night a couple of years ago and caught the tail end of Mass, and said, "This will never do, I'm not into this kind of stuff, it's too loose." A friend of mine said, "Well, give it another shot, come in on time for a change," which I did. I liked that they addressed the AIDS issue, praying for them. I was very touched by that.

In 1968 the Rev. Troy Perry, a former minister in the fundamentalist Church of God who was excommunicated for being gay, started the Metropolitan Community Church with a handful of worshipers in a private home in Los Angeles. Within a year, more than three hundred members were meeting each Sunday in a movie theater. Thirty-two years later, MCC has fifty-two thousand members in 314 congregations around the world.

MCC was the first of many efforts to provide an environment where gay men could reclaim the holy ground from which we'd been ejected. "I don't look at organized religion as our enemy. In some ways, I think our long-term deliverance will come through organized religion. But we don't have to wait for religion to do anything for us," the Rev. Perry told *The Advocate*. "The most important thing is that gay people not allow organized religion to steal their spirituality from them. I say up front, homosexuality is a gift from God. And I believe that with all my heart."

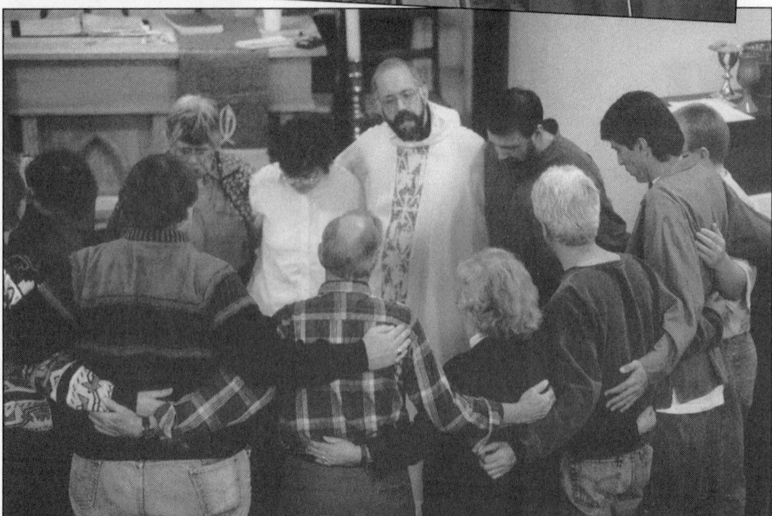

Unwrapping that particular gift and sharing it in a sacred space can be a healing experience, and not just for gay men. "The pastor of our pretty conservative church asked Gerard and me if we could wait a year," says Stephen, forty-two, of his commitment ceremony with his lover of twenty years. "She wanted time to take the congregation along. They came along in force, for a celebration with a big musical element and all the ceremony." At the Unity church in Brooklyn, New York, primarily for members of the Black gay, lesbian, bisexual, and transgendered community, straight attendance has steadily climbed. Apparently, hymns rewritten to include women and prayers reworked to accommodate brothers and sisters of all sexual orientations speak to parts of the straight soul other churches rarely reach. Melissa, a happily married heterosexual and the mother of a two-year-old, says the local gay and lesbian synagogue was the "only congregation I found where I didn't have to fight the distraction of sexist language. I'd go to other congregations that called themselves 'egalitarian' and that would mean that women would get to read the same male-centered prayers as the men. That was an absurd definition of egalitarian. Plus, the gay synagogue didn't charge for high holidays seats, and the inclusive atmosphere and ethics meant that all kinds of people felt like going there: interracial couples, people who didn't like to dress up, parents of gay people."

There are still many deserts to wander through and rivers to cross. Fundamentalist congregations of many varieties continue to hoist up gay men and lesbians for spiritual stoning and crucifixion, dismissing us as criminal, diseased, disgusting, immoral, and deserving of punishments such as AIDS and syphilis. The Rev. Stan Craig, pastor of the Choice Hills Baptist Church in Greenville, South Carolina, observed in 1998 that homosexuals were "a stench in the nostril of God," and his community cheered. Even liberal religious congresses continue to be divided over whether or how to ordain gay men and lesbians as priests, pastors, and rabbis. Arguments frequently occur over why or whether to bless our unions, name our babies, or perform any of the other ceremonies that are ordinarily cause for congregational celebration. "There's a desire for institutional self-preservation in the church that I would have to call evil," says John, a forty-four-year-old psychotherapist in Atlanta who recently parted ways with his church. "Aside from ordaining gay people, the big controversy right now is blessing relationships. The Episcopal Church is big on blessing animals. They even bless houses! But blessing gay relationships is enough to get somebody put on trial. Most Protestant churches now have said that gay people are people of sacred worth but that homosexuality is intrinsically flawed. That's like saying, 'You can be left-handed, but don't use your left hand.'"

Those of us turning to Eastern religions for more flexibility may discover that you don't necessarily need a patriarchal authority or large Western institutions to create homophobia. In *Queer Dharma* (Gay Sunshine Press, 1998), a collection of essays by gay Buddhists, psychiatrist and meditation teacher Robert Hall recalls a disciple asking an Indian master whom he had considered the "embodiment of unconditional love" about homosexuality. "There is nothing to discuss," the teacher interrupted. "It is condemned." When the questioner tried again, the teacher interrupted more harshly. "Do your meditation! It is condemned!"

Searching out a broader, more inclusive definition of spiritual practice has been the project of individuals and individual congregations since the time of Stonewall. New Yorkers and right-wing politicians can mock Los Angeles as an image-driven, empty place, but for gay spiritual movements, it's the heart of soul. MCC's early meetings were an inspiration for gay Protestants, but also a refuge for many Jews who felt unwelcome in their synagogues. In 1972 a group of them founded Beth Chayim Chadashim, the first of what would become sixty-five gay and gay-friendly synagogues now spread across cities from Boston to Minneapolis. Unity church, started in the city of angels to welcome gay, lesbian, bisexual, and transgendered people of all colors, now has branches in Washington, DC, Detroit, Newark, Brooklyn, Atlanta, Seattle, and other locations. Gay Buddhist meditation groups, bolstered by the Dalai Lama's gay-friendly attitude and by growing American interest in Buddhist practice, have spread from San Francisco and Los Angeles and are found in an increasing number of cities across the country.

And the Wall Came Tumbling Down: Neil's Story

"My family has always been a bit more traditional than most American Jews, though not Orthodox. Both my parents were European—my father was sent to England as part of the *kindertransport* and lost his family—and I grew up with the classic child-of-Holocaust-survivors messages. Number one was getting married and having kids. That was the biggest difficulty for me. If I wasn't going to get married and have kids, I'd be 'doing Hitler's job for him,' and how would my family react?

"For a long time I couldn't get close to naming myself as a homo. I was very committed from a Jewish standpoint. Perhaps the insecurity I felt being a fag caused me to look for something really solid to tie myself to. In college I joined an Orthodox Jewish youth group. I started keeping kosher and observing the Sabbath strictly. I got a lot of pleasure from that. An older man befriended me and pushed me to attend the gay synagogue in New York, Congregation Beth Simchat Torah, so I went to a Saturday morning service. I was studying at Columbia and living in Washington Heights. I bought tokens in advance and allowed myself to take the subway—it was the first time I broke the Sabbath, but this was important.

"My first time at the gay synagogue, there was a very dramatic moment. There's a line in the service about God knowing your most secret thoughts. Saying that line, in a synagogue with a group of gay men and lesbians, blew me away. Totally blew me away. That's when I began to take down the wall between these two identities. Going to CBST became a major thing in my life. I became involved in service projects and at different times would give the *d'var torah,* the sermon. Whenever I gave one, it was always about interpreting coming out in religious terms.

"When I came out to my parents, their response—which I've found common among Jewish parents—was, 'Well, you're still my child.' There was a definite post-Holocaust sense of 'There's enough in this world to destroy families. This is not enough.' They conveyed that in a very special way. My mother's father was wealthy, and we had some of his valuable things around the house. One of them was a beautiful leather-bound edition of the first Hebrew Bible printed in the Netherlands. It was always known that this was my favorite thing and that when my parents died I would inherit this Bible. On the weekend I came out to my parents, my mother came in when I was packing to return to New York and gave me this Bible. She said, 'Why should you wait until we're dead to have this? We want to have the pleasure of giving you this now.'"

Working Within Mainstream Churches

Not all gay men and lesbians interested in gay-sensitive theology have found it necessary to leave their traditional denominations. Dignity, the organization of gay Catholics, was founded in 1969 by San Diego–based priest and psychologist Father Patrick Nidorf and seeks to work within the Catholic church. Integrity, for gay Episcopalians, followed quickly. By now, nearly every denomination has a gay group with names that sound like Calvin Klein fragrances from some kind of kinder, gentler parallel universe: Honesty, for gay Baptists; Emergence, for gay Christian Scientists; Affirmation, for gay Mormons; and so on.

Tired of videotaping S/M contingents at Gay Pride marches, or perhaps just armed with all the footage they need, the radical right in America has struck back, spending much of the 1990s going to pulpits of local churches to preach the evils of gay men. Particularly divine has been their efforts to pit the Black civil rights struggle against our work for gay rights. For far longer, though, other, sweeter voices have been raised in support of tolerance and harmony. In 1964 the Rev. Cecil Williams, the African-American "minister of liberation" at San Francisco's Glide Memorial Church, founded the Council on Religion and the Homosexual to help launch a gay-positive theology in socially progressive churches. Nominally a Methodist Church, Glide has built such a strong reputation for inclusiveness that guidebooks (though most gay ones do not list churches) steer tourists to its Sunday morning celebrations. At Cincinnati's Grace Episcopal Church, New York City's Riverside Church, and elsewhere, Black leaders are preaching affirmation for gay and lesbian brothers and sisters. "As long as we keep America divided, then we don't have to talk about economic equality, and we don't have to talk about human equality. As long as we can say this person's bad, this group's bad, let's keep this group out, then we don't even have to talk about the kingdom of God," Cincinnati's Rev. Dr. Wayland E. Melton told Sylvia Rhue, codirector of the award-winning documentary *All God's Children*. "We can always say, 'We've got to purify first,' and somehow it's amazing who always has the answer about what is pure." His words, and the documentary, are reminders that the church is not one place but many.

Even the best of liberal tolerance, though, has not been enough to woo many of us back into a relationship with religion. It's not just the umpteenth round of "We Are a Gentle, Loving People" that creates impatience, but the suspicion that the vast majority of the religious groups in question will never practice what is preached. "I just don't think it makes sense to go where you're not wanted, and pretend you are," says Robert, twenty-four, a waiter in Louisiana. For others, even gay-sensitive theology can seem too unexamined. "Black church for me was motivational and inspirational, but it wasn't informational," says David, thirty-five, a former member of the clergy of Unity church in New York. "So many of us, when you ask us why are we Baptist or Apostolic or Pentecostal, there's a silence. Or when some fundamentalist gets up in your face insisting that Leviticus 2:18 says that man should not lie with man as a woman, you freak out, because you don't know the context or how to work with that."

Or perhaps it's the form, not the substance, that's the problem. "Preaching is public speaking and it's a skill," says David. "But it's easy to get confused between authentic healing and inspirational speaking, between the work of spirit and of the human ego. You may hear something and feel transformed, so much better, but that's not healing. Healing is something that's internal and ongoing. It doesn't just happen on Sunday morning."

For Tom, forty-two, it was Buddhism—as much a philosophy as a religion, and one that invites you to accept the truth of your own experience—that called louder than the church of his childhood. "I read a book called *Crazy Wisdom,* and it talked about, instead of searching for a path, that you are the path," he says. "That made a lot of sense to me. I was always looking outside of myself and trying to decide what I wanted by comparing, as opposed to accepting that what I did was me." With its emphasis on the experience of human suffering, and its teachings about cultivating kindness, compassion, and self-forgiveness, Buddhism has great resonance for anyone who has gone through the confusion of coming out. But as Kobai Scott Whitney points out in *Queer Dharma,* Buddhism's counsel that attachment is the cause of all suffering, and that you should try to strike a middle path between clinging to things you desire and avoiding things you can't stand, can be hard when so much of gay culture is about wanting and being wanted.

"It is much easier for us to be kind and helpful and cheerful with someone who attracts us physically, than with someone who does not fit our stereotype of the sexually desirable," Whitney writes. "If we somehow judge another person to be dumb or ugly or unpleasant, we are unlikely to give them much time or emotional attention. The American sexual marketplace (not just in the gay world) is very clear about who is attractive and who is not. The more we, as gay practitioners, buy into this fleshy consumerism, the more we violate the basic imperative to equanimity. He is not better than she. Blond is not better than brown. Young is not better than old."

"Each one is best," as the old Zen refrain goes. Now *there's* a spiritual challenge.

"This Is Love, and It Doesn't Make Me Separate from God": Jim's Story

"I took drugs and alcohol as far as they could go. As a result, I was rushed to an emergency room on Long Island one Friday night and declared clinically dead. I found myself surrounded by these spiritual entities telling me that I had to go back. I refused. I said, 'I've made a mess of that life. I'll do another one, but I'm not going back.' They said, 'You must go back, there's work for you to do. But we'll make this promise: If you go back, it'll never be as bad again.' That was the beginning of my recovery.

"I didn't immediately embrace the spiritual. I tried to do it by myself, but after a couple of years of white-knuckle sobriety, I realized I needed some assistance. One thing that kept me from embracing the spirituality of the twelve steps was that I felt because of my sexuality there wouldn't be a place for me. I remember my first counselor in treatment, when I finally worked up the courage to tell him I'm gay, he said, 'That's something that will go away as you work the steps.' My first sponsor was an older German guy who was okay with it when I told him. He did say, 'You have to be careful, because there are meetings in the Village that are exclusively gay, and people will take advantage of you.' I was on the next train downtown.

"I walked into a gay AA meeting, and my life changed. It was everything I needed: love, acceptance, humor, the ability to laugh in the face of pain. I remember going over to someone's apartment after a meeting to play hearts. People were carrying on like queens, with jokes and insults and outrage, playing the game as if their lives depended on it. I did this for weeks. I said hardly anything, but it was the most healing experience I could remember up to that time. For years that was my spiritual family. I wouldn't be alive today if it weren't for that community.

"For me AA reframed spirituality. And it educated me about homophobia and revealed other ways of being gay. There's a difference between coming out and saying, 'This is wrong and evil and I'm going to do it anyway,' and coming out and saying, 'This is love, and it doesn't make me separate from God.'"

Twelve-Step Programs: Church Basements and Higher Powers

For some gay men, spirituality's been found not at the altar, minbar, or bema, but below them, at the meetings held in the basements of churches, mosques, temples, and anywhere else that twelve-step programs get space for free or next to nothing. Alcoholics Anonymous and its many offshoots (among them Sexual Compulsives Anonymous, Overeaters Anonymous, Narcotics Anonymous, and Adult Children of Alcoholics) offer concrete advice on conquering particular addictions and crippling habits, but it's often the fellowship and accessible, flexible spirituality of the programs that keep so many coming back. "I'd tried Zen Buddhism in my twenties, was baptized a Catholic in my thirties, but that was all external stuff," says Ralph, forty-five, originally a Jew from Queens, New York. "It wasn't until I sat down with other people who were doing what I couldn't, saw how much they'd gotten by giving over to God, that I got something internal. It's strange, but I had to give up before I started to grow." Ryan, twenty-nine, says that 540 days (each day counts) in AA and NA have taught him what sixteen years of Catholic education never could: to pray. "I could only think of a judging, punishing God who wouldn't hear me," he says. "But that's not what people in the AA rooms were describing. I know my 'higher power' is different from the guy's next to me, and his is different from the woman's next to him. But it's that humanness that seems—I can't believe I'm saying this, it's so gay—divine!"

If a skeptical raising of the eyebrows is your highest power, or the idea of God's humanity seems like inanity, there *is* something called Rational Recovery (see page 278), as well as twelve-step meetings for agnostics. And have faith: Some say those who can walk the edge between belief and doubt have some of the strongest spirits of all (see box below).

SPEAKING OUT: TONY KUSHNER "IF YOU'RE NOT AFRAID, YOU'RE NOT BRAVE"

"I've always had a certain affinity for the spiritual or the supernatural. Since I was a very little kid, I've always been attracted to those things that exist on the boundary between the real and the not-real. Most little kids do. I never lost it. I believe that's the side of me that's attracted to theater. I feel very comfortable expressing a certain spirituality in the theater, because the spiritual dimension is in constant interaction with the material world. That angel, in *Angels in America,* has all those wires attached to her, and you can see that it's unreal and hokey and rigged up at the same time that it feels like a vision. You can't just say, 'Oh, that's a lady in a fancy dress with fake wings and wires.' And you also can't say, 'I've just seen an angel.'

"I don't have a spiritual practice. I'm feeling more and more like I need one, just the way an alcoholic needs AA. There's a lack of inner structure that I'm very eager to acquire and haven't acquired yet. After my mother died, I really began to feel connected to something not bounded by the temporal world. I don't know if that's an ardent desire for her that can't accept her real loss. I do feel a need to make some connection with that.

"The real agnostic position is the one I'm comfortable with, when you allow yourself to suffer the tension of not knowing. It's not a shrug and an 'I don't know,' because then you're really an atheist. The cloud of unknowing has to be part of the deal of spirituality. You can't completely penetrate it. You have to be willing to live in the unknowing. Part of faith is leaping over the chasm of doubt. If you're not afraid, you're not brave."

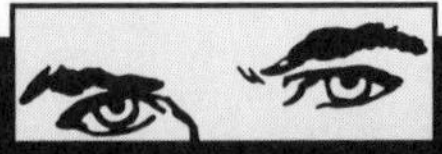

TURNING A GAY GAZE ON SHAME

Why do I think shame is a big issue for me? The usual reasons: the church and other men.

I pushed my lover right out of bed after sex, because I was convinced, absolutely, that God hated me.

Sexual pleasure and the body have rarely fared well in organized religions, at least in traditional, father-knows-best, Judeo-Christian varieties. President Clinton fired Surgeon General Joycelyn Elders for talking about masturbation, that baby step toward sexual self-knowledge, but it was the weight of thousands of years of religious dogma that really brought her down. In *Wrestling with the Angel,* novelist Andrew Holleran recalls the terror of having to step into the confessional booth and admit to the mortal sin of pleasuring himself. "That single phrase . . . 'obscene acts, alone or with others'—was literally breathtaking, heart-constricting, to the child who heard the screen slide open and knew he was about to say these words to the priest," writes Holleran. "'Alone' meant you had jerked off in the bathroom. 'With others' meant you'd compared penises with the boy next door (the son of a Protestant minister, in my case). Either one was terrifying; a new order of guilt—so great one started to postpone, and fear, a sacrament which till then had been eagerly sought."

Catholics by no means have the monopoly on body shame. Neil, thirty-nine, a Jewish doctor from Hartford, Connecticut, remembers knowing that "somehow, from a religious standpoint, anything below my neck was bad. The worst thing I could do was masturbate. When I was fourteen, in 1973, I made a vow that for the ten days between Rosh Hashanah and Yom Kippur I wouldn't do it at all. I made it through day nine. On day ten there was an announcement about Egypt invading Israel, and I knew it was because I'd jerked off."

Double your pleasure, double your shame. Sexual union with another God-fearing man may have sent your youthful erection rising, but for many of us self-doubt quickly followed. Dwight, twenty-seven, a Jamaican raised in Washington, DC, says his first experiences with boys, after choir practice and in the church, left him "confused that the house of worship that wanted to throw gay men out seemed to hold so many of us." Joseph, thirty-nine, had his first gay sex with a priest who masturbated him for two years. "I liked it in the afternoon," says Joseph, "but

"Gay Men as Holy Fools": Sister Missionary Delight's Story

"I was raised in a small working-class town in Pennsylvania and commuted by bus every day to the Catholic school ten miles away. We were taught that to be priests and nuns was the highest calling you could have. By sixth or seventh grade I had decided to become a priest. Starting in eighth grade, I went to the St. Fidelis Seminary, forty miles north of Pittsburgh. I very much enjoyed that. I was attracted to the all-male environment, and I was very happy there. If I was teased about being a sissy, I'd go to the spiritual counselors and they would assuage me: 'You're not a sissy!' The counselors were often sissies, too.

"In my freshman year in college, I started counseling with a psychiatrist on the staff of the seminary. He said I needed to leave and make a heterosexual adjustment, that I couldn't be a priest and be gay. I left the seminary very sadly and told my family and friends that I had lost my vocation, though I still felt called to the spiritual life.

"My friend Kenny in San Francisco had a bunch of nuns' habits in his closet that he'd used once for a drag show. (They'd gotten them from a convent by saying they were doing a

by evening I was beside myself with worry. What was God thinking?" Larry, thirty-six, whose real father was a minister, says he soothed his own burning embarrassment about being gay by going away from the church, taking long walks alone through the woods, and spending nights naked in the ocean.

That there are so many sex-in-church stories, or that so many of us turned to solitude for solace, raises all kinds of questions about the complicated relationship between gay men and God. Perhaps some of us have, in the words of the Rev. Malcolm Boyd, traveled to "hell and back," and gained wisdom in that journey from shame to strength. Perhaps some of us, in the words of Edward Carpenter, have become "intermediates," teachers, priests, and medicine men (see "Homospirituality," below). If you feel as though the closest you'll get to a medicine man is during your next trip to the doctor, don't despair. Getting to hell and back is a lifelong process.

One crucial part of that process, says University of California at Berkeley cultural studies professor Elias Farajaje-Jones, Ph.D., is what he calls the process of "unlearning." "We have to stop playing certain cassettes that have been played to us all our lives to make us feel bad," says Farajaje-Jones, who taught at Howard University Divinity School for twelve years. "This dichotomy—spirituality good, sexuality bad—is false. For a lot of people, sex is spirituality, a source of transcendence." Authors (and boyfriends) Gershen Kaufman and Lev Raphael, both Ph.D.'s, explore some of the same themes of unlearning in their book *Coming Out of Shame* (Doubleday, 1996). Among their suggestions for moving from "gay shame to gay pride" and undoing the feelings that keep gay men divided against ourselves: careful observation of the moments of our own intolerance, "rewriting" certain scripts we use to shame ourselves, and willfully focusing on things outside ourselves at moments we feel most embarrassed (for more on cognitive methods of this type, see "Mind Fields," in Chapter 11). Other exercises include "storing self-esteem," deciding what we value in ourselves and noting when we've been able to accomplish it, and "reowning" exactly those needs and desires we imagine to be unacceptable. Recognizing that the power to forgive lies within yourself, rather than from some external force, is a crucial step in coming out of shame.

production of *The Sound of Music.*) One day in 1979 Kenny and I and another friend donned those habits, went out into the Castro, and just manifested Nun. We got such a great reception that we started finding other ways of doing it. Meanwhile, some friends went to that first spiritual conference for radical faeries in the desert of Arizona. They came back and told us about it and said, 'We want to keep the spirituality we felt in the desert alive in the city.' So five of us went to the Castro Street Fair and passed out cards saying, 'Wanna be in the men's nuns group?' We ended up with fourteen people. In March 1980 we participated in our first community event under the name of the Sisters of Perpetual Indulgence.

"From the very first day that I put on the habit, I was aware of the spiritual tradition of gay men as holy fools. Finally, things started coming together. I knew I had a calling for the spiritual life. I thought for years it was to be a Catholic priest. It turns out I was to be a nun."

Homospirituality

The non-warlike man and the non-domestic woman, in short, sought new outlets for their energies. They sought different occupations from those of the quite ordinary man and woman—as in fact they do today; and so they became the initiators of new activities. They became students of life and nature, inventors and teachers of arts and crafts, or wizards as they would be considered and sorcerers; they became diviners and seers or revealers of the gods and religion; they became medicine men and healers, prophets and prophetesses; and so ultimately laid the foundation of the priesthood and of science, literature and art.

—*Edward Carpenter, Intermediate Types Among Primitive Folk*

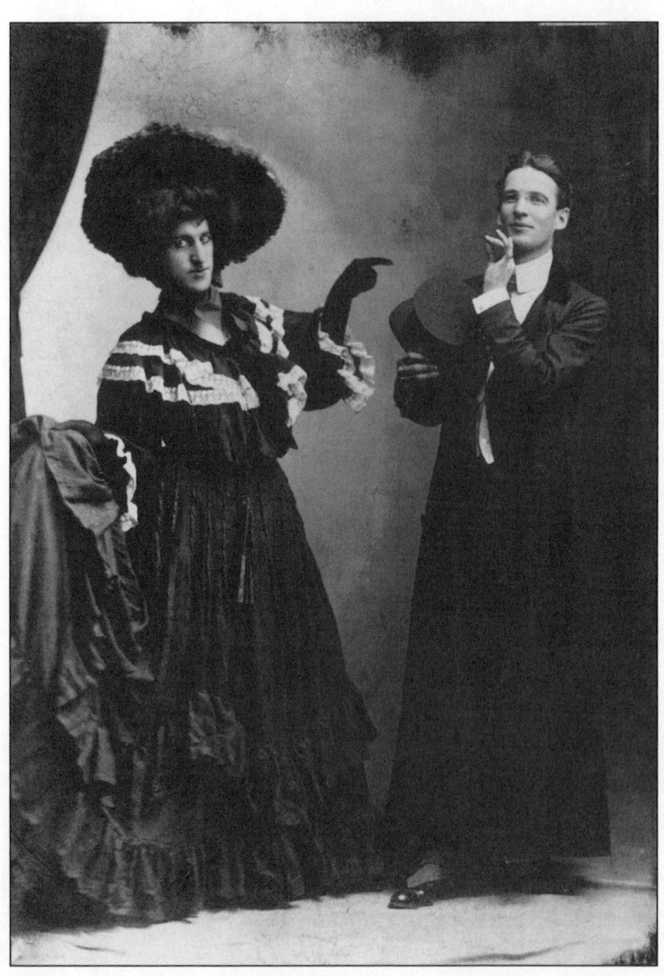

Had he lived long enough to hear the famous 1970s motto "Gay is good," early-twentieth-century author and protogay social historian Edward Carpenter might well have offered an amendment: "Gay is God" (or at least close). He wrote more than seven generations before Stonewall, but even then saw the nelly queen and butch dyke as "intermediates," not just between "quite ordinary" men and women, but between the spirit world and the more mundane one. It's one explanation for why so many gay men take refuge in the church, or even the theater. "Church was my first theater, a show we were always rehearsing for," says Don, forty-four, a former Catholic altar boy who's now a therapist in New York. "Unlike in my family's trailer, things there were maintained with reverence and wonder and mystery. People wore special clothes and used a different language. Incense and candle wax dressed the air. I learned that behind the solemn ceremony there was humor and humanity, and that kindness was available to a boy like me."

"Two-spirit" is the name Native Americans gave to men who guided their audiences into other worlds even as they walked between the worlds of men and women. Often two-spirited men wore women's clothes, lived in women's tents, and did women's work, though they sometimes were the first to ride off into battle. "In most earth-based religions or beliefs, including the Indian tribes of North America, the two-spirited people always had a place of respect," says Clyde Hall, a member of the Shoshone Bannock tribe who works as an openly gay attorney and magistrate on the Fort Hall reservation in southeast Idaho. "They were shamans, the dreamers, the visionaries, and the movers and shakers of the culture."

Other cultures have similar traditions. West African teacher Malidoma Some says that among his people, the Dagara, the *da-po,* or "man-woman," "uses energy as a force to take care of all the spiritual and physical disturbances that affect the people in the village." Among the Kwanyama-speaking people of southern Angola, priests who have sex with other men conduct such spiritual tasks as performing ritual sacrifices, healing with herbs, and divining by way of palmistry. They and their female counterparts are the only members of the culture allowed to play the musical instrument used to summon deities during the sacred ceremonies.

Drag queens in more modern times and cultures—such as San Francisco in the 1970s—

have also worked to raise spirits and be a powerful force for social transformation. On Christmas Day 1971, George Harris, aka Hibiscus, dressed as Mary and joined other self-proclaimed "Angels of Light" to stage an alternative Nativity scene to that of the local church. Dozens of other drag extravaganzas by the Angels—always free, and always outrageous—followed. Poet Allen Ginsberg, Hibiscus's sex buddy at the time, donned drag for the first time for *Blue Angel Cabaret* in 1972. "We were creating mythic figures," Hibiscus told Mark Thompson of his work with the Angels, the Cockettes, and other high-glitter, low-budget radical drag troupes of the era.

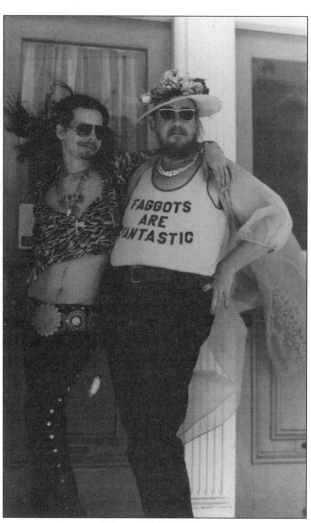

Cross-dressing, of course, is not restricted to gay men or lesbians. Transgender people, whatever their sexual orientation, are probably the ones who most clearly carry the legacy of Carpenter's witches, wizards, and prophets, or the two-spirit people of the Native Americans. In our world, though, not all transgender people, or all femme-y men or butch dykes, are able to use their two-spirited energy to take care of the spiritual disturbances of others, or even their own. Rather than being awarded instruments of leadership or divine mediation, society (including gay society) gives them the short end of the stick, exposing transpeople to psychic and physical violence. Hibiscus recalled to Mark Thompson a visit to the gay disco, the Saint, where the men there recoiled from him as if he were part of some other world they didn't wish to visit. "I felt like Jezebel when she came into the room with a scarlet dress," he said. "Everyone was so afraid to be different."

Mightn't there be in your wiggling walk, giggling talk, or delicate gestures an underappreciated trace of the divine? Perhaps those heartfelt songs you sang in junior-high-school musicals, long lost to bitter memories of cater waitering, were actually edging your eighth-grade teacher and your best friends toward a higher level. Even now, you may not need false eyelashes to find the femme within, or your role as a teacher and intermediary. Shut out the voices of those who told you difference wouldn't do. Listen to the music of your good gay soul instead, and follow. Follow, follow, follow, follow.

Earth to Gay Men: Pagan Passions

"Throw off the ugly green frog skin of heteroimitation to find the shining Faerie Prince beneath!" urged Mattachine Society founder and gay liberationist Harry Hay. The occasion was the opening-night talk at the 1979 Spiritual Conference for Radical Faeries, held in a remote desert retreat center in Arizona at the instigation of Hay, community leader Don Kilhefner, and Jungian psychologist Mitch Walker. This first faerie gathering was the product of a consciousness that had been growing through the 1970s, though the impulse behind it was more

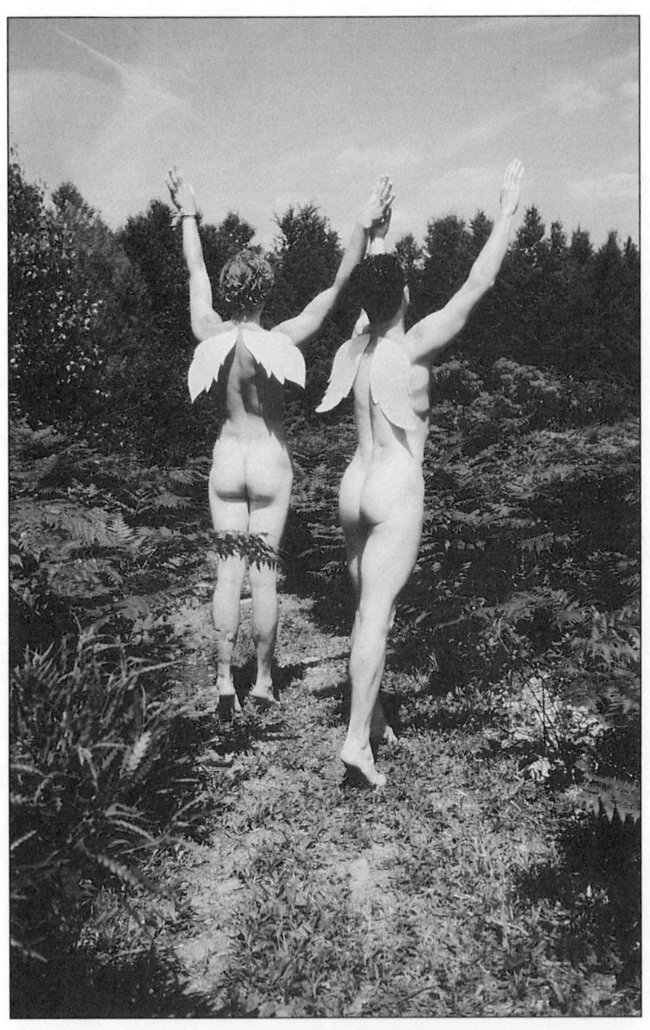

Stonehenge than Stonewall. Men have been gathering for rituals that keep them dancing all night for centuries, long before the Saint, the Stud, or Tracks were glimmers in some party promoter's mascara-laden eye.

Pagan practices, with their emphasis on spirits and earth worship, have always had an uncomfortable relationship with religions seeking to pave that earth to build temples to a single God. In the Middle Ages, Christians tore down pagan ritual sites, built cathedrals over them, or simply burned the practitioners. "Faggot," that charming word, is thought (probably incorrectly) to have come from the fact that gay men were burned like faggots, or kindling, in fires where other witches or wizards were burned at the stake. Today's dynamics are less fiery but not always less hostile. Many traditionally religious gay men look askance at the ragtag, scantily clothed, wing-adorned and often impish fairies, whose Gay Pride contingents scamper naughty and near-naked among the more respectable.

Rather than competing for territory in the cities, radical faeries tend to gather in greener pastures, woods, and wilds. While most think of gay movements as urban and political, this one explores other terrain, both physical and spiritual. The name "radical faerie" was carefully chosen: *radical* meaning both "politically extreme" and "root," and *faerie* (or *fairy* or *faery* or *fairie* or *faierie*) invoking the mythological figures who danced in circles in the moonlight and performed good deeds at will. Those rituals continue to form the heart of faerie spiritual practice, with faeries celebrating solstices and equinoxes as well as the highest of their holy days, Samhain (also known as Halloween).

Many faeries practice Wicca (that's witchcraft to you), though there's no specific doctrine or dogma involved, thank Goddess. Most live in towns and cities, and dance in fields and moonlight only rarely. And although circling a bonfire chanting "Isis, Astarte, Diana, Hecate, Demeter, Kali, Inanna!" is something that happens a lot at faerie gatherings, the essence of faerie spirituality may be as neatly captured by the zeal with which men named "Trixie" and "Lightning" (you usually choose a faerie name) descend upon the church rummage sale to score the perfect gingham frock.

RFD, a magazine "for rural gay men," is the root of the faerie grapevine, and has been for the twenty-five continuous years of its publication. Homespun and proud, *RFD*'s pages feature photos and lists of upcoming faerie gatherings, as well as contact information (including, now, Web sites—see www.rfdmag.org) for the several dozen faerie communities across the world, including those in Oregon, New Mexico, and Tennessee (see "Retreat!," page 540). Like the faeries and their friends, the magazine's form has less gloss and polish than those in gay urban centers. Looking at it, you can almost remember that paper—and pleasure, if your mind is ready for it—comes from the earth.

AIDS and Spirituality

The death of my best friend changed the direction of my life. Nursing him for the last six months of his life (especially after a brain tumor robbed him of the ability to walk, talk, write, or feed himself) called on resources of love and care I didn't know existed within me. Since then nothing has seemed so important as cultivating those inner resources.

I couldn't go for the white-light, spiritual-peace bullshit while Gordon was dying. I couldn't keep sitting there pretending that something like a peaceful departure was taking place. I couldn't keep sitting there. So I didn't. I stopped visiting the hospital. But I took up AIDS activism with a ferocity that I think must have resembled the wrath of God.

When he was dying, Jay asked me if I would call a priest. I had never even heard him mention a priest before. But that's the lesson of AIDS for me: It wasn't about me, it wasn't about us. He was leaving me, just as I was getting ready to leave him. It strained me, but I wanted to imagine that somehow, both directions would lead us to a place, sometime, where we could feel some kind of togetherness, maybe like the kind we'd had when we first met and fell in love.

Beyond the disgusting self-righteousness of it, there's an irony in fundamentalist Christian claims that AIDS is God's punishment for the sin of homosexuality. The colossal dimensions of the losses we've suffered from the epidemic seem to have brought gay men closer to our gods—however we define them—than at any other time in gay history. Even as deaths from AIDS slow, the symptoms of spiritual growth are still detectable: the "healing circles" that provide an environment of supportive prayer and meditation for people facing life-threatening illnesses, the crystals worn as commonly as freedom rings, the yoga classes bursting at the seams with young gay men. AIDS service organizations, from large ones such as GMHC to smaller outfits such as AIDS, Medicine and Miracles in Boulder, Colorado, still run on the compassionate, spirit-driven energy of volunteers. Gurus like Louise Hay and Marianne Williamson, and their numerous books, tapes, workshops, and affirmations, have become the stuff of gay history (and occasionally, of parody). Many men have found in these teachers' work, or their own, new insights into the strength of the spirit in the face of terrible hardship.

"It still rattles my nerves when I hear people say that AIDS has been their greatest gift," says Krishna Stone, outreach coordinator for volunteers at GMHC and an ordained minister at Beloved Sanctuary, a nondenominational church in Conesus, New York. "But there's no question that AIDS brings us right smack up against questions of spirit in all the places and moments we've been told God isn't present: in the bedroom, using drugs, when we're feeling despised or vulnerable. And when people reclaim those places as sacred and worthy, that's powerful. When people admit their vulnerability, voice it honestly and move forward with it, that's powerful." The power is spiritual, adds Dr. Elias Farajaje-Jones, but it's also political. "The undergirding of Western Christian theology, and I use the singular intentionally, has been a discourse that's anti-body, anti-poor, anti-color, anti-sex, and anti-pleasure," says Farajaje-Jones. "Traditionally, the poor and sick have been seen as a source of redemption for the rich and powerful—poor souls suffering for the rest of us—or avoided as a source of disease or filth. But when those souls start speaking for themselves, things change. AIDS has made it impossible for the church to do business as usual."

Has our gayness helped us remake history as we meet the challenges of AIDS? In the introduction to *The Color of Light* (HarperSanFrancisco, 1988), his book of meditations for people living with AIDS, Perry Tilleraas referred to the Native American tradition of the *heyoehkah,* or sacred clown, who walked backward, danced backward, and did everything contrary to the norm. The *heyoehkah*'s role in the tribe was to shake things up and keep people from getting stuck in rigid ways of thinking and living. Perhaps gay men and drug users and those who love us, long used to swimming against the tide of social standards, have all provided a *heyoehkah* response to AIDS. "When the normal response was to react with fear and panic, there were people dancing backward, responding with love and confidence," wrote Tilleraas. "When, every day, the world began repeating a death mantra, our sacred clowns danced the dance of life. They talked about living with AIDS, surviving, healing, recovering. When the normal reaction to a diagnosis was isolation, our *heyoehkahs* dragged us into a community. When the world wanted us to be victims, they drew circles of light around themselves and stood in their power." Whether thriving with AIDS, dying from it, or helping others do both, gay men have both challenged ideas of God and reinvigorated them.

AIDS is a paradox, focusing enormous attention on gay men's bodies, and in the process highlighting our spirits. "I want to share with you the great secret," said AIDS activist Michael Callen in an extraordinary interview published in *Spin* magazine and read at his memorial, "which is that dying can be an amazingly sensual, almost erotic experience because it's very much about the body. I sometimes wake up and the sun is pouring in and the birds are chirping. It sounds so clichéd, so trite, but my brain just repeats like a mantra: Life is good. Life is good, I'm glad I had life, life is wonderful. And because I feel that, I am not at all anguished about it ending. What I say to my friends who are New Age or religious is that perhaps I'm of limited imagination, but the taste of a tomato or Cris Williamson's voice—whatever she's singing—makes my cells vibrate. I cannot imagine anything more beautiful than this."

The Rev. Peter Laarman, senior minister of Judson Memorial Church in New York's Greenwich Village, acknowledges that AIDS has created a crisis of faith for many religiously inclined gay men. No matter how much we might want to believe in God's goodness, he says, the epidemic has forced us to question what so many awful deaths might say about divine compassion. "What sustains and gives me hope," says Rev. Laarman, "is the way in which so many people living with AIDS and so many survivors and mourners have managed to find their way through this with a stronger faith and with more life wisdom rather than with their faith incinerated and their cynicism triumphant. In other words, I don't know what the AIDS experience tells us about God. What it says about the human spirit is very encouraging."

Staying Focused in Your Faith: Kevin's Story

"Up until I was eight or ten, I went to church with my parents. Then I started playing hooky, 'cause I said, 'Ain't no spirit of God up in that church.' I always had an internal sense of spirit, of there being something greater than I was, and I knew I was okay with it on all levels. That's partly why I moved in the direction of Orisha, the worship of ancestral deities practiced in Yoruba culture.

"My lover Hal was involved with it and took me to a spiritual ceremony where they were playing drums. I thought, 'Hmm. This feels good. This feels real good.' Later I started taking classes and got more deeply involved. This isn't a religion you pick up or put down. It's similar to Buddhism—a way of living, not a religious practice. Unlike Christianity, which is a sin-based culture in which by nature of being gay you are an abomination, Orisha doesn't have a concept of sin. Our focus is on maintaining balance. It assumes that you will get out of balance and guides you to get it back. Even with the big ol' taboo subject of sex, the idea is to be conscious of the energy. Be conscious of who you're with. What energy does that person bring to your experience and is that the energy you want to interact with?

"In terms of HIV/AIDS, my spiritual journey has kept me healthy and helped me make decisions based on my internal sense of what I should do rather than simply following whatever medical advice I've been given. I've lost over 150 friends and acquaintances who've had HIV. I can't say they all died of HIV. I think fear kills people, too. I have no fear of death. We're all going to die, not necessarily of HIV. My spiritual culture confirms the importance of staying focused in your faith, in your practices, in your understanding, and not letting other people tell you who or what you are."

Community

Remember when Barbara Walters said about people who get AIDS, "Haitians, drug users, and homosexuals"—"that group"—and we all jumped down her throat because it was so ridiculous to lump us all together? That's the same thing I feel when I hear "gay, lesbian, bisexual, and transgendered."

For several years I spent week after week with all these people with whom I seemed to have nothing in common. Some of them were drag queens; I was a suit. They were piercing their faces, I was in the closet in my job. They had their skills. I had mine. We were working for each other, not because we knew each other or even liked each other, exactly, but because we were part of the same world that needed tending, because people were sick and weren't being cared for. That was a gift. That was inspiring. That made me so proud of them, and myself. For the first time, when I thought about myself and being gay, I thought the word we. Not just-my-friends-"we," or people-like-me-"we." A "we" that was much bigger.

Every year at the Gay Games, the swim teams do a drag event on the last day. You know, a campy thing, like putting dry ice in the pool and having one guy dressed as the dead Judy Garland being ferried across the pool while other swimmers dressed like drag queens act out the Stonewall riot. It's always fun. But I remember one year where the Montreal team did this skit where one swimmer was dressed up as HIV, the virus, and the other team members were in costume rounding up the virus, and vanquishing it. It sounds really hokey, but when they did it, it just totally tapped into the crowd in a way I don't think anyone could have predicted. We were all standing, cheering, crying, screaming with emotion, allowing ourselves at that moment to imagine something in a way we couldn't possibly imagine in normal life.

The word *religion* comes from the same root as *ligament,* the term for the connective tissue that ties together different limbs and muscles and allows them to experience coordinated movement. See yourself as part of a movement—gay, human, cosmic, whatever—and you'll see that spirituality, whatever its particular form, is about reaffirming connection, "re-tying" yourself not just to some idea of God, but to other living beings. God, in fact, may not be the object at all. In Mahayana Buddhism, for example, the student on the verge of enlightenment faces a dilemma: end the cycle of reincarnation and dissolve into the ecstatic nothingness of Nirvana, or decide to continue on the path with the rest of us less enlightened beings and become a *boddhisatva*. The latter is the higher, more exalted choice. Jesus commanded that we should love our neighbors as ourselves. Muslims, Jews, and Christians all pray for collective redemption and guidance: "Give *me* this day *my* daily bread" doesn't have the right ring to it. And if you take that feeling of service and commitment as one of the highest goals of spirituality, you can take it one step farther and realize that you definitely don't have to be sitting on a pew in a church or cross-legged in a Buddhist zendo to feel communion.

Where does the gay community begin and end? For all the talk of gay newspapers, gay institutions, this gay group or that one, the way gay men feel connected to each other is more complicated than who you march with on Gay Pride day or what magazines you get in the mail. Not that there's even a single "group" to be a part of. Trying to define gay community is a little like opening one of those Russian wooden boxes, finding one inside another, each feeling smaller and smaller until hardly anything fits. You may not be conscious of community at all until you bump up against the side of some pigeonhole or other. "I remember this man who came to an ACT UP meeting to beg us not to protest the high price of AIDS drugs," says Joey, thirty-five, in New York. "He said that gay members of the Wall Street community would be put in a difficult position. And I remember I got stuck on this idea of the 'Wall Street community.' I mean, what is that?" If you're on Castro Street rather than Wall Street, or partying with a hundred thousand of your brothers and sisters during a march on Washington, you may still be hard pressed to figure out a way to knit together Gay Armenians Against Genocide, Accountants for a Change, Gay Men Clean and Sober, transgender S/M activists, and go-go boys in hula skirts. Boston-based writer Michael Bronski dismisses the idea of a single-minded or consolidated gay community as "so far from reality as to be, depending upon one's frame of mind, either a myth or a joke."

Myths, though, like all fantasies, enrich as well as disappoint. Thousands of gay and bisexual men stream to urban centers to look for a place where they, quietly or not, can feel part of a greater gay whole. The young wrestlers practicing in gay community centers are moving to put locks not just on each other but on that moment when they feel part of a team. The elderly Scrabble players in the room upstairs may be doing the same, piecing together a vocabulary to speak of themselves as united, on the same board. Some of the greatest political and personal achievements of gay men have been fueled by those moments when gay men and lesbians, bisexuals, transgendered people, and our straight allies have all been able to see ourselves as greater than the sum of our self-interests.

An awareness of collective being is one of community's most precious dividends. Malidoma Some, writing in *Ritual: Power, Healing, and Community* (Viking Penguin, 1997), describes what he calls "supportive presence," the moment where "others in community become the reason that one feels the way one feels. The elder cannot be an elder if there is no community to make him an elder. The young boy cannot feel secure if there is no elder whose silent presence gives him hope in life." If talk of children and elders seems uncomfortably people-of-the-village and not Village People enough for your taste, you might want to look at how you're thinking about aging (see Chapter 8). Or you can adopt a more generation-free description. "I think a lot of community making is about falling in love with each other," Keith, a San Francisco–based performer and activist, says. "Somehow, everything your community does interests you. You let their style rub off on you a little bit. You want to wear their clothes and copy their dance moves. Someone will tell me who they're interested in sexually, and I'll start to find that type sexy, too."

Yearning for community gone by, or disappointment with the one we have, may be as common as feeling its embrace. "Sometimes I look at the local gay newspaper and see endless ads for beer busts, performances by drag queens, and phone sex, and I think, "Is this *really* what I came out for?" says Don, forty-four. Watching reruns of *Ellen* at a bar—is that community? Bowling with a gay league one night a week—is that community? Dancing at a circuit party—is that community? The same Gay Pride march that can set you bubbling when you first move from South Dakota can seem as flat as old champagne ten years later. But not to worry. Having one foot in and one foot out, struggling to recommit, is part of most religious narratives.

Women and Gay Men

I brought my friend Tamar to the beach house I share with a bunch of friends on Fire Island. One of the guys in a nearby house grabbed my wrist as I was walking along the boardwalk. "Let me smell your fingers," he said. "I want to see if they smell like your friend's cunt."

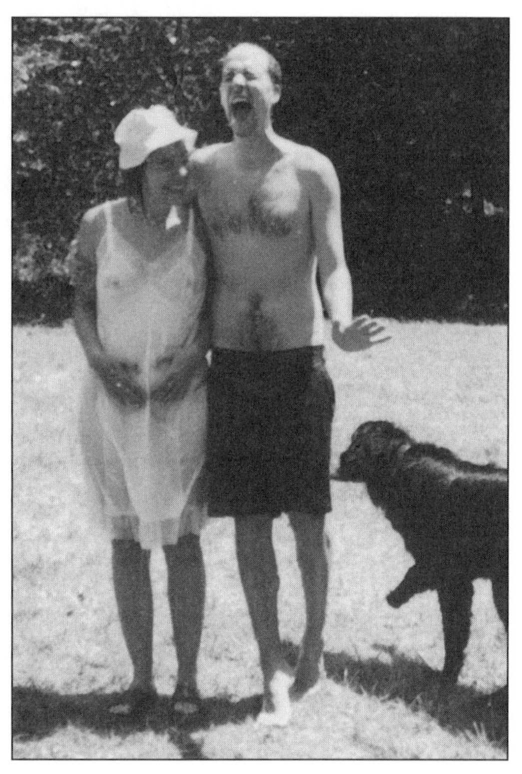

I like sex with women. It's just that my desire to be with a man is stronger, and I find it easier to relate to men in intimacy. My relationships with women always tend to this brotherly-sisterly kind of thing and unless there's some help on her part, it never gets sexual. I know being with a woman is something my family would like. But I recognize that the reality is I am gay. Just like I'm five-ten and would love to be six-three.

Tina has a sexual life of her own, but she understands the ironies of the fag hag role. The other day a bunch of us were talking about anal sex and she got up from the table to go to the bathroom, saying "This isn't the part of gay life I like. I like the part where you scream about my hair and my outfit and tell me how pretty I look."

Everyone who knows us thinks we're married. She knows all my friends. I say, "Marilyn, how would you like to . . ." and she says, "Yep." I don't have to complete the sentence. She can read my thoughts to know when I need to be with someone, and she can also read them and say, "I think you need to be alone." I've developed a family through her: her two sons with their wives and children have become like mine, her grandchildren call me Grandpa. Michael's my lover, but she's my significant other. She knows Michael, Michael knows Marilyn, and there's time in my life for both.

TURNING A GAY GAZE ON THE GAY NEIGHBORHOOD

Every once in a while you'll see someone being totally out there, like a really fabulous drag queen or a man in some outrageous leather outfit, something you know would have no place in another neighborhood. Sometimes it's embarrassing. But if you're in a good mood, especially if they're doing it with a sense of humor, there's this feeling, this fantasy, of a world where behavior like that doesn't have repercussions, and isn't going to be punished.

Better window shopping, greater cruising opportunities, the feeling that everyone there has something in common with you even though they look different, and feeling safe. Oh, and the flea markets are especially good.

All the relationships I have, my own version of family, are contained in this neighborhood. It's like village life, it has that "Howdy, neighbor" feeling. I like running into two friends as they're driving by, having someone intercept you on the way to the gym and convince you to come to dinner instead, doing a little business on your lunch hour. All of that is marked and contained by something as vague, and as powerful, as a few street corners.

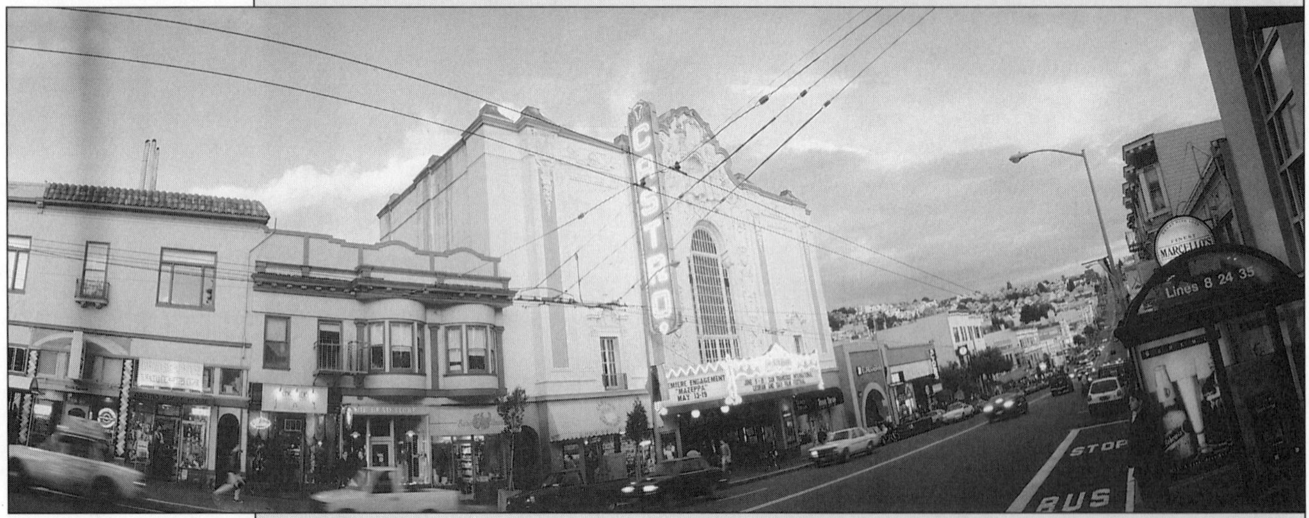

Ask gay men about their local gay neighborhoods, and their answers may vary depending on their age, weight, length of time they've spent there, or even their mood. "When I feel good, I look in the mirror and see a gay man with as much to offer as any Chelsea boy," says John, twenty-five, whose youth may match the ideal of Chelsea 2000, but whose heavy frame (and heavy-framed glasses) doesn't. "I love seeing people, hanging out in those cafés with all those incredible men, being part of the scene. But when I'm down, I just think, 'Oh, God, I'm another ugly old troll, and I don't want to be seen in public! I mean, no way will I walk down Eighth Avenue when I'm feeling that way."

Gay people have often flocked to big cities to escape the loneliness, boredom, disapproval, or danger they experience in small towns and rural areas. If they re-create that small-town feeling in a gay urban neighborhood, at least it's a small town where they feel welcome. "For me, there's a sense of security and connectedness," says Giuliano, fifty-one, a program manager for the San Francisco Department of Health, of life in the Castro, arguably the world's most famous gay neighborhood. "I like the sweet little acknowledgments from the people I see all the time. We smile or wink or flirt with each other. And I appreciate having a gay doctor, a gay cardiologist, a gay barber, a gay garbage collector, and a gay cop (who is cute and will flirt) in the neighborhood."

Outlaw writer and unrepentant queer William Burroughs, in Mark Thompson's *Gay Spirit,* discerned a less sweet, but equally important, potential in gay neighborhoods: protection. Burroughs fantasized about the gay neighborhood as a kind of city-state, supported by gay gangs in the order of Chinese tongs or a gay Mafia. "Greg arrives in a strange town and goes to his [gay] Tong," he wrote of the gay state that never was. "He is immediately eligible for all the services and directed to a gay rooming house or hotel. He can get a job, medical and legal aid. He will be protected from violence by patrols operating around the clock. In the event of a blackmail attempt he can take his complaint to the protection department for legal advice." Burroughs's fantasy—of gay associations able to form a single voting bloc, bring down boycotts on businesses hostile to gay men, and protect their own—is one lived out in limited degree by many men who take up residence in gay urban centers. "Living here makes it safe and easy to find sex, friends, fellow activists, and possibly lovers," says twenty-nine-year-old Tony of his residence near the Hill Crest district of San Diego. "I suppose it also makes it easy to keep away from people different from myself. But at this point in my life I don't mind much. After eleven years of HIV trauma, I'm rebuilding my understanding of gay male solidarity and finding there's a lot to uncover."

But when does gay sweetness begin to sour? When does the need for security become an excuse for ignoring people who remind you in any way of the world outside? What's going on within or without, when a twenty-five-year-old describes himself as "an ugly old troll"? Mark Thompson is among those who see "gay ghettos" as part of our problems rather than part of the solution, a demonstration that "gay people can be as banal, myopic, and prejudiced as anyone else." For him and others who wish we would do more "coming out inside," the strength of being gay lies in using our awareness of difference to expand our options. Gay ghettos, goes the argument, are places where gay men open our wallets and flies more than we do our hearts, where we take pride without taking responsibility. "I think we should close them down," says Stephen, who is fifty-four. "We're only holding ourselves back. If we want to be accepted, we've got to stop acting like everything's a sex party. Get outside. Move out. Move on."

The term "coming out" originally was less about the closet you left behind than about the fabulous world you were coming into. Making that world into someplace where gay men, including fifty-four-year-old or non-White or non-buff or non-rich-and-stylish gay men, feel safe clearly doesn't end with walking the dog down New York's Eighth Avenue or tending garden in San Francisco's "Swish Alps." It might mean politics, or activism, or simply working to keep communication alive with people who aren't part of your gay gang, however you define that. "I've been in *Newsweek,* local papers and am internationally, 'media-atically' out," says Dr. Farajaje-Jones. "That doesn't mean that when I go to the grocery store and the straight cashier asks me, 'What does that T-shirt mean?' that I can toss my head and give a pat answer. We need to talk."

Exhortations to "shut gay neighborhoods down" or "get outside," however, sound suspiciously like attempts to destroy someone else's identity so that you can feel better about your own. Many gay men do choose to live among straight people and see that choice as political without feeling the need to lecture. "It's great to visit Montreal or Boston or New York and feel the erotic energy of the city itself and of a concentrated gay population, but I always love coming home to what feels like a more rooted, more easily accessible, less stratified, and definitely less judgmental population of gay people," says Stan, in Burlington, Vermont. "There are lots of potluck dinners and weekend volleyball picnics here, and almost to an obnoxious degree, people talk about their gardens, wood supply, and home building. But that's true of everyone in Vermont." Dee, a forty-six-year-old librarian who left "the counterculture, folkie, food co-op crowd" of Cambridge, Massachusetts, for Champaign-Urbana, Illinois, found the change—and the fact that the one gay bar in town catered to men, women, leather folk, drag queens, and just about everyone else in the "LGBT community"—refreshing. "College was so specialized, with a gay Jewish campus group, an older Black men's group," he says. "You never met other people." Especially women. "I love gay men," agrees Harry, fifty-one, from Seattle. "But not enough to spend all my time with them. All-male environments, even when they're gay, are scary."

Film critic B. Ruby Rich, looking at *Clueless, My Best Friend's Wedding, As Good as It Gets, The Object of My Affection,* and a host of other 1990s films, termed the relationship between gay men and straight women "the love that wouldn't shut up." But as much as a woman pining after a gay man may seem like a familiar theme, what gay men get out of the relationship—the ways in which we relish the dynamic or retreat from it—remains undiscussed. "It's a marriage of way more than convenience," says Tim of his relationship with his best straight women friends. "I love women and kind of wish I were one. And there's those moments when you think, 'I have everything with this person except the sexual. Why?' It's like an ache." The stereotype of the fag hag—the woman who hangs out with gay men she can't have because it's less painful than lusting after straight men she can't get—is no more psychologically insightful than the stereotype of the dick-crazy, woman-hating gay man.

Nor, contrary to the beliefs of the screenwriters and armchair psychoanalysts, are all gay men's connections with women about romantic connections gone slightly awry, or mothering dynamics reconfigured. Among the things AIDS helped blur were the boundaries of lesbian separatism and gay male independence. "Because it was so often lesbians who were there cleaning up our shit, it made me look at some of my own about women," says Donald, age thirty-five. "Many of these women were activists a hundred times more experienced and aware than the men. They were tough, they liked gay men, but had no intention of having sex with us or being our mothers. I've learned way more about the best side of macho from butch lesbians than from my gay friends or my father."

What do women say? Many different things, of course, but here are a few of the choice items offered up by women who love gay men.

BE THERE FOR WOMEN'S ISSUES

"I remember at an ACT UP meeting when they were talking about how a promising new medication for AIDS that had no women in the trial and I thought, 'Oh, my God, what if they found a cure that only worked for men? Would this room suddenly be empty?'" says Monica, thirty-five. "That was such an unbearably painful thought. The way I've been there for AIDS issues, I want to see my gay friends there for breast cancer and reproductive rights and women with AIDS."

THINK OF LESBIAN BODIES, NOT JUST THE BODY POLITIC

"The comments about the shirtless lesbians with less-than-perfect breasts, the 'Ew, really—I don't want to think about that,' or worse, the fish jokes, say more about you than they do about me," says Hilary. "And don't do the routine about how lesbians represent the model, domestic, best parts of gay life." Adds Lisa: "Lesbians do have sex and nasty breakups and superficial lusts, just like gay men. And we *don't* want to domesticate you. That's why we're lesbians."

ALL-MALE ALL RIGHT?

"I hate it when everyone gets up from the table to go out and they're like, 'Bye,' as if it goes without saying that I won't be going to the club and that's fine," says Debbie. "I know it's not appropriate for me to go. But it's nice when someone acknowledges that, or suggests going someplace I can join."

BAG THE "FAG HAG" TERMINOLOGY

"If we're good enough to entertain you and listen to you talk about boy problems, we're good enough to not be disrespected by you calling us fag hags or fruit flies," says Tanya. "Or else there needs to be a name for all you gay boys who like playing Barbie with real people. Fish fag? Dolly dick?"

Is That All There Is? Five Ways to Break the Bar/Bathhouse Blues

People call it AIDS activism, but for me it was activism about a whole number of gay and gay-related issues. You could go into the street and be arrested and so what? That whole fear of authority was broken. The worst thing that you could imagine happening happened, and so what? Instead of feeling beaten, we felt more powerful. There was momentum, and yes, there was a mob quality too, but it helped you take a lot of liberties. Like kiss-ins. I would never participate. I'm not a big fan of public displays of affection. But I knew there was something important about it, not just for me but for all of us.

People say to me, "Oh, you don't complain because you have all those meetings to go to, but I can't go to that kind of thing. I can't go to meetings, I can't stand those people." And I say, "Well, if you want to do what I do, do what I did." You have to start somewhere.

We all know the tune. Men are pigs, the gay community has nothing to offer except snarky queens with attitude, and you wouldn't consider going to a community center and sitting somewhere with all the rest of the losers with bad shoes and hair on their backs. But if West Hollywood makes you hateful or Chelsea makes you churlish—if bars and bathhouses seem both irresistible and totally unnourishing—perhaps it's time to reread the menu. Sure, doing volunteer work is cliché. But whining about the emptiness of sex or the snottiness of men you can't seem to tear your eyes away from isn't exactly breaking the mold. Besides, working for a change is hip. If Linda Evangelista and friends can form DISHES (Determined Involved Supermodels Helping to End Suffering), can't you get up offa that thing, onto the runway, and into a new flight pattern? Here are five suggestions:

1. *Help another gay man or lesbian by volunteering your time at a local gay organization that you admire.* Anti-violence projects all over the country need volunteers. Many churches and AIDS service organizations operate on volunteer energy. Offer whatever professional skills you have. If you're a massage therapist, you might offer massages to homebound people with AIDS. If you're an accountant, you might offer tax advice. If you're a lawyer, you might assist people with wills and other legal documents. If you're the president of your company, you might volunteer to walk someone's dog.

2. *Check out the nearest gay and lesbian center.* (See "A Room of Our Own," page 564). Just looking over the list of groups that meet there may give you some ideas. The LGBT Community Center in Tallahassee has on its monthly calendar a writers' group, a bowling league, a classic horror movie night potluck, a "polyamorous" chat group, and a gay outdoors group that goes tubing at Ichetucknee Springs.

3. Call your nearest gay switchboard and get a listing of every gay event next Friday night that's not cruising. All over the country men are joining volleyball teams, reading groups, gardening clubs, and cooking classes. "For instance, there is a group of gay men that meets monthly to eat pasta and speak Italian to each other, mio amore," says Giuliano in San Francisco. "There is a branch of the Sierra Club that is queer, and they organize hikes and other outdoor events. If you're looking for community, I would advise you to join clubs, take classes, or hang out at a gay café. Of course, if you live in Omaha or Little Rock, I would advise you to move to San Francisco."

4. Go online. Cyberspace is an invaluable resource, especially for people who live outside metropolitan areas. Dwight, a clock repairman in Hinton, West Virginia, considers the Internet a "fabulous tool." It used to be that his only way to meet up with a guy was to drive forty miles to a gay bar. Thanks to a site called Rural Gay (www.ruralgay.com) he has joined a group called Mountain State Bears who have monthly meetings and plan camping trips together. Personal ads on such Web sites make it possible to meet other people for "alternative" holiday dinners or river-rafting trips. And of course, do-it-yourself sites are an oasis for guys who find body hair, a big belly, and being older than thirty-two better than Viagra for rousing the slumbering beast.

5. Push the envelope. If you don't find what you need, start something yourself. After a television appearance on the *Phil Donahue Show*, Lidell Jackson got a phone call from a twenty-three-year-old Black gay man in Boise, Idaho. "He was struck by my saying on TV that my Blackness was as important to me as my gayness," says Lidell. "I sent him some gay community publications from New York and information about Gay Men of African Descent. The following year he came up to me at the National Gay and Lesbian Task Force conference and introduced himself. He said he placed an ad in the local community newspaper saying, 'I want to start a lesbian and gay group. Let's meet at such-and-such a restaurant.' Over twenty people showed up, and half of them came to the national conference."

Nor is organizing the only way to take initiative. "You don't have to have done X number of things in order to be able to say, 'Okay, I'm an activist,'" says Dr. Farajaje-Jones. "Your work may be something like finally being able to be talk about your male partner like he's a 'he' instead of saying 'they.' That's important." Context is everything. "Here, gay activism is two men getting together and having dinner downtown," says Michael in South Carolina.

Somewhere out of the Rainbow: Men of Color and Gay Community

There was a whole group of us that went to the Million Man March. We went in marching and chanting that we were gay. And we were applauded.

W.E.B Du Bois, founder of the NAACP, described the struggle to achieve things as a Black man in a White-controlled world as a crisis of "double consciousness." Trying to keep from being torn apart by the "twoness," he said, could be met only with "dogged strength." Add homosexuality to the mix, and you are definitely talking multiple personalities. "White gay men in Silverlake or Chelsea may feel like they're coming home to gay neighborhoods, but those of us in Compton or Harlem are leaving ours to get there," says Larry Abrams, assistant director of GMHC's Black gay men's HIV prevention program, Soul Food. Poet Essex Hemphill called having to choose between Black and gay identities like being asked to choose between "my left ball and my right." For Elias Farajaje-Jones, Ph.D., for twelve years "the only out queer professor—correction, the only out queer person"—at Howard University's Divinity School, the question "Are you Black first or gay first?" has always received the answer "Does not compute." "It's kept on not computing for me," says Farajaje-Jones, "primarily because I don't think in either/or ways. People have tried to make us think that having a politicized sexual identity means that you have to move to White gay space, whether that's geographic space or psychic space. But it's essential to come home as well as to come out, to be present in the Black community with all of our pieces. If we are in a community meeting on urban violence and Black teens, we can bring issues of sexuality and homophobia into that meeting, because we were also Black gay teens. The reaction is going to be, 'We're not here to talk about gay stuff, we're here talking about Black stuff.' But this *is* our stuff. This *is* our reality. We live at this intersection."

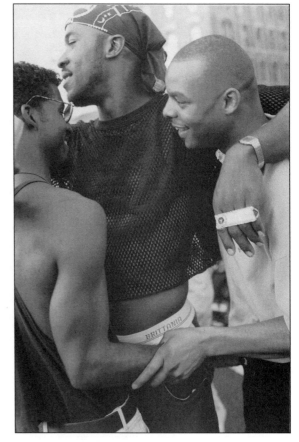

The late video maker and writer Marlon Riggs left the intersection, traveling from the halls of Hepsibah High in Augusta, Georgia, to the promised land of San Francisco's Castro. "I avoided the question," said Riggs in his exquisite video exploration of Black and gay identity, *Tongues Untied*. "Pretended not to notice the absence of black images in this new gay life, in bookstores, poster shops, film festivals, my own fantasies. Tried not to notice the few images of Blacks that were most popular: joke, fetish, cartoon caricature, or disco diva adored from a distance. Something in Oz, in me, was amiss, but I tried not to notice." *Trying* was the word that came to describe Castro life for Riggs, as it has for many manchildren in the promised land whose bodies aren't the hue of milk or honey. "I was an alien, unseen, and seen, unwanted," wrote Riggs of his later decision to quit the Castro. "Here, as in Hepsibah, I was a nigga, still."

Coming home means making peace with first steps. "I tried to get a bunch of us together to talk to the bars about the fact that we were always the ones to get carded," says James E. Miles, an HIV educator and community organizer from Pittsburgh. "We turned out not to be ready for the politics, but it was powerful to meet each other, to see what we looked like as Black gay men together outside of bars." Seeing what you look like as gay men together is one of the most important pieces of coming home, says Miles, though it doesn't have to start at home. "I remember the first time I went down to DC for Memorial Day, which is one of the stops on the Black gay party circuit," says Miles. "I stayed with a friend. We didn't go to the party, but we went to the big picnic at the end, and there were thousands and thousands of men from around the country. I still remember thinking 'Oh, my God, there *is* a larger Black gay community. This is some of what it looks like.' Back in Pittsburgh, and later when I moved to New York, I carried that image with me."

Keith Boykin, former director of the National Lesbian and Gay Black Leadership Forum, sees the fragility of that image—the relative lack of symbols, media outlets, organizations, or

A ROOM OF OUR OWN: GAY AND LESBIAN (AND SOMETIMES BISEXUAL AND TRANSGENDER) COMMUNITY CENTERS

In 1971 a handful of gay men and lesbians in Los Angeles got together to create an organization to provide social services for the local community. They started with a bank account of $35. Since then, the L.A. Gay & Lesbian Center has grown into a major institution with over two hundred staff members, three thousand volunteers, fourteen thousand clients per month, and an annual budget of over $16 million, with a four-story headquarters in Hollywood and satellite offices throughout the greater metropolitan area.

Some version of this story has been repeated in major cities across the country. There are now more than a hundred lesbian and gay community centers in thirty-three states, from the modest Up the Stairs Community Center in Fort Wayne, Indiana, and the Panhandle Gay & Lesbian Support Services in Scottsbluff, Nebraska, to much larger centers serving the gay communities of Los Angeles, Chicago, and New York. Many centers provide meeting space for every conceivable variety of gay organization, and some offer counseling and support for youth, the elderly, people living with HIV and AIDS, people struggling with substance abuse, and survivors of antigay violence. Some of them are attached to community health projects that offer counseling, addiction recovery groups, testing and treatment for sexually transmitted diseases, and so forth. Their cultural programs range from showing weekly movies to hosting speaking engagements by prominent gay writers and thinkers. Most of all, they provide safe space to hang out, meet other gay people, and cure your sense of isolation.

The Web site for the New York City community center (www.gaycenter.org) provides information on other centers in the country as well as links to those with Web sites. (Click on "National Center Directory" and then "Centers by State.") Not all of these serve gay men, or lesbians, or transgender people, or bisexuals. A short list of locations is found below.

ARIZONA
Phoenix
Tucson

CALIFORNIA
Berkeley
Chico
Eureka
Fremont
Garden Grove
Long Beach
Los Angeles
Pleasant Hill
Sacramento
San Anselmo
San Bernadino
San Diego
San Francisco
San Jose
San Luis Obispo
Santa Barbara
Santa Cruz
Ventura

COLORADO
Denver
Fort Collins

CONNECTICUT
East Norwalk
Hartford
New Haven

FLORIDA
Fort Lauderdale
Key West
Miami
North Miami
Orlando
Tallahassee
West Palm Beach

GEORGIA
Atlanta

HAWAII
Honolulu

IDAHO
Boise

ILLINOIS
Champaign
Chicago

INDIANA
Fort Wayne
Indianapolis

IOWA
Cedar Rapids
Iowa City

KANSAS
Wichita

KENTUCKY
Louisville

LOUISIANA
New Orleans

MAINE
Caribou
Limestone

MARYLAND
Baltimore

MASSACHUSETTS
Boston

MICHIGAN
Ferndale
Grand Rapids
Kalamazoo

MINNESOTA
Duluth
Minneapolis

MISSOURI
St. Louis
Springfield

NEBRASKA
Omaha
Scottsbluff

NEVADA
Las Vegas

NEW JERSEY
Asbury Park
New Brunswick
Northfield
Woodbury

NEW YORK
Albany
Brooklyn
Queens
New York
Rochester
Syracuse
White Plains

OHIO
Cincinnati
Cleveland
Columbus
Dayton
Mentor

OKLAHOMA
Oklahoma City
Tulsa

OREGON
Ashland
Portland

PENNSYLVANIA
Harrisburg
Philadelphia
Pittsburgh

SOUTH CAROLINA
Columbia

TENNESSEE
Memphis
Nashville

TEXAS
Austin
Dallas
El Paso
Houston
San Antonio

UTAH
Salt Lake City

VIRGINIA
Harrisonburg

WASHINGTON
Seattle
Tacoma

WISCONSIN
Madison
Milwaukee

annual celebrations for Black gay men and lesbians—as one of the challenges of coming home to Black gay community. Yes, the color purple and the term "same-gender-loving" are making slow but steady appearances at Black gay events, and yes, there is a range of small magazines and Internet sites where Black gay men exchange ideas. But Boykin sees the need for faster change, greater support for men struggling to come out, and greater recognition of how little nourishment can come from living off what he calls "the crumbs of other, mostly White gay notions of community."

Though issues change with their cultures and the stereotypes to which they are subjected, many gay men of color—Latino, Asian, and Native American as well as Black—describe the power of coming together in groups where they don't have to waste time explaining. The journey may mean leaving the country you were born in, or wrestling with a feeling of confusion about whether the neighborhood you live in, or the group you may want to join, really has space for you. "The first time I remember being part of a group of gay Latino men was when I was living in Atlanta," says Daniel Castellanos, a Colombian immigrant and the organizer of GMHC's Proyecto P.A.P.I. (Poder, Apoyo, Prevencion e Identidad). "It was the day of the Gay Pride parade, and my partner and I wanted to go to the parade, but we didn't know anyone. We just stood on the sidewalk, watching the parade go by. And when the Latino group came by, we jumped in. We were having fun and everything, but when it came to the end, where people gathered in the park, I just went away, back to White friends and a different world. I didn't really know the Latino group. I didn't know if I could think about what it meant to be Latino and gay, if that was something I was really ready for."

Paradoxically, leaving the places where people of color live and returning to them, emigrating over and over, is a part of coming home for gay men. "For a lot of us, commuting to a gay neighborhood is like a reenactment of the leaving-home process," says Castellanos, now seven years away from Colombia. "Where I live now, in Queens—that could be downtown Bogotá or downtown Lima. Most gay men near me get on the train and go to Chelsea or the Village, the Manhattan gay neighborhoods, and walk down the street holding hands with their boyfriends. But holding hands in Jackson Heights? For a lot of people, that's doing it too close to home." Castellanos and other volunteers organized a dinner at La Pequeña Colombia, a restaurant in their neighborhood. "Lots of people said it was the first time they could remember sitting down in a restaurant with a large group that was clearly gay," he says. "It was a little uncomfortable, but it also felt so good. Not for something dramatic to happen. Just to be together, and be served, and for everything to be smooth." Sitting together is a literalization of what other of Castellanos's projects spend a lot of time exploring: the moments where the Latino and gay parts of oneself are both present. "We spent three months before the gay parade in Jackson Heights talking about why, since all of us always marched in Manhattan, it was so hard to imagine marching in the parade in Queens—fears that we'd be seen as flamboyant, that someone would tell our neighbors or our relatives, that one man's drag outfit might make people think differently about one of the others of us," says Castellanos. "And we'd review, over and over, that being Latino and gay meant being able to tolerate being them both at the same time, to feel comfortable holding both. And that's a struggle."

Coming home also means coming to terms with the fact that certain people still think white's the only color in the rainbow, and moving past them. "My generation was all about getting the White people to see what we're talking about," says Lidell Jackson about the growing force, and numbers of groups, for young gay men and lesbians of color. "Nowadays the attitude is if they get it, fine; if not, we're not going to spend an inordinate amount of doing their work for them."

After only two men of color attended one of the GaySpirit conferences in Atlanta, a number of White men did some work of their own, engaging in a lengthy questioning on racial segregation in gay society generally and spiritual conferences like theirs in particular. Conversation posted on their Web site (gayspirit.home.mindspring.com) ranged from discussions of disposable income to the "mountain-to-Mohammed" question of why White men would sit back, place a few advertisements, and expect men of color to feel welcome. Perhaps the best summary of the conversation was convener Jonathan Lerner's reminder, long obvious to gay men whose skin is not white, that racism doesn't end with coming out. "Overcoming racism and its effects is not just the job of people of color," he offered. "It's really hard work, and it makes everybody tired, and it won't be finished in our lifetimes." "True enough," says James E. Miles Jr., not content to have that be the last word. "But it's only getting to work on racism today that will get us to tomorrow."

As If

If you don't feel you have an activist's knowledge or conviction, use someone else's. The late Vito Russo, author of *The Celluloid Closet* (HarperCollins, 1987) and champion of grassroots politics, was on his deathbed when David Dinkins, then the mayor of New York City, paid him a call. Vito's voice was reduced to a whisper—he could hardly breathe—but somehow he pulled himself together to offer a last exhortation to political action. "In 1776, Edmund Burke of the British Parliament said of the slavery clause, 'A politician owes the people not only his industry, but his judgment,'" Vito intoned. "'And if he sacrifices his judgment to their opinions, then he has betrayed them.'" Mayor Dinkins left impressed, and later, at Russo's memorial, said he'd remember the moment for the rest of his life. Another speaker at the memorial was Vito's friend Arnie Kantrowitz. "Vito loved that speech, too," he said. "It was from the Broadway musical version of *1776*."

Vito Russo died of AIDS in 1992, having promised to kick the shit out of the epidemic and then to kick the shit out of the system that let things get this bad. His death was a huge loss, but not enough to dim the vital spirit of his promises. "The best way to cause a revolution is to live as openly as you possibly can in your own life," he said in 1980, before we even knew what AIDS would do to him or to our ideas of gay community. "Do it openly so that other people can see that the sky doesn't fall on you and try to affect their lives some way like that. Be open everywhere you go, and don't let people force you into hiding. One of the things that disturbs me most is gay people who try to tell people, if you're going to be openly gay in public, you better conform to the party line, you better say the things that the movement is saying, otherwise you're betraying us. And that's not true at all. A guy is not betraying anybody by being himself. In fact he's helping the gay movement by being himself, because he's showing the people that not every gay person is political, not every gay person is into the kind of things that people think they are—he's breaking stereotypes in his own way. There are as many different kinds of gay people as there are different kinds of straight people."

Viva Vito. Those are some last words we all can live with.

FURTHER READING

Boulder, Brian (ed.). (1995) *Wrestling with the Angel: Faith and Religion in the Lives of Gay Men*. New York: Riverhead Books. Twenty-one personal accounts by gay men reflecting on their spiritual journeys.

Bronski, Michael. (1996) *Taking Liberties: Gay Men's Essays on Politics, Culture and Sex*. New York: Masquerade Books, Inc. Thoughts on where gay community begins and ends, and what delineates the boundaries.

Conner, Randy P. (1993) *Blossom of Bone: Reclaiming the Connections between Homoeroticism and the Sacred*. San Francisco: HarperSanFrancisco. A review of many spiritual roles played by androgynous and gender-bending individuals across history and time.

De La Huerta, Christian. (1999) *Coming Out Spiritually*. New York: Putnam. The founder of Q-spirit offers suggestions on how to get in touch with your spirituality.

Desert Moon Periodicals. *RFD: Gay Men's Magazine for the Rural Lifestyle and Beyond*. Call (505) 474-6311 for subscriptions. The root of the Radical Faerie grapevine, this magazine has been in continuous publication for more than two decades.

Dossey, Larry, MD. (1993) *Healing Words*. New York: HarperPaperbacks. A (slightly) critical survey of the many studies linking healing to the power of prayer, with lots of references and suggestions for further reading.

Kaufman, Gershen, and Lev Raphael. (1996) *Coming Out of Shame*. New York: Doubleday. How to reclaim your pride, inside.

Leyland, Winston (ed.). (1998) *Queer Dharma: Voices of Gay Buddhists*. San Francisco: Gay Sunshine Press Inc. Voices of Black, White, and Asian Buddhists, from monks to weekend workshop warriors, all gay and proud.

McNeill, John J. (1996) *Taking a Chance on God: Liberating Theology for Gays, Lesbians and their Lovers, Families and Friends*. Boston: Beacon Press. A priest's arguments for a Catholic Church tolerant of homosexuality and a homosexuality able to embrace Catholicism.

Raphael, Lev. (1996) *Journeys and Arrivals: On Being Gay and Jewish*. Winchester: Faber and Faber. "Greatest hits" from a leading explorer of the intersection of Jewish and gay identity.

Riggs, Marlon. (1991) "Tongues Untied." In *Brother to Brother*, Essex Hemphill, (ed.) Los Angeles: Alyson Books. Poems, stories, and essays by Black gay writers, including those now lost to AIDS, such as Marlon Riggs and Essex Hemphill.

Rotes, Eric. (1998) *Dry Bones Breathe: Gay Men Creating Post-AIDS Identities and Cultures*. New York: Harrington Park Press. How gay men connect and commune in the post–protease inhibitor era, from an veteran community organizer and cultural critic.

Some, Malidoma. (1997) *Ritual: Power, Healing and Community*. New York: Blue Water/Viking Penguin. A West African spiritual teacher's thoughts on the order of things.

Thompson, Mark (ed.). (1987) *Gay Spirit: Myth and Meaning*. New York: St. Martin's Press. The "classic" exploration on the roots and branches of homospirituality from the former culture editor of *The Advocate*, full of history and essays on everything from Native American gay spirituality to drag queens.

Tilleraas, Perry. (1988) *The Color of Light: Meditations for All of Us Living with AIDS*. San Francisco: Harper SanFrancisco. Inspiration for all people touched by AIDS.

Appendix A

Help: I Need Somebody

Gay-Specific Clinics and Referral Help • Body • Mind • Soul and Spirit • Community • Working the System

Contents

For Transgender resources, please see page 587.

I. Gay-Specific Clinics and Referral Help

Gay and Lesbian Medical Association
459 Fulton Street, Suite 107, San Francisco, CA 94102
(415) 255-4547
www.glma.org

National Lesbian and Gay Health Association
1407 S Street NW, Washington, DC 20009
(202) 939-7880
Fax: (202) 234-1467
www.nlgha.org

Michael Callen/Audre Lorde Community Health Center
356 West 18th Street, New York, NY 10011
Patient care: (212) 271-7200
Administration: (212) 271-7250
Fax: (212) 271-8111
www.callen-lorde.org

Fenway Community Health Center
7 Haviland Street, Boston, MA 02115
(617) 267-0900
Fax: (617) 267-3667
www.fchc.org

Hartford Gay and Lesbian Health Collective
1841 Broad Street, Hartford, CT 06114
(860) 278-4163
Fax: (860) 724-3443
www.hglhc.org

Chase-Brexton Health Services, Inc.
1001 Cathedral Street, Baltimore, MD 21201
(410) 837-2050
Fax: (410) 837-2071
www.chasebrexton.org

Whitman-Walker Clinic, Inc.
1407 S Street NW, Washington, DC 20009
(202) 797-3500
www.whitman-walker.org

Howard Brown Health Center
945 West George Street, Chicago, IL 60657
(773) 871-5777
Fax: (773) 871-5843
www.howardbrown.org

Montrose Clinic
215 Westheimer Boulevard, Houston, TX 77006
(713) 520-2000
Fax: (713) 528-4923
www.montrose-clinic.org

Nelson-Tebedo Clinic (Foundation for Human Understanding)
4012 Cedar Springs Road, Dallas, TX 75219
(214) 528-2336
Fax: (214) 528-8436
www.resourcecenterdallas.org

First Family Medical Group
1444 West Bethany Home Road, Phoenix, AZ 85013
(602) 242-4843
Fax: (602) 433-7712

Jeffrey Goodman Clinic
Los Angeles Gay and Lesbian Center
1625 N. Schrader Blvd., Los Angeles, CA 90028
(213) 993-7400, (213) 993-7640
Fax: (213) 993-7699
Anti-Violence hot line: (213) 993-7673
www.gay-lesbian-center.org

II. Body

Staying Well

SPORTS AND FITNESS

Aerobics and Fitness Foundation of America
(800) YOUR-BODY

American College of Sports Medicine
PO Box 1440, Indianapolis, IN 46206-1440
(317) 637-9200
Fax: (317) 634-7817
www.a1.com/sportsmed

Federation of Gay Games
584 Castro Street, Suite 348, San Francisco, CA 94114
(415) 695-0222
Fax: (415) 695-9222
www.gaygames.org

International Gay and Lesbian Outdoor Organization (IGLOO)
www.radix.net/~erewhon/igloo/rindex.htm

National and local gay sports teams
www.kwic.net/lgb-sports/clubs.html

North American Gay Amateur Athletic Alliance
www.nagaaa.com

President's Council on Physical Fitness and Sports
707 Pennsylvania Avenue NW, Suite 250, Washington, DC 20004
(202) 272-3430
www.os.dhhs.gov/progorg/ophs/pcpfs/htm

QSports: An electronic quarterly newsletter about gay sports
www.qsports.org

NUTRITION

AIDS and Nutrition Resource Library
926 J Street, Suite 408, Sacramento, CA 98154
(916) 443-1721

American Dietetic Association National Nutrition Consumer Hot Line
(800) 366-1655
Call for a referral to a registered dietitian.

American Institute of Cancer Research Nutrition Hot Line:
(800) 843-8114, (202) 328-7744

EPA Safe Drinking Water Hot Line
(800) 426-4791, (202) 269-7943
TDD/TTY: (800) 877-8339
Fax: (202) 260-8072
www.epa.gov/safewater/crypto.html.

Food and Nutrition Information Center
National Agricultural Library/FNIC
10301 Baltimore Boulevard, Room 304, Beltsville, MD 20705-2351
(301) 504-5719

Human Nutrition Information Service
Department of Agriculture
6505 Belcrest Road, Hyattsville, MD 20782
(301) 436-7725

National AIDS Nutrient Bank
PO Box 2187, Guernville, CA 95446
(707) 869-1996
Fax: (707) 869-2562

National Center for Nutrition and Dietetics American Dietetic Association
216 West Jackson Boulevard, Chicago, IL 60606-6995
(800) 366-1655
TTY: (800) 366-1655

OVERALL HEALTH MAINTENANCE

American Institute for Preventative Medicine
30445 Northwestern Highway, Suite 350, Farmington Hills, MI 48334
(800) 345-AIPM

Immunization Information Page
www.cdc.gov/diseases/immun.html

Department of Health and Human Services
National Health Information Center
(800) 336-4797
Clearinghouse for information and referrals.

Immunization Action Coalition
1573 Selby Avenue, St. Paul, MN 55104
(612) 647-9009
Fax: (612) 647-9131
www.immunize.org

National Heart, Lung and Blood Institute Education Programs
Information Center
National Heart, Lung, and Blood Institute
PO Box 30105, Bethesda, MD 20824-0105
(800) 575-WELL
www.nhlbi.nih.gov

SEXUAL HEALTH

American Social Health Association (ASHA)
PO Box 13827, Research Triangle Park (RTP), North Carolina 27709
(919) 361-8400
ASHA Herpes Resource Center: (800) 230-6039
www.ashastd.org

CDC Hepatitis Hot Line: (404) 332-4555
See also "Liver," page 577

CDC National STD Hot Line: (800) 227-8922

Hepatitis Foundation International
30 Sunrise Terrace, Cedar Grove, NJ 07009
Hot line: (800) 891-0707
www.hepfi.org

Hepatitis B Foundation
700 East Butler Avenue, Doylestown, PA 18901
(215) 489-4900
www.hepb.org

Kink Aware Professionals
www.bannon.com/kap/index.htm
Referrals to psychotherapeutic, medical, dental, complementary healing, and legal professionals.

Safer SM Education Project
www.alternate.com

Sex Information and Education Counsel of the United States (SIECUS)
130 West 42nd Street, Suite 350, New York, NY 10036
(212) 819-9770
www.sierus.org

AIDS PREVENTION INFORMATION

Center for AIDS Prevention Studies (CAPS)
University of California, San Francisco
74 New Montgomery, Suite 600, San Francisco, CA 94105
(415) 597-9100
Fax: (415) 597-9213
www.caps.vcsf.edu

Centers for Disease Control (CDC) Prevention Information Network
National Prevention Information Network
PO Box 6003, Rockville, MD 20849-6003
(800) 458-5231, (301) 217-0023
Fax: (301) 738-6616
www.cdcnpin.org

Condom Resource Center
PO Box 30564, Oakland, CA 94604
(510) 891-0455

Gay City Health Project
123 Boylston Avenue East, Suite A, Seattle, WA 98102
(206) 860-6969
Fax: (206) 860-0195
www.gaycity.org

GMHC HIV Prevention Department
119 West 24th Street, 6th Floor, New York, NY 10011
(212) 367-1353
www.gmhc.org

Stop AIDS Project
2128 15th Street, San Francisco, CA 94114-1213
(415) 575-0150
Fax: (415) 575-0166
www.stopaids.org

DIABETES

American Diabetes Association
1660 Duke Street, Alexandria, VA 22314
(800) 232-3472
www.diabetes.org

National Diabetes Information Clearinghouse
PO Box NDIC, 9000 Rockville Pike, Bethesda, MD 20892-3560
(301) 654-3327
www.aoa.dhhs.gov/aoa/dir/153.html

Seeking Treatment

AIDS TREATMENT INFORMATION

There are literally thousands of local organizations offering many different kinds of help, from buddy programs to hot meals, policy information to legal support. The Centers for Disease Control National AIDS hot line, (800) 342-2437 (English) or (800) 344-7432 (Spanish), can refer you to the one nearest you. Some of the larger ones among them are:

AIDS Action Committee of Massachusetts, Inc.
131 Clarendon Street, Boston, MA 02116
(617) 437-6200
TTY: (617) 450-1423
www.aac.org

AIDS Project Los Angeles
1313 North Vine Street, Los Angeles, CA 90028
(213) 993-1600
Fax: (213) 993-1598
California HIV/AIDS hot line: (800) 367-AIDS
www.apla.org

Gay Men's Health Crisis
Treatment Education Department
119 West 24th Street, New York, NY 10011
(212) 807-6664
www.gmhc.org

Northwest AIDS Foundation
127 Broadway East, Seattle, WA 98102
(206) 329-6923
Fax: (206) 325-2689
TDD: (206) 323-2685
www.nwaids.org

Project Inform
1965 Market Street, Suite 220, San Francisco, CA 92103
(415) 558-8669
Hot line: (800) 822-7422 Monday-Friday 9 A.M.–5 P.M. PST
www.projectinform.org

San Francisco AIDS Foundation
995 Market Street, #200, San Francisco, CA 94103
(415) 487-3000 (English)
(415) 487-3004 (Spanish)
TDD: (415) 864-6606
Fax: (415) 487-3009
www.sfaf.org

Whitman-Walker Clinic, Inc.
1407 S Street NW, Washington, DC 20009
(202) 797-3500
www.wwc.org

Other local and national treatment organizations include:

AIDS Clinical Trials Information Service (ACTIS)
(800) 874-2572
www.actis.org
ACTIS can tell you which drug studies are open, their location and eligibility requirements, and how to reach their contact people. It is a cooperative project of several government agencies, including the CDC.

AIDS Treatment Information Service (ATIS)
(800) 448-0440 Monday-Friday, 9–7 EST
www.hivatis.org
Trained ATIS staffers can answer your questions about federally approved treatments and send you information. Like ACTIS, it is a cooperative project of several government agencies, including the CDC.

AIDS Treatment and Data Network
611 Broadway, Suite 613, New York, NY 10012-2809
(800) 734-7104 Monday-Friday, 10–6 EST
www.AIDSinfonyc.org

Critical Path AIDS Project
2062 Lombard Street
Philadelphia, PA 19146
Hot line: (215) 545-2212
www.critpath.org

Direct AIDS Alternative Information Resources
See Complementary and Alternative Medicine, below.

National AIDS Treatment Advocacy Project
580 Broadway, Suite 403, New York, NY 10012
(888) 26-NATAP, (212) 219-0106
Fax: (212) 219-8473
www.natap.org

PWA Health Group
See Complementary and Alternative Medicine, below.

CAREGIVING AND SUPPORT

Kairos Support for Caregivers
www.the-park.com/kairos

LA Shanti
1616 North Labrea Avenue, Los Angeles, CA 90028
(323) 962-8197
Fax: (213) 962-8299
www.LAShanti.org

National Self-Help Clearinghouse
25 West 43rd Street, Room 620, New York, NY 10036
(212) 354-8525
www.selfhelpweb.org

Pets Are Wonderful Support (PAWS) National Headquarters
7327 Santa Monica Boulevard, West Hollywood, CA 90046-6614
(213) 876-PAWS
Fax: (213) 876-0511
E-mail: pawsla7327@aol.com

COMPLEMENTARY AND ALTERNATIVE MEDICINE

The American Foundation of Traditional Chinese Medicine
1280 Columbus Avenue, Suite 302, San Francisco, CA 94133
(415) 776-0502

The American Holistic Health Association
PO Box 17400, Anaheim, CA 92817
(714) 779-6152

American Massage Therapy Association
820 Davis Street, Suite 100, Evanston, IL 60201-4444
(847) 864-0123
Fax: (847) 864-1178
www.amtamassage.org

The Biofeedback and Psychophysiology Clinic
The Menninger Clinic
PO Box 829, Topeka, KS 66601-0829
(913) 273-7500

Critical Path AIDS Project
See AIDS Treatment Information, page 574

Direct AIDS Alternative Information Resources, NYC (DAAIR)
31 East 30th Street, #2A, New York, NY 10016
(212) 725-6994
Fax: (212) 689-6471
www.daair.org

Healing Alternatives Foundation (HIV-specific)
1748 Market Street, #204, San Francisco, CA 94102
(415) 626-4053
Order line: (800) 219-2233
Fax: (415) 626-0451

International Association of Yoga Therapists
4150 Tivoli, Los Angeles, CA 90066
(213) 306-8845

The Mind-Body Medical Institute
185 Pilgrim Road, Boston, MA 02215
(617) 732-7000

Office of Alternative Medicine
National Institutes of Health
Building 31, Room 5B-38, MS-2182
9000 Rockville Pike, Bethesda, MD 20892
(888) NIH-OCAM

People With AIDS Health Group
150 West 26th Street
New York, NY 10001
(212) 255-0520
Fax: (212) 255-1080
www.aidsinfonyc.org/pwahg

END-OF-LIFE ISSUES

Choice in Dying National Office
1035 30th Street NW, Washington, DC 20007
(800) 989-WILL, (202) 338-9790
Fax: (202) 338-0242
www.choices.org

Hospice Education Institute
190 Westbrook Road, Essex, CT 06426
(800) 331-1620

National Hemlock Society
PO Box 101810, Denver, CO 80250-1018
(800) 247-7421
www.hemlock.org

National Hospice Organization
1901 North Moore Street, Suite 901, Arlington, VA 22209
(800) 658-8898
Zen Hospice Project Home Page:
www.zenhospice.org

YOUR BODY, PIECE BY PIECE

Bladder

Incontinence Information Line
(800) 622-9010
National Association for Continence
PO Box 8310, Spartanburg, SC 29305-8310
(864) 579-7900, (800) BLADDER

Bowels and Colon

Alliance for Food and Fiber Hot Line
(800) 266-0200
Fax: (310) 476-1896

Anal Fissure Self-Help Page
http://faf6arc.nasa.gov/af.

Colon Cancer Online Information Library
www.meds.com/mol/colon/Index.html

Crohn's Disease/Colitis Homepage
http://qurlyjoe.bu.edu/cduchome.html
Hot Line: (800) 932-2423

Crohn's Disease and Colitis Foundation of America, Inc.
444 Park Avenue, 11th floor, New York, NY 10016-7374
(800) 932-2423, (212) 685-3440
www.ccfa.org

Digestive Disease National Coalition
507 Capitol Court NE, Suite 200, Washington, DC 20002
(202) 544-7497

Intestinal Disease Foundation, Inc.
1323 Forbes Avenue, Suite 200, Pittsburgh, PA 15219
(412) 261-5888

National Digestive Diseases Information Clearinghouse
2 Information Way, Bethesda, MD 20892-3570
Fax: (301) 907-8906
www.niddk.nih.gov

Ears

The Better Hearing Institute
5021-B Backlick Road, Annandale, VA 22003
(800) EAR-WELL
www.betterhearing.org/index.htm
Will send you a list of possible state and federal sources for financial aid in your area.

Hear Now
9745 East Hampton Avenue, Suite 300, Denver, CO 80231-4923
(800) 648-HEAR
www.leisurelan.com.~hearnow/

Hair

American Hair Loss Council
401 North Michigan Avenue, Chicago, IL 60611
(312) 321-5128
Fax: (312) 245-1080
www.ahlc.org

Bald-Headed Men of America
102 Bald Drive, Morehead City, NC 28557
(919) 726-1855

Hair Replacement Web site
www.newyork.bbb.org/library/publications/sub0046.html

Heart

American Heart Association
(800) AHA-USA (242-8721)
www.amhrt.org

Liver

See also "Sexual Health," page 573.

American Liver Foundation
1425 Pompton Avenue, Cedar Grove, NJ 07009-1000
(201) 256-2550, (800) GO-LIVER
Fax: (201) 256-3214

American Liver Foundation Hepatitis B and C Information Line
(800) 223-0179

Hepatitis C Research Foundation
RR2, Box 12, Verbank, NY 12585
(914) 677-0622
(914) 677-3688
www.hcrf.org

HIV and Hepatitis
www.hivandhepatitis.com

Lungs

American Lung Association
1740 Broadway, New York, NY 10019-4374
(800) LUNG-USA, (212) 315-8700
www.lungusa.org

Penis (and Impotence)

American Urological Association
11512 Allecingie Parkway, Richmond, VA 23235
(804) 379-1306
www.auanet.org/index.html
E-mail: Webmaster@auanet.org

American Foundation of Urologic Disease
1128 North Charles Street, Baltimore, MD 21201
(800) 242-2383
www.afud.org

National Organization of Restoring Men (NORM)
3205 Northwood Drive, Concord, CA 94520-4506
(510) 827-4077
Fax: (510) 827-4119
www.norm.org

Geddings Osbon Association
PO Box 1593, Augusta, GA 30903-1593
(800) 433-4215

Impotence Institute of America
119 South Ruth Street, Maryville, TN 37801-5746
Hot line: (800) 669-1603

Impotence Information Center
PO Box 9, Minneapolis, MN 55440
(800) 843-4315

Impotence World Association
PO Box 410, Bowie, MD 20718-0410
(800) 669-1603
www.impotenceworld.org

Prostate

American Prostate Society
7188 Ridge Road, Hanover, MD 21076
(410) 859-3735
www.ameripros.org

Gay Men's Prostate Cancer Support Network on the Net
www.mindspring.com/~jerryh/prosttop.htm

NIH Web Page on prostatitis
http://www.niddk.nih.gov/health/urolog/summary/prstitis

Cancer Care
275 7th Avenue, 22nd floor, New York, NY 10001
(212) 221-3300
www.cancercare.org

Prostatitis Foundation
1063 30th Street, Box 8, Smithshire, IL 61478
(888) 891-4200
Fax: (309) 325-7184
www.prostatitis.org

Prostatitis Home Page
www.prostate.org

Us Too Prostate Cancer Support Groups (and newsletter)
930 North York Road, Hinsdale, IL 60521
(630) 323-1002
Fax: (630) 323-1003
Hot line: (800) 80-US-TOO
www.ustoo.com

Skin

National Cancer Institute
Building 31, Room 10A03,
31 Center Drive, MSC 2580,
Bethesda, MD 20892
(800) 4-CANCER

Skin Cancer Foundation
245 5th Avenue, New York, NY 10016
(212) 725-5176, (800) SKIN-490
Fax: (212) 725-5751
www.skincancer.org

Skin Cancer Information
www.cancernet.nci.nih.gov

PHYSICAL SAFETY

Gay Bashing and Domestic Violence

Community United Against Violence (CUAV)
Gay Men's Domestic Violence Project
973 Market Street, #500, San Francisco, CA 94103
(415) 777-5500
Fax: (415) 777-5565
24-hour hot line: (415) 333-HELP
www.cuav.org

Family Violence Prevention Fund (not gay-specific)
1001 Potrero Avenue, Building One, Suite 200, San Francisco, CA 94110
(415) 821-4553
Fax: (415) 824-3873
www.fvpf.org

National Coalition of Anti-Violence Programs
c/o New York City Gay and Lesbian Anti-Violence Project
647 Hudson Street, New York, NY 10014
(212) 807-6761
Fax: (212) 807-1044
Hot Line: (800) 807-0197
www.avp.org

National Domestic Violence/Abuse Hot Line
(not gay-specific)
(800) 799-SAFE
www.ndvh.org

Office for Victims of Crime Resource Center (not gay-specific)
PO Box 6000, Rockville, MD 20849-6000
(800) 627-6872

Sexual Assault and Incest

Men Overcoming Sexual Assault
357 MacArthur Boulevard, Oakland, CA 94610
24-hour crisis line: (510) 845-7273

Men Assisting, Leading and Educating, Inc. (MALE), National Organization on Male Sexual Victimization
PMB 103, 5505 Connecticut Avenue NW, Washington, DC 20015-2601
(800) 738-4181
www.malesurvivor.org

Rape, Abuse and Incest National Network (RAINN)
(202) 544-1034
Fax: (202) 544-1401
Hot line: (800) 656-HOPE
www.pcola.gulf.net/~peter/onezeroseven/rainn.html
Connects callers to trained counselors from the rape crisis center closest to you 24 hours a day.

VOICES in Action, Inc.
PO Box 148309, Chicago, IL 60614
(773) 327-1500, (800) 7-VOICE-8
www.voices-action.org
E-mail: voices@voices-action.org

III. Mind

General Resources

The National Institute of Mental Health
National Institutes of Health
Room 17-99, 5600 Fishers Lane, Rockville, MD 20857-8030
www.nimh.nih.gov
Information and links to organizations dedicated to specific problems such as obsessive-compulsive disorder, depression, bipolar disorder, Alzheimer's disease, seasonal affective disorder, eating disorders, and learning disabilities.

Gay-Specific Resources

The Alliance of Psychological Healthcare Professionals
106 Thorn Street, San Diego, CA 94013
(619) 683-8000
www.allianceprofessionals.com
Gives referrals to LGBT psychologists all over the country.

Association of Gay and Lesbian Psychiatrists
4514 Chester Avenue, Philadelphia, PA 19143-3707
(215) 925-5008
Fax: (215) 925-9309
Gives referrals to GLBT psychiatrists all over the country.

Concerned Counseling
24-hour hot line: 1-888-415-TALK
www.concernedcounseling.com
Provides counseling (by licensed professionals, some of whom specialize in GLBT concerns) to both individuals and couples by phone, over e-mail, or in private online chat rooms.

Gay and Lesbian National Hot Line: (888) THE-GLNH
Provides nationwide, toll-free peer counseling, information, and referrals Monday-Friday, 6 P.M.–10 P.M., Saturday 12 P.M.–5 P.M. EST.
www.glnh.org

Alcohol, Tobacco, and Substance Abuse

Al-Anon and Alateen Family Groups Headquarters, Inc.
1600 Corporate Landing Parkway, Virginia Beach, VA 23454
(800) 356-9996

Adult Children of Alcoholics (ACOA) World Service
PO Box 3216, Torrance, CA 90510
(310) 534-1815
www.adultchildren.org

Alcoholics Anonymous (AA) Worldwide Services Office
PO Box 459, Grand Central Station, New York, NY 10163
(212) 686-1100, or see your local telephone book
www.alcoholics-anonymous.org

American Cancer Society Stop Smoking Office
(212) 582-2118

Coalition of Lavender Americans on Smoking and Health/The Last Drag
1748 Market Street, Suite 201, San Francisco, CA 94104
(415) 565-7676

Cocaine Anonymous (CAWSO)
PO Box 2000, Los Angeles, CA 90049-8000
(310) 559-2554 Fax: (310) 559-2554
www.ca.org

National Clearinghouse for Alcohol and Drug Information
Drug Abuse Information and Treatment Referral Line
Box 2345, Rockville, MD 20847-2345
(800) 662-4357/6686 (English), (800) 662-9832 (Spanish).
www.health.org

National Council on Alcoholism and Drug Dependence
12 West 21st Street, New York, NY 10010
(800) 662-HELP, (212) 206-6990
Fax: (212) 645-1690
www.ncadd.org

National Drug and Alcohol Treatment Referral Hot Line
(800) 662-HELP (English), (800) 662-9832 (Spanish)
TDD: (800) 228-0427

National Institute on Drug Abuse Helpline
(800) 843-4971

Narcotics Anonymous World Service Office
PO Box 9999, Van Nuys, CA 91409
(818) 773-9999
Fax: (818) 700-0700

The Pride Institute
14400 Martin Drive, Eden Prairie, MN 10010
(800) 54-PRIDE
www.pride-institute.com
Provides addiction treatment for the GLBT community, and has branches in many cities.

Rational Recovery
http://rational.org/recovery
(530) 621-4374, (530) 621-2667, weekdays 8 A.M.–4 P.M. PST

Smokenders, Inc.
666 11th Street NW, Washington, DC 20001
(800) 828-HELP
www.smokenders.com

Eating Disorders

The American Anorexia/Bulimia Association, Inc.
165 West 46th Street, #1108, New York, NY 10036
(212) 575-6200
www.aabainc.org

Males & Eating Disorders
www.primenet.com/~danslos/males

National Association to Advance Fat Acceptance (NAAFA)
PO Box 18862, Sacramento, CA 95818
(916) 558-6880
Fax: (916) 558-6881
www.naafa.org
Works to eliminate discrimination based on body size and provide fat people with the tools for self-empowerment.

Overeaters Anonymous World Service Office
6075 Zenith Court NE, Rio Rancho, NM 87124
(505) 891-2664
Fax: (505) 891-4320
www.overeatersanonymous.org

Sexual Issues

American Association of Sex Educators, Counselors and Therapists (AASECT)
PO Box 238, Mount Vernon, IA 52314-0238
(319) 895-8407
Fax: (319) 895-6203
Contact this organization for a list of certified sex therapists and counselors.
www.aasect.org

National Council on Sexual Addiction and Compulsivity
1090 Northchase Parkway, Suite 200, South Marietta, GA 30067
(770) 989-9754
www.ncsac.org

Sexual Compulsives Anonymous (SCA)
(800) 977-HEAL
www.sca-recovery.org
Anonymous e-mail: anon-7901@anon.twwelss.com
New York: Old Chelsea Station, PO Box 1585, New York, NY 10113
(212) 439-1123
Chicago: New Town Alano Club, 4407 North Clark Street, Chicago, IL 60640
(312) 589-5856
Los Angeles: 4470-107 Sunset Boulevard, #520, Los Angeles, CA 90027
(310) 859-5585

Sex Addicts Anonymous (SAA)
ISO of SAA
PO Box 70949, Houston, TX 77270
(713) 869-4902
www.sexaa.org

Sex and Love Addicts Anonymous (SLAA)
PO Box 119, New Town Branch, Boston, MA 02258
(617) 332-1845

Sexaholics Anonymous
PO Box 111910, Nashville, TN 37222
(615) 331-6230 Fax: (615) 331-6901
www.sa.org

Sleep Disorders

American Sleep Disorders Association
1610 14th Street, #300, Rochester, MN 55901
www.asda.org

National Sleep Foundation
729 15th Street NW, 4th floor, Washington, DC 20005
www.sleepfoundation.org

Stress Reduction

American Institute of Stress
124 Park Avenue, Yonkers, NY 10703
(800) 24-RELAX
www.stress.org

Suicide Prevention

American Foundation for Suicide Prevention
120 Wall Street, 22nd floor, New York, NY 10005
(888) 333-AFSP
Fax: (212) 363-6237
www.afsp.org
Offers referrals to other organizations.
There is no national suicide crisis hot line. For a listing of local hot lines and centers that aren't funded by private clinics (many in each state), contact:

The American Association of Suicidology
4201 Connecticut Avenue NW, Suite 310, Washington, DC 20008
(202) 237-2280
Fax: (202) 237-2282
www.suicidology.org

Some major suicide hot lines (all open 24 hours a day, 7 days a week) are:

Atlanta: (404) 730-1600
Boston: (617) 247-0220
Chicago: (773) 728-2255
Los Angeles: (310) 391-1253
New York: (212) 727-4008
San Francisco: (415) 781-0500
Seattle: (206) 461-3222

IV. Soul and Spirit

Affirmation (Gay and Lesbian Mormons)
PO Box 46022, Los Angeles, CA 90046
(213) 255-7251
www.affirmation.org/~affadmin

Affirmation: United Methodists for Lesbian, Gay and Bisexual Concerns
PO Box 1021, Evanston, IL 60204
(708) 475-0499

AIDS Medicine and Miracles
PO Box 20650, Boulder, CO 80308-3650
(303) 447-8777 or (800) 875-8770
Fax: (303) 447-3902
www.csd.net/~amm
amm@inspirational.org

AIDS National Interfaith Network
110 Maryland Avenue NE, Room 504, Washington, DC 20002
(202) 546-0807

American Gay and Lesbian Atheists
PO Box 66711, Houston, TX 77266
(713) 862-3283

Axios: Eastern and Orthodox Christians
328 West 17th Street, #4-F, New York, NY 10011
(212) 989-6211; (718) 805-1952

Body Electric School
6527A Telegraph Avenue, Oakland, CA 94979-2512
(415) 488-9883
Fax: (510) 653-1594
www.bodyelectric.org

Dignity (Gay and Lesbian Roman Catholics)
1500 Massachusetts Avenue NW, #11, Washington, DC 20005
(202) 861-0017
Fax: (202) 429-9898
www.dignityusa.org
Also see: LGB Catholic Handbook (www.bway.net/~halsall/lgbh.html)

Emergence International: Christian Scientists Supporting Lesbians, Gay Men, and Bisexuals
PO Box 6061-423, Sherman Oaks, CA 91413
(800) 280-6653

Erospirit Resource Institute
PO Box 3893, Oakland, CA 94609
(510) 428-9063
www.erospirit.org

Gay Christians
www.gaychristians.org
Contains links to numerous sites on gay and lesbian spirituality, both pro and con.

Honesty: Southern Baptists Advocating Equal Rights for Gays and Lesbians
PO Box 2543, Louisville, KY 40201
(502) 637-7609

Integrity, Inc. (Gay and Lesbian Episcopals)
PO Box 19561, Washington, DC 20036-0561

Maitri Dorje (Gay and Lesbian Buddhists)
(718) 384-6136

Metropolitan Community Churches
www.trends.ca/~ufmcc

National Gay Pentecostal Alliance
PO Box 1391, Schenectady, NY 12301-1391
(518) 372-6001

Presbyterians for Lesbian and Gay Concerns
www.epp.cmu.edu/~riley/PLGC.html

People with AIDS Coalition NY/AIDS Medicine and Miracles/Body Positive
19 Fulton Street, Suite 3083
New York, NY 10038
(212) 566-7333
Local hot line: (212) 647-1420
National hot line: (800) 566-6599
www.csd.net/~amm

Radical Faeries
(212) 625-4505
www.sfo.com

San Francisco Zen Center
300 Page Street, San Francisco, CA 94102
(415) 863-3136

Unitarian Universalist Association, Office of Lesbian, Bisexual and Gay Concerns
25 Beacon Street, Boston, MA 02108-2800
(617) 742-2100

Witches/Pagans for Gay Rights
PO Box 4538, Sunnyside, NY 11104-4538

World Congress of Gay and Lesbian Jewish Organizations
PO Box 3345, New York, NY 10008-3345

V. Community

A wealth of gay links can be found at www.planetout.com, www.gay.com, and www.qrd.org. Also see Jeff Dawson's *Gay and Lesbian Online: The Travel Guide to Digital Queerdom on the World Wide Web* (Berkeley, CA: Peachpit Press, 1997) for a nearly exhaustive list of relevant Web sites and descriptions.

Community Centers and Cultural Organizations

Lesbian and Gay Community Services Center (NYC)
208 West 13th Street, New York, NY 10011
(212) 620-7310
www.gaycenter.org
There are over 100 other GLBT centers in 33 states. The New York City center can give referrals to all of them.

Asians and Friends
Box 18974
Washington, DC 20036
(202) 387-ASIA
http://members.aol.com/afwash/afw.htm

LLEGO (National Latino/a Lesbian and Gay Organization)
703 G Street SE, Washington, DC 20003
(202) 454-0092
www.llego.org

National Association of Black and White Men Together
Box 73796 Washington, DC 20056
(800) 624-2968
Fax: (202) 462-3690
www.nabwmt.com

National Black Lesbian and Gay Leadership Forum (NBLGLF)
1436 U Street NW, Suite 200, Washington, DC 20009
(202) 483-6786
www.nblglf.org

Trikone (South Asian Lesbians and Gays)
PO Box 21354, San Jose, CA 95151-1354
(408) 270-8776
Fax: (408) 274-2733
www.trikone.org

Family Organizations

GAY COUPLES

Partners Task Force for Gay and Lesbian Couples
PO Box 9685, Seattle, WA 98109
(206) 935-1206
www.buddybuddy.com

Domestic Partnerships and Same-Sex Marriages
www.qrd.org/family/marriage

Lambda Legal Defense and Education Fund Marriage Project
www.lambdalegal.org

National Freedom to Marry Coalition
www.freedomtomarry.org

GAY PARENTS

Adoption
www.adopting.org/gaystate.htm

Alternative Family Project
425 Divisadero Street, Suite 203
San Francisco, CA 94117
(415) 436-9000
www.queer.org/afp

Center Kids
New York City Lesbian and Gay Community Center
208 W. 13th Street
New York, NY 10011
(212) 741-2247
Fax: (212) 366-1947

Family Pride Coalition
PO Box 34337, San Diego, CA 92163
(202) 583-8029
Fax: (619) 296-0699
www.familypride.org

Gay and Lesbian Family Values Home Page
www.geocities.com/wallstreet/8794

Gay Dads
www.milepost1.com/~gaydad/

Lavender Families Resource Network
PO Box 21567, Seattle, WA 98111
(206) 325-2643

Rainbow Flag Health Services
543A 30th Street
Oakland, CA 94609
(510) 763-SPERM
www.gayspermbank.com

CHILDREN AND PARENTS GROUPS

Children of Lesbians and Gays Everywhere (COLAGE)
2300 Market Street, #165, San Francisco, CA 94114
(202) 583-8029
kidsofgays@aol.com

Parents, Families, and Friends of Lesbians and Gays (PFLAG)
1101 14th Street NW, Washington, DC 20005
(202) 638-4200, (800) 432-6451
Fax: (202) 638-0243
www.pflag.org

Youth

Gay, Lesbian, and Straight Education Network (GLSEN)
121 West 27th Street, Suite 804, New York, NY 10001
(212) 727-0135, (212) 727-0254

Hetrick-Martin Institute for Protection of Lesbian and Gay Youth
2 Astor Place, New York, NY 10003-8650
(212) 674-2400 Fax: (212) 674-8650
www.hmi.org

We Are Family
www.waf.org

Senior Citizens

American Association of Retired Persons
(800) 424-3410, (206) 517-2322
www.aarp.org

Gay and Lesbian Association of Retired Persons (GLARP)
10940 Wilshire Boulevard, Suite 1600, Los Angeles, CA 90024
(310) 966-1500
www.gaylesbianretiring.org

Gray Panthers
733 15th Street NW, Washington, DC 20005
Information and referral service: (800) 280-5362 Fax: (202) 466-3133

Lesbian and Gay Aging Issues Network, American Society on Aging
833 Market Street, Suite 511, San Francisco, CA 94103-1824
(415) 974-9600
www.asaging.org/lgain.html

Lesbian and Gay Informal Interest Group, Gerontological Society of America
1275 K Street NW, Suite 350, Washington, DC 20005
(202) 408-3375
www.geron.org

National Senior Citizen's Law Center
1815 H Street NW, Washington, DC 20006
(202) 887-5280

Pride Senior Network
1756 Broadway, Suite 11H, New York, NY 10019
(212) 757-3203
www.pridesenior.org

Prime Timers Worldwide
Box 436, Manchaca, TX 78652
www.primetimers.org

Senior Action in a Gay Environment (SAGE)
305 7th Avenue, 16th floor, New York, NY 10001-6008
(212) 741-2247
www.sageusa.com
Social, political, and assistance group for gay seniors, with listings of sister organizations nationwide.

Listing of local groups for older gays and lesbians
www.gayscape.com/gayscape/mature.html

Differently Abled People

ABLE-TOGETHER
PO Box 460053, San Francisco, CA 94146-0053
(415) 522-9091
Magazine for gay and bisexual men with and without disabilities.
www.well.com/user/blaine/abletog.html

Americans with Disabilities Act Information Line
(800) 514-0301
TDD: (800) 514-0383

Disabled links
www.ability.org.uk/disabled.html

Job Accommodation Network (JAN)
(800) 526-7234
An information network and consulting network helping qualified workers with disabilities to be hired or retained. Services provided free.

The President's Committee on Employment of People with Disabilities
1331 F Street NW, Washington, DC 20004
(202) 376-6200
TDD: (202) 376-6205
Works to increase employment opportunities for disabled people in the public and private sectors.

The U.S. Equal Employment Opportunity Commission
1801 L Street NW, Washington, DC 20507
Americans with Disabilities Act Helpline: (800) 669-EEOC
TDD: (800) 800-3302

Rural Areas

RFD: Gay Men's Magazine for the Rural Lifestyle and Beyond
1226-A Calle de Comercio, Santa Fe, NM 87505
(505) 474-6311 Fax: (505) 474-6317
www.rfdmag.org
See Radical Faeries in "Soul and Spirit" section.

Rural Gay Men's Network
www.ruralgay.com

International Gay Community

Amnesty International Members for Gay and Lesbian Concerns
www.qrd.org/qrd.orgs.AIMLGC

International Gay and Lesbian Human Rights Commission
540 Castro Street, San Francisco, CA 94114
(415) 255-8680
www.iglhrc.org

International 24-hour Lesbian and Gay Switchboard
(011-4471) 837-7324

VI. Working the System

AIDS Policy

ACT UP National Headquarters
www.actupny.org

AIDS Action Council
1875 Connecticut Avenue NW, Washington, DC 20009
(202) 986-1300
Fax: (202) 986-1345
www.aidsaction.org

GMHC Public Policy Department
119 West 24th Street, New York, NY 10011
(212) 367-1239
www.gmhc.org

National Association of People with AIDS (NAPWA) Education and Advocacy
143 K Street NW, Washington, DC 20005
(202) 898-0414
Fax: (202) 898-0435
www.napwa.org

National Minority AIDS Council
1931 13th Street NW, Washington, DC 20009
(202) 483-6622
Fax: (202) 483-1135
www.nmac.org

Health Insurance and Quality of Care

NONGOVERNMENTAL

American Board of Medical Specialists
(800)776-2378
www.certifieddoctor.org
Contact this organization to see if your doctor is board-certified in the specialty.

Caredata.com
www.caredata.com
Databases on healthcare plans and quality, both free and for a fee.

Consumer Coalition for Quality Health Care
1275 K Street NW, Suite 602
Washington, DC 20005
(202)789-3606
www.consumers.org

Medical Information Bureau
PO Box 105, Essex Station, Boston, MA 02112
(617) 426-3660
Keeps insurance data about your medical history.

Medicare Rights Center
1460 Broadway, New York, NY 10036
(212) 869-3850
Fax: (212) 869-3532
Medicare hot line: (800) 638-6833
www.medicarerights.org
Information on Medicare.

National Committee for Quality Assurance
2000 L Street NW, Suite 500, Washington, DC 20036
(800) 839-6487
www.ncoa.org
Access and reports on the quality of managed care plans.

National Viator Representatives
(800) 932-0050, (212) 586-5600
www.nvrnvr.com
Information on selling your life insurance.

People's Medical Society
462 Walnut Street, Allentown, PA 18102
(610) 770-1670
Fax: (610) 770-0607
www.peoplesmed.org

Public Citizen Health Research Group
1600 20th Street NW, Washington, DC 20009
(202) 588-1000
www.citizen.org/hrg

GOVERNMENTAL

COBRA, ELISA, and Self-funded Insurance Plans
Division of Technical Assistance and Inquiries
Pension and Welfare Benefits Administration
U. S. Department of Labor
200 Constitution Avenue NW
Washington, DC 20210-0999
202-219-8766
Only written complaints are accepted.

Health Care Financing Administration National Headquarters
(410) 786-3000
Call for a referral to your state Medicaid agency.

Medicare Health Care Financing Administration Hot Line
(800) 638-6833

Social Security Administration
Baltimore, MD 21235
(800) 772-1213
Call with questions about SSA programs, eligibility, and how to file for benefits.

Law

American Civil Liberties Union Lesbian and Gay Rights Project
25 Broad Street, 18th Floor, New York, NY 10004-2400
(212) 549-2500
Fax: (212) 869-9061
www.aclu.com

Lambda Legal Defense and Education Fund National Headquarters
120 Wall Street, New York, NY 10004
(212) 809-8585
www.lambdalegal.org

Politics

Gay and Lesbian Alliance Against Defamation (GLADD)
150 West 26th Street, #503, New York, NY 10001
(212) 807-1700
Fax: (212) 807-1806
www.glaad.org

Human Rights Campaign (HRC)
1101 14th Street NW, Washington, DC 20005
(202) 628-4160
Fax: (202) 347-5323
www.hrc.org

National Gay andLesbian Task Force (NGLTF)
2320 17th Street NW, Washington, DC 20009
(202) 332-6483
Fax: (202) 332-0207
www.ngltf.org

Appendix B

Transgender, Transvestite and Intersex Resources

In many minds, a book about gay men is no place for discussing transgender health. Plenty of transgender individuals, whether male-to-female (M-T-F) or female to male (F-T-M), do not consider themselves gay. Many, whether hermaphrodites or transitioning, do not consider themselves men. Increasingly, transgender activists suggest that we'd be better off ditching the concept of men and women altogether, or at least expanding the male/female binarism to include five genders: M, F, M-T-F, F-T-M, and intersex individuals. It might make for a few more boxes on application forms or your driver's license, they argue, but would also free us all from the narrow roads we've been traveling in the journey toward self-definition.

The complexities of gender stereotypes, and the many questions of mental and physical health confronted by those who wish to challenge them, can easily fill books of their own. While this volume has touched on a few such issues, many more of them have been explored far better elsewhere. There are now dozens of newsletters, books, and organizations devoted to exploring different aspects of transgender well-being. This appendix refers readers to some useful sources. It is offered with the recognition that, even for transgender people who do not wish their concerns to be obscured by gay men's issues, books for gay men are a likely place for transgender people of all genders and sexual orientations to turn for information.

As for gay men who insist that transgender people are not "like us," that's right and wrong. Some transgenders do identify as gay men, and many live as gay before they find their way across the gender boundary. Talk to transgendered individuals about their feelings and experiences, and you'll hear themes familiar to students of gay history: A conviction that you're somehow different, a search for self-definitions in dictionaries and textbooks, the struggle to sort out what's you and what's your sexual desire, and the process of coming out (if you're lucky) into a community of people whose savvy and sense help you to recognize your options. Not that the struggle ends there: Gender dysphoria is still classified as a mental illness, transgender people have to hide their identities for fear of loss of employment, large numbers can only pursue sexual partners in bars and networks that exist largely underground, and many are victims of violence at the hands of bashers and murderers as well as a discriminatory legal system that refuses to protect them. Ring a bell?

Internet Resources

The Web has made resources on transgender issues abundant, so if you have interest and access to the Internet, let your fingers do some walking. In addition to the resources below, check out the Web sites of the organizations at night concerned with transgender and intersex issues. Most have extensive links to other programs and sources of information.

Above and Beyond Gender Resources
www.abma.com/cb/tg/resnew.html
This shopping mall/resource center is a strange and wonderful blend, with links to more than twenty different transgender newsletters, more than thirty different newsgroups or chat rooms, hundreds of resources, and more than a thousand personal pages of interest.

Gender Education and Advocacy
Formed in 1998 through the merger of the American Educational Gender Information Service and the advocacy group It's Time, America! (both of whose addresses can be found under "organizations," below). Extensive resources, media monitoring, press releases, and information on surgeons, gender identity programs, voice programs, employment law, political analysis and much, much more. www.gender.org

Lavender Links
www.lavenderlinks.com/topics/trans.html.
Extensive list of multilingual links to TG/TV resources.

TransBoy Resource Network
www.geocities.com/WestHollywood/Park/6484/index.html
More links for the transgendered and those who love them.

Transgender Forum
http://www.tgforum.com/
Includes free and pay features, links, resources, pix, and more.

Organizations of Interest

American Educational Gender Information Service, Inc.
P.O. Box 33724
Decatur, GA 30033-0724
(770) 939-2128 Business
(770) 939-0244 Information & Referrals
Fax (770) 939-1770
www.gender.org/aegis

FTM International
1360 Mission Street
Suite 200
San Francisco, CA 94103
(415) 553-5987
www.ftm-intl.org

Gender Identity Project
The New York City Lesbian & Gay Community Services Center
One Little West 12th Street
New York, NY 10014
(212) 620-7310
www.gaycenter.org/gip.html

Gender Public Advocacy Coalition (GenderPAC)
274 West 11th Street, Suite 4R
New York, NY 10014
www.gpac.org

International Conference on Transgendered Law and Employment Policy
PO Drawer 1010, Cooperstown, NY 13326
(607) 547-4118 ictlephdq@aol.com

International Foundation for Gender Education
PO Box 229 Waltham, MA 02254-0229
(781) 899-2212
Fax (781) 899-5703
www.ifge.org
Quarterly newsletter: Transgender Tapestry

Intersex Society of North America (ISNA)
PO Box 31791
San Francisco, CA 94131
(415) 575-3885
www.isna.org
Newsletter: Hermaphrodites with Attitude

It's Time, America!
Political Action for the Transgendered Community
PO Box 65, Kensington, MD 20895
www.gender.org/ita

Renaissance Transgender Association, Inc.
987 Old Eagle School Road, Suite 719
Wayne, PA 19087
(610) 975-9119
www.ren.org
Monthly publication: Transgender Community News

Gender Programs

These provide a structured approach to sex reassignment, with services ranging from counseling to hormonal therapy, plastic surgery, and sex reassignment surgery (SRS). While gender programs performing sex reassignment surgery may be more expensive than a do-it-yourself approach to finding electrologists, endocrinologists, plastic surgeons, and surgeons, they are also more thorough and careful than individual practitioners, using a multidisciplinary team approach to track each person's progress through the transition.

Center for Gender Reassignment
330 W. Brambleton Avenue
Suite 203
Norfolk VA 23510
(804) 625-7622
(804) 625-7649

Transsexual Program
University of Kentucky
800 Rose Street
Lexington, KY 40536-0084
(606) 233-6677 (office)
(606) 233-3533 (appointments)

Central Ohio Gender Dysphoria Program
PO Box 02008
Columbus, OH 43202
(614) 451-0111

University of Michigan Comprehensive Gender Program
1500-E Medical Center Drive
Office No. 1H223
Ann Arbor, MI 48109-0050
(313) 936-7067

Transgender Identity Group
c/o Ivanoff & Ivanoff
Suite 1810, Clark Building
633 W. Wisconsin Avenue
Milwaukee, WI 53203-1918
(414) 271-3323

Pathways Counseling Center
2645 N. Mayfair Road, Suite 230
Wauwatosa, WI 53226-1304
(414) 774-4111

University of Minnesota Program
1300 South 2nd Street
Minneapolis, MN 55454
(612) 625-1500
(612) 626-8311

Chicago Gender Society
Box 578005
Chicago, IL 60657
(708) 863-7714

Gender Dysphoria Program of Orange County
32148 Camino Capistrano
Suite 203
San Juan Capistrano, CA 92675

Gender Dysphoria Program, Inc.
1515 El Camino Real
Palo Alto, CA 94306
(415) 326-4645

Institute for Psychosexual Health
5594 North Hollywood Avenue
Suite 204
Whitefish Bay, WI 53217

Los Angeles Gender Center
1923½ Westwood Boulevard
Suite 2
Los Angeles, CA 90025
(310) 475-8880

Gender Community Advocates
PO Box 6333
Santa Maria, CA 93454
(805) 922-1309
Fax (805) 549-0961

Center for Special Problems
2107 Van Ness Avenue
San Francisco, CA
(415) 292-2261

Sexual Identity Center
PO Box 3224
Honolulu, HI 96801-3224
(808) 926-1000

Ingersoll Gender Center
1812 E. Madison Street
Suite 106
Seattle, WA 98122-2843
(206) 329-6651

BOOKS

Bornstein, Kate. (1998) *My Gender Workbook: How to Become a Real Man, a Real Woman, the Real You, or Something Else Entirely.* New York: Routledge.

Brown, Mildred L., et al. (1996) *True Selves: Understanding Transsexualism—For Families, Friends, Coworkers, and Helping Professionals.* San Francisco: Jossey-Bass Publishers.

Dreger, Alice. (1998) *Hermaphrodites and the Medical Invention of Sex.* Cambridge: Harvard University Press.

Kessler, Suzanne. (1998) *Lessons from the Intersexed.* New Brunswick, NJ: Rutgers University Press.

Kirk, Sheila. (1995) *Feminizing Hormonal Therapy for the Transgendered.* Blawnox, PA: Together Lifeworks.

Kirk, Sheila. (1997) *Masculinizing Hormonal Therapy for the Transgendered.* Blawnox, PA: Together Lifeworks.

Kirk, Sheila. (1995) *Medical, Legal and Workplace Issues for the Transsexual.* Blawnox, PA: Together Lifeworks.

Ramsey, Gerald. (1996) *Transsexuals: Candid Answers to Private Questions.* Freedom, CA: Crossing Press.

Wilchins, Riki Anne. (1997) *Read My Lips: Sexual Subversion and the End of Gender.* Ithaca: Firebrand Books.

Appendix C

Citations and References

Chapter 1

Alter, Gary A. (1995) "Penile Enhancement," *Advances in Urology* 9. 225.

Bechtel, Stefan, and Laurence Roy Stains. (1995) *Sex: A Man's Guide*. Emmaus, PA: Rodale Books.

Berkow, Robert, MD. (1992) "Anal Fissure." In his *Merck Manual of Diagnosis and Therapy*. Rahway. NJ: Merck Research Laboratories. 856–57.

Bigelow, Jim. (1995) *The Joy of Uncircumcising!* Aptos, CA: Hourglass Book Publishing.

Bullough, Vern L., and Bonnie Bullough. (1994) *Human Sexuality: An Encyclopedia*. New York: Garland Publishing, Inc.

Coxon, Anthony P. M. (1996) *Between the Sheets: Sexual Desire and Gay Men's Sex in the Era of AIDS*. New York: Cassell.

Devine, C. J., Jr. (1997) "International Conference on Peyronie's Disease Advances in Basic and Clinical Research," *Journal of Urology* 157 (1). 272–75.

Gilbaugh, James H., Jr. (1988) *Men's Private Parts: An Owner's Manual*. New York: Crown Trade Paperbacks.

Gould, Stephen Jay. (1987) "Freudian Slip," *Natural History* 96 (2). 14–21.

Gui, D., et al. (1994). "Botulinum Toxin for Chronic Anal Fissure," *The Lancet* 344. 1127–28.

Hitzig, Gary S. (1997) *Help and Hope for Hair Loss*. New York: Avon.

Hsu, Karen. (August 13, 1997) "For Men with Breast Cancer, Loneliness Follows Surprise," *The New York Times*. C8.

Jamison, P. L., and P. H. Gebhard. (1988) "Penis Size Increases Between Flaccid and Erect States: An Analysis of the Kinsey Data," *Journal of Sex Research* 24. 177–83.

Jeffries, Noah. (1993) "Turn for the Worse," *Men's Health* 8 (7). 28.

Kinsey, Alfred C., Wardell B. Pomeroy, and Clyde E. Martin. (1948) *Sexual Behavior in the Human Male*. Philadelphia: W. B. Saunders.

Klein, Randy Sue. "Penile augmentation surgery." Publication pending.

Ladas, Alice Kahn, et al. (1982) *The G Spot and Other Recent Discoveries About Human Sexuality*. New York: Holt, Rinehart and Winston.

Laumann, E.O. (1997) "Circumcision in the United States: Prevalence, Prophylactic Effects and Sexual Practice," *Journal of the American Medical Association* 277 (13). 1052–57.

Lever, Janet. August 29, 1994. "Sexual Revelations," *The Advocate*. 21.

Lund, J., and J. Scholefield. (1997) "A Randomised, Prospective, Double-Blind, Placebo-Controlled Trial of Glyceryl Trinitrate Ointment in Treatment of Anal Fissure," *The Lancet* 349 (9044). 11–14.

Men's Fitness Magazine and Kevin Cobb. (1996) *Men's Fitness Magazine's Complete Guide to Health and Well-Being*. New York: HarperPerennial.

Miles, A. J., et al. (1990) "Surgical Management of Anorectal Disease in HIV-Positive Homosexuals," *British Journal of Surgery* 77 (8). 869–71.

Morganstern, Steven, and Allen Abrahams. (1993) *The Prostate Sourcebook*. Los Angeles: Lowell House.

Morgentaler, Abraham, MD. (1993) *The Male Body: A Physician's Guide to What Every Man Should Know About His Sexual Health*. New York: Fireside.

Morin, Jack, Ph.D. (1998) *Anal Pleasure and Health*. San Francisco: Down There Press.

Murray, Frank. (1994) "Therapy and Treatment with Aloe Vera," *Better Nutrition for Today's Living* 56 (3). 52.

Nagier, Harris M., and Carl A. Wisson. (1989) "Prostate," in *The Columbia University College of Physicians and Surgeons Complete Home Medical Guide*. New York: Crown Publishers.

National Institutes of Health. (1995) "Peyronie's Disease." Bethesda, MD: NIH Publication No. 95–3902.

Neufeld, David M., et al. (1995) "Outpatient Surgical Treatment of Anal Fissure," *European Journal of Surgery*. 161.

Parsons, Alexandra. (1989) *Facts and Phalluses: A Collection of Bizarre and Intriguing Truths, Legends and Measurements*. New York: St. Martin's Press.

Petros, James G., et al. (1993) "Clinical Presentation of Chronic Anal Fissures," *The American Surgeon* 59 (10). 666–68.

Philips, William. (1987) "Foreskin Hygiene," *Australian Family Physician* 15 (5). 661.

Pump It Up! Spring, 1997. 6 (1).

Rabkin, Judith, Robert Remien, and Christopher Wilson. (1994) *Good Doctors, Good Patients: Partners in HIV Treatment*. New York: NCM Publishers, Inc.

Regadas, F.S.P., et al. (1993) "Internal Anal Sphincter in Patients with Chronic Anal Fissure," *British Journal of Surgery* 80 (6). 799–801.

Reinisch, June M., with Ruth Beasley. (1992) *Kinsey Institute New Report on Sex*. New York: HarperPerennial.

Rowen, Robert L., and Paul J. Gillette. (1978) *The Gay Health Guide: A Modern Medicine Book*. Boston: Little, Brown & Co.

Shimberg, E. (1988) *Relief From IBS*. New York: M. Evans and Company.

Silverstein, Charles, and Felice Picano. (1992) *The New Joy of Gay Sex*. New York: HarperPerennial.

Sobel, D. (1996) "What Causes Anal Fissure?" *Gastroenterology* 111 (4). 1154–55.

Taguchi, Yosh, MD. (1996) *Private Parts: An Owner's Guide to the Male Anatomy,* 2nd edition. Ontario: McClelland and Stewart.

Taylor, J. R., et al. (1995) "The Prepuce: Specialized Mucosa of the Penis and Its Loss to Circumcision," *British Journal of Urology* 77. 291–95.

Tiefer, Leonore. (1995) *Sex Is Not a Natural Act and Other Essays*. Boulder, CO: Westview Press.

Townsend, Larry. (1985) *The Leatherman's Handbook*. New York: Carlyle Communications.

Trockman, Brett A., et al. (1994) "Complication of Penile Injection of Autologous Fat," *Journal of Urology* 151. 429–30.

Walker, Mitch. (1977) *Men Loving Men*. San Francisco: Gay Sunshine Press.

Walsh, Patrick C., MD, and Janet Farrar Worthington. (1997) *The Prostate: A Guide for Men and the Women Who Love Them*. New York: Warner Books, Inc.

Weidner, Shroeder W., et al. (1997) "Sexual Dysfunction in Peyronie's Disease," *Journal of Urology* 157 (1). 325–28.

Wessells, Hunter, et al. (1996). "Penile Length in the Flaccid and Erect States: Guidelines for Penile Augmentation," *Journal of Urology* 156. 995-997.

Westheimer, Ruth K. (1994) *Dr. Ruth's Encyclopedia of Sex*. New York: Continuum.

White, Edmund. (1983) *States of Desire*. New York: E.P. Dutton.

Wilkson, Steven K., and John R. Delk, II. (1994) "A New Treatment for Peyronie's Disease: Modeling the Penis Over an Inflatable Penile Prosthesis," *Journal of Urology* 152. 1121–23.

Zilbergeld, Bernie. (1992) *The New Male Sexuality*. New York: Bantam Books.

Internet

http://faf6.arc.nasa.gov/af. "Anal Fissure Self-Help Page."

http://www.menshealth.com/noframes/features/mensconf/belt/doc27.html. "Feed Your Prostate Right."

http://www.netpoint.nte/prostate/index.htm. "Prostate Center of Florida."

http://nq.guardian.co.uk. "The Body Beautiful: Why Do Males of the Human and Related Species Have Nipples?" Stephenson, Matthew. 1997.

Chapter 2

Ames, Lynda J., et al. (1995) "Love, Lust and Fear: Safer Sex Decision Making Among Gay Men," *Journal of Homosexuality* 30 (1). 53–73.

Anonymous. (May 1995) "How Reliable Are Condoms?" *Consumer Reports*. 320–25.

Anonymous. (September 1998) "Hip-Hop Condoms?" *HIV Plus*. 48.

Berzon, Betty. (1988) *Permanent Partners: Building Gay and Lesbian Relationships That Last*. New York: NAL/Dutton.

Bochow, M., et al. (1994) "Sexual Behaviour of Gay and Bisexual Men in Eight European Countries," *AIDS Care* 6 (5). 533–49.

Buchbinder, Susan P., et al. (1996) "Feasability of Human Immunodeficiency Virus Vaccine Trials in Homosexual Men in the United States: Risk Behavior, Seroincidence, and Willingness to Participate," *Journal of Infectious Diseases* 174. 954–61.

Campsmith, Michael L., et al. (1995) "Demographic and Behavioral Differences Among Participants, Nonparticipants and Dropouts in a Cohort of Men Who Have Sex with Men," *Sexually-Transmitted Diseases* 22 (5). 312–16.

Carballo-Dieguez, Alex, and Curtis Dolezal. (1995) "Association Between History of Childhood Sexual Abuse and Adult HIV-Risk Sexual Behavior in Puerto Rican Men Who Have Sex with Men," *Child Abuse and Neglect* 19 (5). 595–605.

———. (1996) "HIV Risk Behaviors and Obstacles to Condom Use Among Puerto Rican Men in New York City Who Have Sex with Men," *American Journal of Public Health* 86 (11). 1619–22.

———. (1994) "Contrasting Types of Puerto Rican Men Who Have Sex with Men (MSM)," *Journal of Psychology and Human Sexuality* 6 (4). 41–67.

Celebrate the Self: The Magazine of Solo Sex. (January-February, 1997) 5 (1) .

Center for AIDS Prevention Studies, University of California, San Francisco. (1994) "Do Condoms Work?" San Francisco: Center for AIDS Prevention Studies.

———. (1994) "What Are Young Gay Men's HIV Prevention Needs?" San Francisco: Center for AIDS Prevention Studies.

———. (1997) "What Is Post-Exposure Prevention (PEP)?" San Francisco: Center for AIDS Prevention Studies.

Centers for Disease Control and Prevention. (1997) "Transmission of HIV Possibly Associated with Exposure of Mucous Membrane to Contaminated Blood," *Morbidity and Mortality Weekly Report* 46 (27). 620–23.

———. (1993) "Facts About Condoms and Their Use in Preventing HIV Infection and Other STD's," *Condoms and STD/HIV Prevention*.

Condom Resource Center. "Condom Educator's Guide." Oakland, CA: Condom Resource Center.

Connet, Skip. July, 1997 "Condom Bust," *Mother Jones*. 11.

Dean, Laura, and Ilan Meyer. (1994) *Journal of Acquired Immune Deficiency Syndromes and Human Retrovirology* 8. 208–11.

Diaz, Rafael M., et al. (1996) "HIV Risk Among Latin Men in the Southwestern United States," *AIDS Education and Prevention* 8 (5). 415–29.

———. (1997) "Trips to Fantasy Island: Contexts of Risky Sex for San Francisco Gay Men," Paper commissioned by the San Francisco AIDS Foundation.

Florida International University. November, 1996. "New Study Reveals High Rate of HIV Infection in South Beach" (news release).

Gluck, Bob. (1987) "Learning to Write." In Fleming, Jim, and Peter Lanborn Wilson (eds.), *Semiotext*. New York: Columbia University Press.

Gold, Ron. (August 1998) "Addressing 'Heat of the Moment' Thinking that Leads to Unsafe Sex." *Focus: A Guide to AIDS Research and Counseling*. 13 (9). 1–4.

Gold, Ron S. (1993) "On the Need to Mind the Gap: On-Line Versus Off-Line Cognitions Underlying Sexual Risk-Taking," In Terry, D.J., et al. (eds.), *The Theory of Reasoned Action: Its Applications to AIDS Preventive Behavior.* Oxford: Pergamon Press. 227–52.

Gold, Ron S., and Doreen A. Rosenthal. (1995) "Preventing Unprotected Anal Intercourse in Gay Men: A Comparison of Two Intervention Techniques," *International Journal of STD and AIDS* 6. 89–94.

Gold, Ron S., et al. (1994) "Unprotected Anal Intercourse in HIV-Infected and Non-HIV-Infected Gay Men," *Journal of Sex Research* 31 (1). 59–77.

Griffin, Gary M., MBA. (1993) *The Condom Encyclopedia*. Los Angeles: Added Dimensions Publishing.

Gross, M., et al. (1996) "Relevance and Feasibility of Clinical Trials of Topical Virucides Designed for Rectal Administration Among U.S. Gay Men," *International Conference on AIDS* 11 (3). 232.

Hays, Robert B., et al. (1990) "High Risk-Taking Among Young Gay Men," *AIDS* 4 (9). 901–07.

Kalichman, Seth C., et al. (1997) "Oral Sex Anxiety, Oral Sexual Behavior, and Human Immunodeficiency Virus (HIV) Risk Perceptions Among Gay and Bisexual Men," *Journal of the Gay and Lesbian Medical Association* 1 (3). 161–68.

Kelly, Jeffrey A., et al. (1992) "Acquired Immunodeficiency Syndrome/Human Immunodeficiency Virus Risk Behavior Among Gay Men in Small Cities: Findings of a 16-City Sample," *Archives of Internal Medicine* 152. 2293–97.

———. (1991) "Situational Factors Associated with AIDS Risk Behavior Lapses and Coping Strategies Used by Gay Men Who Successfully Avoid Lapses," *American Journal of Public Health* 81 (10). 1335–38.

Lambda Legal Defense and Education Fund. (1993) *The Little Black Book*. New York: Lambda Legal Defense and Education Fund.

Laumann, Edward O., et al. (1994) *Social Organization of Sexuality: Sexual Practices in the United States*. Chicago: University of Chicago Press.

Liuzzi, Giuseppina, et al. (1996) "Analysis of HIV-1 Load in Blood, Semen and Saliva: Evidence for Different Viral Compartments in a Cross-Sectional and Longitudinal Study," *AIDS* 10. F51–F56.

Love, Brenda. (1992) *Encyclopedia of Unusual Sexual Practices*. Fort Lee, NJ: Barricade Books.

Maurer, Harry. (1994) *Sex: An Oral History*. New York: Viking.

Mayne, Tracy J., and Ross W. Buck. (1997) "Sex, Emotion and the Triune Brain," *Health Psychology* 19 (3). 8–14

Mays, Vickie M., et al. (1992) "The Language of Black Gay Men's Sexual Behavior: Implications for AIDS Risk Reduction," *Journal of Sex Research* 29 (3).

Morris M., and L. Dean. (1994) "Effects of Sexual Behavior Change on Long-Term Human Immunodeficiency Virus Prevalence Among Homosexual Men," *American Journal of Epidemiology* 140 (3). 217–32.

National Highway Traffic Safety Administration. (1997) *Traffic Safety Facts Overview*.

Nelson, Craig. (1996) *Finding True Love in a Man-Eat-Man World: The Intelligent Guide to Gay Dating, Romance, and Eternal Love*. New York: Dell Publishing.

Odets, Walt. (1994) "AIDS Education and Harm Reduction for Gay Men: Psychological Approaches for the 21st Century," *AIDS and Public Policy Journal* 9 (1). 2–15.

Ostrow, David G., MD, Ph.D., et al. (1995) "A Case-Control Study of Human Immunodeficiency Virus Type 1 Seroconversion and Risk-Related Behaviors in the Chicago MACS/CCS Cohort, 1984–1992," *American Journal of Epidemiology* 142 (8). 875–83.

Peterson, John L., et al. (1995) "Help-Seeking for AIDS High-Risk Sexual Behavior Among Gay and Bisexual African-American Men," *AIDS Education and Prevention* 7 (1). 1–9.

Penkower, Lili, et al. (1991) "Behavioral Health and Psychosocial Factors and Risk for HIV Infection Among Sexually Active Homosexual Men: The Multicenter AIDS Cohort Study," *American Journal of Public Health* 81 (2). 194–96.

Phillips, D. M., and V. R. Zacharopoulos. (1998) "Nonoxynol-9 Enhances Rectal Infection by Herpes Simplex Virus in Mice," *Contraception* 57 (5). 341–348.

Prochaska, James O. (1994) "Strong and Weak Principles for Progressing from Precontemplation to Action on the Basis of Twelve Program Behaviors," *Health Psychology* 13 (1). 47–51.

Richters, Juliet, MPH, et al. (1995) "Why Do Condoms Break or Slip Off in Use? An Exploratory Study," *International Journal of STD and AIDS* 6. 11–18.

Robbins, Jim. (January 29, 1997) "Rubber Gloves Peril for Some," *The New York Times*. C7.

Robins, Anthony G., et al. (1994) "Psychosocial Factors Associated with Risky Sexual Behavior Among HIV-Seropositive Gay Men," *AIDS Education and Prevention* 6 (6). 483–92.

Rubin, Gayle. (1989) "Thinking Sex," In Carole Vance (ed.), *Pleasure and Danger*. London: Pandora Books. 267–320.

Sacco, William P., and Richard Rickman. (1996) "AIDS-Relevant Condom Use by Gay and Bisexual Men: The Role of Person Variables and the Interpersonal Situation," *AIDS Education and Prevention* 8 (5). 430–43.

Sanderson, Terry. (1994) *A to Z of Gay Sex: An Erotic Alphabet*. London: Other Way Press.

Spenser, Colin. (1996) *The Gay Kama Sutra*. New York: St. Martin's Press.

Thompson, John L., et al. (1993) "Estimated Condom Failure and Frequency of Condom Use Among Gay Men," *American Journal of Public Health* 83 (10). 1409–14.

Thompson, Michael. (1994) "Gay and Bisexual Men of Color: HIV Prevention Needs and Issues, Summary of Current Findings and Bibliography." Unpublished paper presented at the Dallas HIV Prevention Summit.

Verlaine, P., and A. Rimbaud. (1986) "Sonnet to the Asshole," Trans. J. Murai and W. Gunn. In Coote, Stephen (ed.), *The Penguin Book of Homosexual Verse*, 2nd edition. New York: Viking Penguin.

Walker, Mitch (1977) *Men Loving Men*. San Francisco: Gay Sunshine Press.

Winkelstein, Warren, Jr., et al. (1987) "Sexual Practices and Risk of Infection by the Human Immunodeficiency Virus," *Journal of the American Medical Association* 257 (3). 321–25.

Chapter 3

Bannon, Race. (1992) *Learning the Ropes: A Basic Guide to Safe and Fun S/M Lovemaking*. San Francisco: Daedelus.

Bean, Joseph W. (1994) *Leathersex: A Guide for the Curious Outsider and the Serious Player*. San Francisco: Daedelus.

———. (1996) *Leathersex Q & A*. San Francisco: Daedelus.

Chia, Mantak, and Douglas Abrams Arava. (1996) *The Multi-Orgasmic Man*. New York: HarperCollins.

Davies, Peter M., et al. (1992) *Sex, Gay Men and AIDS*. London, New York: The Falmer Press.

Dawson, Jill M. (1994) "Awareness of Sexual Partners' HIV Status as an Influence upon High-Risk Sexual Behavior Among Gay Men," *AIDS* 8 (6). 837–41.

Elovich, Richard. (1999) "Beyond Condoms: Toward a Culture of Gay Male Sexual Health." New York: Gay Men's Health Crisis.

Hickson, Ford, and Project SIGMA. February, 1993. "Gay Men and Fucking." London: Project SIGMA Working Paper No. 36.

Hickson, Ford, C.I., et al. (1994) "Gay Men as Victims of Nonconsensual Sex," *Archives of Sexual Behavior* 23 (3). 281–94.

———. (1994) "Perceptions of Own and Partner's HIV Status and Unprotected Anal Intercourse Among Gay Men." Paper presented at AIDS Impact, Second Conference of Biopsychosocial Aspects of HIV/AIDS (Brighton), and European Conference on Methods and results of Psycho-Social AIDS Research (Berlin).

In the Family. (January 1996) 1 (3).

Isenee, Rik. (1990) *Love Between Men: Enhancing Intimacy and Keeping Your Relationship Alive*. New York: Prentice Hall Press.

———. (1997) *Reclaiming Your Life: The Gay Men's Guide to Love, Self-Acceptance and Trust*. Los Angeles: Alyson Publications, Inc.

Jacques, Trevor. (1993) *On the Safe Edge: A Manual for SM Play*. Toronto: Whole SM Publishing.

Jordan, Reed. (1997) "Everything You Always Wanted to Know About Three-Ways," *Genre*. 65–67.

Kalichman, Seth C., and David Rompa. (1995) "Sexually Coerced and Noncoerced Gay and Biesexual Men: Factors Relevant to Risk for Human Immunodeficiency Virus (HIV) Infection," *Journal of Sex Research* 32 (1). 45–50.

Kessler, Gil. (1997) "Safe, Sane, Consensual," *GMSMA Newslink*. 38.

Klinger, Rochelle L., MD, and Terry S. Stein, MD. (1996) "Impact of Violence, Childhood Sexual Abuse, and Domestic Violence and Abuse on Lesbians, Bisexuals and Gay Men." In Cabaj, Robert P., MD, and Terry S. Stein (eds.) *Textbook of Homosexuality and Mental Health*. Washington, DC: American Psychiatric Press.

Lew, Mike. (1990) "Focus: Finding Your Voice." In his *Victims No Longer: Men Recovering From Incest and Other Sexual Child Abuse*. New York: HarperCollins.

McWhirter, David P., MD, and Andrew M. Mattison, MSW, Ph.D. (1985) *The Male Couple: How Relationships Develop*. Englewood Cliffs, NJ: Prentice Hall, Inc.

Mezey, Gillian C., and Michael B. King. (1993) *Male Victims of Sexual Assault*. New York: Oxford University Press.

Morin, J. (1995) *The Erotic Mind*. New York: HarperCollins.

Odets, Walt. (1997) "Gay Male Couples: Psychological and Social Issues," *GLMA Reporter* 1 (1). 13–14.

Scarce, Michael. (1997) *Male on Male Rape*. New York: Insight Books.

Chapter 4

Adams, V., et al. (1995) "Detection of Several Types of Human Papilloma Viruses in AIDS-Associated Kaposi's Sarcoma," *Journal of Medical Virology* 46 (3). 189–193.

Alter, Miriam. (1997) "Epidemiology of Hepatitis C11," *Hepatitis Foundation International Washington Report, Excerpts from Hepatitis C Consensus Conference*. 1–2.

Altman, Lawrence, MD. (October 23, 1990) "Tiny Mite Causes Overwhelming Itch: Elusive Scabies," *The New York Times*. C3.

American Urological Association. (1996) *Treatment of Organic Erectile Dysfunction: A Patient's Guide*. Baltimore: American Urological Association.

Anonymous. (1987) *Hope and Recovery: A Twelve-Step Guide for Healing From Compulsive Sexual Behavior*. Center City, MN: Hazelden Foundation.

Beck, E. J., et al. (1996) "Case-Controlled Study of Sexually Transmitted Diseases as Cofactors for HIV-1 Transmission," *International Journal of STD and AIDS* 7 (1). 34–38.

Bielski, Vince. (November 19, 1996) "Erection Results," *The Village Voice*. 37–40.

Brody, Jane E. (January 22, 1997) "Personal Health: There Is Bad News and Good About a Hidden Viral Epidemic: Hepatitis C," *The New York Times*. C9.

Centers for Disease Control and Prevention. (September 15, 1995) "Certain STD's Associated with Faster HIV Progression," *Infectious Disease Weekly*. 13–14.

———. (1997) "Gonorrhea Among Men Who Have Sex With Men—Selected Sexually Transmitted Disease Clinics, 1993–1996," *Morbidity and Mortality Weekly Report* 46 (38).

———. (1997) "The Role of STD Testing and Treatment in HIV Prevention," *CDC Update*.

Cohen, Myron, et al. (1997) "Reduction of Concentration of HIV-1 Semen After Treatment of Urethritis: Implications for Prevention of Sexual Transmission of HIV-1," *The Lancet* 349. 1868–73.

Dambro, Mark R. (1997) *Griffith's 5-Minute Clinical Consult*. Baltimore, MD: Williams & Wilkins.

Dover, Jeffrey S., and Kenneth A. Arndt. (1997) "Valaciclovir and Famciclovir, 2 New Agents for Varicella Zoster and Herpes Simplex," *Journal of the American Medical Association* 227 (23). 1848–50.

Food and Drug Administration. (1995) "New Choices for Coping with Genital Warts," *FDA Consumer*.

Fenwick, R. D. (1978) *The Advocate Guide to Gay Health*. New York: E. P. Dutton.

Fleming, Douglas T., et al. (1997) "Herpes Simplex Virus Type 2 in the United States, 1976 to 1994," *New England Journal of Medicine* 337 (16). 1105–11.

Fisher, Lawrence M. (June 13, 1997) "Schering-Plough and Lilly Sign Liver Drug Deals." *The New York Times*. D6.

Frank, E., C. Anderson, and D. Rubinstein. (July 20, 1978) "Frequency of Sexual Dysfunction in 'Normal' Couples," *New England Journal of Medicine* 299 (3). 111–15.

Frisch, Morten, et al. (1997) "Sexually Transmitted Infection as a Cause of Anal Cancer," *New England Journal of Medicine* 337 (19). 1350–58.

Geddings-Osbon Foundation. (1993) *Male Impotence: A Treatment Guide*. Augusta, GA: Geddings-Osbon Foundation.

Giuliani, M., et al. (1997) "Incidence and Determinants of Hepatitis C Virus Infection Among Individuals at Risk of Sexually Transmitted Diseases Attending a Human Immunodeficiency Virus Type I Testing Program," *Sexually Transmitted Diseases* 24 (9). 533–37.

Glück, Robert. (1996) "The Purple Men," *Lingo* 6. 28.

Goldberg, Ken, MD. (1993) *How Men Can Live as Long as Women: Seven Steps to a Longer and Better Life*. Fort Worth, TX: The Summit Group.

Gordon, Steven M., et al. (1994) "The Response of Symptomatic Neurosyphilis to High-Dose Intravenous Penicillin G in Patients with Human Immunodeficiency Virus Infection," *New England Journal of Medicine* 331 (22). 1471–1473.

Groopman, Jerome. (May 11, 1998) "The Shadow Epidemic: Why Does the Surgeon General Want Letters Sent to Hundreds of Thousands of People Informing Them That They Might Be Dying?" *The New Yorker*. 48–60.

Guerrant, Richard, et al. (1990) "Intestinal Protozoa: *Giardia lamblia, Entamoeba histolytica* and *Cryptosporidium*." In Holmes, King, et al. (eds.), *Sexually Transmited Diseases*. New York: McGraw Hill. 493–514.

Hellstrom, Wayne J. G., et al. (1996) "A Double-Blind, Placebo-Controlled Evaluation of the Erectile Response to Transurethral Alprostadil," *Urology* 48 (6). 851–56.

Hepatitis B Foundation. (Spring 1997) "B Informed." Jenkintown, PA: Hepatitis B Foundation.

Impotence Institute of America. (1997) "Knowledge Is the Best Medicine." Columbia, MD: Impotence Institute of America.

Kassler, Jeanne. (1983) *Gay Men's Health: A Guide to the AIDS Syndrome and Other Sexually Transmitted Diseases*. New York: Harper & Row.

Keusch, Gerald T. (1990) "Enteric Bacterial Pathogens: Shigella, Salmonella, Campylobacter. In Holmes, King, et al. (eds.), *Sexually Transmitted Diseases*. New York: McGraw Hill. 295–303.

Laumann, Edward, et al. (1999). "Sexual Dysfunction in the United States: Prevalence and Predictors," JAMA 281 (3). 537-544.

Levine, William C., et al. (1995) "Texas Syphilis Related to HIV Infection," abstract presented at 11th Annual Meeting of the International Society for Sexually Transmitted Disease Research (August 27–30).

The Lighthouse, Inc. (1998) "The Lighthouse National Survey on Vision Loss: The Experience, Attitudes and Knowledge of Middle-Aged and Older Americans." New York: The Lighthouse, Inc.

Meinking, Terri L., et al. (1995) "The Treatment of Scabies with Intervention," *New England Journal of Medicine* 333 (1). 26–29.

Morbidity and Mortality Weekly Report Recommendations and Reports. (1998) *1998 Guidelines for Treatment of Sexually Transmitted Diseases*. Atlanta, GA: U.S. Department of Health and Human Services Center for Disease Control and Prevention.

Ndimbie, O. K., et al. (1996) "Hepatitis C Virus Infection in a Male Homosexual Cohort: Risk Factor Analysis," *Genitourinary Medicine* 72 (3).

O'Neill, Joseph P., and Peter Shalit. (1992) "Health Care of the Gay Male Patient," *Primary Care* 19 (1). 191–201.

Oriel, David. (1990) "Genital Human Papillomavirus Infection," In Holmes, King, et al. (eds.), *Sexually Transmitted Diseases*. New York: McGraw-Hill. 433–41.

Padma-Nathan, Harin, MD, et al. (1997) "Treatment of Men with Erectile Dysfunction with Transurethral Alprostadil," *New England Journal of Medicine* 336. 1–7.

Palefsky, Joel. (1994) "Anal Human Papillomavirus Infection and Anal Cancer in HIV-positive Individuals: An Emerging Problem," *AIDS* 8. 283–95.

———. "Human Papillomavirus Infection Among HIV-Infected Individuals: Implications for Development of Malignant Tumors," *Hematology/Oncology Clinics of North America: Hematologic and Oncologic Aspects of HIV Disease* 5 (2). 357–70.

Palefsky, Joel, et al. (1998) "Anal Squamous Intraepithelial Lesions in HIV-positive and HIV-negative Homosexual and Bisexual Man: Prevalence and Risk Factors," *Journal of Acquired Immune Deficiency Syndrome and Human Retrovirology* 17(4). 320-26.

———. (1997) "Anal Cytology as a Screening Tool for Anal Squamopus Intraepithelial Lesions," *Journal of Acquired Immune Deficiency Syndrome and Human Retrovirology* 14 (5). 415–22.

Phelps, William C., and Kenneth Alexander. (1995) "Antiviral Therapy of Human Papilloma viruses: Rationale and Prospects," *Annals of Internal Medicine* 123. 368–82.

Pinsky, Laura, and Paul Harding Douglas. (1993) *The Essential HIV Treatment Fact Book*. New York: Pocket Books.

Reed, Sharon L. (1992) "Amebiasis: An Update," *Clinical Infectious Diseases* 14. 385–93.

Reinisch, June M., and Ruth Beasley. (1991) *Kinsey Institute New Report on Sex*. New York: St. Martin's Press.

Rompalo, Anne, and H. Hunter Handsfield. (1989) "Overview of Sexually Transmitted Diseases in Homosexual Men," In Ma, Pearl, and Donald Armstrong (eds.), *AIDS and Infections of Homosexual Men*. Boston: Butterworths.

Rowen, Robert L., and Paul J. Gillette. (1978) *The Gay Health Guide: A Modern Medicine Book*. Boston: Little, Brown & Co.

San Francisco AIDS Foundation. (1995) "Behind Our Backs." San Francisco: San Francisco AIDS Foundation.

Shlegel, Peter N., MD. (1995) "Examining the Mechanics of Ejaculation," *Contemporary Urology*. 45–52.

Seeff, Leonard. (1997) "Natural History of Hepatitis C." Hepatitis Foundation International Washington Report, Excerpts from Hepatitis C Consensus Conference.

Shute, Nancy. (June 22, 1998) "Hepatitis C: A Silent Killer," *U.S. News and World Report*. 60–66.

Skolnick, Andrew A. (1997) "Guidelines for Treating Erectile Dysfunction Issued," *Journal of the American Medical Association* 277 (1). 7–8.

Spraycar, Marjory (ed.). (1995) *Stedman's Medical Dictionary*, 26th edition. Baltimore, MD: Williams and Wilkins.

Vernon, Suzanne D., et al. (1995) "Human Papillomavirus Infection and Associated Disease in Persons Infected with Human Immunodeficiency Virus," *Clinical Infectious Diseases* 21. S121–S124.

Weinke, Thomas, et al. (1990) "Prevalence and Clinical Importance of *Entamoeba histolytica* in Two High-Risk Groups: Travelers Returning from the Tropics and Male Homosexuals," *Journal of Infectious Diseases* 161. 1029–31.

Wikstrom, A. (1995) "Clinical and Serological Manifestations of Genital Human Papillomavirus Infection," *Acta Dermato-Venereologica* 193. 1–85.

Internet

http://www.unspeakable.com. "Nothing But the Facts: Hepatitis B." Pfizer, Inc.

http://cure.medinfo.org. "The Association of Cancer Online Resources, Inc."

Chapter 5

Anderson, Arnold E., ed. (1990) *Males with Eating Disorders*. New York: Brunner/Mazel.

Anonymous. (June 4, 1997) "Proposed Rules," *Federal Register* 62 (107), 30677–724

Atkins, Dawn. (1998) *Looking Queer: Body Image and Identity in Lesbian, Gay and Transgender Communities*. New York: Harrington Park Press.

Bailey, Covert. (1994) *Smart Exercise: Burning Fat/Getting Fit*. New York: Houghton Mifflin.

Beren, Susan, et al. (1996) "The Influence of Sexual Orientation on Body Dissatisfaction in Adult Men and Women," *International Journal of Eating Disorders* 20 (2). 135–41.

Clark, Janie. (1992) *Full Life Fitness: A Complete Exercise Program for Mature Adults*. Champaign, IL: Human Kinetics Publishers.

Conant, Marcus A. (n.d.). "Skin Care & You...The HIV Connection." San Francisco, CA: Conant Foundation.

Connors, T. J., et al. (1990) "Australian Trial of Topical Minoxidil and Placebo in Early Male Pattern Baldness," *Australian Journal of Dermatology* 31 (1). 17–25.

Crowden, Craig R., and Patricia B. Koch. (1995) "Attitudes Related to Sexual Concerns: Gender and Orientation Comparisons," *Journal of Sex Education and Therapy* 21 (2). 78–87.

France, David. (1996) "There's No Such Thing as a Free Crunch," *Smart Money*. 132–36.

Franks, B. Don, and Edward T. Howley. (1989) *Fitness Facts: The Healthy Living Handbook*. Champaign. IL: Human Kinetics Books.

Freeman, R. J. (1990) *Bodylove: Learning to Like Our Looks—and Ourselves*. New York: Perennial Library.

Gawande, Atul. (March 30, 1998) "No Mistake—The Future of Medical Care: Machines That Act Like Doctors, and Doctors Who Act Like Machines," *The New Yorker*. 75–81.

Gettelman, Thomas E., and J. Kevin Thompson. (1993) "Actual Differences and Stereotypical Perceptions in Body Image and Eating Disturbance: A Comparison of Male and Female Heterosexual and Homosexual Samples," *Sex Roles* 29 (7–8). 545–62.

Katz, H. I., et al. (March, 1987) "Long-term Efficacy of Topical Minoxidil in Male Pattern Baldness." *Journal of the American Academy of Dermatology* 16 (3) Pt. 2. 711–18.

Men's Fitness Magazine and Kevin Cobb. (1996) "Exercise: How Intense?" In *Men's Fitness Magazine's Complete Guide to Health and Well-Being*. New York: HarperPerennial. 168.

———. (1996) "Body Image." In *Men's Fitness Magazine's Complete Guide to Health and Well-Being*. New York: HarperPerennial. 131–77.

Men's Health Magazine Editors. (1996) *Get Rid of That Gut*. Emmaus, PA: Rodale Press.

Merck and Co. (December, 1997) *Propecia (Finasteride) Tablets: Patient Information about Propecia*. West Point, PA: Merck and Co.

National Institutes of Health. (1996) "Statistics Related to Overweight and Obesity." Bethesda, MD: NIH Publication No. 96–4158.

Nieman, David C. (1998) *The Exercise Health Connection*. Champaign, IL: Human Kinetics.

Olsen, E.A., et al. (April, 1990) "Five-year Follow-up of Men with Androgenetic Alopecia Treated with Topical Minoxidil," *Journal of the American Academy of Dermatology* 22 (4). 643–46.

Onstott, Michael. (March, 1998) "Say Chi," *POZ*. 75.

Pinsky, Laura, et al. (1992) "Skin Problems." In their *The Essential HIV Treatment Fact Book*. New York: Pocket Books. 185–90.

Pope, Harrison G., Jr., et al. (1997) "Muscle Dysmorphia: An Underrecognized Form of Body Dysmorphic Disorder," *Psychosomatics* 38. 548–57.

Prevention Magazine Editors. (1990) "Psoriasis." In *The Doctor's Book of Home Remedies*. Emmaus, PA: Rodale Press. 511–17.

Puhn, Adele. (1998) *The 5 Vital Secrets for a Healthy Life*. New York: Ballantine Books.

Siever, Michael D. (1994) "Sexual Orientation and Gender as Factors in Socioculturally Acquired Vulnerability to Body Dissatisfaction and Eating Disorders," *Journal of Consulting and Clinical Psychology* 62 (2). 252–60.

Silberstein, Lisa R., et al. (1989) "Men and Their Bodies: A Comparison of Homosexual and Heterosexual Men," *Psychsomatic Medicine* 51 (3). 337–46.

Signorile, Michelangelo. (1997) *Life Outside*. New York: HarperCollins.

Stringer, JoAnn Altman. (1990) "Igor, Throw the Switch," *The Transsexual's Survival Guide: To Transition and Beyond, Vol. I*. King of Prussia, PA: Creative Design Services. 26–29.

Thompson, Wend, and Jerry Shapiro. (1996) *Alopecia Areata: Understanding and Coping with Hair Loss*. Baltimore, MD: Johns Hopkins University Press.

Tschachler, Erwin, et al. (1996) "HIV-Related Skin Diseases," *The Lancet* 348 (9028). 659–63.

Ulene, Art. (1996) *Really Fit Really Fast*. Encino, CA: HealthPOINTS.

Vanderveen, E. E., et al. (September 1984). "Topical Minoxidil for Hair Regrowth," *Journal of the American Academy of Dermatology* 11 (3). 416–21.

Vaughn, Lewis. (1998) "Better Blood Pressure," In *Prevention* Magazine Editors (ed.), *Everyday Health Tips: 2000 Practical Hints for Better Health and Happiness*. Emmaus, PA: Rodale Press. 8–9.

Westcott, Wayne. (1994) *Strength Fitness: Psychological Principles and Training Techniques*, 4th edition. Madison, WI: William Brown Publishers.

Whitman, Walt. (1998) *Leaves of Grass*. New York: Oxford University Press.

Yealis, C. E. (1993) "Anabolic-Androgenic Steroid Use in the United States," *The Journal of the American Medical Association* 270 (5). 1217.

Internet

http://www.shaolin-wahnam.org/chikung.html. "Chi Kung."

http//members.tripod.com/~SifuWong/taiji-faq-cthtml. "Frequently Asked Questions of Taijiquan—Clear Text."

http:/www.newyork.bbb.org/library/publications/sub0046.html. "Hair Replacement." The Better Business Bureau.

http://webcom.com/bkm/ifr/calendar/priderun98.html. "Pride Runs."

http://www.ABCNews.com. (March 27, 1998) "Sniffing Out a Mate." Ritter, Bill.

http://pridefest.org/sportsfest.htm. "Sportsfest."

http://www.healthy.net/library/articles/westcott/twelvereasons.htm. Westcott, Wayne. "Twelve Reasons Every Adult Should Do Strength Exercise." 1998.

CHAPTER 6

Bagasra, Omar, and Roger Pomerantz. (1993) "Human Immunodeficiency Virus Type 1 Replication in Peripheral Blood Mononuclear Cells in the Presence of Cocaine," *Journal of Infectious Diseases* 168 (5). 1157–64.

Bock, Kenneth, and Nellie Sabin. (1997) *The Road to Immunity: How to Survive and Thrive in a Toxic World*. New York: Pocket Books.

Bredenberg, Jeff, et al. (1996) *Food Smart: A Man's Plan to Fuel Up for Peak Performance*. Men's Health Improvement Guides. Emmaus, PA: Rodale Press.

Brody, Jane E. (October 26, 1997) "In Vitamin Mania, Millions Are Taking a Gamble on Their Health," *The New York Times*. A1, A28.

———. (1997) *The New York Times Book of Health*. New York: Random House.

Brucker, Emily L. (1995) *Out and Free: Sexual Minorities and Tobacco Addiction*. Seattle, WA: Group Health Cooperative.

Burns, David N., et al. (1996) "Cigarette Smoking, Bacterial Pneumonia, and Other Clinical Outcomes in HIV-1 Infection," *Journal of Acquired Immune Deficiency Syndrome and Human Retrovirology* 13 (4). 374–83.

Bux, Donald A., Jr. (1996) "The Epidemiology of Problem Drinking in Gay Men and Lesbians: A Critical Overview," *Clinical Psychology Review* 16 (4). 277–98.

Conley, Lois J., et al. (1996) "The Association Between Cigarette Smoking and Selected HIV-Related Medical Conditions," *AIDS* 10 (10). 1121–26.

Crawford, D. (1990) *Easing the Ache: Gay Men Recovering from Compulsive Behaviors*. New York: Dutton.

Dax, E.M. (1991) "Amyl Nitrate Alters Human In Vitro Immune Function," *Immunopharmacology and Immunotoxicology* 13 (4). 577–87.

Duffum, John, and Charles Moser. (1986) *Journal of Psychoactive* Drugs 18 (4).

Gay Council on Drinking Behavior. (1981) *The Way Back: The Stories of Gay and Lesbian Alcoholics*. Washington, DC: Whitman-Walker Clinic.

Hellman, Ronald E. (1989) "Treatment of Homosexual Alcoholics in Government-Funded Agencies: Provider Training and Attitudes," *Hospital and Community Psychiatry* 40 (11). 1163–68.

Hilts, Philip J. (August 2, 1994) "Is Nicotine Addictive? It Depends on Whose Criteria You Use," *The New York Times*. C3.

Hollis, Judi. (1985) *Fat Is a Family Affair*. Center City, MN: Hazelden Educational Materials.

Hurt, Richard D., et al. (October 23, 1997) "A Comparison of Sustained-Release Bupropion and Placebo for Smoking Cessation," *New England Journal of Medicine* 337 (17). 1195–202.

Institute for the Study of Drug Dependency. (1995) "Anabolic Steroids." London: Institute for the Study of Drug Dependency.

James, John S. (July 10, 1998) "Successful Treatment of 'Buffalo Hump' with Growth Hormone," *AIDS Treatment News* 298. 5.

Judell, Brandon. (1997) *The Gay Quote Book*. New York: Dutton.

Lamm, Steven, and Gerald Secor Couzens. (1997) *Younger at Last: The New World of Vitality Medicine*. New York: Simon & Schuster.

Lehmann, Robert H. (1997) *Cooking For Life: A Guide to Nutrition and Food Safety for the HIV-Positive Community*. New York: Dell Publishing.

Layzell, S. (1993) *Staying Safe: HIV and Drug Abuse*. London: Standing Conference on Drug Abuse.

Lisker, Jerry. (July 6, 1969). "Homo Nest Raided, Queen Bees Are Stinging Mad," *Daily News*.

Lugliani, Greg. (June 1997) "Smoking," *POZ*. 86–87.

Mangweth, Barbara. (1997) "Eating Disorders in Austrian Men: An Intracultural and Crosscultural Comparison Study," *Psychotherapy Psychosomatics* 66. 214–21.

Massing, Michael. (March 22, 1998) "Why Beer Won't Go Up in Smoke," *The New York Times*. A36.

Monte, Tom, and the Editors of *Natural Health* Magazine. (1997) *The Complete Guide to Natural Healing*. New York: Berkeley Publishing Group.

Moss, A., et al. (1987) "Risk Factors for AIDS and HIV Seropositivity in Homosexual Men," *American Journal of Epidemiology* 125 (6). 1035–47.

Olivardia, Roberto, et al. (1995) "Eating Disorders in College Men," *American Journal of Psychiatry* 152. 1279–85.

———. (1996) "Substance Abuse, HIV, and Gay Men," *Focus: A Guide to AIDS Research and Counseling* 11 (7). 2–8.

Paris, Bob. (1991) *Beyond Built: Bob Paris' Guide to Achieving the Ultimate Look*. New York: Warner Books.

Peterson, Anne. (May 4, 1998) "Eating Disorders and HMO's," The Associated Press.

Prochaska, James O., et al. (1994) *Changing for Good: A Revolutionary Six-Stage Program for Overcoming Bad Habits and Moving Your Life Positively Forward.* New York: Avon Books.

Ricaute, George. (1995) "Reorganization of Ascending 5–HT Projections in Animals Previously Exposed to the Recreational Drug (+/-) 3,4-Methylene-dioxymethamphetamine," *Journal of Neuroscience* 15 (8). 5476–85.

Royce, Rachel A., and Warren Winkelstein, Jr. (1990) "Smoking . . . Counts: Preliminary Results from the San Francisco Men's Health Study," *AIDS* 4. 327–33.

Rustim, Terry A. (1996) *Get Ready: Clean and Free Workbook 1. Get Set: Clean and Free Workbook 2. Go: Clean and Free Workbook 3*. Center City, MN: Hazelden.

Seage G., et al. (1992) "The Relation Between Nitrite Inhalants, Unprotected Receptive Anal Intercourse, and the Risk of Human Immunodeficiency Virus Infection," *American Journal of Epidemiology* 135 (20). 1–11.

Silberstein, L. R., et al. (1990). "Men and Their Bodies: A Comparison of Homosexual and Heterosexual Men," *Psychosomatic Medicine* 51 (3). 337-46.

Sonberg, Lynn. (1995) *The Health Nutrient Bible: The Complete Encyclopedia of Food as Medicine*. New York: Fireside.

U.S. Department of Agriculture. (Summer, 1988) "Food News for Consumers." Washington, DC: U.S. Department of Agriculture.

van Griensven, G., et al. (1987) "Risk Factors and Prevalence of HIV Antibodies in Homosexual Men in the Netherlands," *American Journal of Epidemiology* 125 (6). 1048–57.

Vizzier, Carol. (January/February 1994) "Medicaid Update: Smoking and HIV, " *The Volunteer* 6.

Washton, Arnold. (1989) *Cocaine Addiction*. New York: Norton.

Wertheimer, Neil (ed.). (1995) *Total Health for Men*. Emmaus, PA: Rodale Press.

Ziebold, T. O., and J. E. Mongeon (eds.). (1982) *Alcoholism and Homosexuality*. New York: Haworth.

Internet

March 9, 1998. "$13B Medicaid Bill From Smoke." ©Reuters. *ABCNews.com*.

May 6, 1998. "Drugs Don't Kill This Salmonella." ©Associated Press. *ABCNews.com*.

http://www.fda.gov/bbs/topics/NEWS/NEW00637.html. U.S. Department of Health and Human Services. "FDA Proposes Rules to Make Claims for Dietary Supplements More Informative, Reliable and Uniform."

http://www.cdc.gov/nchswww/faq/hpdp1.htm. NCHS, CDC "Health Promotion and Disease Prevention."

Sandok, Mary A. (April 29, 1998) "Smokers' Minds May 'Go' Quicker." ©Associated Press. *ABCNews.com*.

Chapter 7

Berkman, Sue, (ed.) (1996) *How to Find the Best New York Metro Doctors: A Castle/Connolly Guide*. New York: Castle/Connolly Medical Ltd.

Bindman, Andrew, et al. (1998). "A Multi-state Evaluation of Anonymous HIV Testing and Access to Medical Care," *JAMA* 280 (16). 1–16.

Brody, Jane. (November 18, 1997) "Acupuncture: An Expensive Placebo or a Legitimate Alternative?" *The New York Times*. F9.

Brooks, D. D. (1991) "Medical Apartheid: An American Perspective," *The Journal of the American Medical Association* 266. 2746–49.

Busch, M. P., et al. (1995) "Time Course of Detection of Viral and Serologic Markers Preceding Human Immunodeficiency Virus Type 1 Seroconversion: Implications for Screening of Blood and Tissue Donors," *Transfusion* 14 (2). 91–97.

Brown, Don. (1997) *Herbal Prescriptions for Better Health: Your Everyday Guide to Prevention, Treatment and Care*. San Francisco: Prima Publishing.

Cabaj, Robet P., and Terry S. Stein. (1996) *Textbook of Homosexuality and Mental Health*. Washington, DC: American Psychiatric Press.

Chase, Marilyn. (October 20, 1997) "Home Testing Kits Get More Reliable, But Beware of Frauds," *The Wall Street Journal*. 17.

"Cholesterol Drugs Revisited." (July, 1998) *Harvard Health Letter* 23 (9). 8.

Chopra, Deepak. (1995) *Ageless Body, Timeless Mind.* New York: Crown Publishers.

Clayman, Charles B. (ed.). (1994) *American Medical Association Family Guide*. New York: Random House.

Cummings, Stephen, and Dana Ullman. (1984) *Everybody's Guide to Homeopathic Medicines*. Los Angeles: Jeremy P. Tarcher, Inc.

Eisenberg, D. M., et al. (1993) "Unconventional Medicine in the United States: Prevalence, Costs, and Patterns of Use," *New England Journal of Medicine* 328 (4). 282–83.

Gilden, David. (1998) "A Further Point About Statins," *GMHC Treatment Issues* 12 (6). 8

Goldberg, Ken, MD. (1993) *How Men Can Live as Long as Women: Seven Steps to a Longer and Better Life.* Fort Worth, TX: The Summit Group.

Green, James. (1991) *The Male Herbalist: Health Care for Men and Boys*. Freedom, CA: The Crossing Press.

Hoffman, David. (1996) *The Complete Illustrated Holistic Herbal: A Safe and Practical Guide to Making and Using Herbal Remedies*. Rockport, MA: Element Books.

Hoffman, Ronald L., MD (1997) *Intelligent Medicine: A Guide to Optimizing Health and Preventing Illness for the Baby-Boomer Generation*. New York: A Fireside Book.

Kalichman, Seth C. (1998) *Preventing AIDS: A Sourcebook for Behavioral Interventions*. Mahwah, NJ: Lawrence Erlbaum Associates.

Kwan, Delbert J., MD, and Franklin C. Lowe, MD, MPH. (1995) "Genitourinary Manifestations of the Acquired Immunodeficiency Syndrome," *Urology* 45 (1). 13–27.

Myss, Caroline. (1996) *The Anatomy of Spirit: The Seven Stages of Power and Healing*. New York: Crown Publishing Group.

National Heart, Lung and Blood Institute. (1996) *Facts About Blood Cholesterol*. National Institutes of Health.

Office of Gay and Lesbian Health Concerns, New York City Department of Health and Community Health Project. (1996) *Giving the Best Care Possible: Unlearning Homophobia in the Health and Social Service Setting.*

Penn, Robert E. (1997) *The Gay Men's Wellness Guide*. New York: Henry Holt and Co., Inc.

Peterson, K. J., DSW (ed.). (1996) *Health Care for Lesbians and Gay Men: Confronting Homophobia and Heterosexism*. New York: Haworth Press.

Rabkin, Judith G., et al. (1994) *Good Doctors, Good Patients: Partners in HIV Treatment*. New York: NCM Publishers.

Rimer, Robert A., and Michael Connolly. (1993) *HIV+ Working the System*. Boston: Alyson Publications.

Robinson. Mike. (May 4, 1998) "Study Finds Increased Steroid Use Among Boys and Girls: Bigger, Stronger, Younger," *Associated Press*.

Rubenstein, William B., et al. (1996) "HIV Testing." In *The Rights of People Who Are HIV Positive*. Carbondale, IL: Southern Illinois University Press. 21–39.

Schatz, Benjamin, and Katherine O'Hanlan. (1994) *Anti-Gay Discrimination in Medicine: Results of a National Survey of Lesbian, Gay and Bisexual Physicians*. San Francisco: American Association of Physicians for Human Rights.

Society for the Scientific Study of Sexuality. (1995) "What Sexual Scientists Know About Rape" 1 (1). Mount Vernon, IA: Society for the Scientific Study of Sexuality.

Weil, Andrew. (1996) *Spontaneous Healing: How to Discover and Enhance Your Body's Natural Ability to Maintain and Heal Itself*. New York: Fawcett Columbine.

Chapter 8

Ahsan, H. et al. (1998). "Family History of Colorectal Adenomatous Polyps and Increased Risk for Colorectal Cancer," *Annals of Internal Medicine* 128 (11). 900-905.

American Cancer Society. (1998) *Cancer Facts and Figures*. New York: American Cancer Society.

American Psychiatric Association. (1998). Depression. Washington, DC: American Psychiatric Association.

Arnos, Kathleen Shaver, Ph.D. (August 18, 1994) "Hereditary Hearing Loss." *New England Journal of Medicine* 31 (7).

Beauvoir, Simone de. (1972) *Coming of Age*. London: W. W. Norton and Co.

Berger, Raymond. (1996) *Gay and Gray*, 2nd edition. New York: Harrington Park Press.

Berman, Claire. (1996) *Caring for Yourself While Caring for Your Aging Parents*. New York: Henry Holt and Company, Inc.

Berkery, Jr., Peter M., and Gregory A. Diggins. (1998) *Gay Finances in a Straight World*. New York: Macmillan Publishing.

Bower, Bruce. (1996). "Gene Pair May Incite Obesity, Depression," *Science News* 150 (12). 181-182.

Brody, Jane E. (January 20, 1998) "For Glaucoma Risk Group, Ignorance Is Blindness," *The New York Times*. F9.

Brody, Jane E., and Reporters of *The New York Times* (1997) *The New York Times Book of Health*. New York: Times Books.

Broyard, Anatole. (1992) *Intoxicated By My Illness and Other Writings on Life and Death*. New York: Clarkson Potter.

Cadoret, Remi J., et al. (1996). "Depression Spectrum Disease, I: The Role of Gene-Environment Interaction," *American Journal of Psychiatry* 153 (7). 892–899.

Clayman, Charles B., MD, (ed.). (1994) *The American Medical Association Family Medical Guide*, 3rd edition. New York: Random House.

D'Augelli, Anthony R., and Charlotte J. Patterson (eds.). (1995) *Lesbian, Gay, and Bisexual Identities Over the Lifespan*. New York: Oxford University Press.

Darby, Sarah C., et al. (1998) "Survival and Progression to AIDS up to 1996 in 13,000 HIV-1 Seroconverters," abstract presented at the 12th World AIDS Conference, Geneva, June 28–July 3.

Dass, Ram. (1992) *Conscious Aging: On the Nature of Change and Facing Death 1 and 2*. Boulder, CO: Sounds True. Audiocassette.

Davis, Karen. (1996) 1996 AHSR Presidential Address: Uninsured in an Era of Managed Care. Speech given at the annual meeting of the Association for Health Services Research, Atlanta, GA, June 10.

Doress, Paula Brown, et al. (1984) "Women Growing Older," in The Boston Women's Health Book Collective, *The New Our Bodies, Ourselves*. New York: Simon and Schuster.

Dunsmuir, William D., and Mark Emberton. (February 1, 1997) "Surgery, Drugs, and the Male Orgasm," *British Medical Journal* 314 (7077). 319–20.

Elias, Marilyn. (October 28, 1996) "Cancer Therapy Impotence Rates Roughly Equal," *USA Today*. 1.

Erikson, Erik H. (1980) *Identity and the Life Cycle*. New York: W. W. Norton & Co.

Garstecki, Dean C., and Susan F. Erler. (1998). "Hearing Loss, Control and Demographic Factors Influencing Hearing Aid Use Among Older Adults," *Journal of Speech, Language and Hearing Research* 41 (3). 527–37.

Goldberg, Ken, MD. (1993) *How Men Can Live as Long as Women*. Fort Worth, TX: The Summit Group.

Goldschmidt, Jane. (1998) Outing Age: A Working Paper on Policy Issues Facing Gay, Lesbian, Bisexual and Transgender Old People. National Gay and Lesbian Task Force Policy Institute.

Inlander, Charles B., and the Staff of the People's Medical Society. (1998) *Men's Health and Wellness Encyclopedia*. New York: Macmillan.

Isensee, Rik, Ph.D. (1999) *Ready or Not! The Gay Men's Guide to Thriving at Midlife*. Los Angeles: Alyson Publications, Inc.

Jaggar, Sarah F. (1996) "Dangerous Prescriptions for the Elderly." *Consumers' Research Magazine* 79 (6).

Kolata, Gina. (April 8, 1997) "Documents Like Living Wills Are Rarely of Aid, Study Says." *The New York Times*.

Lacan, Jacques. (1982) *Ecrits: A Selection*. New York: W. W. Norton & Co, Inc.

Larson, Per. (1997) *Gay Money*. New York: Dell Publishing, Inc.

Lesko, S. M., et al. (1996) "Family History and Prostate Cancer Risk," *American Journal of Epidemiology* 144 (11). 1041-7.

Levinson, Daniel J., et al. (1978) *The Seasons of a Man's Life*. New York: Ballantine.

Kertzner, Robert M. (June, 1997) "Entering Midlife: Gay Men, HIV, and the Future," *Journal of the Gay and Lesbian Medical Association* 1 (2). 87–95.

Margolis, Simeon, MD, Ph.D., and H. Ballentine Carter, MD. (1998) "Prostate Disorders," *The Johns Hopkins White Papers*. Baltimore, MD: Medletter Associates, Inc.

McCann, Jean. (February 5, 1997) "Impotence Is Not Inevitable After Prostate Cancer Treatment," *Journal of the National Cancer Institute* 89 (3). 194–96

McDonald, Ann, et al. (1988) "HIV Disease Progression Following Newly Acquired HIV Infection in Australia, 1991–1997," abstract presented at the 12th World AIDS Conference, Geneva, June 28–July 3.

Men's Fitness Magazine and Kevin Cobb. (1996) "The Aging Process." In *Men's Fitness Magazine's Complete Guide to Health and Well-Being*. New York: HarperPerennial. 300–07.

Morgenstern, Steven, MD (1993) *The Prostate Sourcebook*. Los Angeles: Lowell House.

National Association of Insurance Commissioners. (1995) *Guide to Health Insurance for People with Medicare*. Washington, DC: Health Care Financing Administration, U.S. Department of Health and Human Services.

National Institutes of Health. (1991) "Prostate Enlargement: Benign Prostatic Hyperplasia." Bethesda, MD: NIH Publication No. 91–3012.

Neergaard, Lauran. (May 11, 1998) "Americans Ignore Colon Cancer Screenings," Associated Press.

———. (November 7, 1997) "Sensor Device May Help Prevent Impotence from Prostate Surgery," *The Advocate*. 10.

Perlman, David. (Feb. 16, 1998) "How Genes Can Define Risk Factors for Heart Disease," *San Francisco Chronicle*. A8.

Peterson, K. Jean, DSW, (ed.). (1996) *Health Care for Lesbians and Gay Men: Confronting Homophobia and Heterosexism*. New York: Haworth Press.

Salwen, Kevin G. (April 12, 1994) "A Special News Report on People and Their Jobs in Offices, Fields and Factories." *The Wall Street Journal*. A1.

Shapiro, Charles E., MD, FACS, and Kathleen Doheny. (1993) *The Well-Informed Patient's Guide to Prostate Problems*. New York: Dell Publishing.

Sheehy, Gail. (1998) *Understanding Men's Passages*. New York: Random House.

Sill, A.M., et al. (June 15, 1994) "Genetic Epidemiologic Study of Hearing Loss in an Adult Population." *American Journal of Medicine* 54 (2). 149–153.

Smeltz, Katie J. (January 21, 1998) "Side Effects of Prostate Cancer Treatment Are Difficult to Discuss, but Manageable," *Journal of the National Cancer Institute* 90 (2). 96–97.

Story, Paula. (June 1, 1998) "Prostate Cancer Deaths Decline." ©Associated Press. *ABCNews.com*.

Talcott, James A., et al. (August 6, 1997) "Patient-Reported Impotence and Incontinence After Nerve-Sparing Radical Prostatectomy," *Journal of the National Cancer Institute* 89 (15). 1117–23.

Walsh, Patrick C., MD, and Janet Farrar Worthington. (1997) *The Prostate: A Guide for Men and the Women Who Love Them*. New York: Warner Books, Inc.

Internet

http://www.cancer.org/cidSpecificCancers/prostate/prstats.html. American Cancer Society. "What Are the Key Statistics About Prostate Cancer?"

http://www.ustoo.com/louis.html. US TOO International, Inc. "Louis Harris Survey: Perspectives on Prostate Cancer Treatments: Awareness, Attitudes and Relationships—A Study of Patients and Urologists."

http://www.resortoncb.com/about.htm. "The Resort on Carefree Boulevard."

Chapter 9

AIDS Treatment Data Network. (n.d.) *Should I Join an AIDS Drug Trial?* New York: ATDN.

Anonymous. (September, 1998) "Give Yourself a Complement," *HIV Plus*. 44–45.

Before I Die: Medical Care and Personal Choices. (1997) Produced by Seminars, Inc. 60 min. PBS Home Video. Videocassette.

Cofrancesco, Joseph, Jr., MD, MPH. (1997) "Testosterone Replacement for Hypognadal Men with HIV Infection and Pharmacological Doses of Anabolic Steroids for Men with Wasting." Paper presented at the annual conference of the Gay and Lesbian Medical Association.

Kearney, Brian, and Project Inform. (1998) *The HIV Drug Book*. New York: Pocket Books.

Levin, Jules. (1997) *New Protease Inhibitor User's Guide: How to Maximize the Benefits of Protease Inhibitors*. New York: National AIDS Treatment Advocacy Project.

Rabkin, Judith, and George Gewirtz. (1992) "Depression and HIV," *Treatment Issues: The GMHC Newsletter of Experimental AIDS Therapies* 6 (11). 12–15.

Romeyn, Mary, MD. (1995) *Nutrition and HIV: A New Model for Treatment*. San Francisco: Jossey-Bass Publishers.

Stephenson, Joan. (1996). "Survival of Patients with AIDS Depends on Physician's Experience Treating the Disease," *JAMA* 275 (10). 745–46.

Tung, Tien-Huei. (1997) *Living with AIDS: A Guide to New York City and Beyond*. 4th edition. New York: Gay Men's Health Crisis.

U.S. Department of Health and Human Services. (December 18, 1992) "1993 Revised Classification System for HIV Infection and Expanded Surveillance Case Definition for AIDS Among Adolescents and Adults," *Morbidity and Mortality Weekly Report* 41. 2–15.

Internet

http://www.thebody.com. "The Body."

http://www.healthcg.com/hiv/nihreport/guide. "Guidelines for the Use of Antiretroviral Agents in HIV-Infected Adults and Adolescents."

http://www.healthcg.com/hiv/nihreport/summary.html. "Report of the NIH Panel to Define Principles of Therapy of HIV Infection."

http://www.healthcg.com: Kotler, Donald, MD, Abby Shevitz, MD, and Marcy Fenton, MS, RD. (1998) "Update on Wasting, Metabolism and Altered Body Shape in HIV/AIDS"

Chapter 10

Bell, L. (1991) *On Our Own Terms: A Practical Guide for Lesbian and Gay Relationships*. Toronto: Coalition for Lesbian and Gay Rights in Ontario.

Berkmen, Sue (ed.). (1997) *How to Find the Best Doctors in the New York Metro Area: A Castle/Connolly Guide*. New York: Castle/Connolly Medical Ltd.

Brown, Paul, and Tess Ayers. (1994) *The Essential Guide to Lesbian and Gay Weddings*. San Francisco: HarperSanFrancisco.

Brown, Walter. (1998). "The Placebo Effect," *Scientific American* 278 (1). 90–95.

Centers for Disease Control. (1998) National Center for Chronic Disease Prevention and Health Promotion. "About Chronic Disease: Definition, Overall Burden, and Cost Effectiveness of Prevention." Fact sheet.

DeCarlo, Pamela, and Susan Folkman. (1996) "Are Informal Caregivers Important in AIDS Care?" UCSF Center for AIDS Prevention Studies. Fact sheet.

Doyle, Derek. (1994) *Caring for a Dying Relative*. New York: Oxford University Press.

Findlay, Steve. (1998) "Making Sense of a Bustling Managed Care Market." *The State of Health Care in America 1998*. Supplement A to *Business and Health* 16 (4).

Firshein, Janet. (1998) "Competing For Professional Turf in Primary Care." *The State of Health Care in America 1998*. Supplement A to *Business and Health*. 6 (4).

Heyman, Jason. (1994) "The Use of Alternative Medicine in the Treatment of HIV Infection and AIDS." *Bulletin of Experimental Treatments for AIDS*. 3–11. No. 21, June 1994.

Isaacs, Stephen L., JD, and Ava C. Swartz, MPH. (1992) *The Consumer's Legal Guide to Today's Health Care: Your Medical Rights and How to Assert Them*. New York: Houghton Mifflin Company.

Kolata, Gina. (April 8, 1997) "Documents Like Living Wills Are Rarely of Aid, Study Says." *The New York Times*, A12.

Kübler-Ross, Elisabeth. (1969) *On Death and Dying*. New York: Collier Books.

Kertzner, Robert M. (June 1997) "Entering Midlife: Gay Men, HIV, and the Future," *Journal of the Gay and Lesbian Medical Association* 1 (2). 87–95.

Mace, Nancy L., MA, and Peter V. Rabins, MD, MPH. (1991) *The 36–Hour Day: A Family Guide to Caring for Persons with Alzheimer's Disease, Related Dementing Illnesses, and Memory Loss in Later Life*. Baltimore: Johns Hopkins University Press.

McFarlane, Rodger. (1997) "We Must Love One Another or Die." In Mass, Lawrence D. (ed.), *We Must Love One Another or Die: The Life and Legacies of Larry Kramer*. New York: St. Martin's Press.

Pinsky, Laura, and Paul Harding Douglas with Craig Metroka, MD, Ph.D. (1992) *The Essential HIV Treatment Fact Book*. New York: Pocket Books.

Project Inform Diagnostics Fact Sheet. (1998) San Francisco: Project Inform.

Quill, Timothy E. *Death and Dignity*. New York: W. W. Norton and Company.

Rees, Alan M. (1998) *Consumer Health Information Source Book*. Phoenix: Oryx Press.

Rubinstein, William B., Ruth Eisenberg, and Lawrence O. Gostin. (1996) "Health Care Decision Making." In their *The Rights of People Who Are HIV Positive*. Carbondale, IL: University of Illinois Press.

Spiegel, D., J. R. Bloom, H. C. Kraemer, and E. Gottheil. (October 14, 1989) "Effect of Psychosocial Treatment on Survival of Patients with Metastatic Breast Cancer," *The Lancet* 2 (8668): 888–91.

Sullivan, Andrew, (ed.) (1997) *Same-Sex Marriage: Pro and Con, A Reader*. New York: Vintage.

Vaughn, Diane. (1988) *Uncoupling*. New York: Oxford University Press.

VOICES in Action. "How to Confront Your Perpetrator: Dead or Alive." Chicago: VOICES in Action.

Weston, Kath. (1991) *Families We Choose*. New York: Columbia University Press.

Woolf, Virginia. (1974) "On Being Ill." In *The Moment and Other Essays*. San Diego: Harcourt Brace and Company.

Internet

http://dairr.immunet.org. "Evaluating Therapies."

Chapter 11

Alexander, Christopher J., Ph.D., (ed.). (1997) *Gay and Lesbian Mental Health: A Sourcebook for Practitioners*. Binghamton, NY: Harrington Park Press.

American Association of Suicidology. (July 1, 1991) *Suicide and How to Prevent It*. Washington, DC: American Association of Suicidology.

Amico, M.Div., CAS, Joseph M. (May-June 1997) "Sharing the Secret: The Need for Gay-Specific Treatment." *The Counselor*.

Anderson, Janis, and Gabrielle I. Weiner. (February, 1996) "Seasonal Depression." *Harvard Health Letter* 21 (4). 7–8.

Andrews, Edmund L. (September 9, 1997) "In Germany, Humble Herb Is a Rival to Prozac," *The New York Times*. C1, C7.

Angier, Natalie. (June 22, 1997) "Drugs for Depression Multiply, and So Do the Hard Questions," *The New York Times*. WH11.

Bell, A.P., and M. Weinberg. (1978) *Homosexualities: A Study of Diversity Among Men and Women*. New York: Simon & Schuster.

Berzon, Betty. (1988) *Permanent Partners: Building Gay and Lesbian Relationships That Last*. New York: NAL/Dutton.

———. (1988) "Telling Your Family You're Gay." *Positively Gay: New Approaches to Gay and Lesbian Life*. Berkeley, CA: Celestial Arts.

———. (1996) *The Intimacy Dance: A Guide to Long Term Success in Gay and Lesbian Relationships*. New York: NAL/Dutton.

BuSpar (buspirone HCl, USP) Pharmaceutical Insert. (April 1996) Princeton, NJ: Bristol-Meyers Squibb Company.

Cabaj, Robet P., and Terry S. Stein. (1996) *Textbook of Homosexuality and Mental Health*. Washington, DC: American Psychiatric Press.

Chauncey, George. (1994) *Gay New York*. New York: Basic Books.

Cohen, Philip. (May 24, 1997) "Can Cutting Out the Trauma Keep AIDS at Bay?" *New Scientist*. 12.

Corbett, Ken, Ph.D. (October 1996) "Homosexual Boyhood: Notes on Girlboys." *Gender and Psychoanalysis: An Interdisciplinary Journal* 1 (4). 429–61.

———. (April, 1997) "It Is Time to Distinguish Gender from Health: Reflections on Lothstein's 'Pantyhose Fetishism and Self Cohesion: A Paraphilic Solution?'" *Gender and Psychoanalysis: An Interdisciplinary Journal* 2 (2). 259–71.

———. (1993) "The Mystery of Homosexuality," *Psychoanalytic Psychology* 10 (3). 345–57.

———. (October, 1997) "Speaking Queer: A Reply to Richard C. Friedman." *Gender and Psychoanalysis: An Interdisciplinary Journal* 2 (4). 495–514.

———. (1999) "Homosexual Boyhood: Notes on Girlyboys." In *Sissies and Tomboys*. Matthew Rottnek, Ed. New York: New York University Press.

Dambro, Mark R. (1998) *Griffith's 5-Minute Clinical Consult*. Baltimore, MD: Williams & Wilkins.

Diagnostic and Statistical Manual of Mental Disorders, 4th edition. (1994) Washington, DC: American Psychiatric Press, Inc.

Eidenberg, David. (May 26, 1998) "It's All in Your Head," *The Advocate*. 49.

Friedman, Richard C. (October, 1997) "Response to Ken Corbett's 'Homosexual Boyhood: Notes on Girlyboys' (Vol. 1, No. 4, 1996)." *Gender and Psychoanalysis: An Interdiscplinary Journal* 2 (4). 487–94.

The Gay Almanac. (1996) New York: Berkeley Books.

Gorman, Jack, MD. (1997) *The Essential Guide to Psychiatric Drugs*, 3rd edition. New York: St. Martin's Press.

Gunderson, E. K., and Richard H. Rahe. (1974) *Life Stress and Illness*. Springfield, IL: Thomas.

Halkitis, Perry N., and Tracy Mayne, Ph.D. (November, 1997) "Helping Clients with HIV Disease Navigate Managed Care." *Focus: A Guide to AIDS Research and Counseling* 12 (12). 1–4.

Hall, Marny. (1985) *The Lavender Couch: A Consumer's Guide to Psychotherapy for Lesbians and Gay Men*. Boston: Alyson Publications.

Hall, Trish. (April 28, 1998) "Seeking a Focus on Joy in Field of Psychology." *The New York Times*. F7.

Hartman, Stephen, Ph.D. (Summer 1997) "Affirming Gay and Lesbian Experience in Psychotherapy." *Carrier Foundation Medical Education Letter*. Carrier Letter No. 198.

Isay, Richard. (1996) *Becoming Gay*. New York: Pantheon.

Jay, J., and A. Young. (1977) *The Gay Report: Lesbians and Gay Men Speak Out About Sexual Experiences and Lifestyles*. New York: Summit.

Jeffrey, Nancy Ann. (July 9, 1997) "HMOs Seek Cures for Costly Psychosomatic Ills," *The Wall Street Journal*. B1, B12.

Kabat-Zinn, Jon. (1995) *Wherever You Go, There You Are*. New York: Hyperion.

King, Mike. (November 12, 1996) "Suicide Watch: A New Study Suggests That Young Gay Men Are at Even Higher Risk for Attempting to Kill Themselves Than Previously Thought," *The Advocate*. 41–42.

Kramer, Peter. (1997) *Listening to Prozac*. New York: Penguin.

Lemonick, Michael D. (September 29, 1997) "The Mood Molecule," *Time*. 74–80.

The PDR Family Guide to Prescription Drugs, 5th edition. (1997) New York: Crown Publishing Group.

The Physician's Desk Reference, 52nd edition. (1998)

Montvale, NJ: Medical Economics Company, Inc.

Pinksy, Laura, et al. (1992) *Essential HIV Treatment Fact Book*. New York: Pocket Books.

Project Inform. (1998) *The HIV Drug Book,* 2nd edition. New York: Pocket Books.

Ridgewood Financial Institute. (May, 1997) "Special Survey Report," *Psychotherapy Finances* 23 (5), issue 277.

Rothblum, Esther D. (1994) "'I Only Read About Myself on Bathroom Walls': The Need for Research on the Mental Health of Lesbians and Gay Men," *Journal of Consulting and Clinical Psychology* 62 (2): 213–20.

Rosenthal, Norm, MD. (1998) *Winter Blues*. New York: Guilford Press.

Ross, Michael W., and B. R. Simon Rosser. (January 1996) "Measurement and Correlates of Internalized Homophobia: A Factor Analytic Study." *Journal of Clinical Psychology* 52 (1). 15–21.

Salzberg, Sharon. (1997) *Loving-Kindness: The Revolutionary Art of Happiness*. Boston: Shambhala Publications, Inc.

Schweizer, Edward, MD, et al. (January, 1990) "What Constitutes an Adequate Antidepressant Trial for Fluoxetine?" *Journal of Clinical Psychiatry* 51 (1). 8–11.

Shernoff, Michael, CSW, ACSW. (1992) *How to Choose a Psychotherapist*. New York: Chelsea Psychotherapy Associates.

Shernoff, Michael, ed. (1997) *Gay Widowers: Life After the Death of a Partner*. New York: The Harrington Park Press.

Smith, R. (October, 1997) "Mixed-HIV Status Couples: Navigating the Challenges of Everyday Life." *Body Positive*. 16–20.

Spada, J. (1979) *The Spada Report: The Newest Survey of Gay Male Sexuality*. New York: Signet.

"States of Consciousness." (1993–1997) *Microsoft® Encarta® Encyclopedia*. Microsoft Corporation.

Tasman, A, et al. (eds.). (1997) *Psychiatry*. Philadelphia: W. B. Saunders.

Ulene, Art. (1996) *Really Fit, Really Fast*. Encino, CA: HEALTHPoints.

U.S. Department of Health and Human Services. (1983) *Plain Talk About Handling Stress*. Washington, DC: U.S. Department of Health and Human Services.

Walters, Karina L., and Jane M. Simoni. (1993) "Lesbian and Gay Male Group Identity Attitudes and Self-Esteem: Implications for Counseling," *Journal of Counseling Psychology* 40 (3). 302.

CHAPTER 12

Bell, A. P., and M. Weinberg. (1978) *Homosexualities: A Study of Diversity Among Men and Women*. New York: Simon & Schuster.

Bell, L. (1991) *On Our Own Terms: A Practical Guide for Lesbian and Gay Relationships*. Toronto: Coalition for Lesbian and Gay Rights in Ontario.

Bernstein, Fred A. (1996) "This Child Does Have Two Mothers . . . and a Sperm Donor with Visitation," *New York University Review of Law and Social Change* 22 (1).

Berzon, Betty. (1988) *Permanent Partners: Building Gay and Lesbian Relationships That Last*. New York: NAL/Dutton.

———. (1992) "Telling Your Family You're Gay," In Berzon, B. (ed.), *Positively Gay: New Approaches to Gay and Lesbian Life*. Berkeley, CA: Celestial Arts. 67–78.

———. (1996) *The Intimacy Dance: A Guide to Long Term Success in Gay and Lesbian Relationships*. New York: E. P. Dutton.

Brown, Paul, and Tess Ayers. (1994) *The Essential Guide to Lesbian and Gay Weddings*. San Francisco: HarperSanFrancisco.

Driggs, J. H., MSW, and S. E. Finn, Ph.D. (1990) *Intimacy Between Men*. New York: Dutton.

Fairchild, Betty, and Nancy Hayward. (1998) *Now That You Know: A Parents' Guide to Understanding Their Gay and Lesbian Children*. San Diego, CA: Harcourt Brace.

Friess, Steve. (December 9, 1997) "Domestic Violence

Behind Closed Doors," *The Advocate*. 48.

Giddens, Anthony. (1992) *The Transformation of Intimacy: Sexuality, Love & Eroticism in Modern Societies.* Berkeley, CA: Stanford University Press.

Green, R. J., et al. (1998) "Are Lesbian Couples Fused and Gay Male Couples Disengaged?" In J. Laird and R. J. Green (eds.), *Lesbians and Gays in Couples and Families*. San Francisco: Jossey Bass.

Hendrix, Harville, Ph.D. (1988) *Getting the Love You Want: A Guide for Couples*. New York: HarperPerennial.

Herek, G. M., et al. (1991) "Avoiding Heterosexist Bias in Psychological Research," *American Psychologist* 46 (9). 957–63.

Holt, Susan. (September 26, 1996) "Ending the Cycle of Domestic Violence," *The Gay and Lesbian Times*. 39.

Isensee, Rik. (1990) *Love Between Men: Enhancing Intimacy and Keeping Your Relationship Alive*. New York: Prentice Hall Press.

Island, David, and Patrick Letellier. (1991) *Men Who Beat the Men Who Love Them*. New York: Harrington Park Press.

Jay, J., and A. Young. (1977) *The Gay Report: Lesbians and Gay Men Speak Out About Sexual Experiences and Lifestyles*. New York: Summit.

Kingston, Tim. (May 17, 1996) "Queer Domestic Violence: The Unspoken Epidemic," *Frontiers*. 65.

Letellier, Patrick. (1994) "Identifying and Treating Battered Gay Men," *San Francisco Medicine*. 18–19.

———. (June 27, 1994) "Stop Gay-Bashing at Home," *The San Francisco Chronicle*. 19.

Levine, M. (1998) *Gay Macho: The Life and Death of the Homosexual Clone*. New York: New York University Press.

Lew, Mike. (1990) *Victims No Longer: Men Recovering From Incest and Other Sexual Child Abuse*. New York: HarperCollins.

Lewin, Tamar. (June 22, 1997) "Seeking Public Health Solution for a Problem That Starts at Home," *The New York Times*. WH19.

Mallon, G. (1998) "Social Work Practice with Gay Men and Lesbians Within Families." In Mallon, G. (ed.), *Foundations of Social Work Practice with Lesbian and Gay Persons*. New York: Harrington Park Press. 145–82.

Marcus, Eric. (1992) *The Male Couple's Guide: Finding a Man, Making a Home, Building a Life*. New York: Harper Perennial.

Martinac, Paula. (1998) *The Lesbian and Gay Book of Love and Marriage*. New York: Broadway Books.

McWhirter, David P., MD, and Andrew M. Mattison, MSW, Ph.D. (1985) *The Male Couple: How Relationships Develop*. Englewood Cliffs, NJ: Prentice Hall, Inc.

———. (1996) "Male Couples." In Cabaj, R., and T. Stein (eds.), *Textbook of Homosexuality and Mental Health*. Washington DC: American Psychiatric Press. 319–38.

National Gay and Lesbian Task Force Policy Institute. (1995) *To Have and to Hold: Arguing for Our Right to Marry*. Washington, DC: National Gay and Lesbian Task Force.

Nelson, Craig. (1996) *Finding True Love in a Man-Eat-Man World: The Intelligent Guide to Gay Dating, Romance and Eternal Love*. New York: Dell Publishing.

Signorile, Michelangelo. (December–January, 1998) "Church and Its Current State." *Out*. 59–60.

Smith, R. (October, 1997) "Mixed HIV-Status Couples: Navigating the Challenges of Everyday Life," *Body Positive*. 16–20.

Spada, J. (1979) *The Spada Report: The Newest Survey of Gay Male Sexuality*. New York: Signet.

Sullivan, Andrew (ed.). (1997) *Same-Sex Marriage: Pro and Con, A Reader*. New York: Vintage.

Weston, Kath. (1991) *Families We Choose*. New York: Columbia University Press.

Internet

http://www.jimhopper.com/male-ab. Hopper, Jim. "Sexual Abuse of Males: Prevalence, Lasting Effects, and Resources." 1997.

Chapter 13

All God's Children. (1996) Produced and directed by Dr. Dee Mosbacher, et al., 26 min. Woman Vision. Videocassette.

Balka, Christie, and Andy Rose (eds.). (1989) *Twice Blessed: On Being Lesbian, Gay, and Jewish*. Boston: Beacon Press.

Barzan, Robert (ed.). (1995) "Sex and Spirit: Exploring Gay Men's Spirituality," *White Crane Journal*.

Bell, Bernard W., et al. (eds.). (1996) *W .E. B. Du Bois on Race and Culture*. New York: Routledge.

Bishop, Clifford. (1996) *Sex and Spirit*. New York: Little Brown.

Boswell, John. (1980) *Christianity, Social Tolerance, and Homosexuality: Gay People in Western Europe from the Beginning of the Christian Era to the Fourteenth Century*. Chicago: University of Chicago Press.

Boulder, Brian (ed.). (1995) *Wrestling with the Angel: Faith and Religion in the Lives of Gay Men*. New York: Riverhead Books.

Boyd, Malcolm, and Nancy L. Wilson (eds.). (1991) *Amazing Grace: Stories of Lesbian and Gay Faith*. Freedom, CA: Crossing Press.

Boyd, Malcolm. (1993) *Take Off the Masks*. San Francisco: HarperSanFrancisco.

Bronski, Michael. (1996) *Taking Liberties: Gay Men's Essays on Politics, Culture, and Sex*. New York: Masquerade Books, Inc.

Carpenter, Edward (1982) *Intermediate Types Among Primitive Folk: A Study in Social Evolution*. Reprint. Darby, PA: Darby Books.

Chamberlain, Claudine. (December 15, 1997) "Could Spirituality Save Money? Mixing Faith and Healing." *ABCNews.com*.

Conner, Randy P. (1993) *Blossom of Bone: Reclaiming the Connections between Homoeroticism and the Sacred*. San Francisco: HarperSanFrancisco.

Desert Moon Periodicals. *RFD: Gay Men's Megazine for the Rural Lifestyle and Beyond*. Call (505) 474–6311 for subscriptions.

Dossey, Larry, MD. (1993) *Healing Words: The Power of Prayer and the Practice of Medicine*. New York: HarperPaperbacks.

Evans, Arthur. (1978) *Witchcraft and the Gay Counterculture*. Boston: Fag Rag Books.

Glaser, Chris. (1996) *Uncommon Calling: A Gay Christian's Struggle to Serve the Church*. Louisville, KY: Westminster Press.

Helminiak, Daniel. (1994) *What the Bible Really Says? Top Scholars Put Homosexuality in Perspective*. San Francisco: Alamo Square Press.

Heyward, Carter. (1989) *Touching Our Strength: The Erotic as Power and the Love of God*. San Francisco: HarperSanFrancisco.

"The History Behind Trent Lott," (July 10, 1998) *The New York Times*. A14.

Johnson, Fenton. (1995) "Gods, Gays and the Geography of Desire," in *Wrestling with the Angel: Faith and Religion in the Lives of Gay Men*. Brian Bouldrey, Ed. New York: Riverhead Books.

Kark, J. D., et al. March 1996. "Does Religious Observance Promote Health? Mortality in Secular vs Religious Kibbutzim in Israel," *American Journal of Public Health*. 341–46.

Kaufman, Gershen, Ph.D., and Lev Raphael, Ph.D. (1996) *Coming Out of Shame*. New York: Doubleday.

Kornfield, Jack. (1993) *A Path with Heart*. New York: Bantam Books.

Leyland, Winston (ed.). (1998) *Queer Dharma: Voices of Gay Buddhists*. San Francisco: Gay Sunshine Press, Inc.

"Making a Place for Spirituality," (February 1998) *Harvard Health Letter* 23 (4). 1–3.

Moore, Thomas. (1992) *Care of the Soul*. New York: HarperCollins.

O'Neill, Craig, and Kathleen Ritter. (1992) *Coming Out Within: Stages of Spiritual Awakening for Lesbians and Gay Men*. New York: HarperCollins.

Ramer, Andrew. (1997) *Two Flutes Playing: A Spiritual Journeybook for Gay Men*. San Francisco: Alamo Square Press.

Raphael, Lev. (1996) *Journeys and Arrivals: On Being Gay and Jewish*. Winchester, MA: Faber and Faber.

Ratzinger, Joseph Cardinal. (1995) "Letter to the Bishops of the Catholic Church on the Pastoral Care of Homosexual Persons." In Bard, Robert M., and M. Katherine Baird (eds.), *Homosexuality: Debating the Issues*. Amherst, NY: Prometheus Books.

Riggs, Marlon. (1991) "Tongues Untied." In Hemphill, Essex (ed.), *Brother to Brother.* Los Angeles: Alyson Publications, Inc. 200–05.

Rotes, Eric. (1998) *Dry Bones Breathe: Gay Men Creating Post-AIDS Identities and Cultures*. New York: Harrington Park Press.

Rinpoche, Sogyal. (1993) *The Tibetan Book of Living and Dying*. San Francisco: HarperSanFrancisco.

Roscoe, Will (ed.). (1988) *Living the Spirit: A Gay American Indian Anthology*. New York: St. Martin's Press.

Russo, Vito. (1987) *The Celluloid Closet*. New York: HarperCollins Publishers, Inc.

Savage, Todd. (December 9, 1997) "Taking It to the People," *The Advocate*. 33.

Some, Malidoma P. (1997) *Ritual: Power, Healing and Community*. New York: Viking Penguin.

Spencer, Collin. (1996) *The Gay Kama Sutra*. New York: St. Martin's Press.

Szymanski, Katie. (September 4, 1998) "Anti-Gay Crime Jumps Sharply: Duane Criticizes City's Response to Recent Killings." *New York Blade* 1, 8.

Thompson, Mark (ed.). (1987) *Gay Spirit: Myth and Meaning*. New York: St. Martin's Press.

———. (1994) *Gay Soul: Finding the Heart of Gay Spirit and Nature*. San Francisco: HarperSanFrancisco.

———. (1994) *Long Road to Freedom: The Advocate History of the Gay and Lesbian Movement*. New York: St. Martin's Press.

Tilleraas, Perry. (1988) *The Color of Light*. San Francisco: HarperSanFrancisco.

Turning Wheel: Journal of the Buddhist Peace Fellowship. (Fall, 1997) Berkeley, CA: Buddhist Peace Fellowship.

Wagner, Glenn, MA, et al. (1994) "Integration of One's Religion and Homosexuality: A Weapon Against Internalized Homophobia?" *Journal of Homosexuality* 26 (4). 91–110.

White, Mel. (1995) *Stranger at the Gate: To Be Gay and Christian in America*. New York: NAL/Dutton.

Williams, Walter L. (1986) *The Spirit and the Flesh: Sexual Diversity in American Indian Culture.* Boston: Beacon Press.

Photo/Art References

CHAPTER 1

p1 Courtesy of International Gay Information Center (IGIC) Archive, Manuscripts & Archives Division, The New York Public Library, Astor Lenox & Tilden Foundations
p4 © Kate Rudin
p8 © Jack Louth
p10 © Stephen Barker
p14 © *Shunga: The Charge, A Phallic Contest,* Private Collection/Bridgeman Art Library
p26 © Paul Teeling

CHAPTER 2

p47 © Nicolas Pages
p52 © George Perkins
p54 © Jack Louth
p55 © Chantal Regnault
p59 © Anja Hinrichsen
p69 © Anja Hinrichsen
p73 © Exum
p75 © Jack Louth

CHAPTER 3

p95 © Exum
p97 Mirror Portrait with John Kelly by John Dugdale (Courtesy of the Wessel + O'Connor Gallery)
p98:
top © John O.
middle © Aaron Cobbett
bottom © Aaron Cobbett
p100 © Allen Frame/Frank Franca
p108 © Jonathan Saunders
p120 © Leonard Fink/National Archive of Gay & Lesbian History, Lesbian & Gay Community Services Center, NY
p121 © Anja Hinrichsen
p125 © Jack Louth
p127 © Loring McAlpin
p129 © Linda Pallotta/Impact Visuals
p131 © Noe Dewitt
p133 © *John, Gary and Kris in Bed,* 1996/ Howard Roffman, courtesy Wessel+O'Connor Gallery, NY
p134 © Linda Pallotta/Impact Visuals

CHAPTER 4

p137 © Loring McAlpin
p142 © Courtesy of International Gay Information Center Archive, Manuscripts & Archives Division, The New York Public Library, Astor Lenox & Tilden Foundations
p176© John O.
p178 © Clay McBride

CHAPTER 5

p189 © UPI/Corbis-Bettmann
p192 © Donna Binder/Impact Visuals
p197 © Dianora Niccolini
p202 © Chantal Regnault
p204 © Tom Haynes
p207 © Stephen Barker
p217 © Jean Kugler/FPG
p220 © Alexis Rodriguez-Duarte
p222 © Leonard Fink/National Archive of Gay & Lesbian History, Lesbian & Gay Community Services Center, NY
p229 © Richard Laird/FPG
p230 (by name):
© Corbis-Bettmann (Alexander the Great)
© Corbis-Bettmann (Oscar Wilde)
© Courtesy of the Bayley-Whitman Collection (Walt Whitman)
© UPI/Corbis-Bettmann (Yukio Mishima)
© CameraPress/Retna Ltd, USA (Jean Genet)
p231 (by name):
(no credit) Liberace
© Max Redferns/Retna (Sylvester)
© Greg Gorman (Quentin Crisp)
© Mathiù Andersen (Ru Paul)

CHAPTER 6

p239 © Jack Louth
p243 © Susan Johann/Outline
p244 © Ken Probst
p247 top © Cori Wells Braun/Outline
p247 bot © Barry Canter
p248 © Courtesy POZ Magazine
p252 © Andrea Marouk
p254 © Robert Fleischauer
p261 © Corbis-Bettmann
p273 © Pascale Willi

CHAPTER 7

p283 © UPI Corbis/Bettmann
p287 © Corbis/Bettmann
p297 © Tom McKitterick/Impact Visuals
p312 © Barry Canter
p319 © Tom Haynes

CHAPTER 8

p329 © Val Shaff
p334 © Anderson Archive/Daniel Gundlach (all photos)
Cliff Anderson lived in San Francisco from 1927–1997, working as a messenger and in the concession stands at the Golden Gate bridge and the Santa Fe railroad. He passed away in 1997.
p337 ©Tom McKitterick
p338 © Donna Binder/Impact Visuals
p341 ©Anja Hinrichsen
p361 ©Donna Binder/Impact Visuals
p368 © A.L. Steiner
p370 © Tom McKitterick/Impact Visuals

CHAPTER 9:

p375 © Pascale Willi
p378 © Peter Lien/LNP
p387 © Rick Gerharter
p394 © Corbis-Bettmann
p406 © Pascale Willi
p414 © Courtesy Gran Fury

CHAPTER 10

p417 © Courtesy of International Gay Information Center (IGIC) Archive, Manuscripts & Archives Division, The New York Public Library, Astor Lenox & Tilden Foundations
p428 © Peter Schaaf
p439 © Pascale Willi
p440 © Lonny Shavelson/Impact Visuals

CHAPTER 11

p459 © Loring McAlpin
p461 © George Perkins
p462 © Tom McKitterick/Impact Visuals
p470 © Laurence Monneret/Tony Stone Images
p473 © Corbis-Bettmann
p477 © Fred McDarrah
p491 © Alison Shirk

CHAPTER 12

p495 Photos © Anja Hinrichsen
p496 © Paul Teeling
p497 © Lee Schy
p498 © Allen Frame/Frank Franca
p502 © George Perkins
p506 © Donna Binder/Impact Visuals
p507 © Rick Gerharter/Impact Visuals
p508 © Carolina Kroon/Impact Visuals
p511 © Corbis/Bettmann
p517 © George Perkins
p522 © Lisa Ross
p524 © Christina Alicino
p527 © Lonny Shavelson/Impact Visuals
p529 © Anja Hinrichsen

CHAPTER 13

p533 © Mojgan Azimi
p536 © Corbis-Bettman
p540 © Rick Gerharter
p542:
Top © Mary Ellen Mark
Mid © Donna Binder/Impact Visuals
Bot © Rick Gerharter
p550 © Courtesy of International Gay Information Center (IGIC) Archive, Manuscripts & Archives Division, The New York Public Library, Astor Lenox & Tilden Foundations
p551 © Daniel Nicoletta
p552 © Peter Lien/LNP
p557 © A.L. Steiner
p558 © Rick Gerharter
p563 © Chantal Regnault

—

All line drawings: Ellen Forney

INDEX

Page numbers for illustrations appear in italic.

ABOUT THE AUTHOR

Daniel Wolfe is GMHC's former Director of Communications and a writer based in New York City. His work has appeared in *The Advocate, The Guardian, The New York Times Book Review,* and numerous other publications.